Pearls and Pitfalls in
PEDIATRIC IMAGING
Variants and Other
Difficult Diagnoses

Pearls and Pitfalls in
PEDIATRIC IMAGING

Variants and Other Difficult Diagnoses

Edited by

Heike E. Daldrup-Link
Lucile Packard Children's Hospital, Stanford University

Beverley Newman
Lucile Packard Children's Hospital, Stanford University

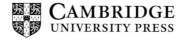

CAMBRIDGE
UNIVERSITY PRESS

CAMBRIDGE
UNIVERSITY PRESS

University Printing House, Cambridge CB2 8BS, United Kingdom

Cambridge University Press is part of the University of Cambridge.

It furthers the University's mission by disseminating knowledge in the pursuit of education, learning and research at the highest international levels of excellence.

www.cambridge.org
Information on this title: www.cambridge.org/9781107017498

First published 2014

Printed in Spain by Grafos SA, Arte Sobre papel

A catalog record for this publication is available from the British Library

Library of Congress Cataloging-in-Publication Data
Pearls and pitfalls in pediatric imaging : variants and other difficult diagnoses / edited by Heike E. Daldrup-Link, Beverley Newman.
     p. ; cm.
Includes bibliographical references.
ISBN 978-1-107-01749-8 (Hardback)
I. Daldrup-Link, Heike E., editor of compilation.   II. Newman, Beverley, editor of compilation.
[DNLM: 1. Diagnostic Imaging–methods–Case Reports.   2. Adolescent.   3. Child.
4. Diagnosis, Differential–Case Reports.   5. Infant. WN 240]
RC78.7.D53
616.07'54–dc23   2013038647

ISBN 978-1-107-01749-8 Hardback

Contents

List of contributors   viii
Preface   xi
Acknowledgment   xii

Section 1 Head and neck

Case 1 Trilateral retinoblastoma *Andreas Rauschecker and Heike E. Daldrup-Link*   1

Case 2 Fibromatosis colli *Siobhan M. Flanagan, Kristen W. Yeom, Patrick D. Barnes, and Beverley Newman*   7

Case 3 Craniopharyngioma *Camilla Mosci and Andrei Iagaru*   10

Case 4 Labyrinthitis ossificans *Lex A. Mitchell and Kristen W. Yeom*   14

Case 5 Branchio-oto-renal syndrome *Lex A. Mitchell and Kristen W. Yeom*   16

Case 6 Medulloblastoma *Neilish Gupta and Kristen W. Yeom*   18

Case 7 Ectopic cervical thymus *Michael Iv and Kristen W. Yeom*   20

Case 8 X-linked adrenoleukodystrophy *Jared Narvid and Kristen W. Yeom*   23

Case 9 Langerhans cell histiocytosis *Vy Thao Tran, Thomas Pulling, Kristen W. Yeom, and Bo Yoon Ha*   25

Case 10 PHACES syndrome (Posterior fossa malformations, Hemangiomas of the face, Arterial anomalies, Cardiovascular anomalies, Eye anomalies, and Sternal defects or supraumbilical raphe) *James Kang and Kristen W. Yeom*   30

Section 2 Thoracic imaging

Case 11 Lipoid pneumonia *Beverley Newman*   33

Case 12 Pleuropulmonary blastoma *Jordan Caplan, Rakhee Gawande, and Beverley Newman*   36

Case 13 Neuroendocrine cell hyperplasia of infancy (NEHI) *Beverley Newman*   40

Case 14 Endobronchial foreign body recognition *Matthew Thompson and Beverley Newman*   44

Case 15 Chronic esophageal foreign body *Beverley Newman*   48

Case 16 Opsoclonus–myoclonus due to underlying ganglioneuroblastoma *Rakhee Gawande and Beverley Newman*   53

Case 17 Lymphoma: pulmonary manifestations *Rakhee Gawande and Beverley Newman*   56

Case 18 Acute and subacute pneumonia in childhood: tuberculosis *Beverley Newman*   62

Case 19 Thymus: normal variations *Beverley Newman*   66

Case 20 Airleak in the neonate *Beverley Newman*   72

Case 21 Bronchopulmonary malformation: hybrid lesions *Beverley Newman*   79

Case 22 Lymphatic abnormality in the pediatric chest *Beverley Newman*   87

Section 3 Cardiac imaging

Case 23 Tetralogy of Fallot with pulmonary atresia *Beverley Newman*   94

Case 24 Left pulmonary artery sling *Beverley Newman*   98

Case 25 Vascular ring *Beverley Newman*   102

Case 26 Scimitar syndrome *Rakhee Gawande and Beverley Newman*   107

Case 27 Portosystemic shunt and portopulmonary syndrome *Beverley Newman*   111

Case 28 Aortic coarctation and interrupted aortic arch *Albert Hsiao and Beverley Newman*   117

Case 29 Ebstein's anomaly *Theo Blake and Beverley Newman*   122

Case 30 Transposition of the great arteries *Beverley Newman*   127

Case 31 Total anomalous pulmonary venous return *Horacio Murillo, Michael J. Lane, Carlos S. Restrepo, and Beverley Newman*   135

Case 32 Aberrant left coronary artery arising from the pulmonary artery *Beverley Newman*   141

Section 4 Vascular and interventional

Case 33 Lower extremity ischemia due to homocystinuria *Edward A. Lebowitz*   147

Case 34 Iatrogenic pathology masquerading as an artifact *Edward A. Lebowitz*   151

Case 35 Fibromuscular dysplasia *Edward A. Lebowitz*   158

Case 36 Traumatic vertebral arteriovenous fistulae *Edward A. Lebowitz*   162

Case 37 Colonic perforation during intussusception reduction *Edward A. Lebowitz*   169

Case 38 Juvenile nasopharyngeal angioma *Edward A. Lebowitz*   173

Case 39 Small bowel fistula complicating perforated appendicitis: successful treatment with tissue adhesive *Edward A. Lebowitz*   177

Case 40 Extrahepatic collateral arterial supply to hepatocellular carcinoma *Edward A. Lebowitz* 181

Case 41 Use of a curved needle to access an otherwise inaccessible abscess *Edward A. Lebowitz* 183

Case 42 Umbilical venous catheter malposition *Rakhee Gawande and Beverley Newman* 188

Case 43 Middle aortic syndrome *Elizabeth Sutton and Heike E. Daldrup-Link* 193

Section 5 Gastrointestinal imaging

Case 44 Ruptured appendicitis mimicking an intussusception *Rakhee Gawande and Beverley Newman* 196

Case 45 Choledochal cyst *Gregory Cheeney and Heike E. Daldrup-Link* 201

Case 46 Henoch–Schönlein purpura *Kriengkrai Iemsawatdikul and Heike E. Daldrup-Link* 205

Case 47 Biliary atresia *Guido Davidzon, Heike E. Daldrup-Link, and Beverley Newman* 207

Case 48 Mesenchymal hamartoma of the liver *Aman Khurana, Fanny Chapelin, and Heike E. Daldrup-Link* 211

Case 49 Lymphoid follicular hyperplasia *Heike E. Daldrup-Link* 215

Case 50 Midgut volvulus *Heike E. Daldrup-Link* 218

Case 51 Foveolar hyperplasia: post prostaglandin therapy *Kriengkrai Iemsawatdikul and Heike E. Daldrup-Link* 222

Case 52 Pneumatosis cystoides intestinalis *Heike E. Daldrup-Link* 226

Case 53 Desmoplastic small round cell tumor *Heike E. Daldrup-Link* 229

Case 54 Post-transplantation lymphoproliferative disorder *Khun Visith Keu and Andrei Iagaru* 231

Case 55 Traumatic pancreatic injury *Matthew Schmitz and Beverley Newman* 234

Case 56 Meconium ileus *Amy Neville and Beverley Newman* 237

Section 6 Urinary imaging

Case 57 Renal cysts in tuberous sclerosis *Heike E. Daldrup-Link* 245

Case 58 Prune belly syndrome *Heike E. Daldrup-Link* 248

Case 59 Renal vein thrombosis *Kriengkrai Iemsawatdikul and Heike E. Daldrup-Link* 252

Case 60 Acute bacterial pyelonephritis *Heike E. Daldrup-Link* 255

Case 61 Ectopic ureterocele *Heike E. Daldrup-Link* 257

Case 62 Nephroblastomatosis *Gregory Cheeney, Rakhee Gawande, Beverley Newman, and Heike E. Daldrup-Link* 260

Case 63 Urachal mass *Rakhee Gawande and Beverley Newman* 264

Case 64 Wilms' tumor *Rakhee Gawande, Kriengkrai Iemsawatdikul, Heike E. Daldrup-Link, and Beverley Newman* 269

Case 65 Ureteropelvic junction obstruction *Rakhee Gawande, Heike E. Daldrup-Link, and Beverley Newman* 276

Case 66 Oxalosis in an 11-year-old boy *Heike E. Daldrup-Link* 281

Section 7 Endocrine – reproductive imaging

Case 67 Pediatric Graves' disease *Sami M. Akram and Andrei Iagaru* 285

Case 68 Thyroglossal duct cyst *Richard A. Barth* 287

Case 69 Thyroid colloid cyst *Richard A. Barth* 289

Case 70 Adrenal hemorrhage *Rakhee Gawande, Rosalinda Castaneda, and Heike E. Daldrup-Link* 291

Case 71 Neuroblastoma *Khun Visith Keu and Andrei Iagaru* 294

Case 72 Ovarian torsion in childhood *Atalie Thompson and Beverley Newman* 297

Case 73 Torsion of the appendix testis *Rakhee Gawande, Heike E. Daldrup-Link, and Beverley Newman* 303

Case 74 Intratesticular neoplasms *Hedieh K. Eslamy and Beverley Newman* 307

Section 8 Fetal imaging

Case 75 Fetal lymphatic malformation *Erika Rubesova* 313

Case 76 Anal atresia with urorectal fistula *Erika Rubesova* 316

Case 77 Cystic dysplasia of the kidneys *Erika Rubesova* 319

Case 78 Gastroschisis *Binh Huynh and Erika Rubesova* 322

Case 79 Fetal osteogenesis imperfecta *Jordan Caplan and Erika Rubesova* 326

Case 80 Congenital diaphragmatic hernia *Vy Thao Tran and Erika Rubesova* 329

Case 81 Hydrops fetalis *Kriengkrai Iemsawatdikul and Heike E. Daldrup-Link* 334

Section 9 Musculoskeletal imaging

Case 82 Clubfoot *Bo Yoon Ha* 336

Case 83 Developmental dysplasia of the hip *Vanessa Starr and Bo Yoon Ha* 339

Case 84 Legg–Calve–Perthes disease *Vy Thao Tran and Bo Yoon Ha* 343

Case 85 Slipped capital femoral epiphysis *Vy Thao Tran and Bo Yoon Ha* 347

Case 86 Langerhans cell histiocytosis: MRI/PET for diagnosis and treatment monitoring *Wolfgang P. Fendler, Eva Coppenrath, Klemens Scheidhauer, and Thomas Pfluger* 350

Case 87 Congenital syphilis *Vanessa Starr and Bo Yoon Ha* 354

Case 88 Medial malleolus avulsion fracture *Vanessa Starr and Bo Yoon Ha* 359

Case 89 Triplane fracture *Bo Yoon Ha* 362

Case 90 Fibrous dysplasia *Vy Thao Tran, Aman Khurana, and Bo Yoon Ha* 365

Case 91 Chest wall sarcoma *Vanessa Starr and Bo Yoon Ha* 370

Case 92 Campomelic dysplasia *Ralph Lachman* 374

Case 93 Type II collagenopathy (hypochondrogenesis) *Ralph Lachman* 377

Case 94 Morel-Lavallée lesions *Justin Boe* 380

Case 95 Infantile myofibromatosis *Justin Boe and Heike E. Daldrup-Link* 384

Case 96 Osteochondritis dissecans of the capitellum *Rakhee Gawande* 387

Index 389

Contributors

Sami M. Akram, MD, MHA
Resident, Department of Radiology, Molecular Imaging/Nuclear Imaging, Stanford University, Stanford, CA, USA

Patrick D. Barnes, MD
Professor of Pediatric Radiology, Lucile Packard Children's Hospital at Stanford University, Stanford, CA, USA

Richard A. Barth, MD
Radiologist-in-Chief, Professor and Associate Chairman of Radiology, Lucile Packard Children's Hospital at Stanford University, Stanford, CA, USA

Theo Blake, MD
Prior Cardiovascular Fellow, Stanford University, Stanford, CA, USA
Staff Radiologist, Division of Cardiovascular Radiology, Royal Columbian Hospital, New Westminster, BC, Canada

Justin Boe, MD
Prior Pediatric Radiology Fellow, Stanford University, Stanford, CA, USA
Radiologist, University of Oklahoma Health Sciences Center, Oklahoma City, OK, USA

Jordan Caplan, MD
Prior Pediatric Radiology Fellow, Stanford University, Stanford, CA, USA
Pediatric Radiologist, Shady Grove Radiology, Rockville, MD, USA

Rosalinda Castaneda
Research Associate, Stanford University Molecular Imaging, Stanford, CA, USA

Fanny Chapelin, MS
Research Associate, Stanford University Molecular Imaging, Stanford, CA, USA

Gregory Cheeney, MD
Prior Visiting Student, Stanford University, Stanford, CA, USA
Radiology Resident, University of Washington, Seattle, WA, USA

Eva Coppenrath, MD
Klinikum rechts der Isar, Technische Universität München, Nuklearmedizinische Klinik und Poliklinik, Munich, Germany

Heike E. Daldrup-Link, MD, PhD
Associate Professor of Radiology, Lucile Packard Children's Hospital at Stanford University, Stanford, CA, USA

Guido Davidzon, MD
Nuclear Medicine Resident, Stanford University, Stanford, CA, USA

Hedieh K. Eslamy, MD
Prior Instructor in Pediatric Radiology at Stanford University and Lucile Packard Children's Hospital, Stanford, CA, USA
Assistant Professor of Pediatric Radiology, Seattle Children's Hospital, Seattle, WA, USA

Wolfgang P. Fendler, MD
University Hospital of the Ludwig–Maximilians–Universität, Munich, Germany

Siobhan M. Flanagan, MD
Prior Pediatric Radiology Fellow, Stanford University, Stanford, CA, USA
Pediatric Radiologist, University of Minnesota, Minneapolis, MN, USA

Rakhee Gawande, MD
Prior Pediatric Radiology Fellow, Stanford University, Stanford, CA, USA
Neuroradiology Fellow, Department of Radiology, University of Minnesota, Minneapolis, MN, USA

Neilish Gupta, M.D.
Prior Neuroradiology Fellow, Stanford University, Stanford, CA, USA
Attending Neuroradiologist, Diversified Radiology of Colorado, Denver, Colorado, USA.

Bo Yoon Ha, MD
Chief of Pediatric Radiology, Santa Clara Valley Medical Center, San Jose, CA, USA

Albert Hsiao, MD, PhD
Cardiovascular Fellow, Stanford University, Stanford, CA, USA

Binh Huynh, MD
Prior Pediatric Radiology Fellow, Stanford University, Stanford, CA, USA
Staff Radiologist, Kaiser Permanente, Oakland, CA, USA

Andrei Iagaru, MD
Assistant Professor of Radiology, Nuclear Medicine, Stanford University, Stanford, CA, USA

Kriengkrai Iemsawatdikul, MD
Instructor in Radiology, Siraraj Hospital, Mahidol University, Nakhon Pathon, Thailand

Michael Iv, MD
Clinical Instructor in Neuroradiology, Stanford University, Stanford, CA, USA

James Kang, MD
Radiology Fellow, Stanford University, Stanford, CA, USA

Khun Visith Keu, MD
Clinical Assistant Professor, Départemente de Médecine Nucléaire et de Radiobiologie, Centre Hospitalier Universitaire de Sherbrooke, Sherbrooke, Québec, Canada

Aman Khurana, MD
Postdoctoral Fellow, Department of Radiology, Stanford University, Stanford, CA, USA

Ralph Lachman, MD
Emeritus Professor, UCLA School of Medicine; Clinical Professor, Stanford University, and International Skeletal Dysplasia Registry, Los Angeles, CA, USA

Michael J. Lane, MD
Chief Cardiovascular CT/MRI, South Texas Radiology Group, San Antonio, TX, USA

Edward A. Lebowitz, MD
Clinical Professor of Radiology, Lucile Packard Children's Hospital at Stanford University, Stanford, CA, USA

Lex A. Mitchell, MD
Fellow, Stanford University, Stanford, CA, USA

Camilla Mosci, MD
Research Fellow, Stanford University, Stanford, CA, USA

Horacio Murillo, MD, PhD
Prior Cardiovascular Radiology Fellow, Stanford University, Stanford, CA, USA
Cardiothoracic Radiologist, Sutter Medical Group, Sacramento, CA, USA

Jared Narvid, MD
Radiology Resident, Stanford University, Stanford, CA, USA

Amy Neville, MD
Radiology Fellow, Stanford University, Stanford, CA, USA

Beverley Newman, MBBCh, FACR
Professor of Radiology, Associate Chief of Pediatric Radiology, Lucile Packard Children's Hospital at Stanford University, Stanford, CA, USA

Thomas Pfluger, MD
Klinikum rechts der Isar, Technische Universität München, Nuklearmedizinische Klinik und Poliklinik, Munich, Germany

Thomas Pulling, MD
Chief of MRI, Dwight David Eisenhower Army Medical Center, Evans, GA, USA

Andreas Rauschecker, MD, PhD
Radiology Resident, Stanford University, Stanford, CA, USA

Carlos S. Restrepo, MD
Associate Professor and Head of MRI Section, Louisiana State University Health Science Center, New Orleans, LA, USA

Erika Rubesova, MD
Clinical Associate Professor of Radiology, Lucile Packard Children's Hospital at Stanford University, Stanford, CA, USA

Klemens Scheidhauer, MD
Senior Physician, Klinikum rechts der Isar, Technische Universität München, Nuklearmedizinische Klinik und Poliklinik, Munich, Germany

Matthew Schmitz, MD
Prior Pediatric Radiology Fellow, Stanford University, Stanford, CA, USA
Radiologist, Diversified Radiology of Colorado, Denver, Colorado, USA

Vanessa Starr, MD
Radiologist, Santa Clara Valley Medical Center, San Jose, CA, USA

Elizabeth Sutton, MD
Assistant Professor of Radiology, Memorial Sloan-Kettering Cancer Center, New York, NY, USA

Atalie Thompson, MPH
Medical Student, Stanford University School of Medicine, Stanford, CA, USA

Matthew Thompson, MD
Prior Medical Student, Stanford University, Stanford, CA, USA
Radiology Resident, University of Texas Southwestern, Dallas, TX, USA

Vy Thao Tran, MD
Clinical Instructor in Radiology, Lucile Packard Children's Hospital at Stanford University, Stanford, CA, USA

Kristen W. Yeom, MD
Assistant Professor of Radiology, Lucile Packard Children's Hospital at Stanford University, Stanford, CA, USA

Preface

This book presents pediatric imaging cases that are easily missed or misinterpreted by trainees or radiologists, who do not see a large volume of pediatric imaging studies and/or do not see pediatric imaging studies on a daily basis. The book is primarily intended as a practicing tool for Radiology residents and fellows, who are preparing for the radiology core exam, the radiology certifying exam, or Certificate of Added Qualification (CAQ) exams. It will also provide a resource for general radiologists, pediatricians, and pediatric surgeons who want to improve their diagnostic proficiency in the interpretation of pediatric imaging studies. Pediatric radiologists may find this book useful for refreshing their knowledge on specific topics in the field. The book covers all relevant pediatric imaging modalities, such as ultrasound, Doppler ultrasound, conventional radiography, fluoroscopy, CT, MR, nuclear/molecular imaging, and interventional radiology.

It is our goal to provide our readers with a tool to recognize and understand common pitfalls in pediatric imaging in order to reduce the likelihood of missed or false diagnoses. This book is dedicated to the children in hospitals worldwide who, hopefully, will receive more accurate diagnoses and enhanced treatment because well-trained physicians have taken the time and effort to educate themselves beyond minimum requirements.

Heike E. Daldrup-Link and Beverley Newman

Acknowledgment

Our heartfelt thanks to our spouses Thomas Link and Paul Michelow for their unwavering support and understanding of the many extra hours of work required to bring this book to fruition. Also thanks to Jocelyn Shaw, Danielle Beecham, and Jennifer Vancil for their expert administrative assistance.

Heike E. Daldrup-Link and Beverley Newman

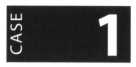

CASE 1

Trilateral retinoblastoma

Andreas Rauschecker and Heike E. Daldrup-Link

Imaging description

A two-year-old boy presented with leukocoria (= white pupil). Ophthalmoscopy demonstrated large masses in both globes. A CT scan showed extensive calcifications of both lesions (Fig. 1.1a). An MR scan better delineated the contrast-enhancing masses in the bilateral globes, both of which demonstrated extraocular extension (Fig. 1.1b).

An axial contrast-enhanced MR scan of the brain in a different patient with retinoblastoma shows an additional, inhomogeneously enhancing mass in the pineal gland (Fig. 1.2).

Importance

Retinoblastoma is the most common intraocular tumor of childhood, occurring in one in 15000 to 20000 live births. Approximately 200 new cases a year are diagnosed in the USA. The disease presents in infancy or early childhood, with the majority of cases diagnosed before the age of 4 years.

A second primary malignancy, most commonly a midline intracranial tumor, is found in 5–7% of patients with bilateral retinoblastoma. Often, these other brain tumors occur weeks or months after the diagnosis of the retinoblastoma, with a median interval of 21 months. Trilateral retinoblastoma has traditionally been nearly universally fatal, although a recent study suggests that intensive chemotherapy may improve survival. Early detection is likely an important factor in survival.

Typical clinical scenario

The most frequent presenting sign of retinoblastoma is leukocoria, a white papillary reflex. Other clinical presentations include strabismus, decreased vision, orbital and/or periorbital inflammation, glaucoma, hypopyon (tumor cells anterior to the iris), or ocular pain. The genetic evolution of retinoblastoma follows the Knudson's two-hit hypothesis: patients who have unilateral unifocal disease have mutations at the retinoblastoma locus in both alleles within a single retinal cell. This is an unlikely event; therefore, these tumors are usually unifocal and unilateral, and are rarely associated with other tumors. By contrast, patients with multifocal and bilateral retinoblastomas harbor an underlying germ-line mutation that results in a mutant *RB* gene in every cell of their bodies. Loss of heterozygosity and loss of the normal allele leads to the development of multiple retinoblastomas in one or both eyes. These patients with germ-line mutations are predisposed to development of additional midline brain tumors and other non-ocular tumors.

A trilateral retinoblastoma is the association of a midline intracranial tumor with familial bilateral retinoblastoma, and has been reported in 6% of children with bilateral retinoblastoma and 10% of those with a family history of retinoblastoma. Classically, the intracranial tumor is located in the pineal region and the most common tumor type is a pinealoblastoma.

On CT scans, a retinoblastoma is recognized as a hyperattenuating intraocular mass, which contains punctate or nodular calcifications in over 90% of cases. The tumor may lead to retinal detachment, subretinal effusion, and/or vitreal hemorrhage.

On MR scans, retinoblastomas are hyperintense to vitreous on T1-weighted and proton density-weighted images, and show marked enhancement after contrast media injection. On T2-weighted MR images, retinoblastomas appear hypointense to adjacent vitreous. Possible extension of the tumor beyond the sclera and along the optic nerve is prognostically important, and needs to be reported.

Pineal gland tumors are delineated as inhomogeneous, contrast-enhancing soft tissue masses in the pineal region. Careful attention has to be paid to possible leptomeningeal metastases and spinal lesions. Of note, the normal pineal gland does not have a blood–brain barrier. Therefore, the presence of contrast enhancement alone should not be confused with a pineal gland mass.

Differential diagnosis

Strongly T2-weighted images (long TE, 120ms) may be useful for differentiating retinoblastoma from Coats' disease (retinal telangiectasis) or a persistent hyperplastic primary vitreous, which are both hyperintense on these scans (Figs. 1.3, 1.4).

Coats' disease represents a congenital, non-hereditary, usually unilateral vascular malformation of the retina, which may eventually lead to retinal detachment. The pathophysiology is breakdown of the blood–retina barrier resulting in a subretinal lipoproteinaceous exudate, which typically does not contain calcifications and does not enhance on imaging studies after contrast media injection (Fig. 1.3). Peak prevalence is later than the typical retinoblastoma population, around six to eight years of age, although it can be seen as early as the first year of life. The typical clinical presentation is progressive vision loss. Local therapies include photocoagulation and cryogenic and laser ablation.

Persistent hyperplastic primary vitreous (PHPV): The primary vitreous represents primitive mesenchymal tissue that occupies the posterior eye chamber during embryonic stages of life. This tissue is gradually replaced by mature vitreous, persisting only at the small central canal between the retina and the posterior aspect of the lens (Cloquet canal). A proliferation of this primary vitreous leads to hyperplastic fibrovascular tissue posterior to the lens and along the Cloquet canal. PHPV is congenital and usually noted at birth or within a few weeks of life with leukocoria and microphthalmos. It is unilateral in 90–98% of cases. Untreated PHPV frequently progresses to pthisis bulbi, due to recurrent intraocular hemorrhage.

Retinal astrocytic hamartomas represent masses in the globe, which may have calcifications as well but are predominantly seen in patients with tuberous sclerosis. They are also seen rarely in patients with neurofibromatosis or in isolation. The majority of cases are asymptomatic and come to attention due to other clinical manifestations. In patients with tuberous sclerosis, the lesions are frequently congenital, usually multiple, bilateral in 25% of cases, and may calcify. The majority are non-progressive and do not require treatment. Imaging is primarily performed to evaluate and follow other manifestations of tuberous sclerosis.

Teaching point

Staging and follow-up MR exams of patients with retinoblastoma requires imaging not only of the orbit, but also a contrast-enhanced MRI of the whole brain in order to evaluate for possible additional brain tumors. The risk of "trilateral" tumors is particularly high in patients with multifocal and bilateral retinoblastomas.

REFERENCES

1. Blach LE, McCormick B, Abramson DH, Ellsworth RM. Trilateral retinoblastoma – incidence and outcome: a decade of experience. *Int J Radiat Oncol Biol Phys* 1994;**29**(4):729–33.

2. Dunkel IJ, Jubran RF, Gururangan S, *et al.* Trilateral retinoblastoma: potentially curable with intensive chemotherapy. *Pediatr Blood Cancer* 2010;**54**(3):384–7.

3. Finger PT, Harbour JW, Karicioglu ZA. Risk factors for metastasis in retinoblastoma. *Surv Opthalmol* 2002;**47**(1):1–16.

4. Kivelä T. Trilateral retinoblastoma: a meta-analysis of hereditary retinoblastoma associated with primary ectopic intracranial retinoblastoma. *J Clin Oncol* 1999;**17**(6):1829–37.

(a)

(b)

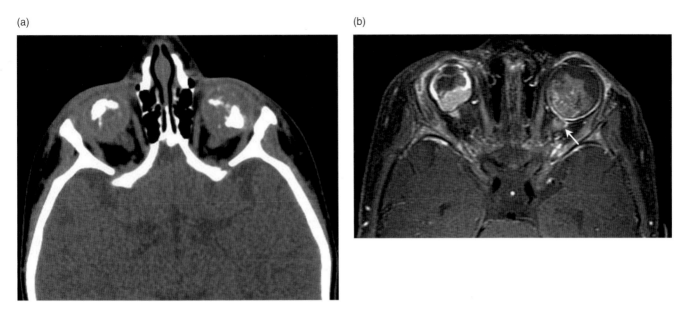

Figure 1.1. (a) An axial CT scan through the orbits shows calcifications in both globes. **(b)** An axial T1-weighted MR scan after injection of Gd-DTPA demonstrates large, contrast-enhancing tumors in the globes bilaterally, with extraocular extension. The tumor in the right globe shows extrascleral extension and the tumor in the left globe shows extension into the optic nerve with associated contrast enhancement of the proximal optic nerve (arrow).

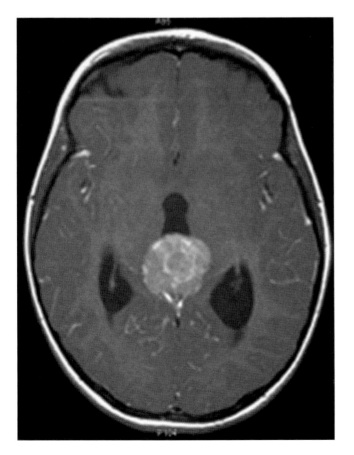

Figure 1.2. Axial T1-weighted MR scan after injection of Gd-DTPA demonstrates a large, inhomogeneously enhancing mass in the pineal gland in a different patient.

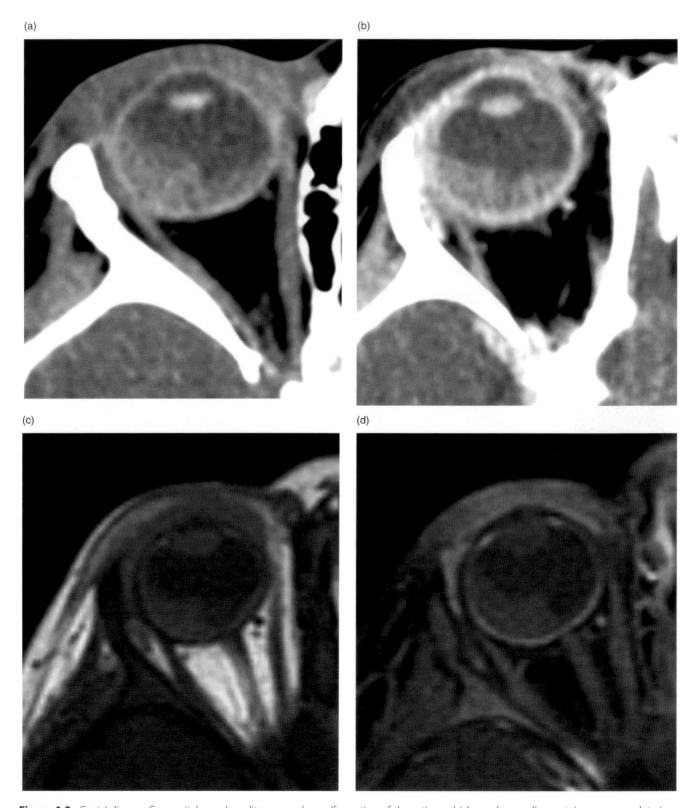

Figure 1.3. Coats' disease. Congenital, non-hereditary, vascular malformation of the retina, which produces a lipoproteinaceous exudate in the subretinal space. Non-contrast and contrast-enhanced CT images of the right orbit **(a, b)** show an intraocular high-density lesion, which represents the lipoproteinaceous exudate. No calcification and no enhancement after contrast media administration are noted. Axial T1-weighted non-contrast **(c)** and T1 postcontrast **(d)** fat-saturated images showing homogeneous intermediate signal of the intraocular lesion without contrast enhancement.

(a)

(b)

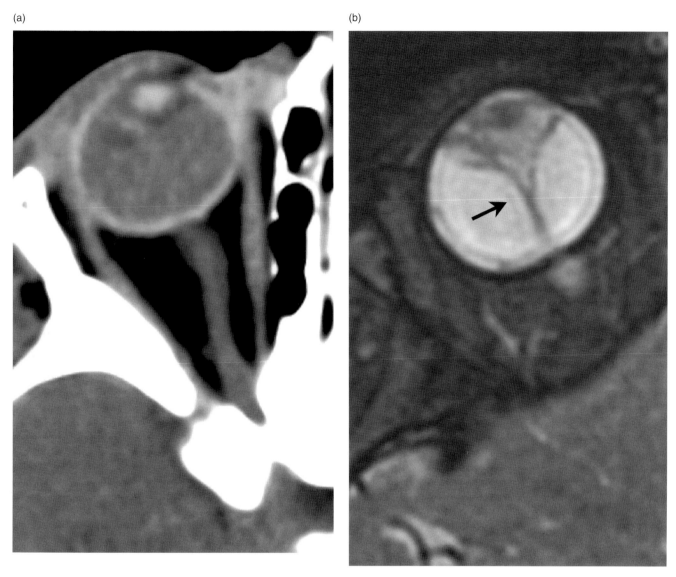

Figure 1.4. Persistent primary hypertrophied vitreous. Axial CT image through the right orbit **(a)** showing uniform high attenuation of the vitreous. T2-weighted image **(b)** shows the Cloquet canal (arrow), very characteristic of this condition.

(c)

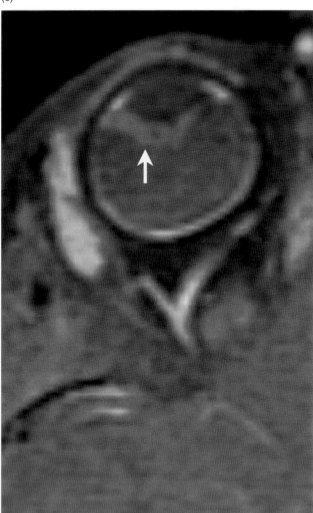

Figure 1.4. (cont.) A postcontrast T1-weighted image **(c)** shows enhancement of the retrolental primary vitreous (arrow)

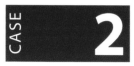

CASE 2 Fibromatosis colli

Siobhan M. Flanagan, Kristen W. Yeom, Patrick D. Barnes, and Beverley Newman

Imaging description

A one-month-old male presented with a palpable right neck mass, which had been noticed 10 days previously. The mass was not perceived to be painful or bothersome to the patient. There was no reported fever or weight loss. He was feeding normally and there was ipsilateral mild torticollis. He was born at 37 weeks by cesarean section due to cardiac decelerations during labor. Imaging evaluation with ultrasound (US) (Fig. 2.1a) demonstrated heterogeneous, mass-like enlargement involving the right inferior sternocleidomastoid muscle (SCM). The mass tapered gently toward the SCM and was surrounded by normal appearing SCM. The fascial planes surrounding the muscle were preserved. There were morphologically normal appearing prominent ipsilateral cervical chain lymph nodes. The lesion did demonstrate moderate internal vascularity on Doppler ultrasound (Fig. 2.1b).

An MRI was also performed in spite of the fact that the US appearance was strongly suggestive of fibromatosis colli. This demonstrated enlargement of the inferior right SCM, with intact surrounding fascial planes. The process was confined to the inferior SCM. There was increased T2 signal and heterogeneous enhancement of the involved muscle (Fig. 2.1c, d, e). There were no calcifications present in the lesion. The MRI findings also supported the diagnosis of fibromatosis colli.

Clinically, the lesion decreased in size over time confirmed by follow-up ultrasound.

Importance

Fibromatosis colli is a form of infantile fibromatosis which is rare and occurs solely in the SCM. Most cases present at two to four weeks of age as a palpable neck mass. They typically occur in the inferior third of the SCM and can occur in either the sternal or clavicular head. Cases are usually unilateral, occur more often on the right, and males are affected slightly more often than females. Torticollis toward the affected side is seen in about 20% of cases and is thought to be due to shortening or contraction of the affected SCM. The precise mechanism is unclear. Suggested etiologies have included birth trauma or an in utero compartment syndrome related to fetal crowding and abnormal head position causing venous obstruction and muscle injury followed by necrosis and fibrosis. Initially, the mass may grow rapidly. Growth, however, slows and eventually ceases. In two-thirds of cases, lesions completely regress by the age of one year.

US is the preferred imaging modality for diagnosis since it is low cost, lacks ionizing radiation, and can well assess superficial lesions. The US appearance, although variable, is usually diagnostic. US can demonstrate heterogeneous enlargement of the SCM, with at times the appearance of a focal mass with variable echogenicity. Extended field of view imaging to show the entire length of the SCM can be useful. Color Doppler imaging may show hyperemia during the acute phase and decreased vascularity during the fibrotic phase. Key findings include confinement within the SCM in the inferior one-third of the muscle and a characteristic spindle-shaped transition to normal muscle. It can be useful to image the contralateral SCM for the purpose of comparison.

MR is not required to make the diagnosis of fibromatosis colli, but is at times obtained during the initial workup of the condition. MRI demonstrates fusiform enlargement of the affected SCM, with variable T2 signal hyperintensity. Signal intensity decreases as the fibrotic stage ensues. There can be hemorrhage in the affected muscle and the lesion can appear very heterogeneous. However, it is not the appearance of the primary lesion that should raise concern for an aggressive neoplastic process such as neuroblastoma or rhabdomyosarcoma, but rather location or extension outside of the SCM and infiltration into surrounding soft tissues. The presence of calcifications in fibromatosis colli is very rare, and should raise concern for neuroblastoma.

Radiographs may be requested by the clinician in cases of torticollis, which will help exclude spinal fusion abnormalities. Rarely, there can be lytic change in the clavicle at the site of attachment of the affected SCM in fibromatosis colli.

Typical clinical scenario

Fibromatosis colli typically presents within the first 8 weeks of life, most often in the first two to four weeks. The affected SCM can continue to enlarge for two to three months. Eventually, the fibrotic phase ensues, after which the size typically decreases over time.

Once confirmed by a combination of clinical assessment and imaging, treatment of fibromatosis colli is conservative, and involves clinical observation and muscle stretching exercises. Most cases resolve by the age of one year. Surgical intervention is necessary in 10–15% of cases, where there is severe refractory disease after 1 year of age. The purpose of surgery is to prevent permanent contracture and plagiocephaly. Surgical treatment consists of proximal or distal release of the SCM. Excision of the fibrous lesion is rarely indicated. More recently, use of *Botulinum* toxin type A has been used for treatment of refractory cases and may further prevent the need for surgical intervention.

Fibromatosis colli has been associated with hip dysplasia, perhaps also related to intrauterine crowding. More recent series have suggested that the association is less important than previously thought. US screening of the hips for dislocation or instability may be useful in the presence of fibromatosis colli and vice versa.

Differential diagnosis

The differential diagnosis for a neck mass in an infant of this age includes cervical lymphadenopathy, congenital neuroblastoma (consider if calcifications are present and involves the paraspinal soft tissues medial to the SCM), and cervical extension of mediastinal thymus (common on the left side, medial and posterior relative to the SCM). Rhabdomyosarcoma and cervical teratoma (consider if fat and calcifications are present) are very uncommon neoplasms in this age group and location.

The presence of torticollis in an infant without a soft tissue mass raises additional diagnostic possibilities. Spinal fusion anomalies are osseous causes that can usually be excluded with cervical spine radiographs. Neurologic causes of torticollis include posterior fossa and cervical spine tumors as well as the Arnold Chiari malformation and syringomyelia. Other miscellaneous causes include ocular deficiency, hearing deficits, and Grisel (C1/C2 subluxation associated with inflammatory conditions such as retropharyngeal cellulitis) and Sandifer (torticollis or unusual neck movement associated with gastroesophageal reflux) syndromes.

Teaching point

Fibromatosis colli is the most common cause of a cervical "mass" during infancy. It presents typically within the first 8 weeks of life. The process is usually confined to the inferior SCM and surrounding fascial planes should be intact. The best imaging modality for diagnosis is US, and that is usually all that is necessary. The appearance can be heterogeneous and variable. If the mass is centered outside of the SCM or there is extension beyond the affected SCM or if there are internal calcifications, consider a neoplastic process such as neuroblastoma.

REFERENCES

1. Do TT. Congenital muscular torticollis: current concepts and review of treatment. *Curr Opin Pediatr* 2006;**18**(1):26–9.
2. Lowry KC, Estroff JA, Rahbar R. The presentation and management of fibromatosis colli. *Ear Nose Throat J* 2010;**89**(9):E4–8.
3. Meuwly JY, Lepori D, Theumann N, *et al.* Multimodality imaging of the pediatric neck: techniques and spectrum of findings. *Radiographics* 2005;**25**(4):931–48.
4. Murphey MD, Ruble CM, Tyszko SM, *et al.* From the archives of AFIP: musculoskeletal fibromatoses: radiologic-pathologic correlation. *Radiographics* 2009;**29**(7):2143–73.
5. Robbin MR, Murphey MD, Temple HT, *et. al.* Imaging of musculoskeletal fibromatosis. *Radiographics* 2001;**21**(3):585–600.

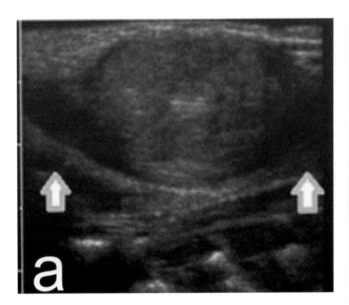
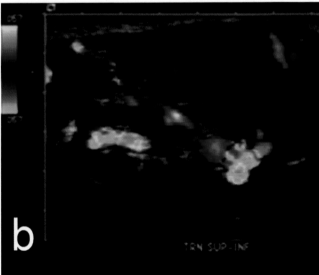

Figure 2.1. Fibromatosis colli, 1-month-old male. **(a)** Longitudinal gray-scale ultrasound image demonstrates a heterogeneous superficial lesion that is contained in the sternocleidomastoid muscle (SCM), with smooth tapering to normal appearing SCM (arrows). Surrounding fascial planes are intact. **(b)** Sagittal color Doppler imaging demonstrates moderate internal vascularity to the lesion.

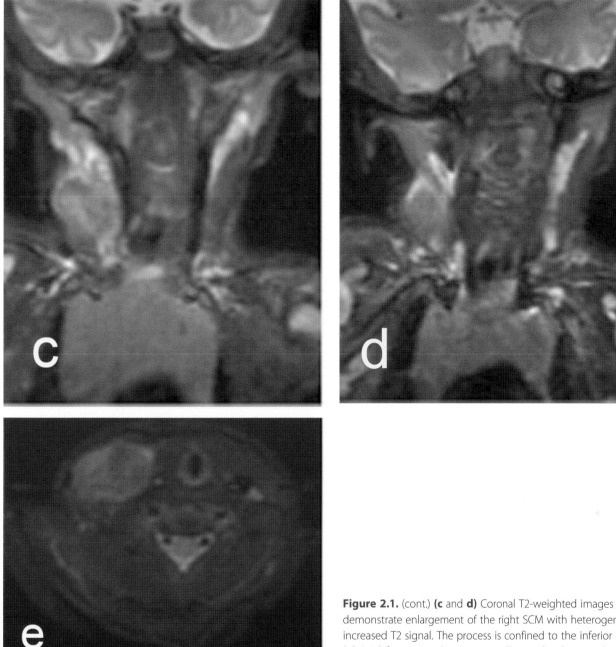

Figure 2.1. (cont.) **(c** and **d)** Coronal T2-weighted images demonstrate enlargement of the right SCM with heterogeneous increased T2 signal. The process is confined to the inferior SCM. **(e)** Axial, fat-saturated, postcontrast T1-weighted image demonstrates heterogeneous enhancement of the involved SCM.

Craniopharyngioma

Camilla Mosci and Andrei Iagaru

Imaging description

A five-year-old girl presented to the emergency room with new onset of nausea, vomiting, and headaches. MRI showed a 36 × 26 × 30 mm multicystic suprasellar mass extending superior to the third ventricle (Fig. 3.1a, b) with areas of calcification and ventriculomegaly. An Ommaya device was placed in the right frontal lobe for cyst drainage. Pathology was consistent with craniopharyngioma. She was followed with serial MRI and CT scans. The imaging studies were stable for one and a half years when an MRI scan demonstrated further increase in the cystic and solid components of the suprasellar mass with increased ventriculomegaly. The patient underwent a right frontal endoscopic fenestration and partial resection of the suprasellar mass, with removal of the blocked Ommaya reservoir and placement of an external ventricular drainage system. Follow-up MRI showed increased size of the cystic mass and ventricles stable in size. However, there was evidence of mass compression of the optic chiasm. The patient underwent MRI-guided placement of a new right frontal Ommaya reservoir into the cystic portion of her tumor. Therapy with ^{32}P (β emitter) colloid chromic phosphate was recommended by the treating physician. A diagnostic ^{99m}Tc sulphur colloid scan of the cystic tumor was performed to evaluate the distribution of the injected material on the inner surface of the tumor and to exclude the presence of a leak from the craniopharyngioma to the cerebrospinal fluid (CSF) space. The ^{99m}Tc sulphur colloid scan showed radiotracer migration from the Ommaya reservoir and coating of the suprasellar mass. However, uptake was also seen into the ventricular system, due to a leak (Fig. 3.1c, d). Due to this leak to the CSF space, the ^{32}P chromic phosphate treatment was aborted in order to avoid excess radiation of normal central nervous system (CNS) structures.

Importance

Craniopharyngioma is a benign tumor that arises along the path of the craniopharyngeal duct. It accounts for 2–5% of all intracranial tumors and 5.6–13% of pediatric intracranial tumors and is classified into cystic, solid, and mixed. Despite its benign histologic appearance, prognosis may often be unfavorable due to mass effect on adjacent structures and the optimal therapeutic approach remains controversial. Total resection is the treatment of choice, but when the tumor localization is unfavorable (proximity and adherence to hypothalamus, pituitary stalk, visual apparatus, circle of Willis, floor of the third ventricle) limited resection followed by local irradiation is recommended. The rate of tumor recurrence is about 10–30% even after total resection. The utilization of radiotherapy can decrease the rate of tumor recurrence in patients who undergo limited resection. However, it also may cause endocrine dysfunction, visual deterioration, radiation-related tumors, and cognitive impairment. In cystic tumors, radionuclide therapy with ^{32}P chromic phosphate colloid is indicated. ^{32}P is a β emitter that has been shown to ablate the epithelial lining of the cyst, effectively reducing the rate of cystic fluid reaccumulation and reducing the cyst size. Compared to conventional external beam radiotherapy, radionuclide therapy delivers a higher dose of radiation directly into the inner surface of the cyst, while reducing the radiation dose to tissues adjacent to the tumor. It is important not only to obtain long-term tumor control but also to preserve the patient's quality of life and stereotactic instillation of ^{32}P chromic phosphate colloid causes minimal risk and is effective as either primary or adjuvant treatment of craniopharyngiomas (Fig. 3.2).

Typical clinical scenario

Clinical presentation is dependent on the size and site of the lesion and can vary from non-specific manifestations of increased intracranial pressure to more specific symptoms as a result of pituitary hormone deficiencies or excess. Symptoms include headache, nausea, vomiting, visual disturbance, seizures, and endocrine dysfunction (diabetes insipidus, amenorrhea, sexual inadequacy, growth retardation).

Differential diagnosis

Craniopharyngioma can be misdiagnosed as a pituitary tumor, metastasis, meningioma, epidermoid or dermoid tumors, hypothalamic-optic pathway glioma, hypothalamic hamartoma, and teratoma. Other differential diagnoses that should be considered include congenital anomalies (arachnoid cyst and Rathke's cleft cyst), infectious/inflammatory processes (eosinophilic granuloma, lymphocytic hypophysitis, sarcoidosis, syphilis, and tuberculosis), and vascular malformations (aneurysm of the internal carotid or anterior communicating artery, arteriovenous malformation).

Teaching point

Despite the benign histologic classification, craniopharyngioma may behave aggressively due to its propensity for recurrence and mass effect on adjacent structures. Radical resection (when possible) or limited resection followed by postoperative irradiation is suggested. In cystic lesions, radionuclide therapy with ^{32}P chromic phosphate colloid may deliver a higher dose of radiation to the inner surface of the cyst than conventional external beam radiotherapy and may prevent recurrence. However, as leaks into the CSF are possible, a diagnostic ^{99m}Tc sulphur colloid scan of the cystic tumor should be conducted before therapy to document distribution to the inner surface of the cystic tumor and the absence of a leak into the CSF. Attention should be paid to administering the correct agent, ^{32}P chromic phosphate colloid and not ^{32}P sodium phosphate as the latter is absorbed in the systemic circulation and may result in death of the treated patient.

REFERENCES

1. Garnett M, Puget S, Grill J, Sainte Rose C. Craniopharyngioma. *Orphanet J Rare Dis* 2007;**2**:18.
2. Hasegawa T, Kondziolka D, Hadjipanayis C, Lunsford LD. Management of cystic craniopharyngiomas with phosphorus-32 intracavitary irradiation. *Neurosurgery* 2004;**54**(4):813–20.
3. Karavitaki N, Brufani C, Warner JT, *et al.* Craniopharyngiomas in children and adults: systematic analysis of 121 cases with long-term follow-up. *Clin Endocrinol* 2005;**62**(4):397–409.
4. Taasan V, Shapiro B, Taren JA, *et al.* Phosphorus-32 therapy of cystic grade IV astrocytomas: technique and preliminary application. *J Nuclear Med* 1985;**26**(11):1335–8.
5. Zhao R, Deng J, Liang X, *et al.* Treatment of cystic craniopharyngioma with phosphorus-32 intracavitary irradiation. *Childs Nerv Syst* 2010;**26**(5):669–74.
6. Zhao X, Yi X, Wang H, Zhao H. An analysis of related factors of surgical results for patients with craniopharyngiomas. *Clin Neurol Neurosurg* 2012;**114**(2):149-55.

(a)   (b)

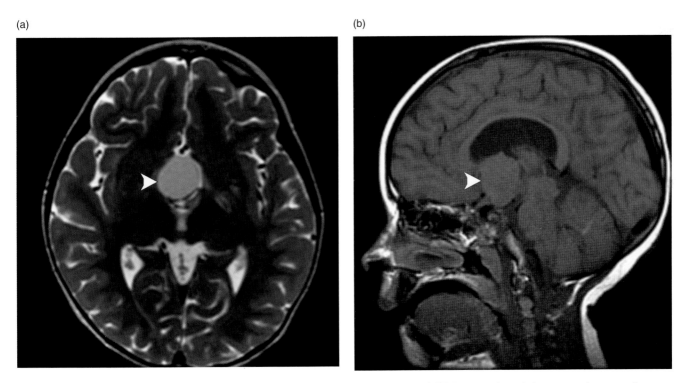

Figure 3.1. A five-year-old girl with craniopharyngioma. MRI [**(a)** T2 transaxial view and **(b)** T1 sagittal view] shows a cystic suprasellar mass extending superiorly to the third ventricle (arrowheads).

(c)

(d)

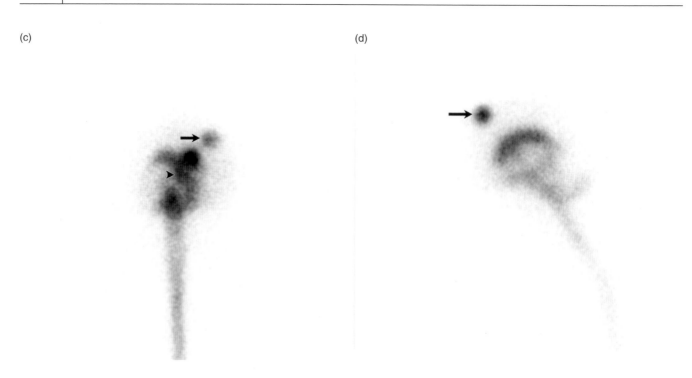

Figure 3.1. (cont.) The ^{99m}Tc sulphur colloid scan [**(c)** anterior view and **(d)** lateral view] showed radiotracer migration from the Ommaya reservoir (arrow) and coating of the suprasellar mass (arrowhead). However, uptake was also seen into the CSF space, due to a leak.

(a)

(b)

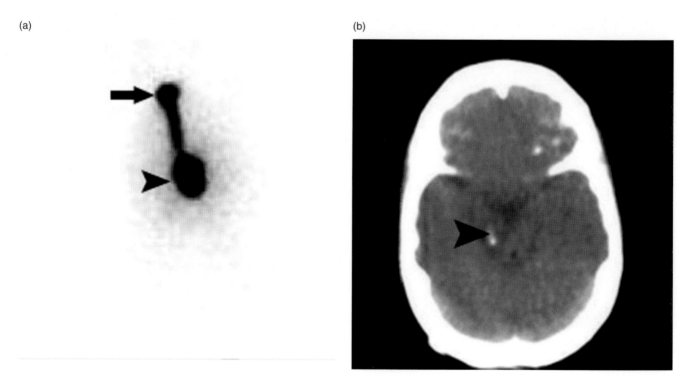

Figure 3.2. A six-year-old girl with craniopharyngioma. Normal distribution of the ^{99m}Tc sulphur colloid from an Ommaya reservoir (arrow) to the tumor (arrowhead), without CSF leak, seen on anterior planar scintigraphy **(a)**, as well as on transaxial images from SPECT/CT **(b, c, d)**. Bremsstrahlung image **(e)** acquired after the administration of ^{32}P chromic phosphate shows accumulation of the radiopharmaceutical in the craniopharyngioma (arrowhead). Bremsstrahlung is electromagnetic radiation produced by the deceleration of a charged particle when deflected by another charged particle. The moving particle loses kinetic energy, which is converted into a photon. The nuclide ^{32}P is a pure β emitter and the particulate radiation by itself cannot be imaged externally. However, the bremsstrahlung emission, resulting from interaction of the β particle with matter, can be utilized to portray an image with gamma cameras.

(c)

(d)

(e)

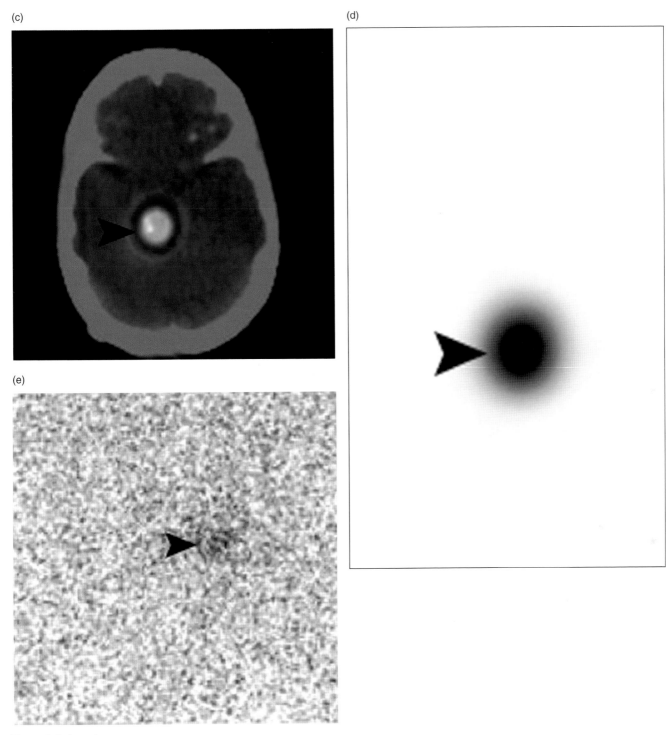

Figure 3.2. (cont.)

Labyrinthitis ossificans

Lex A. Mitchell and Kristen W. Yeom

Imaging description

A six-year-old male with a prior history of meningitis presented with recent onset of bilateral sensorineural hearing loss (SNHL). CT imaging showed developing calcification within the vestibule (Fig. 4.1a, c) as well as within the cochlea (Fig. 4.1b). The history and imaging findings were consistent with labyrinthitis ossificans (LO).

Importance

LO is characterized by new bone formation in the cochlea, classically involving the scala tympani of the basal turn of the cochlea, and vestibule during the end-stage of bacterial/purulent labyrinthitis. In bacterial/purulent labyrinthitis, infection reaches the inner ear from the subarachnoid space via the cochlear aqueduct or the internal auditory meatus. Labyrinthine infection can also occur as a result of bacterial middle ear infections, from direct spread through the oval or round windows or by hematogenous seeding of the labyrinth. *Haemophilus influenzae*, *Streptococcus pneumoniae*, and *Neisseria meningitidis* are the most common organisms causing bacterial meningitis and SNHL in children. Other etiologies of LO include vascular obstruction of the labyrinthine artery, temporal bone trauma, autoimmune ear disease, otosclerosis, leukemia, or tumors of the temporal bone. Treatment by cochlear implantation may mitigate speech and language deterioration in children with LO and SNHL.

Typical clinical scenario

LO associated with purulent meningitis most often presents two months or longer after the onset of infection with bilateral, symmetrical hearing loss of a flat or gradually sloping configuration and is usually irreversible.

Differential diagnosis

LO is defined as pathologic new bone formation within the otic capsule in response to an inflammatory and/or destructive process. Other potential etiologies of increased density in the labyrinth include osteopetrosis and post-traumatic hemolabyrinth, and in adults, Paget's disease.

Teaching point

LO is most often due to bacterial labyrinthitis accompanying meningitis and has a characteristic CT imaging appearance. The timing of cochlear implantation is critical as the incidence of LO in the cochlea is high, the onset and rate of progression are unpredictable, and advanced cochlear basal turn LO may prevent adequate insertion of the cochlear electrode.

REFERENCES

1. Chan CC, Saunders DE, Chong WK, *et al.* Advancement in post-meningitic lateral semicircular canal labyrinthitis ossificans. *J Laryngol Otol* 2007;**121**:105–9.

2. Mukerji SS, Parmar HA, Pynnonen MA. Radiology quiz case 1. Labyrinthitis ossificans (LO)-stage of fibrosis. *Arch Otolaryngol Head Neck Surg* 2007;**133**:298, 300.

3. Westerlaan HE, Meiners LC, Penning L. Labyrinthitis ossificans associated with sensorineural deafness. *Ear Nose Throat J* 2005;**84**:14–15.

4. Xu HX, Joglekar SS, Paparella MM. Labyrinthitis ossificans. *Otol Neurotol* 2009;**30**:579–80.

(a) (b)

(c)

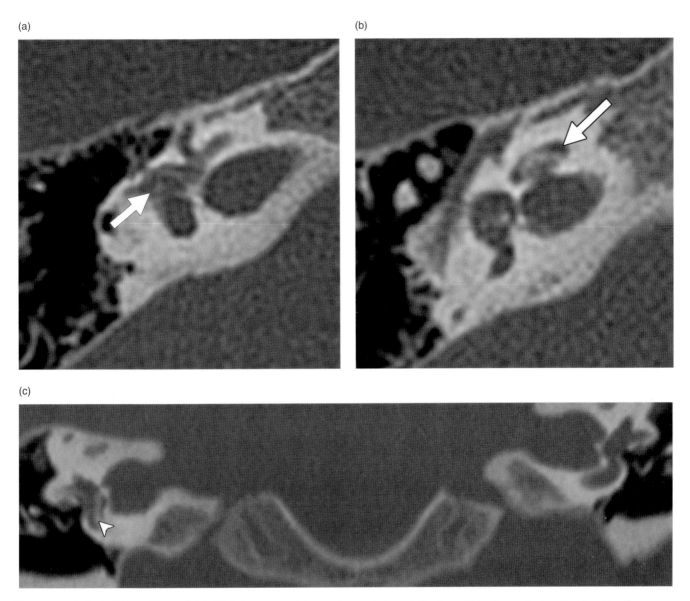

Figure 4.1. Labyrinthitis ossificans. Axial CT of the temporal bones demonstrates calcification within the vestibule extending into the semicircular canal, arrow **(a)** and arrowhead **(c)**, as well as within the cochlea, arrow **(b)**. No calcification was seen in the contralateral inner ear structures **(c)**.

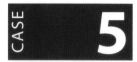

CASE 5

Branchio-oto-renal syndrome

Lex A. Mitchell and Kristen W. Yeom

Imaging description

A five-year-old male presented with left sensorineural hearing loss, bilateral pre-auricular pits, and a draining right neck sinus. Initial audiometry demonstrated bilateral hearing loss. CT of the temporal bones was remarkable for bilateral enlargement of the internal auditory canals, dysmorphic appearance of the cochlea bilaterally, and hypoplasia of the lateral semicircular canals (Fig. 5.1). The imaging appearance, in conjunction with the clinical findings, was suggestive of branchio-oto-renal (BOR) syndrome.

Importance

BOR syndrome is an autosomal dominant disorder occurring in approximately 1:40000 births, although the true incidence may be difficult to establish because not all affected individuals undergo imaging evaluation. Despite the relatively common presentation, the severity of the syndrome is hard to predict given the variable penetrance. The presence of one or more features of the syndrome should prompt clinical and imaging investigation for associated anomalies.

Typical clinical scenario

BOR patients will typically present in the infant/toddler age group with history of hearing loss and pre-auricular pits. Physical examination may show a long, narrow face, pre-auricular pits, mis shaped ears, lacrimal duct aplasia or stenosis, high arched or cleft palate, branchial cleft fistula, or clefts. Imaging features have classically been described to include a calcified or shortened anterior malleolar ligament, narrowed malleoincudal joint, ossicular displacement, hypoplastic apical and basal turns of the cochlea, medial deviation of the facial nerve, underdevelopment of the vestibule, enlarged vestibular aqueduct, and funnel-or ellipsoid-shaped internal auditory canal. Renal malformations are common and can be unilateral or bilateral and occur in any combination. Some of the more common anomalies seen on renal ultrasound or intravenous pyelography are renal agenesis (29%), hypoplasia (19%), dysplasia (14%), ureteropelvic junction obstruction (10%), calyceal cyst or diverticulum (10%), and caliectasis, pelviectasis, hydronephrosis, and vesico-ureteral reflux (all at 5%). There are even documented cases of renal dysplasias not presenting until adulthood.

Differential diagnosis

BOR syndrome is a syndrome that is difficult to diagnose early because of the cost of genetic testing and variable expressivity and penetrance. Positive imaging evaluation and correlative findings on physical exam allow clinicians to test more specifically for a potential genetic etiology, in the case of BOR, EYA1. Other entities that may be differential considerations include dysmorphic pinna-polycystic kidney syndrome, dysmorphic pinna-hypospadias-renal dysplasia syndrome, or oto-renal-genital syndrome.

> ### Teaching point
> BOR is a genetic disease that is primarily suggested by imaging and confirmed with focused genetic testing.

REFERENCES

1. Millman B, Gibson WS, Foster WP. Branchio-oto-renal syndrome. *Arch Otolaryngol Head Neck Surg* 1995;**121**(8):922–5.

2. Misra M, Nolph KD. Renal failure and deafness: branchio-oto-renal syndome. *Am J Kidney Dis* 1998;**32**(2):334–7.

3. Propst EJ, Blaser S, Gordon KA, Harrison RV, Papsin BC. Temporal bone findings on computed tomography imaging in branchio-oto-renal syndrome. *Laryngoscope* 2005;**115**(10):1855–62.

4. Rodriguez Soriano J. Branchio-oto-renal syndrome. *J Nephrol* 2003;**16**(4):603–5.

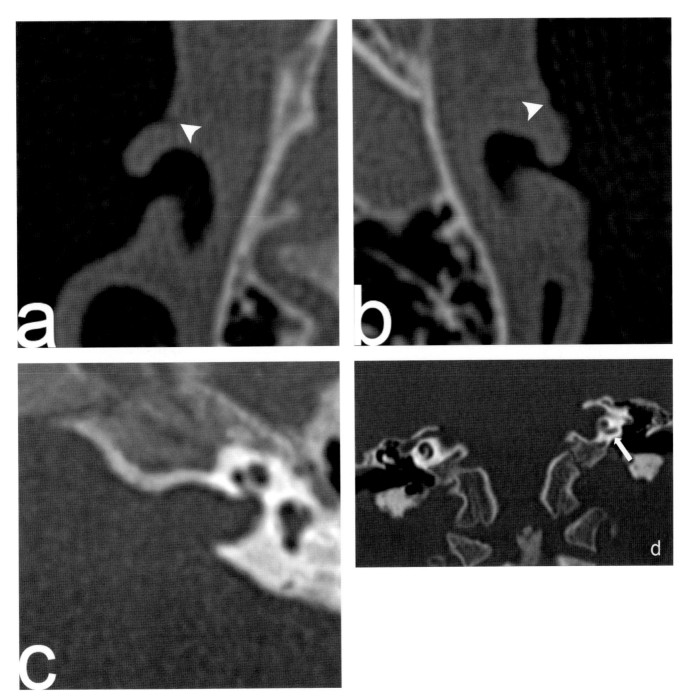

Figure 5.1. Branchio-oto-renal syndrome. CT of the temporal bones in a child with bilateral hearing loss and bilateral pre-auricular draining pits revealed bilateral pre-auricular pits [**(a, b)** white arrowheads], a flared appearance of the internal auditory canal **(c)**, and dismorphic cochlea with elongated basal turn [**(d)** white arrow].

Medulloblastoma

Neilish Gupta and Kristen W. Yeom

Imaging description

A three-year-old girl presented with back pain, vomiting, lethargy, and ataxia over a 1-month period. The non-contrast head CT demonstrates a hyperdense midline posterior fossa mass with obstructive hydrocephalus (Fig. 6.1a). MRI examination demonstrates a heterogeneous mass predominantly iso-intense to gray matter on both T1- and T2-weighted images with moderate enhancement post contrast (Fig. 6.1b–d). Additional nodules of similar signal characteristics are seen within the lateral ventricle as well as along the spinal column consistent with cerebrospinal fluid (CSF) metastatic spread.

Importance

Medulloblastomas are the most common posterior fossa tumors in children (30–40%) and comprise 15–20% of intracranial neoplasms in children. They comprise up to 1% of adult brain tumors. The tumors can arise in the cerebellar vermis or hemispheres.

Medulloblastomas are highly malignant tumors and may be composed of classic undifferentiated primitive small round cells, although histologic variants such as desmoplastic, extensive nodular, and large cell histologies may be seen, the latter of which imparts a worse prognosis. The case presented here is of the large cell histology with extensive spread and rapid growth. On CT, medulloblastomas are hyperdense due to their high nuclear to cytoplasmic ratio. On MRI, they are variable in signal although usually isointense to gray matter on T1 and hypo- to isointense on T2-weighted images and associated with reduced diffusion due to the highly cellular nature of the tumor. Cysts and calcifications are possible within the tumor and enhancement is variable.

Typical clinical scenario

The duration of symptoms is typically short prior to diagnosis (<3 months), including nausea, vomiting, and headaches. In children less than one year of age, increasing head size and lethargy may be the presenting symptoms while in older children and adults, ataxia may predominate. Spinal tumor seeding is present in approximately 30% of initial diagnoses and symptoms referable to spinal involvement may be present.

Differential diagnosis

Ependymoma, atypical teratoid/rhabdoid tumor, and astrocytoma are differential considerations for a posterior fossa neoplasm in childhood. A hyperdense appearance of the posterior fossa mass on CT and low diffusion on MRI are key imaging features suggesting medulloblastoma.

Teaching point

The most common malignant posterior fossa tumor in children is medulloblastoma, an aggressive neoplasm which often disseminates along the subarachnoid spaces without proper treatment. This tumor is typically hyperdense on CT, which is a major distinguishing factor from pilocytic astrocytoma.

REFERENCES

1. Barkovich AJ. *Pediatric Neuroimaging*, 4th edition. Philadelphia: Lippincott Williams & Wilkin, 2005.
2. Koeller KK, Rushing EJ. From the archives of the AFIP: medulloblastoma: a comprehensive review with radiologic-pathologic correlation. *Radiographics* 2003;**23**(6):1613–37.

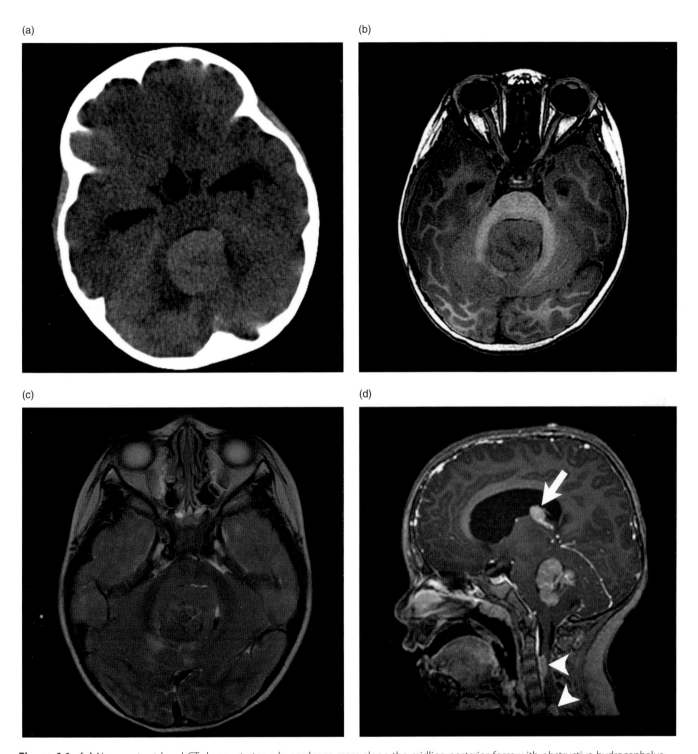

Figure 6.1. **(a)** Non-contrast head CT demonstrates a hyperdense mass along the midline posterior fossa with obstructive hydrocephalus. **(b, c)** T1- (b) and T2- (c) weighted MR images demonstrate the posterior fossa mass with heterogeneous signal predominantly isointense to gray matter. **(d)** Sagittal postcontrast T1-weighted MR image demonstrates enhancement of the primary posterior fossa mass as well as additional enhancing nodules along the lateral ventricle (arrow) and spinal column (arrowheads) consistent with metastatic disease.

Ectopic cervical thymus

Michael Iv and Kristen W. Yeom

Imaging description

A five-month-old boy presented with a palpable left neck mass. MRI shows a left parapharyngeal mass that is isointense to muscle on T1-weighted imaging (Fig. 7.1a) and hyperintense to muscle and homogeneous in signal on T2-weighted imaging (Fig. 7.1b). A coronal contrast-enhanced T1-weighted image (Fig. 7.1c) shows mild enhancement of this mass and again shows homogeneous signal. The MR imaging characteristics are similar to intrathoracic thymus but there is not definite contiguity. The diagnosis of normal thymic tissue was confirmed following CT-guided fine-needle aspiration.

Importance

The primordial thymus arises from the third and fourth pharyngeal pouches during the sixth week of gestational life. During the seventh week, thymic primordia migrate medially and caudally, forming the thymopharyngeal duct, to their final anatomic location in the anterior mediastinum. Ectopic and accessory thymic tissue may occur anywhere along the descending pathway of the thymopharyngeal duct (from the angle of the mandible to the superior mediastinum) due to arrest in migration, sequestration, or failure of involution. Ectopic thymic tissue and remnants are congenital lesions that may be solid and/or cystic in nature. Most ectopic cervical thymic tissue is unilateral and usually on the left for reasons that are unclear. Manifestation of ectopic thymic tissue as a neck mass may be mistaken for a pathologic process.

Typical clinical scenario

Clinically apparent ectopic cervical thymus is a rare condition and usually presents as an asymptomatic mass or neck swelling on routine physical examination. In 50% of cases, this condition occurs in children between two and 13 years of age and is more common in males. These lesions may be large in size and can cause compression and displacement of neighboring structures resulting in symptoms of stridor, hoarseness, or dysphagia. Although these lesions are ultimately diagnosed by histopathology obtained from fine-needle aspiration or surgical excision, radiologic imaging using ultrasound, CT, and/or MRI plays a significant role in evaluation. The sonographic appearance of thymus is unique, with hypoechoic cortex and echogenic medulla containing linear and echogenic septae. Additionally, vessels between septae are seen as discrete, high level echoes. A small clinically inapparent superior extension of thymic tissue into the neck is commonly seen in pediatric neck and chest cross-sectional imaging. It is important not to mistake this for tumor or adenopathy. The imaging appearance, homogeneity, and contiguity with mediastinal thymic tissues are often helpful in defining this tissue as normal thymus. Thymic cysts also occur with some regularity both within the mediastinal thymus and particularly within ectopic thymic tissue in the neck (Fig. 7.2). They may present acutely due to hemorrhage or secondary infection.

Differential diagnosis

The differential diagnosis of ectopic cervical thymus includes branchial cleft cyst, cystic hygroma, cystic teratoma, thyroglossal duct cyst, esophageal duplication cyst, reactive adenopathy, lymphoproliferative disorders, neoplasms, and lipoblastoma.

Teaching point

Ectopic cervical thymus may present as a neck mass or cyst, most often left sided, and may be easily mistaken for pathology. The role of ultrasound, CT, and/or MRI with or without histopathology is important in the diagnosis of this condition. As in many other situations, knowledge of the variations in location and appearance of normal tissues is essential to suggest likely or possible differential considerations and direct or curtail further investigation.

REFERENCES

1. Ahsan F, Allison R, White J. Ectopic cervical thymus: case report and review of pathogenesis and management. *J Laryngol Otol* 2010;**124**(6):694–7.
2. Nasseri F, Eftekhari F. Clinical and radiologic review of the normal and abnormal thymus: pearls and pitfalls. *Radiographics* 2010;**30**(2):413–28.
3. Tunkel DE, Erozan YS, Weir G. Ectopic cervical thymic tissue: diagnosis by fine needle aspiration. *Arch Pathol Lab Med* 2001;**125**(2):278–81.
4. Wang J, Fu H, Yang H, Wang L, He Y. Clinical management of cervical ectopic thymus in children. *J Pediatr Surg* 2011;**46**(8):e33–6.

(a)

(b)

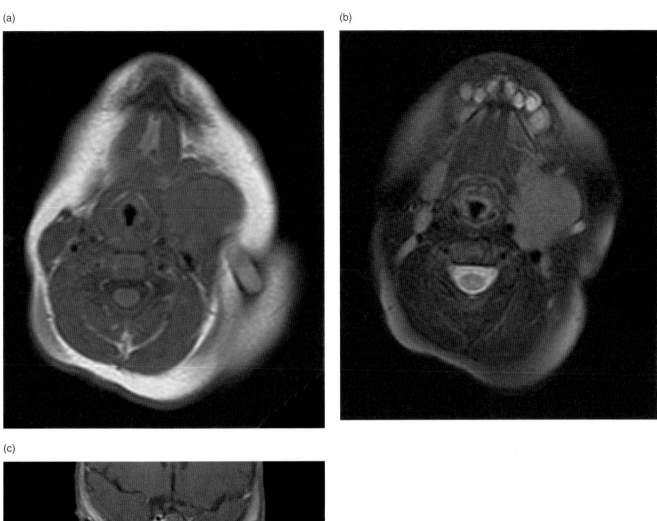

(c)

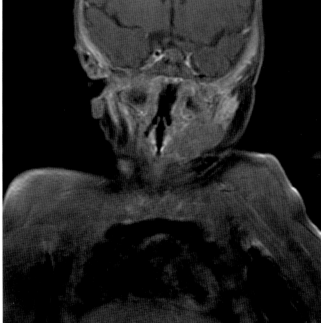

Figure 7.1. Ectopic cervical thymus. A five-month-old boy presented with a palpable left neck mass. MRI shows a left parapharyngeal mass that is isointense to muscle on T1-weighted imaging **(a)** and isointense to fat on T2-weighted imaging **(b)**. Coronal contrast-enhanced T1-weighted image **(c)** shows mild homogeneous enhancement within this mass, similar to mediastinal thymic tissue but without definite contiguity. The diagnosis of thymic tissue was confirmed following CT-guided fine-needle aspiration.

(a)

(c)

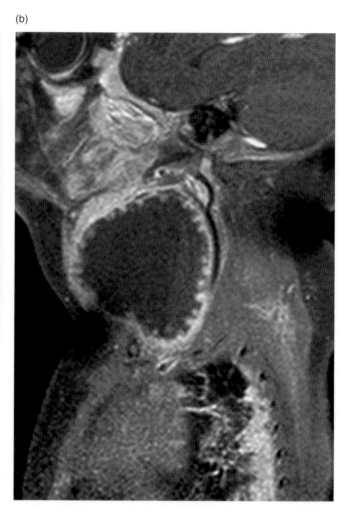

(b)

Figure 7.2. Thymic cyst in the neck. A one-month-old girl with an acutely enlarging left neck mass and respiratory distress. Transverse color Doppler ultrasound of the left neck demonstrates a large cyst with a thickened hyperemic wall containing dependent echogenic debris **(a)**. Sagittal T1 postcontrast **(b)** and coronal STIR **(c)** MRI reveal corresponding findings to the ultrasound, with a large cyst (dark T1, bright T2) demonstrating thick, irregular, and enhancing wall as well as dependent debris. The cyst is immediately contiguous with the mediastinal thymic tissue. Turbid fluid, which was thought to be related to acute infection, was found in the cyst at the time of surgical removal. Pathology confirmed a thymic origin. (Case courtesy of Ron Cohen, MD, Oakland Children's Hospital.)

X-linked adrenoleukodystrophy

Jared Narvid and Kristen W. Yeom

Imaging description

A six-year-old male presented with hyponatremia and hyperpigmentation. MRI of the brain was obtained which showed abnormal FLAIR signal within the splenium of the corpus callosum (Fig. 8.1a). Sagittal and axial postcontrast T1-weighted images demonstrated prominent zonal enhancement along the anterior margin of the lesion (Fig. 8.1b, c). The findings were strongly suggestive of adrenoleukodystrophy.

Importance

X-linked adrenoleukodystrophy (XALD) is a genetic disorder affecting the adrenal cortex and the central nervous system (CNS) with wide phenotypic variability. XALD is caused by mutations in the ABCD1 gene located on chromosome Xq28 which encodes a peroxisomal membrane transporter protein (XALDP). This mutation causes accumulation of saturated very long chain fatty acids in all tissues, especially CNS white matter and adrenal cortex. As such, XALD is considered within the general category of peroxisome disorders.

The pathologic abnormalities in the brain consist of widespread demyelination of the white matter. In most cases, the process starts in the splenium of the corpus callosum and spreads bilaterally to the occipital and parietal periventricular regions. Histopathologic examination reveals different zones of demyelination within the affected brain, with anterior zones demonstrating active inflammatory demyelination, while posterior zones appear destroyed and burnt out.

MR imaging of the brain in XALD often mirrors the histopathologic appearances. Namely, signal abnormalities on T2 or FLAIR images are seen within the splenium of the corpus callosum as well as parieto-occipital white matter, reflecting demyelination. In fact, in 80% of cases, imaging shows abnormalities in the occipital white matter. After administration of contrast, a zone of enhancement can be seen where the active demyelinating front advances into unaffected areas. More posterior regions often do not enhance, indicating a more complete, quiescent demyelination. In general, the end-stage demonstrates significant atrophy of large portions of affected white matter in a typical symmetrical pattern.

In addition to its role in diagnostics, MRI has a major role in monitoring disease progression. There are currently two treatments of XALD, dietary modification and bone marrow transplantation. Diets enriched in monounsaturated fatty acids have been found to lower long chain fatty acids levels and are accordingly employed in XALD patients. Nevertheless, only bone marrow transplant has been found to alter the clinical disease course. When employed early in the course of XALD, bone marrow transplant has been found to mitigate further deterioration. In this context, MRI plays a significant role in determining patient eligibility for bone marrow transplant and evaluating treatment response. Loes et al. have developed a 34-point MR scoring system to make these determinations. Most significantly, contrast enhancement has important predictive value; an absence of enhancement predicts stable disease in 85% of patients.

Typical clinical scenario

The childhood cerebral form accounts for one-third of cases, usually developing between five and nine years of age. Symptoms related to adrenal insufficiency may precede neurologic impairment, with many such cases receiving the initial diagnosis of Addison disease. More commonly, neuropsychiatric symptoms dominate early. Behavioral changes include hyperactivity, aggressive behavior, and worsening school performance, often initiating diagnostic evaluation for attention-deficit/hyperactivity disorder. Nonetheless, these early features ultimately give way to a relentless progressive neurocognitive impairment, blindness, and spastic quadriplegia. The pace of deterioration is highly variable.

The most common clinical symptoms are sensorineural hearing loss (90%), pyramidal tract symptoms (50%), visual deficits (40%), behavioral abnormalities (33%), and seizures (6%).

Differential diagnosis

Differential considerations include acute demyelinating encephalomyelitis, multiple sclerosis, toxic or treatment-related leukoencephalopathy, and infection. The notable symmetrical, contiguous, posterior, and enhancing demyelination is the hallmark of XALD in contrast to more patchy findings in other demyelinating processes. In adults, gliomas and lymphomas may be included as well but are less commonly as symmetrical. Focal splenial lesions have also been described in the context of seizures and mild encephalitis in children, but do not typically demonstrate zonal enhancement.

> ### Teaching point
>
> XALD is often initially misdiagnosed as psychiatric disease or adrenal insufficiency. Progressive neurologic impairment and characteristic symmetric MRI findings are hallmarks of the disease.

REFERENCES

1. Ferrer I, Auborg P, Pujol A. General aspects and neuropathology of X-linked adrenoleukodystrophy. *Brain Pathol* 2010;**20**(4):817–30.
2. Loes DJ, Hite S, Moser H, *et al.* Adrenoleukodystrophy: a scoring method for brain MR observations. *AJNR Am J Neuroradiol* 1994;**15**(9):1761–6.
3. Moser HW, Mahmood A, Raymond GV. X-linked adrenoleukodystrophy. *Nat Clin Pract Neurol* 2007;**3**(3):140–51.

(a)

(b)

(c)

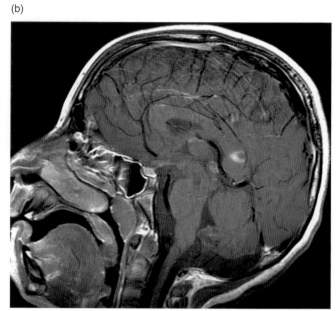

Figure 8.1. (a) Axial FLAIR MR image demonstrates signal abnormality in the splenium of the corpus callosum, a typical location of early adrenoleukodystrophy (ALD) involvement. **(b)** Sagittal postcontrast T1 MR image demonstrates zonal phenomenon. **(c)** Axial postcontrast T1 MR image shows leading edge enhancement to better advantage.

Langerhans cell histiocytosis

Vy Thao Tran, Thomas Pulling, Kristen W. Yeom, and Bo Yoon Ha

Imaging description

A 10-year-old boy presented with pain and soft tissue swelling of the left cheek. A CT scan demonstrated an extensive soft tissue mass centered in the left maxilla with associated cortical erosion of the left alveolar ridge and left maxillary sinus walls. Contralateral involvement of the right alveolar ridge and anterior maxillary sinus wall was also noted. Several teeth appeared to be "floating" within the maxilla. There was absence of adjacent soft tissue fat stranding (Fig. 9.1a–c).

A five-month-old infant presented with bi-parietal scalp swelling. CT of the head showed bi-parietal calvarial lytic lesions with associated soft tissue masses and a characteristic "beveled edge" appearance with greater destruction of the outer table of the calvarium relative to the inner table (Fig. 9.2a, b). On MRI, mixed T1 and T2 intensities and heterogeneous enhancement of the soft tissue mass was seen (Fig. 9.2c–e).

Langerhans cell histiocytosis (LCH) was confirmed pathologically in both cases.

Importance

LCH is an idiopathic multisystem disorder, which is characterized by abnormal immune regulation and clonal proliferation of histiocytes (activated dendritic cells and macrophages). The characteristic Langerhans cells in LCH lesions are immature dendritic cells that express the monocyte marker CD14. The estimated annual incidence in the USA is 0.05–0.5/100000 children. The mean age at presentation is five to seven years, with almost all patients presenting before the age of 30. LCH can affect any organ, but has a predilection for the reticuloendothelial system including the bone, skin, lymph nodes, liver, and spleen as well as the chest and brain. A definitive diagnosis can only be made by histologic examination, which demonstrates CD14 and CD1 positivity on immunohistochemistry, or visualization of Birbeck granules by electron microscopy. Classically, LCH was divided into three clinical groups: (1) Letterer–Siwe disease, a severe, fulminant, frequently fatal multisystem disease, encountered in infants and very young children; (2) Hand–Schuller–Christian syndrome, a multisystem, more chronic form of the disease, intermediate in clinical severity, affecting older children; and (3) eosinophilic granuloma (EG), a localized form of the disease in bone. This former classification is less relevant to current clinical practice as affected patients are categorized and treated according to risk stratification parameters such as age of presentation, focal versus multifocal disease, single organ system versus multiple organ system involvement, and involvement of specific "high-risk" organ systems such as the liver, spleen, and lungs. The extent of disease and the age of presentation are very important prognostic factors. Children under two years of age with vital organ dysfunction tend to have a very poor prognosis. However, EG, which represents 70% of LCH cases, responds to minimal therapy and portends an excellent prognosis. Treatment of LCH varies from observation and spontaneous remission, curettage for localized isolated lesions, direct injection of intralesional methylprednisolone, and rarely chemotherapy for systemic high-risk patients.

The radiographic appearance of LCH depends on the location and the stage at presentation. Generally, LCH has a predilection for flat bones and ribs (Fig. 9.3). The lesions typically are lytic with ill-defined margins, which later become more demarcated with increasing sclerosis. LCH can mimic infection as well as benign or malignant tumors. In the skull, LCH tends to produce lytic lesions with beveled edges, due to differential involvement of the inner and outer tables of the calvarium (Fig. 9.2a, b). In the maxilla and mandible, LCH tends to destroy alveolar bone, which produces the radiologic appearance of "floating teeth" (Fig. 9.1a–c). The classic spine lesion is the "vertebra plana" (flat vertebra), which is seen as complete collapse of the vertebral body (Fig. 9.4). In the long bones and ribs, LCH typically presents as an ill-defined medullary lytic lesion (Fig. 9.3) in the diaphysis and sometimes metaphysis. Periosteal reaction and an adjacent soft tissue mass may be present. In the early stages, these lytic lesions can appear aggressive with ill-defined borders and a moth-eaten appearance. As the lesions enlarge, endosteal scalloping with better defined margins can occur. Infiltration of the bone marrow can be readily detected with MRI and associated soft tissue masses can also be seen. Lesions typically appear T2-hyperintense and T1-hypointense to normal bone marrow. "Active" lesions show marked enhancement on postgadolinium MR sequences while contrast enhancement may be less pronounced or absent during the healing phase. Because of the overlap and variability of imaging features, LCH usually requires biopsy for final diagnosis. Some authors suggest combining bone scintigraphy with a plain film skeletal survey for the initial staging, because of the overlap of false negatives and false positives that occur with either imaging technique. However, conventional radiographic survey remains the single most cost-effective diagnostic study and the mainstay for evaluating LCH at most centers. Whole body MR imaging and FDG PET imaging are in the investigational phases to evaluate extent of disease, assess response to treatment, and for re-staging, as these modalities identify more skeletal lesions than plain film or bone scintigraphy and provide additional information about the metabolic activity of individual lesions.

MRI is most useful in evaluating for the presence and extent of intracranial disease, which is less common in patients with

LCH. The most common intracranial manifestation of LCH is an enhancing mass or thickening of the pituitary infundibulum, often with absence of the normal T1-hyperintensity in the posterior pituitary. Other intracranial manifestations of LCH, such as T2-hyperintense lesions in the brain parenchyma with or without associated enhancement are less commonly seen, and when present predominate in the choroid plexus, brainstem, and cerebellum. MRI may also provide better delineation of the soft tissue masses and adjacent soft tissue structures in focal bone lesions including skull, orbit, mastoid, maxilla, and mandible.

Typical clinical scenario

Given the heterogeneity of the disease, LCH may present with great variability in symptomatology and physical findings. Focal pain or swelling over the bone is typical when LCH presents in an extremity or in the maxillofacial region. A characteristic patient from the perspective of a radiologist is a three-year-old presenting with a painful, enlarging soft tissue mass in the scalp, "recalcitrant oto-mastoiditis," proptosis, and polyuria-polydypsia. These features encompass the common features of the disease with lytic bone lesions, particularly of the temporal bone, and the less common manifestation of diabetes insipidus caused by disease within the central nervous system involving the hypothalamus and/or pituitary infundibulum.

Differential diagnosis

The differential diagnosis of LCH varies depending on the stage of disease, the age of patients, and the site. However, due to the variable aggressive appearance of LCH, osteomyelitis or malignancies such as Ewing's sarcoma, lymphoma, leukemia, or metastatic disease are considered in the differential diagnosis in the long bones.

The finding of a mass or thickening of the pituitary infundibulum on MRI should generate a differential diagnosis including LCH, germ cell tumor (particularly germinoma), lymphocytic hypophysitis, and optic-hypothalamic astrocytoma. The differential diagnosis of a lucent lesion of the skull base or calvarium in a child includes both benign and malignant etiologies such as LCH, metastatic disease, dermoid/epidermoid, hemangioma, leukemia, lymphoma, infection, post-traumatic (i.e., leptomeningeal cyst), or fibrous dysplasia. Isolated lytic disease of the temporal bone should include additional potential etiologies unique to this structure to include rhabdomyosarcoma and aggressive coalescent mastoiditis.

Teaching points

LCH is a mimicker of many benign and malignant diseases. Pain, swelling, and presence of one or more lytic bony lesions in a younger patient should lead to the inclusion of LCH in the differential diagnosis. Most children have monoostotic EG, which has an excellent prognosis. The central nervous system manifestations of LCH, while typical, remain non-specific and most commonly present as an enhancing mass or thickening of the pituitary infundibulum in a child with diabetes insipidus. Knowledge of the variable presentations and determining the extent of vital organ involvement is critical in order to facilitate an early diagnosis, stratify patients into risk groups, and initiate appropriate treatment. Initial imaging should start with a bone survey. The value of cross-sectional imaging studies such as whole body MRI and FDG PET is currently being investigated.

REFERENCES

1. Azouz EM, Saigal G, Rodriguez MM, et al. Langerhans' cell histiocytosis: pathology, imaging and treatment of skeletal involvement. Pediatr Radiol 2005;35(2):103–15.

2. Demaerel P, Van Gool S. Paediatric neuroradiological aspects of Langerhans cell histiocytosis. Neuroradiology 2008;50(1):85–92.

3. Hoffbrand AV, Arceci RJ, Hann IM, Smith OP. Pediatric Hematology. Malden, Massachusetts: Blackwell Publishing, Inc., 2006.

4. Johnson K, Hobin D. Langerhans cell histiocytosis. In: Davies AM, Sundaram M, James SLJ, eds. Imaging of Bone Tumors and Tumor Like Conditions. Heidelberg: Springer, 2009; 447–59.

5. Stull MA, Kransdorf MJ, Devaney KO. From the archives of the AFIP Langerhans cell histiocytosis of bone. Radiographics 1992;12(4):801–23.

(a)

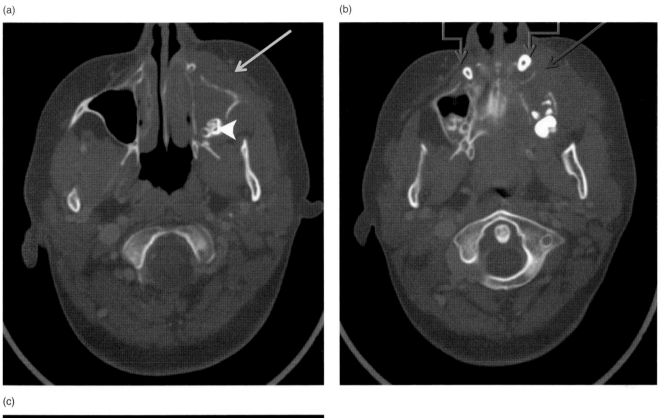

(b)

(c)

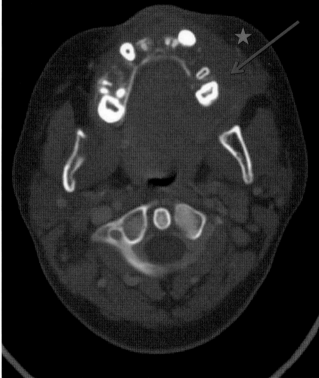

Figure 9.1. A 10-year-old boy with cheek pain, Langerhans cell histiocytosis (LCH). **(a)** An axial CT scan of the facial bones demonstrated a soft tissue mass centered in the left maxilla (arrow) with associated cortical erosion of the left alveolar ridge and left maxillary sinus walls. A "floating tooth" was seen adjacent to the left maxillary sinus wall (arrowhead). **(b)** Axial image at a slightly lower level than **(a)**. The soft tissue mass was again seen with associated cortical destruction involving the left maxillary bone and alveolar ridge (arrow). "Floating teeth" were again noted (stepped arrows). **(c)** Lower axial scan at the level of the maxilla demonstrated the soft tissue mass with cortical bony erosion and a prominent lytic process of the maxilla (arrow). The lack of inflammatory fat stranding suggested that this was unlikely to be an infectious process (star).

(a)

(b)

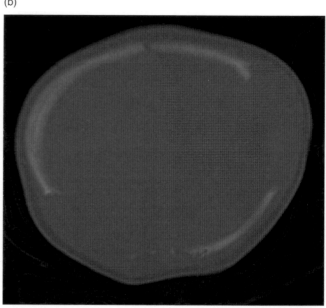

(c)

Figure 9.2. A five-month-old infant with LCH who presented with bi-parietal soft tissue swelling. **(a)** Axial CT image of the brain (brain window) demonstrating bi-parietal calvarial lytic lesions with associated soft tissue masses. **(b)** Axial CT image of the brain (bone window) at the same level as Figure 9.2a demonstrating bi-parietal lytic lesions, lack of associated sclerosis at the margins, absence of significant periosteal reaction, and a characteristic "beveled edge" appearance with greater destruction of the outer table of the calvarium relative to the inner table.

(d)

(e)

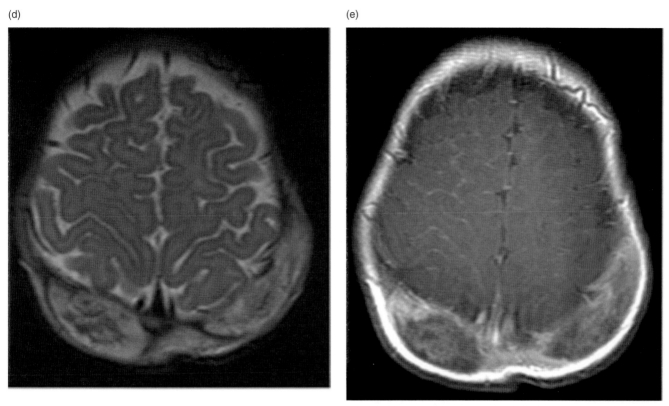

Figure 9.2. (cont.) Axial T1- **(c)** and T2- **(d)** weighted MR images of the brain revealed bilateral expansile soft tissue masses centered within the posterior parietal calvaria, with internal mixed signal intensity ranging from isointense to hypointense relative to brain parenchyma. **(e)** Axial T1-weighted MR image of the brain after IV administration of gadolinium-based contrast reveals heterogeneous enhancement of the bilateral parietal soft tissue masses.

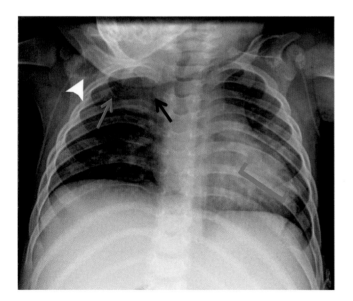

Figure 9.3. A 15-month-old boy with LCH and multiple lytic bone lesions originally thought to be metastatic neuroblastoma. There is marked bone destruction of the posterior right 4th rib with an associated ill-defined soft tissue mass (arrows). There is also an expansile lytic lesion of the left mid posterior 7th rib (bracket) and a lytic lesion of the right scapula (arrowhead).

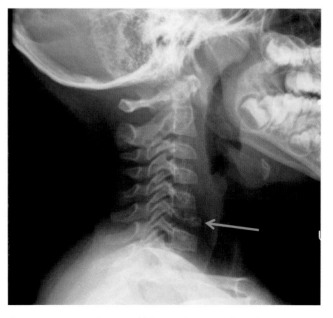

Figure 9.4. An eight-year-old boy with C6 vertebra plana (arrow), a classic finding for EG. In isolation without other clinical information, the differential would also include metastasis, lymphoma, or trauma.

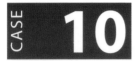
PHACES syndrome (*Posterior fossa malformations, Hemangiomas of the face, Arterial anomalies, Cardiovascular anomalies, Eye anomalies, and Sternal defects or supraumbilical raphe*)

James Kang and Kristen W. Yeom

Imaging description

A neonate presented with multiple facial hemangiomas. Multiple enhancing lesions were seen in right facial and extraconal spaces of the right orbit (Fig. 10.1a), as well as in bilateral masticator and parapharyngeal spaces (Fig. 10.1b). Multiple flow-voids were seen in these lesions, suspicious for hemangiomas. Additionally, evaluation of the brain showed dysplastic right cerebellum (Fig. 10.1c), additional enhancing lesion in the right auditory canal (Fig. 10.1d), and steno-occlusive disease of the right internal carotid artery along the petrous and cavernous segments (Fig. 10.1e).

Importance

PHACES syndrome is an under-recognized syndrome. In addition to a thorough cutaneous, cardiac, and ophthalmologic evaluation, patients with cervicofacial hemangiomas should undergo a full neurologic evaluation, including an MRI of the brain and an MR angiogram of the head and neck. Patients with severe cerebrovascular disease may benefit from revascularization and/or aggressive medical therapy to prevent ischemic injury.

Typical clinical scenario

A typical clinical presentation is a young infant with a facial hemangioma and developmental delay. Structural abnormalities of the brain on imaging most commonly involve the posterior fossa. Posterior fossa anomalies include a Dandy–Walker malformation and its spectrum, including hypoplasia of the cerebellar vermis or cerebellar hemispheres. Other malformations are less common and include cortical dysplasia, heterotopia, and polymicrogyria. Corpus callosal abnormalities, including agenesis or hypoplasia, have also been described.

Vascular abnormalities are commonly associated, and can involve not only the cervical carotid and vertebral arteries, but also the circle of Willis intracranially. The most significant findings include arterial hypoplasia or agenesis, and focal stenoses or occlusions that may lead to a moyamoya-like vasculopathy and infarction. The intracranial arteries may be dysplastic, predisposing to saccular aneurysms. Additional abnormalities include persistent embryonic arteries, most commonly a persistent trigeminal artery, as well as aberrant origins or courses of the arteries.

Orbital abnormalities that may be detected by imaging include microphthalmos, which is ipsilateral to the facial hemangioma, along with optic nerve atrophy.

Intracranial hemangiomas are uncommon, but are becoming increasingly recognized, particularly in the internal auditory canal, associated with facial nerve hemangioma.

Differential diagnosis

Sturge–Weber syndrome. While PHACES syndrome is associated with abnormalities of the intracranial arterial system, Sturge–Weber syndrome primarily involves the capillaries and veins (Fig. 10.2).

> ### Teaching point
>
> PHACES syndrome presents with a constellation of intracranial findings readily detectable by imaging. The most important and characteristic findings include posterior fossa anomalies and cerebrovascular anomalies, which may guide therapeutic goals and counseling in the care of the patient.

REFERENCES

1. Frieden IJ, Reese V, Cohen D. PHACE syndrome. The association of posterior fossa brain malformations, hemangiomas, arterial anomalies, coarctation of the aorta and cardiac defects, and eye abnormalities. *Arch Dermatol* 1996;**132**(3):307–11.
2. Hartemink DA, Chiu YE, Drolet BA, *et al.* PHACES syndrome: a review. *Int J Pediatr Otorhinolaryngol* 2009;**73**(2):181–7.
3. Heyer GL, Dowling MM, Licht DJ, *et al.* The cerebral vasculopathy of PHACES syndrome. *Stroke* 2008;**39**(2):308–16.

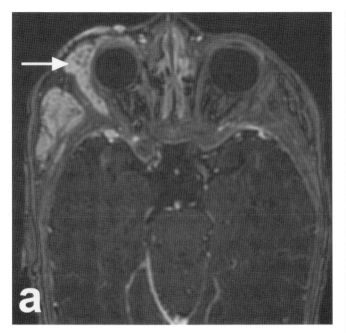

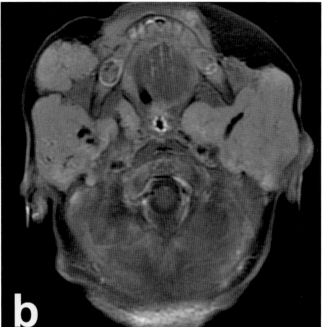

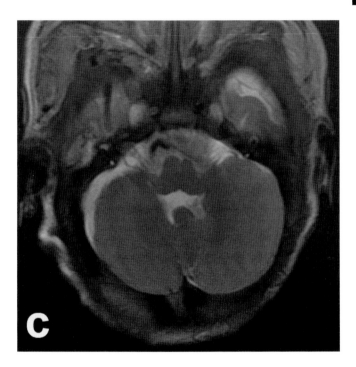

Figure 10.1. **(a)** An axial T1 SPGR (spoiled gradient recalled acquisition) postcontrast image demonstrates a right facial hemangioma with involvement of the extraconal space of the right orbit (arrow). **(b)** An axial T1 postcontrast image with fat saturation demonstrates extensive hemangiomata in the neck, involving bilateral masticator and parapharyngeal spaces. **(c)** An axial T2-weighted image demonstrates an asymmetrically small and dysplastic right cerebellar hemisphere.

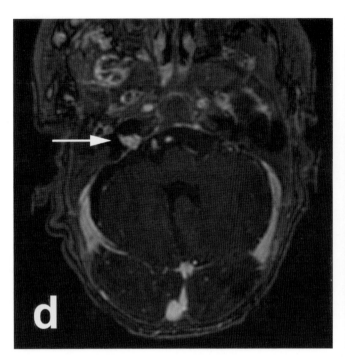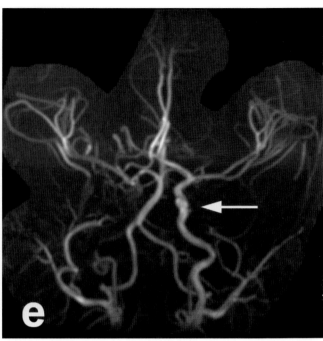

Figure 10.1. (cont.) **(d)** An axial T1 SPGR postcontrast image demonstrates an enhancing right internal auditory canal mass (arrow), representing an internal auditory canal hemangioma. **(e)** MR angiogram demonstrates severe steno-occlusive disease of the right internal carotid artery along the petrous and cavernous segments. The left internal carotid artery is normal (arrow). Flow within the right internal carotid artery is not seen due to the severe steno-occlusive disease.

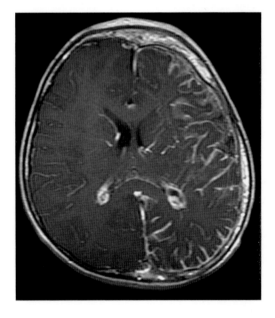

Figure 10.2. Axial T1 postcontrast image demonstrates diffuse leptomeningeal enhancement, representing pial angiomatosis, within an asymmetrically small left cerebral hemisphere. These findings are characteristic of Sturge–Weber syndrome.

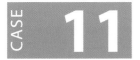

Lipoid pneumonia

Beverley Newman

Imaging description

This two and a half-month-old female infant presented with persistent tachypnea and abnormal chest radiographs with no response to antibiotics. Frontal and lateral chest radiographs over a two-month period demonstrated persistent patchy bilateral upper and lower confluent opacities, predominantly perihilar and posterior on the lateral view (Fig. 11.1a–c). A contrast-enhanced CT scan demonstrated low-density confluent consolidation in a perihilar and posterior distribution (Fig. 11.1d, e). On the basis of the combination of prolonged mild clinical symptoms and the location and appearance of the consolidated lung, the possibility of chronic lipoid pneumonia was raised. The family was questioned and confirmed that they adhered to a Hispanic cultural practice of giving the baby a teaspoonful of olive oil daily as a general health booster. The baby underwent bronchoalveolar lavage (BAL), which yielded milky fluid containing many lipid-laden macrophages typical of lipoid pneumonia; no organisms were present.

Importance

Oral administration of various oils is a relatively common cultural practice; these include mineral oil, olive oil, shark liver oil, cod liver oil, coconut oil, and ghee. These materials are poorly handled by the swallowing mechanism of infants or older children with swallowing dysfunction and readily slide into the airway, often without eliciting a cough reflex. They are poorly removed by cilia and accumulate in the distal airways and alveoli, producing consolidation and surrounding local inflammatory response. The diagnosis is often very delayed as parents are usually not aware of the harmful effects of these agents and physicians rarely think to question this practice in a child with respiratory symptoms. Key imaging findings are marked radiographic findings in the face of mild clinical distress as well as the perihilar and posterior distribution of consolidation, typical of aspiration. Low-density consolidation on CT is a suggestive imaging finding but is quite uncommonly present due to the accompanying inflammatory response which masks the low-density lipid. Patchy confluent opacity is often surrounded by ground glass opacity, similar to other consolidative processes. Prominent interlobular septal thickening has also been described in children with lipoid pneumonia.

Typical clinical scenario

Lipoid pneumonia typically occurs in infants fed lipid materials as well as older children with swallowing dysfunction or reflux and presents with indolent, usually mild, respiratory symptoms. Persistent lipid material in the lung is associated with superimposed infection, particularly due to atypical

mycobacteria. Treatment consists of cessation of lipid administration and is usually accompanied by slow recovery. Additional therapy may include steroids, antibiotics, and repeated BAL. Complete recovery is typical, especially with administration of vegetable oils. Animal oils tend to incite a more vigorous inflammatory response and may result in chronic scarring or pulmonary fibrosis.

Differential diagnosis

From a radiographic standpoint the combination of marked prolonged consolidative changes with mild clinical findings raises the spectrum of atypical, more chronic pulmonary infections that include viral agents, mycoplasma, chlamydia, mycobacteria, and fungal disease. A posterior and perihilar predominance is quite suggestive of aspiration, raising the spectrum of causes of aspiration in children that include swallowing dysfunction, loss of normal oropharyngeal defenses, reflux, fistula, esophageal obstruction, and inappropriate feeding. The most commonly aspirated materials in children include oropharyngeal secretions, gastric contents, water, hydrocarbon, foreign bodies, and lipid materials. When the child aspirates in a supine position, the aspirated material may extend into the upper rather than lower lungs.

> ### Teaching point
>
> Lipoid pneumonia, although uncommon, should be promptly considered in the differential diagnosis of an infant with mild respiratory symptoms accompanying persistent radiographic lung consolidation. The radiologist may be the first person to suggest this diagnostic possibility.

REFERENCES

1. Eslamy HK, Newman B. Pneumonia in normal and immunocompromised children: an overview and update. *Radiol Clin North Am* 2011;**49**(5):895–920.
2. Hadda V, Khilnani GC, Bhalla AS, *et al.* Lipoid pneumonia presenting as non resolving community acquired pneumonia: a case report. *Cases J* 2009;**16**(2):9332.
3. Lee KH, Kim WS, Cheon JE, *et al.* Squalene aspiration pneumonia in children: radiographic and CT findings as the first clue to diagnosis. *Pediatr Radiol* 2005;**35**(6):619–23.
4. Ridaura-Sanz C, Lopez-Corella E, Salazar-Flores M. Exogenous lipoid pneumonia superinfected with acid-fast bacilli in infants; a report of nine cases. *Fetal Pediatr Pathol* 2006;**25**(2):107–17.
5. Zanetti G, Marchiori E, Gasparetto TD, *et al.* Lipoid pneumonia in children following aspiration of mineral oil used in the treatment of constipation: high resolution CT findings in 17 patients. *Pediatr Radiol* 2007;**37**(11):1135–9.

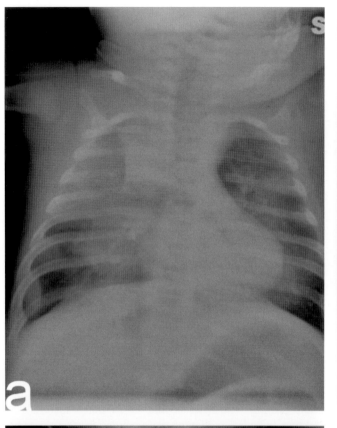

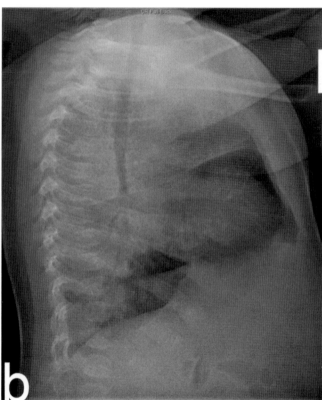

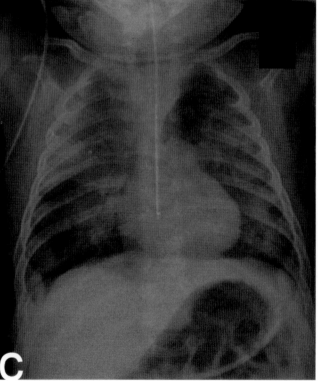

Figure 11.1. Lipoid pneumonia. A two and a half-month-old female with persistent tachypnea. (a–c) Three chest radiographs over a 2-month period demonstrating extensive patchy consolidation in the lungs that does not change substantially. The lateral view best demonstrates the striking posterior and perihilar location of the consolidation.

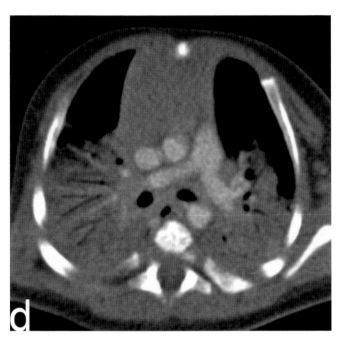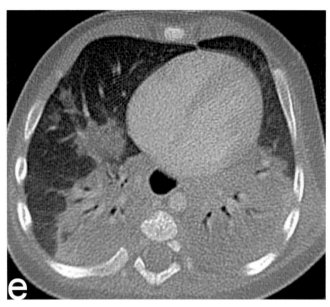

Figure 11.1. (cont.) Axial contrast-enhanced CT scan, soft tissue **(d)** and lung **(e)** windows at age two and one-half months confirms the poorly enhancing predominantly posterior lung consolidation with air bronchograms. Houndsfield units were negative (–60) in some areas raising the question of lipid material.

CASE 12

Pleuropulmonary blastoma

Jordan Caplan, Rakhee Gawande, and Beverley Newman

Imaging description

A three-year-old previously healthy male presented with 1 week of progressive respiratory distress, fever, and lethargy. He was being treated for a viral upper respiratory tract infection.

The frontal chest radiograph (Fig. 12.1a) shows complete opacification of the left hemithorax with marked tracheal and mediastinal shift to the right and compressive atelectasis of the right lung. The differential diagnosis includes a large left pleural effusion, which could be related to infection/pneumonia/empyema, versus a large mediastinal or intrapulmonary mass such as lymphangioma, teratoma, neuroblastoma, pleuropulmonary blastoma, or lymphoma.

Axial contrast-enhanced CT (Fig. 12.1b) and coronal reformat (Fig. 12.1c) show a large hypodense heterogeneous largely intrapulmonary mass with irregular enhancing areas, causing mediastinal shift and inversion of the left hemidiaphragm. It was uncertain whether the mass was partially cystic or if there was some component of pleural effusion. The mass did not extend behind the aorta or encase the mediastinal vessels, making a diagnosis of a primary mediastinal mass such as neuroblastoma or lymphoma less likely.

Ultrasound of the chest (longitudinal view) revealed a largely solid lesion with heterogeneous echogenicity with some cystic components (Fig. 12.1d). There was no evidence of pleural effusion.

Based on imaging this was thought to be a large cystic/solid intrapulmonary neoplasm with pleuropulmonary blastoma the most likely diagnosis in a child of this age. Subsequent biopsy of the lesion confirmed a type II pleuropulmonary blastoma.

Interestingly, the patient had undergone a CT scan of the abdomen and pelvis two years previously for abdominal pain. Limited images of the lung bases show no solid mass, but a small cyst is noted in the left lower lobe (Fig. 12.1e, arrow). This may have been the precursor of the current lung mass.

Importance

Pleuropulmonary blastoma (PPB) is a rare malignant embryonal mesenchymal neoplasm arising from primitive pleuropulmonary mesenchyme. It is the pulmonary anlage of hepatoblastoma, neuroblastoma, and nephroblastoma. PPB occurs almost exclusively in young children less than 5 years of age and may present as a large mass occupying an entire hemithorax, a small mass with rapid growth, a small or large thin-walled cystic lesion, or a mixed cystic and solid lesion.

In conjunction with its varied imaging appearances, the classification system for PPB describes three subtypes: purely cystic (type I) (Fig. 12.2), mixed solid and cystic (type II), and purely solid (type III). PPB may be solitary or multiple (approximately 50% of cases), and multiple lesions may present synchronously or metachronously in the same patient.

Type I cystic PPB can subsequently progress and acquire a solid appearance, also thereby becoming more aggressive. Likewise, tumor recurrences tend to be more solid and aggressive. Histology consists of malignant blastema with mesenchymal sarcomatous components, especially rhabdomyosarcoma and chondrosarcoma, with the result that many lesions that are now considered PPB were previously diagnosed as other mesenchymal tumors. In up to 40% of cases there is a hereditary tumor predisposition with other associated lesions present including cystic nephroma, rhabdomyosarcoma, medulloblastoma, Hodgkin's lymphoma, leukemia, and thyroid and germ cell tumors. A *DICER1* gene mutation has been found in some families with these lesions.

These neoplasms can be aggressive, with possible involvement of the pulmonary, pleural, mediastinal, and chest wall compartments. Metastasis may occur to the central nervous system, bone, and liver. Treatment is primarily surgical for the type I lesions, with adjuvant chemotherapy in cases of incomplete resection. The type II and type III lesions require adjuvant chemotherapy after resection and radiation therapy in cases of positive surgical margins. Close clinical follow-up is recommended due to the potential for recurrence, metastasis, multifocality, and associated extrapulmonary lesions.

Prognosis correlates with lesion type and histology, with a five-year survival of 83% in type I and 46% in types II and III.

Typical clinical scenario

Type I PPBs usually occur in infants and toddlers (Figs. 12.2, 3). Types II and III are more commonly diagnosed in toddlers (Fig. 12.1).

Spontaneous pneumothorax may occur in cystic PPBs since the lesions tend to be peripheral (Fig. 12.2). Cystic pulmonary airway malformation (CPAM) and other bronchopulmonary malformations probably do not degenerate into PPB. PPB likely arises de novo and may mature over time from a cystic to a more aggressive solid neoplasm.

Prenatal occurrence of PPB is unusual but has been described as early as 19–21 weeks with progressive increase in size over time, unlike the more typical decrease in size of bronchopulmonary malformations prenatally.

Differential diagnosis

Based on imaging features alone type I (cystic) PPB is difficult to distinguish from large cystic CPAM, in particular, but also other lung cystic lesions. PPB may even be a difficult histologic diagnosis, especially type I, and careful histologic evaluation is required to distinguish PPB and CPAM. Imaging findings that raise the question of PPB include: a cystic pulmonary lesion (especially peripheral) without clear etiology (Fig. 12.3); lack of prenatal diagnosis with a normal second trimester anatomic survey; a cystic lesion with solid nodule/s; rapid growth; pneumothorax; multiplicity; other lesions related to PPB; and/or positive family history.

Type II (cystic and solid) and type III (solid) PPB need to be differentiated from primary sarcomas of the lung such as rhabdomyosarcoma, synovial sarcoma, and mesothelioma, other lung neoplasms such as lymphoma and squamous cell carcinoma, benign lung lesions including inflammatory pseudotumor and lymphangioma, mediastinal masses such as neuroblastoma, lymphoma or germ cell tumor, and chest wall masses such as Ewing's sarcoma and Askin tumor.

Other cystic lesions in the pediatric lung include: cystic congenital bronchopulmonary malformations (CPAM, hybrid lesions, bronchogenic cyst); infectious cystic changes including pneumatocele, infarct, cavitation, abscess, septic emboli, hydatid cyst, cystic bronchiectasis; autoimmune/inflammatory/vasculitic disease with cavitation including Wegener's granulomatosis, rheumatoid arthritis, and Behçet disease; neoplastic conditions including Langerhans cell histiocytosis, papillomatosis, lymphangioma, lymphoproliferative diseases, lymphoma and cavitating metastases, and collagen/soft tissue abnormalities including Marfan, Proteus, Down syndrome, and tuberous sclerosis. In addition, other lesions can masquerade as pulmonary cystic change, including artifacts, diaphragmatic hernia, hiatal hernia, loculated pneumothorax, pulmonary interstitial emphysema, bronchopleural fistula, traumatic lung injury, and cystic bronchopulmonary dysplasia.

Teaching point

- PPB is a rare primary lung tumor that may mimic benign lung cysts in young children and should be kept in mind in the differential diagnosis of cystic or solid lung masses in older children.
- The pleuropulmonary blastoma registry (http://www.ppbregistry.org) recommends that young children with unexplained lung cysts should have careful surveillance until at least 5 years of age.

REFERENCES

1. Dishop MK, Kuruvilla S. Primary and metastatic lung tumors in the pediatric population: a review and 25-year experience at a large children's hospital. *Arch Path Lab Med* 2008;**132**:1079–103.
2. Hill DA, Jarzembowski JA, Priest JR, *et al.* Type I pleuropulmonary blastoma: pathology and biology study of 51 cases from the International Pleuropulmonary Blastoma Registry. *Am J Surg Pathol* 2008;**32**(2):282–95.
3. Manivel JC, Priest JR, Watterson J, *et al.* Pleuropulmonary blastoma: the so-called pulmonary blastoma of childhood. *Cancer* 1988;**62**:1516–26.
4. Miniati DN, Chintagumpala M, Langston C, *et al.* Prenatal presentation and outcome of children with pleuropulmonary blastoma. *J Pediatr Surg* 2006;**41**:66–71.
5. Newman B, Effmann E. Lung masses. In: Slovis T, ed. *Caffey's Pediatric Diagnostic Imaging*, 11th edition. Mosby: Elsevier, 2008; 1294–323.
6. Priest JR, Williams GM, Hill DA, Dehner LP, Jaffé A. Pulmonary cysts in early childhood and the risk of malignancy. *Pediatr Pulmonol* 2009;**44**(1):14–30.

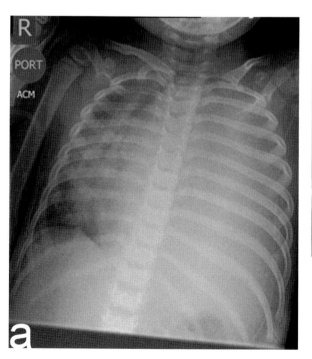
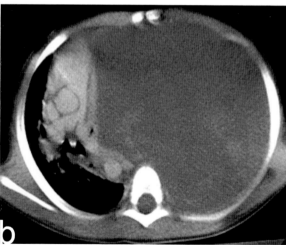

Figure 12.1. Type II pleuropulmonary blastoma (PPB) in a three-year-old male. **(a)** Frontal chest radiograph demonstrates complete opacification of the left hemithorax with mass effect on the trachea and right lung. **(b)** Axial CT image shows a large hypodense, heterogeneous mass occupying the left hemithorax, causing severe mediastinal shift to the right with compression of the heart and compressive atelectasis of both lungs.

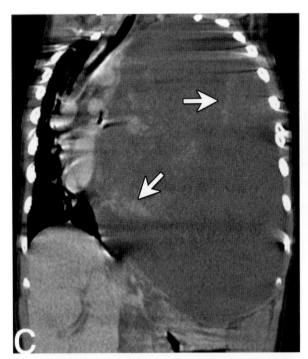

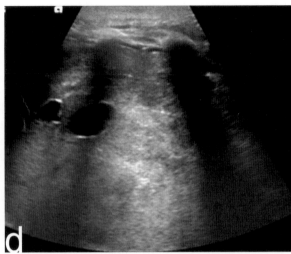

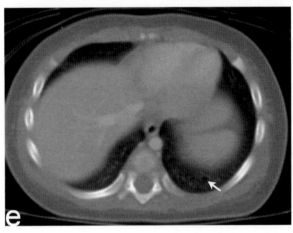

Figure 12.1. (cont.) **(c)** Coronal CT reformat demonstrates the extent of the left pulmonary mass and shows scattered enhancing elements (arrows). Note the marked mass effect on the heart, central airways, and right lung, including inversion of the left hemidiaphragm. **(d)** Longitudinal gray-scale ultrasound image of the left hemithorax shows a predominantly solid mass of heterogeneous echotexture with several cystic elements. **(e)** Axial CT image from unrelated CT scan performed at 1 year of age shows a small pulmonary cyst in the left lower lobe (arrow), possibly a precursor to the PPB.

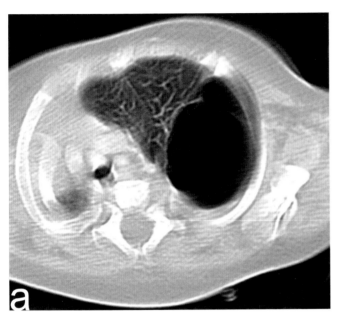
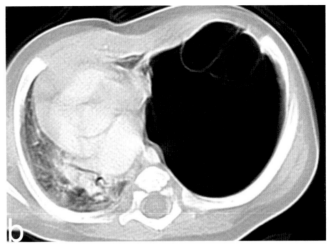

Figure 12.2. Cystic (type I) PPB in a one-month-old male. **(a)** Axial CT image in a one-month-old male shows a purely cystic peripheral lesion of the left lung, proven to be a type I PPB. **(b)** More inferior image of the same study demonstrates the PPB to be complicated by a large left tension pneumothorax with contralateral mediastinal shift.

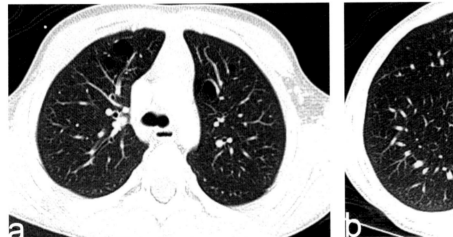
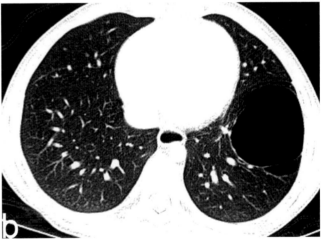

Figure 12.3. Cystic PPB. CT lung window–2 axial slices **(a and b)** in a three-year-old child with incidental finding of multiple cysts scattered in the lungs, some with multicystic components. No pre- or postnatal history, familial or clinical findings to explain the cysts. Excisional biopsy of the largest left lower lobe lesion revealed type I PPB.

Neuroendocrine cell hyperplasia of infancy (NEHI)

Beverley Newman

Imaging description

This 16-month-old girl presented with a year-long history of persistent cough and tachypnea. On physical examination she had sternal retractions and widespread crackles on auscultation. A chest radiograph (Fig. 13.1a) demonstrated bilateral overinflation and increased perihilar markings. A controlled ventilation inspiratory/expiratory low dose CT (Fig. 13.1b, c, d) was performed and showed perihilar and anterior (right middle lobe and lingula) ground glass opacity (GGO) as well as patchy lower lobe air trapping in expiration. On the basis of the CT appearance in conjunction with the clinical findings, the diagnosis of neuroendocrine cell hyperplasia of infancy (NEHI) was suggested. Infant pulmonary function tests confirmed the presence of an obstructive lung abnormality. Biopsy was considered unnecessary and the child was followed clinically and has been stable with slow improvement in clinical symptoms.

Importance

NEHI, also known as persistent tachypnea of infancy or chronic idiopathic bronchiolitis of infancy, is an idiopathic interstitial lung condition in infants. While the only definitive diagnostic test is lung biopsy that demonstrates prominent immunostaining with bombesin of an increased number of bronchiolar neuroendocrine cells, the CT appearance is typical in a high percentage of cases. The reason for the increased number of neuroendocrine cells is uncertain (perhaps a non-specific response to injury); these cells are known to mediate bronchiolar vasoconstriction. GGO distributed in the lingula, right middle lobe, and perihilar regions along with mosaic perfusion and air trapping are the most characteristic CT findings (Fig. 13.1). This CT appearance has been shown to be approximately 78% sensitive and 100% specific for NEHI. CT findings are atypical and non-diagnostic in approximately 20% of cases. Correct diagnosis has both prognostic and therapeutic implications.

Controlled ventilation CT is a useful technique in infants like this so that true inspiration and expiration images can be obtained with suspended respiration. Various controlled ventilation techniques have been described including sedation with mask hyperventilation along with cricoid pressure (to prevent air entering the esophagus) to produce a brief apneic period for scanning. We have found anesthesia with intubation, lung recruitment to prevent atelectasis, and a specific inspiratory and expiratory breathhold at 25 cm and 0 cm of H_2O (disconnect from ventilator) respectively to be a more reliable method.

Typical clinical scenario

NEHI typically presents in infants less than two years of age; symptoms often begin at one to three months of age with tachypnea, retractions, crackles, and hypoxia. Many affected infants develop failure to thrive. Children with NEHI do not show a sustained response to steroids, bronchodilators, or antibiotics. While they may require prolonged oxygen therapy, the long-term prognosis is usually favorable although many have persistent symptoms, reactive airways disease, and relapse with respiratory infections.

Differential diagnosis

While interstitial lung disease in infants is relatively rare overall, NEHI is one of the more frequent conditions encountered. There has been a recent classification scheme of interstitial lung disease in infants that is unique and distinct from the diseases encountered in older children as well as adults. The classification includes diffuse developmental disorders (acinar/alveolar dysgenesis or dysplasia, alveolar/capillary dysplasia); growth abnormalities (neonatal chronic lung disease, pulmonary hypoplasia, chromosomal and cardiac abnormalities); specific idiopathic conditions (NEHI, pulmonary interstitial glycogenosis [PIG]); surfactant dysfunction disorders; disorders of the previously normal (immune intact) host (infectious and post-infectious conditions, environmental exposure, aspiration); disorders of the immune compromised host (opportunistic infections); disorders related to systemic disease (Langerhans cell histiocytosis, immune-mediated and metabolic diseases); and arterial, venous, and lymphatic abnormalities that may masquerade as interstitial lung disease. The idiopathic interstitial pneumonias, especially usual interstitial pneumonia (UIP), commonly seen in adults, are very uncommon in children. Non-specific interstitial pneumonia (NSIP) may be seen in children in association with surfactant abnormalities as well as autoimmune disorders; desquamative interstitial pneumonitis (DIP) is typically associated with surfactant disorders.

The major differential diagnostic considerations for GGO on CT in an infant with chronic lung disease include the surfactant disorders where the characteristic early CT appearance is that of alveolar proteinosis with very widespread GGO and prominent interlobular septal thickening (Fig. 13.2). Bronchiolitis obliterans may have GGO (typically patchy); it also shows patchy air trapping and often bronchiectasis (Fig. 13.3). PIG (a histologic diagnosis) may be diffuse or patchy (associated with many of the lung growth abnormalities) and has a varied appearance on imaging, often with GGO and increased linear opacities.

Teaching point

NEHI is an idiopathic chronic interstitial lung disease of infancy that tends to have a characteristic CT imaging appearance consisting of central and anterior (middle lobe and lingula) GGO as well as hyperinflation and patchy air trapping. Recognition of this pattern by the radiologist and correlation with the clinical history and obstructive changes on pulmonary function tests can provide a confident diagnosis, reassurance to the family, and obviate the need for lung biopsy. There is a separate distinct classification scheme for interstitial lung disease in infants based on pathologic findings with clinical and radiologic correlation. Radiologists should be familiar with this schema and the imaging appearance of these entities.

REFERENCES

1. Brody AS. Imaging considerations: interstitial lung disease in children. *Radiol Clin North Am* 2005;**43**:391–403.

2. Brody AS. New perspectives in imaging interstitial lung disease in children. *Pediatr Radiol* 2008;**38**(S2):S205–7.

3. Brody AS, Guillerman RP, Hay TC, *et al.* Neuroendocrine cell hyperplasia of infancy: diagnosis with high-resolution CT. *AJR Am J Roentgenol* 2010;**194**:238–44.

4. Dasa S, Langston C, Fan LL. Interstitial lung disease in children. *Curr Opin Pediatr* 2011;**23**:325–31.

(a) (b)

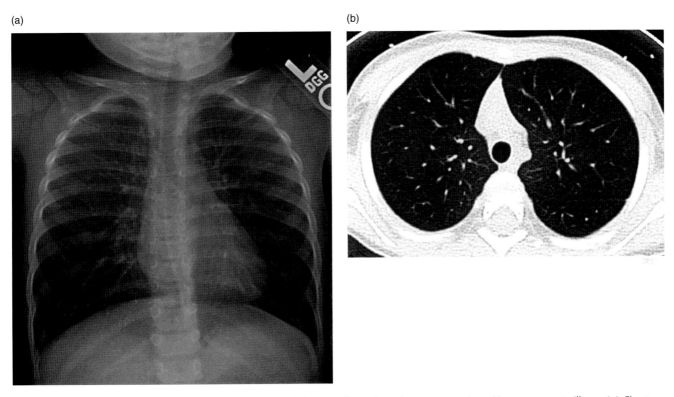

Figure 13.1. NEHI. A 16-month-old female with a 13-month history of cough, tachypnea, retractions. No current acute illness. **(a)** Chest radiograph demonstrates bilateral overinflation and increased perihilar markings. **(b)** Axial inspiratory (25 mm H$_2$O) upper lobe image from a controlled ventilation chest CT. 2 mm thick 100 kVp, 40 mAs. Note subtle perihilar ground glass opacity. **(c)** Axial inspiratory (25 mm H$_2$O) lower lobe image. There is perihilar and anterior right middle lobe and lingula ground glass opacity.

(c)

(d)

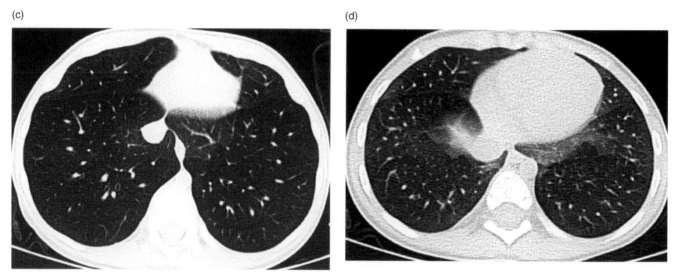

Figure 13.1. (cont.) **(d)** Axial expiratory (0mm H$_2$O) lower lobe image from controlled ventilation chest CT. 2mm thick 100kVp, 40mAs. Note slightly greater conspicuity of perihilar and anterior ground glass opacity as well as patchy lower lobe air trapping.

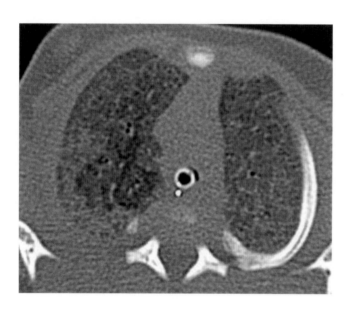

Figure 13.2. Congenital surfactant deficiency (absent protein B). A 20-day-old with persistent severe respiratory distress, post-ECMO at birth. 1-mm-thick axial HRCT image demonstrates the typical appearance of alveolar proteinosis, diffuse ground glass opacity, and interlobular septal thickening (crazy paving). There is also patchy air trapping in the posterior right lung. This is a typical early CT appearance of congenital surfactant deficiency. With less severe mutations survival is possible; the later CT appearance may be less characteristic, with more patchy changes and areas of distorted architecture and scarring resembling bronchopulmonary dysplasia present also.

(a) (b)

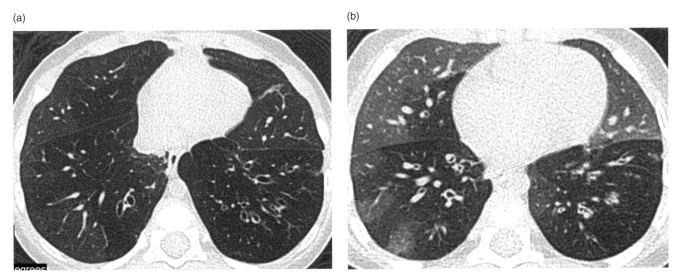

Figure 13.3. **(a)** A one-year-old with post adenovirus bronchiolitis obliterans. Inspiratory controlled ventilation CT image with bilateral lower lobe bronchiectasis and subtle central hyperlucency with mosaic perfusion. **(b)** Expiratory controlled ventilation CT demonstrates deflation of normal peripheral lung and patchy hyperlucency with air trapping centrally.

Endobronchial foreign body recognition

Matthew Thompson and Beverley Newman

Imaging description

This previously healthy 10-month-old infant presented with coughing and wheezing. The frontal chest radiograph demonstrated subtle hyperlucency of the right lung compared to the left side (Fig. 14.1a).

Right and left lateral decubitus views of the same child (Fig. 14.1b, c) show that the left lung inflates and deflates normally in the up and down position respectively, while the right lung field does not change due to air trapping on that side. A right mainstem foreign body was diagnosed and food material was removed at a subsequent bronchoscopy.

Importance

Endobronchial foreign body aspiration most often occurs in children between the ages of one and three years. Peanuts, seeds, and beans are the most common foreign bodies aspirated.

Since most endobronchial foreign bodies are radiolucent (80%), the foreign object itself is rarely visible radiographically (Fig. 14.2); therefore, diagnosis based on imaging often depends on the secondary effects produced by the foreign body (Fig. 14.1). If an inhaled foreign body is suspected, inspiratory/expiratory films (in a cooperative child) or lateral decubitus films (in a child unable to hold his/her breath) are useful in aiding in the detection of air trapping of the affected lung (Fig. 14.1b, c).

In normal respiration, negative intrathoracic pressure expands the intrathoracic airways slightly upon inhalation, with relatively decreased caliber upon expiration. A partially obstructive intraluminal airway foreign body may form a one-way valve since air may be able to move past it on inspiration when the airway expands, but not on expiration. This produces the chest radiographic appearance of air trapping (hyperlucency) in the affected lung (Figs. 14.1, 14.2). If the trapped object causes complete airway obstruction such that air movement is prevented in both inspiration and expiration (no-way valve), the affected lung tends to become atelectatic (Fig. 14.3a). A foreign body that is too small to affect air movement in either inspiration or expiration (two-way valve) may be missed radiographically, resulting in delayed diagnosis until secondary findings such as associated infection manifest.

Typical clinical scenario

The pediatric patient with foreign body aspiration classically presents with a triad of coughing, choking, and wheezing (often unilateral), but a history of choking is the most reliable clue for diagnosis. In many cases there is no clear-cut history of aspiration, and non-specific symptoms can make early diagnosis difficult. In infants and young children, an inhaled foreign body tends to become lodged in the mainstem bronchi, right slightly more common than left; distal airways are less frequently affected. If diagnosis is delayed, the patient may present with hemoptysis or pneumonia.

Plain chest radiographs with the addition of inspiratory/expiratory or decubitus films as needed are often the only imaging studies required in the evaluation of a suspected endobronchial foreign body. Radiographic findings depend on the location, size, duration, and nature of the foreign body (Figs. 14.1–14.3). The spectrum of findings includes normal; visible foreign body or interruption of the air column; asymmetry with air trapping or atelectasis; lung consolidation; and airleak, both pneumomediastinum and pneumothorax. Fluoroscopic observation of lung inflation/deflation along with diaphragmatic and mediastinal motion may be helpful in some cases. Esophagrams are rarely utilized in foreign body evaluation currently but may occasionally be useful in differentiating between an endobronchial or esophageal foreign body, tracheobronchomalacia, or an impinging mediastinal lesion such as vascular ring or sling. Contrast-enhanced CT is used in select instances such as prolonged or unresolving symptoms, suspected complications, and the possibility of other diagnoses such as an underlying mass. CT is much more sensitive in visualizing airway foreign bodies not apparent on chest radiographs and evaluating airway or lung complications related to the foreign material (Fig. 14.3). Airway foreign bodies are usually removed via bronchoscopy.

Differential diagnosis

The differential diagnosis of an endobronchial foreign body is quite large. Considerations include other intraluminal, mural, and extraluminal lesions that can impinge on the intrathoracic airway. Consideration of the age of the patient and anatomic location of the lesion help in further narrowing the likely diagnoses. Possible differential considerations include common childhood respiratory conditions, such as tracheobronchomalacia and acute airway inflammation (bronchiolitis and bronchitis), as well as pneumonia and asthma. Less common entities include an endobronchial granuloma or neoplasm (carcinoid is most common), tracheobronchial stenosis, bronchial atresia, vascular compression (including vascular ring), extrinsic mass (including infectious adenopathy, especially tuberculosis), congenital malformation (e.g. bronchogenic cyst), esophageal lesion, or neoplasm (lymphoma most common).

The differential diagnosis of an asymmetric hyperlucent lung on a chest radiograph includes ipsilateral air trapping, interstitial emphysema, pneumothorax, congenital lobar emphysema, bronchiolitis obliterans and hypoplastic lung. The latter two conditions are associated with a smaller rather than increased lung volume, hyperlucency, and oligemia rather than air trapping or airleak. Inspiratory and expiratory high-resolution CT imaging is useful in differentiating airway (air trapping) from vascular (oligemia) abnormalities.

Teaching point

Foreign body aspiration in the pediatric population is a common occurrence and may present with subtle and non-specific symptoms. The diagnosis may be difficult and imaging findings subtle. Asymmetric aeration, particularly focal hyper-inflation, is a key finding. A normal inspiratory chest radiograph should not rule out foreign body aspiration. Expiratory films are important in eliciting air trapping. Similarly, lateral decubitus films can be used for the same purpose in an unco-operative pediatric patient. Prompt diagnosis and treatment can obviate prolonged symptoms, superimposed infection, and other long-term complications. In difficult cases, where complications are suspected or other lesions are being considered, CT imaging is very useful for detailed anatomic evaluation.

REFERENCES

1. Eslamy HK, Newman B. Imaging of the pediatric airway. *Pediatr Anesth* 2009;**19**(Suppl 1):9–23.
2. Koplewitz BZ, Bar-Ziv J. Foreign body aspiration: imaging aspects. In Lucaya J, Strife JL, eds. *Pediatric Chest Imaging: Chest Imaging in Infants and Children.* Heidelberg: Springer, 2007; 195–213.
3. Ludwig BJ, Foster BR, Saito N, *et al.* Diagnostic imaging in nontraumatic pediatric head and neck emergencies. *Radiographics* 2010;**30**(3):781–99.
4. Yadav SPS, Sign J, Aggarwal N, Goel A. Airway foreign bodies in children: experience of 132 cases. *Singapore Med J* 2007;**48**(9): 850–3.

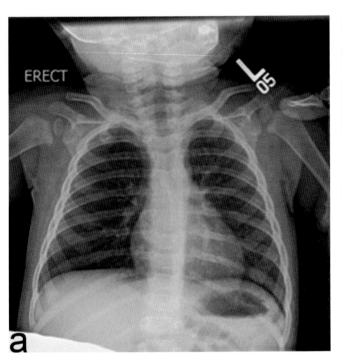
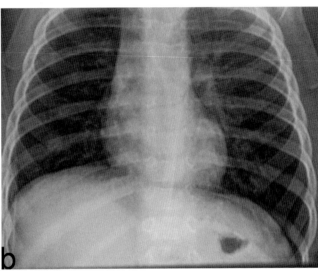

Figure 14.1. **(a)** A 10-month-old infant with cough and wheezing–right-sided endobronchial foreign body. Frontal chest radiograph demonstrates subtle hyperlucency of the right lung compared to the left side.

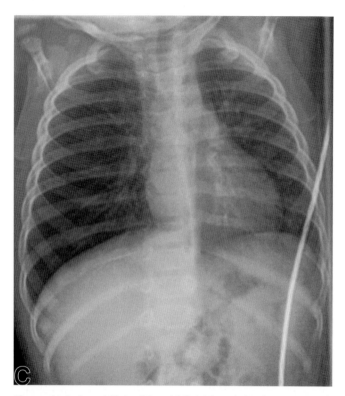

Figure 14.1. (cont.) Right **(b)** and left **(c)** lateral decubitus views of the same child. The right lung remains hyperinflated on both decubitus views while the left lung deflates appropriately on the left down decubitus view **(c)** and inflates on the opposite decubitus view.

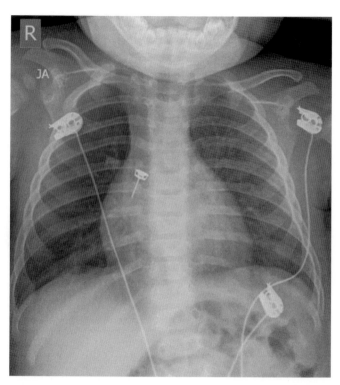

Figure 14.2. An eight-year-old female presented with a choking episode–aspiration of an earring. The right lung is hyperlucent with a flattened hemidiaphragm. A metallic earring foreign body is lodged in the right mainstem bronchus.

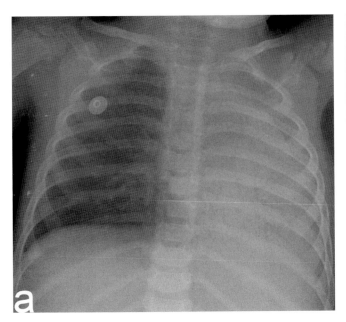
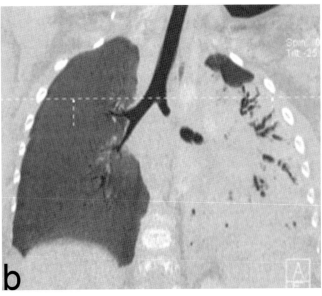

Figure 14.3. An 18-month-old with chronic endobronchial foreign body (peanuts) and three-week history of cough and low grade fever.
(a) Frontal chest radiograph shows complete opacification of the left hemithorax with volume loss and leftward cardiomediastinal shift.
(b) Coronal minimum intensity projection (MINIP) reconstructed CT image of the same patient demonstrating focal complete obstruction of the left mainstem bronchus with left lung atelectasis and postobstructive consolidation with air bronchograms. Fragments of peanuts were later removed from the left bronchus at bronchoscopy. (Originally published as Figures 22 A–B. Eslamy HK, Newman B. Imaging of the Pediatric Airway, *Pediatric Anesthesia* 2009;**19**(Suppl. 1):9–23. © 2009 HK Eslamy, MD and B Newman, MD. *Pediatric Anesthesia* © 2009 Blackwell Publishing Ltd.)

Chronic esophageal foreign body

Beverley Newman

Imaging description

A 16-month-old male infant presented with persistent symptoms of croup, unresponsive to treatment. Frontal and lateral chest radiographs (Fig. 15.1a, b) demonstrated widening of the superior mediastinum with marked attenuation of the lower extrathoracic and intrathoracic airway, displaced rightward and anteriorly. A mediastinal mass was suspected, therefore a contrast-enhanced chest CT scan was ordered. The anesthesiologist was extremely reluctant to give this child any sedation or anesthesia for CT; the risk was considered to be very high because of his compressed airway. Therefore the CT scan was obtained with the child fed, swaddled, and breathing quietly.

The CT examination (Fig. 15.1c–e) demonstrated smooth diffuse low-density tissue in the mediastinum, more suggestive of edema or infiltration rather than a focal mass or confluent adenopathy. No focal fluid or abscess collection was present. There was marked tracheal narrowing and displacement. In addition there was a thin linear density on the axial image (Fig. 15.1c) that appeared rounded on the coronal image (Fig. 15.1e, arrow) behind and to the left of the trachea; several central small rounded well-defined lucencies appeared to be part of this structure. This density did not correspond to any anatomic landmark but was located in the area of the esophagus. The overall appearance led to the suggestion by the radiologist that there was likely a chronically impacted esophageal foreign body with surrounding mediastinal inflammation, probably resulting from penetration or perforation of the esophagus. At a subsequent endoscopy an upper esophageal foreign body was found to be embedded in the esophageal wall with marked surrounding inflammation and granulation tissue. This was removed endoscopically with great difficulty. The object removed proved to be a plastic clamp from a mylar balloon. The child did well post operatively on antibiotic treatment with rapid improvement of respiratory symptoms.

An esophagram obtained a few days later (Fig. 15.1f) demonstrated mild narrowing of the upper esophagus with widening of the soft tissues between the esophagus and trachea (residual inflammatory tissue). There was a small anterior esophageal diverticulum at the thoracic inlet, likely the site of perforation/penetration of the esophageal wall by the foreign body.

Importance

An esophageal foreign body should be included in the differential diagnosis of a child with respiratory symptoms. A chronic esophageal foreign body, while relatively uncommon, can mimic other lesions including chronic asthma or a mediastinal mass, as in this case. Recognition may be difficult and is often delayed (weeks, months, or even years). On plain chest radiographs the presence of a radiopaque esophageal foreign body along with widening of the soft tissues between the esophagus and trachea (Fig. 15.2) with or without tracheal displacement or narrowing suggests that the foreign body is subacute or chronic and that removal may be more difficult. This finding may not be apparent when the foreign body is not radiographically visible. If a chronic esophageal foreign body is suspected, a contrast esophagram is typically diagnostic of the location of the foreign body, extent of airway narrowing, and condition of the esophagus (e.g. narrowing, irregularity, or perforation). CT may not be necessary but can provide more detailed information on the appearance of the trachea, esophagus, and mediastinum (inflammation or abscess) as well as the nature and location of the foreign body.

Typical clinical scenario

Esophageal foreign bodies may be either acute or chronic (approximately 10%) and typically occur in young preschool age children. Acute esophageal foreign bodies account for the majority of cases and may be asymptomatic or present with drooling or swallowing difficulty. Foreign bodies tend to lodge at the level of the cricopharyngeus, thoracic inlet, level of the aortic arch, gastroesophageal junction, or in areas of pathologic esophageal stenosis. The most commonly ingested items are swallowed coins, batteries, small toys, pieces of household items, or bulky food material. Smaller foreign bodies can become lodged in the esophagus but may not produce swallowing difficulty and can escape notice in small children who eat a largely liquid or soft solid diet, particularly if the ingestion was not witnessed. Over time, a more chronic esophageal foreign body incites adjacent inflammation and granulation tissue forms. The foreign body tends to become surrounded by granulation tissue and incorporated into the esophageal wall. Erosion of the esophagus with contained or free perforation may occur with extensive surrounding mediastinal inflammation or abscess formation. A tracheoesophageal (Fig. 15.3) or aortoesophageal fistula may result with serious or disastrous consequences. The extensive periesophageal inflammation displaces and compresses the trachea with the result that respiratory symptoms (stridor or wheezing depending on location) are often more prominent than dysphagia. Additionally the nature of the foreign body may contribute to inflammatory changes. In particular, ingested batteries may leak corrosive chemicals that injure and produce rapid inflammation of surrounding tissues (Figs. 15.2, 15.3). Radiographs should be carefully scrutinized to establish the location, nature, and number of foreign bodies present and any possible secondary complications.

Most esophageal foreign bodies can be extracted endoscopically; occasionally thoracotomy is required for removal. Even when there is pre-existing esophageal perforation or esophageal tear associated with foreign body extraction, treatment is usually conservative, with a good outcome in most cases. Since esophageal foreign bodies are more common when there is underlying esophageal abnormality, such as prior repair of a tracheoesophageal fistula and congenital or acquired esophageal stenosis, a contrast esophagram may be helpful after removal to evaluate the integrity of the esophageal wall and presence of underlying abnormality.

Differential diagnosis

Differential diagnostic considerations are those entities that produce subacute or chronic respiratory or swallowing symptoms. These include croup, asthma, airway foreign body, middle mediastinal masses (common entities include bronchogenic or esophageal duplication cyst and inflammatory or neoplastic adenopathy), vascular ring/sling, and other obstructive esophageal lesions (stenosis, diverticulum, and achalasia). Both esophagram and contrast-enhanced CT can usually distinguish these entities.

Teaching point

Lesions of the esophagus in children, especially a chronic esophageal foreign body, tend to present clinically with respiratory rather than esophageal symptoms due to displacement and narrowing of the adjacent airway. The radiologist should be vigilant regarding this possibility; making the correct diagnosis has important therapeutic and prognostic implications. Chronic esophageal foreign bodies are associated with significant morbidity and even mortality. Anesthesia for CT is extremely dangerous when there is significant airway compromise. Although the examination may not be optimal, a rapid diagnostic CT study can often be obtained without sedation or anesthesia.

REFERENCES

1. Eslamy HK, Newman B. Imaging of the pediatric airway. *Pediatr Anesth* 2009;**19**(Suppl 1):9–23.
2. Gilchrist BF, Valerie EP, Nguyen M, *et al.* Pearls and perils in the management of prolonged, peculiar, penetrating esophageal foreign bodies in children. *J Pediatr Surg* 1997;**32**:1429–31.
3. Haegen TW, Wojtczak HA, Tomita SS. Chronic inspiratory stridor secondary to a retained penetrating radiolucent esophageal foreign body. *J Pediatr Surg* 2003;**38**:e6.
4. Miller RS, Willging JP, Rutter MJ, Rookkapan K. Chronic esophageal foreign bodies in pediatric patients: a retrospective review. *Int J Pediatr Otorhinolaryngol* 2004;**68**:265–72.
5. Naidoo RR, Reddi AA. Chronic retained foreign bodies in the esophagus. *Ann Thorac Surg* 2004;**77**:2218–20.

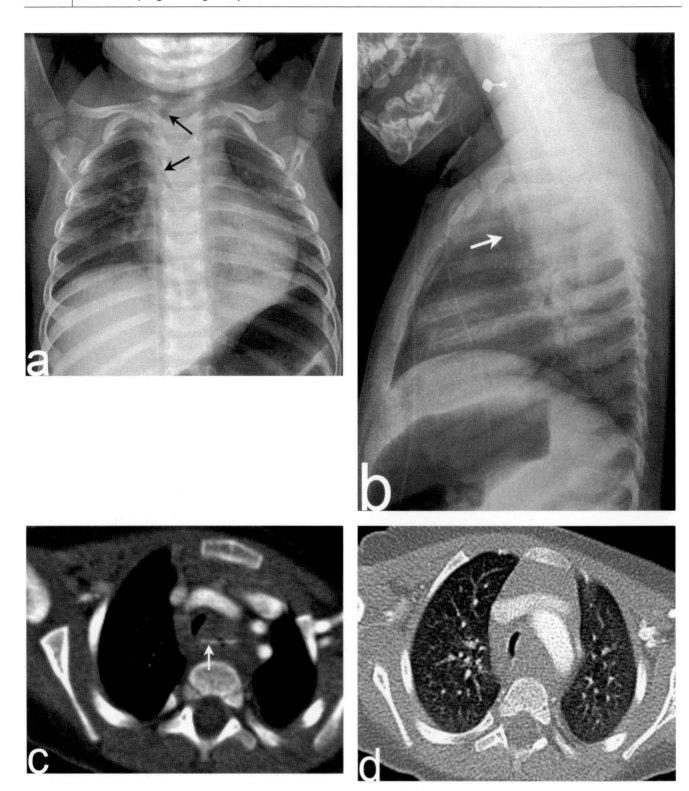

Figure 15.1. Chronic esophageal foreign body. A 16-month-old male with a history of persistent symptoms of croup. **(a, b)** Frontal and lateral chest radiographs demonstrate widening of the superior mediastinum with marked rightward and anterior displacement and narrowing of the intrathoracic trachea (arrows). **(c–e)** Images from a CT scan obtained to evaluate for a possible mediastinal mass. Because of airway compression, anesthesia was considered a very high risk in this infant. The study was therefore obtained with the infant fed, swaddled, and breathing quietly. Parts (c) (axial mediastinal window), (d) (axial lung window), and (e) (coronal reconstruction, mediastinal window) demonstrate increased low-density tissue in the mediastinum with marked tracheal narrowing along with rightward and anterior displacement. In addition there is a thin linear density on the axial image (c, arrow) that is rounded on the coronal image [(e) arrow] behind and to the left of the trachea. Central small rounded lucencies appear to be part of this lesion. **(f)** Lateral view of esophagram after removal of esophageal foreign body (plastic clip from mylar balloon) shows mild narrowing of the upper esophagus, widening of the soft tissues between the esophagus and trachea (residual inflammatory tissue), and a small anterior esophageal diverticulum at the thoracic inlet.

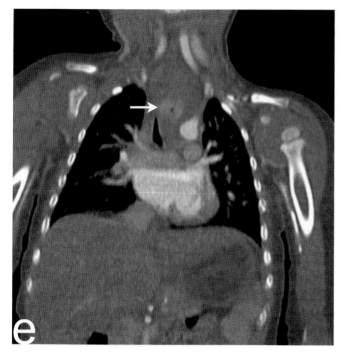

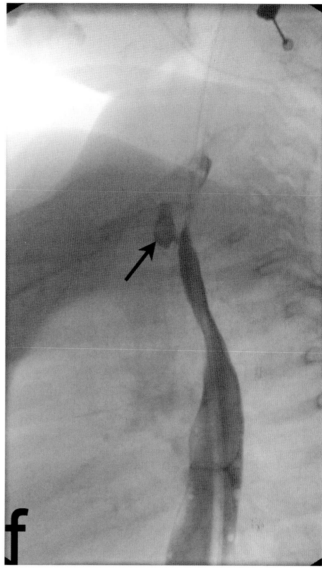

Figure 15.1. (cont.)

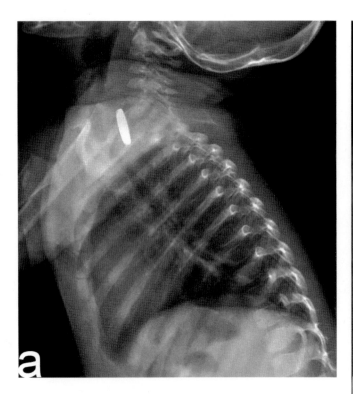
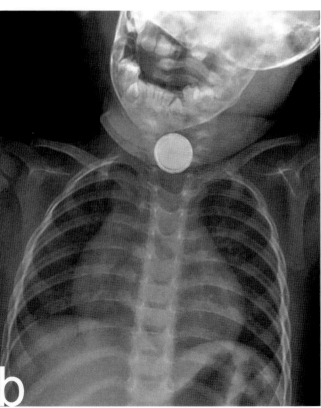

Figure 15.2. Battery ingestion. This 15-month-old boy was brought to the pediatrician with a 24-hour history of drooling and emesis. In retrospect, he and his older brother had been playing with a flashlight the day before but no ingestion was witnessed. **(a)** Lateral chest radiograph demonstrates a rounded metallic foreign body lodged at the thoracic inlet. Note widening of the soft tissues between the trachea and esophagus and focal upper tracheal narrowing indicative of adjacent inflammatory changes. This appearance suggests that the foreign body is subacute or chronic and predicts that removal may be difficult and should not be attempted without direct visualization of the esophagus and foreign body. The foreign body could easily be mistaken for a coin in this view although it is somewhat thick. **(b)** In the frontal view, the etched nature of the foreign body is much more obvious, identifying it as a battery rather than a coin. The marked inflammatory changes that were present in this case were likely due to leakage of the battery as well as the subacute nature of the foreign body. The battery was extracted endoscopically with great difficulty and there was an extensive burn and possible perforation of the esophagus. Subsequent follow-up on endoscopy and esophagram showed good healing without evidence of stricture or diverticulum.

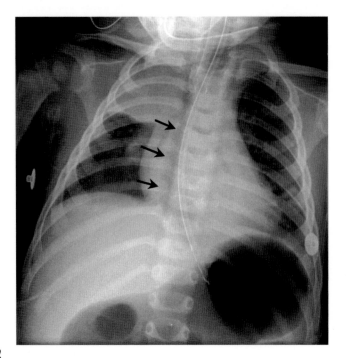

Figure 15.3. A 13-month-old male with aspiration pneumonia in the right upper lobe and left lower lobe status post removal of an ingested esophageal button battery that had eroded through the esophagus to form a traumatic tracheoesophageal fistula just above the carina. The fistula and lower esophagus are distended with air (arrows). There is also a large amount of air in the bowel. The child was very difficult to ventilate and had to be placed on ECMO because of marked fistulous airleak into the gastrointestinal tract.

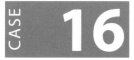

Opsoclonus–myoclonus due to underlying ganglioneuroblastoma

Rakhee Gawande and Beverley Newman

Imaging description

A 19-month-old child presented with symptoms of difficulty in walking, abnormal eye and limb movements, and irritability. MRI of the brain for suspected cerebellar ataxia was unremarkable (Fig. 16.1a, b). CT scan of the neck and chest revealed a small left paraspinal soft tissue lesion at the level of T1 and T2 (Fig. 16.1c–e) and a diagnosis of neuroblastoma-associated opsoclonus–myoclonus syndrome (OMS) was suggested. Metaiodobenzylguanidine scintigraphy (MIBG) scan was negative (Fig. 16.1f). Excision biopsy of the mass confirmed the diagnosis of a ganglioneuroblastoma.

Importance

OMS, also known as dancing eye syndrome, is a rare disorder that presents in early childhood with involuntary rapid eye movements, myoclonic limb jerking, ataxia, and behavioral changes. It can be idiopathic, postinfectious, or a paraneoplastic manifestation of neuroblastoma. OMS is associated with neuroblastoma in 40% of patients and occurs between the ages of six months and three years in these patients. Conversely, only about 2% of patients with neuroblastoma present with OMS. In children, OMS may occur as a paraneoplastic manifestation of all neural crest tumors, including neuroblastoma, ganglioneuroblastoma, and ganglioneuroma. The pathogenesis of OMS is thought to be immune-mediated, with a cross-reactive autoimmunity between neuroblastoma cells and the central nervous system. Neuroblastomas associated with OMS tend to be low grade, thoracic in location, and have a more favorable outcome than non-OMS neuroblastomas. Neuroblastomas associated with OMS are usually very small in size and present a diagnostic challenge as they are less metabolically active and urinary catecholamines or MIBG scans can be negative. CT and/or MRI of the neck, chest, abdomen, and pelvis are the most sensitive studies to detect these occult neuroblastomas (Fig. 16.1).

Typical clinical scenario

OMS presents in children between six months and three years of age with acute to subacute ataxia and inability to sit or walk. This is accompanied by severe irritability, involuntary rapid eye movements, myoclonic limb jerking, and behavioral changes such as sleep problems and developmental regression. While removal of the tumor may result in reversal of clinical symptoms and signs, chronic neurologic sequelae including motor, speech, and cognitive deficits occur in as many as 70% of cases and may result in long-term steroid dependence. Patients with severe initial symptoms and young age at onset are at greater risk of developing chronic neurologic sequelae. One-third of the patients present with atypical symptoms, which results in delayed diagnosis.

Differential diagnosis

OMS is often misdiagnosed as postinfectious acute cerebellar ataxia, which is a more common disorder. The main distinguishing feature is the usual presence of abnormal eye and limb movements with OMS, which are not seen in cerebellar ataxia. The outcome of OMS is more disabling than acute cerebellar ataxia.

Other (less common) syndromes associated with neuroblastoma include intractable diarrhea caused by vasoactive intestinal peptide (VIP) tumor secretion and neurocristopathy, a term applied to the association of Hirschsprung's disease, Ondine's curse (congenital hypoventilation), and congenital neuroblastoma. Another very rare association of ganglioneuroblastoma is ROHHADNET syndrome (rapid-onset obesity with hypothalamic dysfunction, hypoventilation, autonomic dysregulation, and neural crest tumors).

> ### Teaching point
>
> OMS is a paraneoplastic syndrome associated with neuroblastoma. The primary tumor is often very small in size, low grade, and quite frequently located in the chest and can be metabolically less active. It can be associated with chronic long-term neurologic sequelae.

REFERENCES

1. Bougnères P, Pantalone L, Linglart A, Rothenbühler A, Le Stunff C. Endocrine manifestations of the rapid-onset obesity with hypoventilation, hypothalamic, autonomic dysregulation, and neural tumor syndrome in childhood. *J Clin Endocrinol Metab* 2008;**93**(10):3971–80.
2. Brunklaus A, Pohl K, Zuberi SM, de Sousa C. Outcome and prognostic features in opsoclonus–myoclonus syndrome from infancy to adult life. *Pediatrics* 2011;**128**(2):e388–94
3. De Grandis E, Parodi S, Conte M, *et al*. Long-term follow-up of neuroblastoma-associated opsoclonus–myoclonus–ataxia syndrome. *Neuropediatrics* 2009;**40**(3):103–11.
4. Lonergan GJ, Schwab CM, Suarez ES, Carlson CL. Neuroblastoma, ganglioneuroblastoma, and ganglioneuroma: radiologic-pathologic correlation. *Radiographics* 2002;**22**(4):911–34.
5. Roshkow JE, Hailer JO, Berdon WE, Sane SM. Hirschsprung's disease, Ondine's curse, and neuroblastoma-manifestations of neurocristopathy. *Pediatr Radiol* 1988;**19**:45–9.
6. Sahu JK, Prasad K. The opsoclonus–myoclonus syndrome. *Pract Neurol* 2011;**11**(3):160–6.

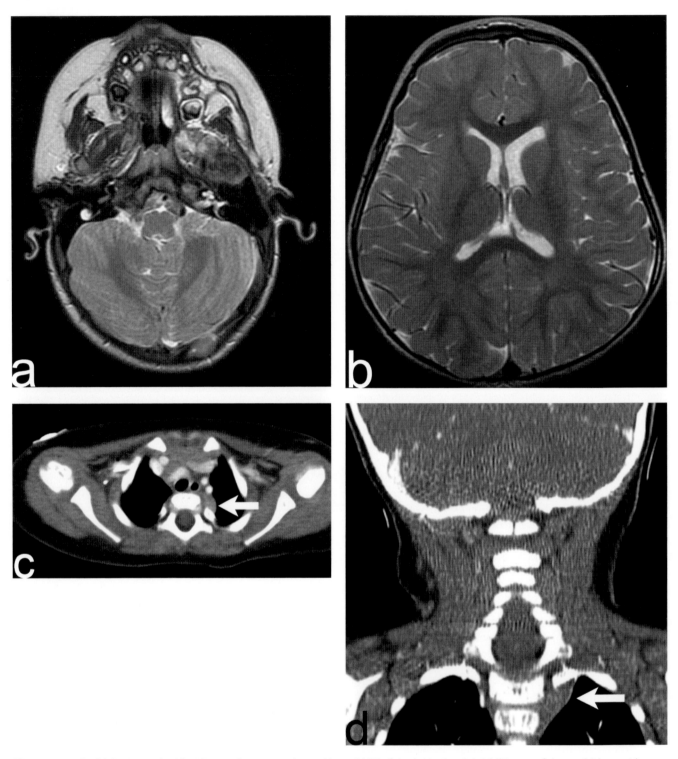

Figure 16.1. (a, b) A 19-month-old with opsoclonus–myoclonus. Normal MRI of the brain. **(c–e)** Axial CT scan of the neck/chest with sagittal and coronal reformats reveals a small left paraspinal soft tissue lesion at the level of T1 and T2 (arrow). Pathologically this was a ganglioneuroblastoma. **(f)** MIBG scan of the thorax reveals no evidence of any abnormal tracer uptake.

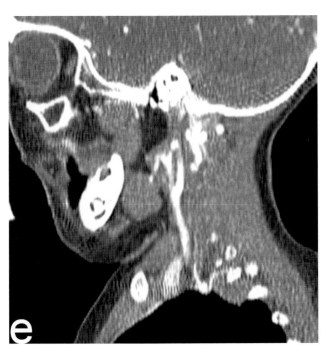

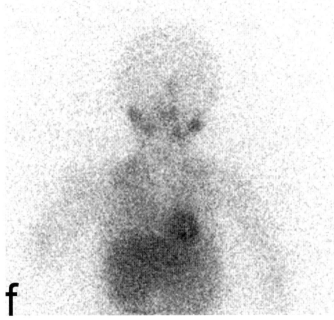

Figure 16.1. (cont.)

Lymphoma: pulmonary manifestations

Rakhee Gawande and Beverley Newman

Imaging description

A 16-year-old girl presented with a two-month history of night sweats, weight loss, and cough. A radiograph of the chest revealed nodules in the right lung and mediastinal widening suggestive of lymphadenopathy (Fig. 17.1a, b). CT scan of the chest (Fig. 17.1c, d) demonstrated multiple nodules of varying sizes in both lungs. Most of the nodules demonstrated air bronchograms. In addition a pleural-based nodule was noted in the right upper lobe. Multiple enlarged mediastinal and hilar lymph nodes were present. The lung nodules and the mediastinal and hilar lymph nodes demonstrated increased FDG uptake on PET/CT (Fig. 17.1e, f). A lymph node biopsy confirmed the diagnosis of Hodgkin's lymphoma, nodular sclerosis.

Importance

Pulmonary parenchymal involvement in children is slightly more common with Hodgkin's disease (HD) than non-Hodgkin's lymphoma (NHL). It is seen in HD in approximately 12% of patients, most at the time of diagnosis and usually associated with mediastinal or hilar lymphadenopathy. Pulmonary involvement in NHL is seen in around 10% of cases and may occur without the presence of associated lymphadenopathy. The mechanism of spread of the disease to the lungs is typically by hematogenous or lymphangitic channels and less commonly by direct or endobronchial spread. On CT imaging, different patterns of involvement can be seen. A nodular pattern is characterized by the presence of single or multiple nodules, which may have irregular borders, air bronchograms, or cavitation (Figs. 17.1 and 17.2). Subpleural nodules or masses can also occur (Fig. 17.1). Lymphoma may also produce a pattern of lobar or segmental consolidation that can be confused with pneumonia (Fig. 17.3).

A reticulo-interstitial pattern can occur due to venous or lymphatic obstruction related to hilar/mediastinal lymphadenopathy or interstitial tumor deposition (Fig. 17.4).

Typical clinical scenario

The most common presentation of childhood lymphoma is with extrathoracic lymphadenopathy or systemic symptoms. Respiratory symptoms are often absent and both mediastinal and lung involvement may be discovered on screening radiographs or CT scans. When the lymphoma is limited to the chest, the most common symptoms are chest pain, fever, dry cough, hemoptysis, dyspnea, and pneumonia.

Both Hodgkin's and non-Hodgkin's lymphoma (especially T-cell lymphoblastic leukemia/lymphoma type) commonly affect the mediastinum (Figs. 17.1–17.5). A large anterior heterogeneous lobulated mediastinal mass involving the thymus and adjacent nodes with contiguous neck adenopathy is typical in Hodgkin's lymphoma. Foci of necrosis within the mass are common. Encasement of adjacent mediastinal vessels and displacement and compression of the airway in children is common in lymphoma and cross-sectional imaging studies requiring sedation or anesthesia must be undertaken with great care. Splenic involvement (Fig. 17.4) may be present in Hodgkin's lymphoma, more common in the mixed cellularity than nodular sclerosing type, but other non-contiguous abdominal disease is uncommon.

NHL is more common in younger children with a similar imaging appearance to Hodgkin's lymphoma, but with more frequent involvement of hilar, subcarinal, posterior mediastinal, and paracardiac nodes as well as concomitant non-contiguous tumor in the abdomen. Acute lymphocytic leukemia (ALL, typically the less common T-cell type) may also present with large mediastinal adenopathy (Fig. 17.5) and is only distinguished from non-Hodgkin's T-cell lymphoma by a greater degree of bone marrow involvement. Diffuse or nodular pulmonary involvement by leukemia is uncommon and most often seen in acute myelocytic or monocytic leukemia.

Differential diagnosis

Pulmonary disease accompanying lymphoma can be confusing. Pleural effusion can occur without pleural tumor and may be due to nodal lymphatic obstruction; pericardial effusion typically denotes tumor involvement. Infection, pulmonary edema, hemorrhage, and drug reactions are all confounding causes of pulmonary abnormality in children with lymphoma, especially after initiation of therapy.

Post-transplant lymphoproliferative disease (PTLD) is more common in pediatric than adult transplant recipients and occurs (most often in the first year) following a variety of solid organ or bone marrow transplants. It is a B-cell lymphocyte proliferation associated with immunosuppression and Epstein–Barr virus infection or reactivation. Lung involvement is quite common, with a similar spectrum of pulmonary manifestations as pulmonary lymphoma including single or multiple pulmonary nodules that may cavitate or pulmonary infiltrate/s with air bronchograms simulating pneumonia (Fig. 17.6). Mediastinal adenopathy may or may not be present (Fig. 17.6). A similar variety of pulmonary imaging appearances to that of pulmonary lymphoma and PTLD may be seen in other benign non-transplant-related lymphoproliferative conditions such as pseudolymphoma, lymphocytic interstitial pneumonitis, follicular bronchiolitis, and lymphomatoid granulomatosis.

Imaging findings of other pulmonary metastatic disease can mimic a wide range of benign, infectious, and non-infectious diseases and both parenchymal nodules and mediastinal adenopathy may occur. However, alveolar infiltration or nodules with air bronchograms is a specific characteristic of lymphoma as opposed to other metastatic lung disease.

Mediastinal and hilar adenopathy are common in bacterial pneumonias in children although the extent is usually not as marked as that seen with lymphoma. Tuberculosis and atypical mycobacterial infection are typified by the presence of prominent adenopathy (usually low-density) and adjacent lung infiltrate, nodules, or masses. Pulmonary nodules and mediastinal lymphadenopathy also occur in other granulomatous diseases such as histoplasmosis. The presence of central calcifications and history of residence in or visit to an endemic area may help to differentiate granulomatous disease from lymphoma. In addition, presence of mediastinal or splenic calcifications may indicate a granulomatous process but does not exclude lymphoma. Langerhans cell histiocytosis may also present with pulmonary nodules and cysts plus mediastinal adenopathy, especially in young children (Fig. 17.7).

FGD PET/CT scanning has a significant role in differentiating benign from malignant disease and has been a major modality in the staging of pediatric lymphoma.

Teaching point

Pulmonary parenchymal involvement is a characteristic of more advanced lymphoma. The finding of pulmonary involvement can significantly alter therapy and prognosis and hence it is important to keep in mind the various manifestations of pulmonary lymphoma involvement and correctly differentiate benign from malignant pulmonary disease. CT and PET/CT are the primary useful cross-sectional imaging modalities for defining location, type, and extent of disease.

REFERENCES

1. Berkman N, Breuer R, Kramer MR, Polliack A. Pulmonary involvement in lymphoma. *Leuk Lymphoma* 1996;**20**:229–37.
2. Kaste SC. Lymphoma: controversies in imaging the chest. In: Lucaya J, Strife JL, eds. *Pediatric Chest Imaging: Chest Imaging in Infants and Children*. Heidelberg: Springer, 2007; 241–62.
3. Lewis ER, Caskey CI, Fishman EK. Lymphoma of the lung: CT findings in 31 patients. *AJR Am J Roentgenol* 1991;**156**:711–14.
4. Maturen KE, Blane CE, Strouse PJ, Fitzgerald JT. Pulmonary involvement in pediatric lymphoma. *Pediatr Radiol* 2004;**34**:120–4.
5. Paes FM, Kalkanis DG, Sideras PA, Serafini AN. FDG PET/CT of extranodal involvement in non-Hodgkin lymphoma and Hodgkin disease. *Radiographics* 2010;**30**:269–91.
6. Toma P, Granata C, Rossi A, Garaventa A. Multimodality imaging of Hodgkin disease and non-Hodgkin lymphomas in children. *Radiographics* 2007;**27**:1335–54.

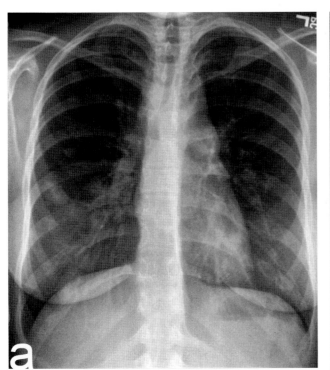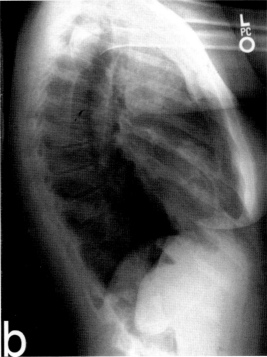

Figure 17.1. Hodgkin's lymphoma in a 16-year-old girl. **(a, b)** Chest radiographs (PA and lateral views) demonstrate multiple ill-defined nodules in the right middle and lower lobe with lobulated superior mediastinal widening, suggestive of lymphadenopathy.

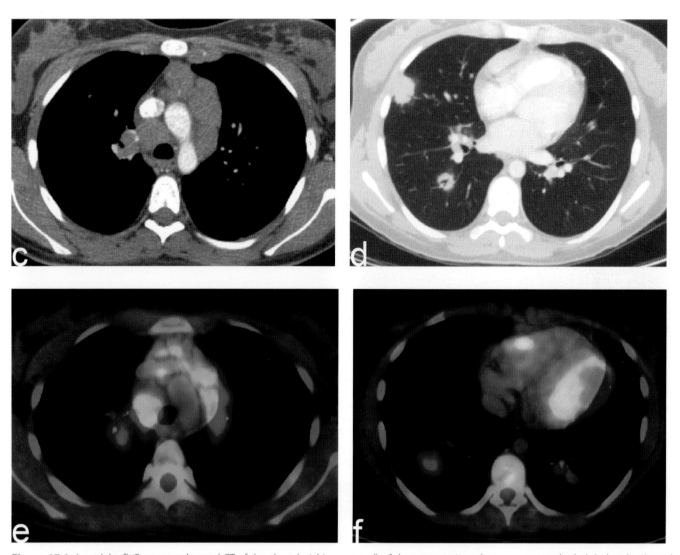

Figure 17.1. (cont.) **(c–f)** Contrast-enhanced CT of the chest (axial images c, d) of the same patient demonstrates multiple lobulated enlarged mediastinal and hilar lymph nodes and irregular nodules with air bronchograms in the right middle and both lower lobes. Axial FDG PET/CT images **(e, f)** demonstrate intense FDG uptake in the mediastinal lymph nodes and lung nodules.

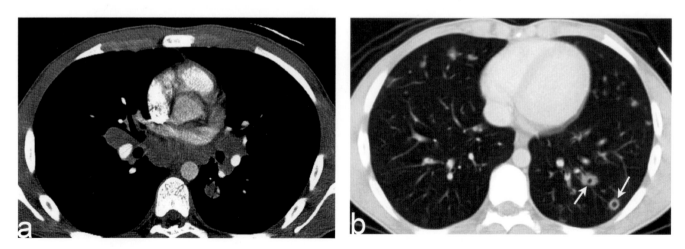

Figure 17.2. A 14-year-old with Hodgkin's lymphoma. **(a, b)** Axial CT scan images [mediastinal window, (a) lung window, (b)] demonstrate multiple enlarged posterior mediastinal and bilateral hilar lymph nodes. Multiple small pulmonary nodules are noted in the right middle lobe, lingula, and left lower lobe. The left lower lobe nodules show cavitation (arrows).

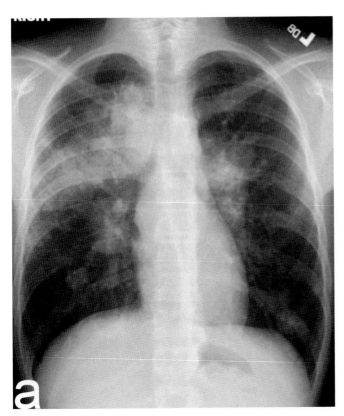
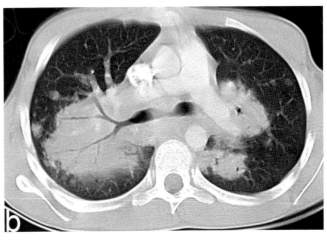

Figure 17.3. A 15-year-old with Hodgkin's lymphoma. Chest radiograph [PA view, **(a)**] demonstrates ill-defined nodular opacities with air bronchograms in both lung fields, predominantly in the perihilar regions and right upper and mid zones. CT chest [**(b)** lung window, axial image] shows enlarged subcarinal lymph nodes and contiguous irregular alveolar infiltrates in both perihilar regions with air bronchograms. Bilateral small peripheral pulmonary nodules are also noted. (Previously published as Fig 78–29A and B in Newman B, Effmann EL. Lung masses. In: Slovis T, editor. *Caffey's Pediatric Diagnostic Imaging*, Vol. 1. 11th edition. Philadelphia: Mosby Elsevier; 2008:1294–323.)

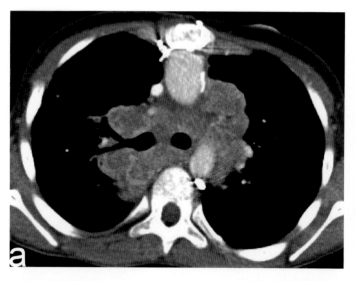

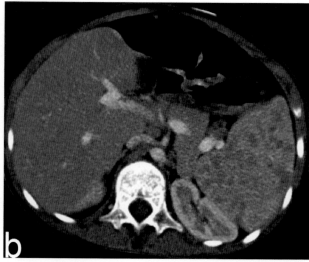

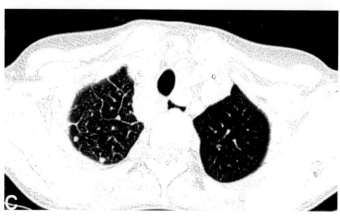

Figure 17.4. An eight-year-old post heart transplant with Hodgkin's disease. **(a–c)** CT scan of the chest [axial sections: (a, b, soft tissue and c, lung windows)] demonstrates marked mediastinal and hilar lymphadenopathy (a) and splenomegaly with diffuse low-density infiltrating lesions (b). Reticular changes are noted in the right upper lobe with interlobular septal thickening and small pulmonary nodules (c).

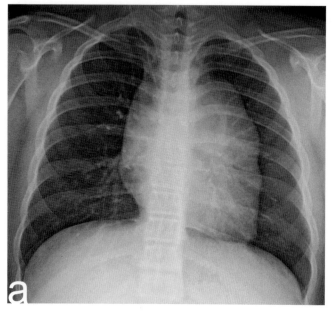

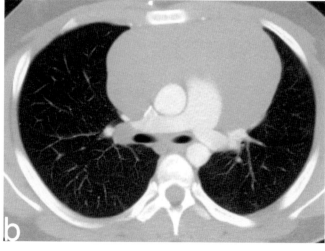

Figure 17.5. A 12-year-old with T-cell acute lymphocytic leukemia (ALL). **(a)** Radiograph of the chest (PA view) demonstrates marked mediastinal widening with lobulated margins. **(b)** CT scan of the chest (axial view) shows a large lobulated anterior mediastinal mass (differentiated from a normal thymus by the presence of lobulated convex margins and large size). Patchy ill-defined ground glass opacities in the lung may represent early infection or leukemic infiltration.

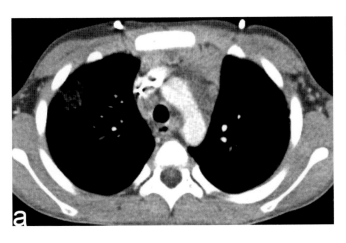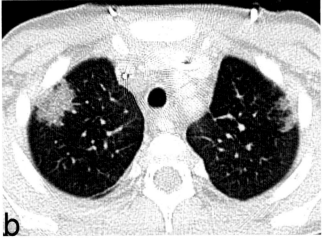

Figure 17.6. Post-transplant lymphoproliferative disorder (PTLD). This eight-year-old boy presented with cough, fever, and rising Epstein–Barr virus titers, 3 months post bone marrow transplant. CT scan of the chest [axial sections: (a) mediastinal and (b) lung window] demonstrates anterior mediastinal lymphadenopathy and irregular peripheral ground glass lung nodules in both upper lobes.

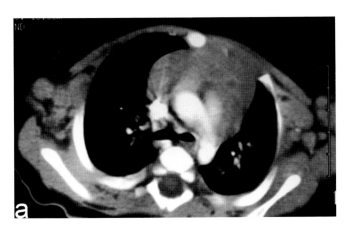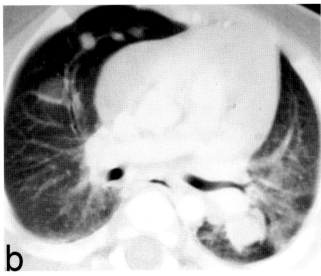

Figure 17.7. Langerhans cell histiocytosis in a one-month-old child. **(a, b)** CT scan of the chest [axial sections: (a) mediastinal and (b) lung window] which demonstrates anterior mediastinal lymphadenopathy, thymic infiltration and multiple pulmonary nodules in the right middle lobe and left lower lobe. Bilateral axillary lymphadenopathy is also noted. (Previously published as Fig. 78-11A and B in Newman B, Effmann EL. Lung masses. In: Slovis T, editor. *Caffey's Pediatric Diagnostic Imaging*, Vol. 1. 11th edition. Philadelphia: Mosby Elsevier; 2008.)

Acute and subacute pneumonia in childhood: tuberculosis

Beverley Newman

Imaging description

This previously healthy seven-month-old boy was brought to a local community hospital with acute fever and cough. A chest radiograph demonstrated extensive opacification of the right upper lung. Pneumonia was diagnosed and the child was admitted and given intravenous antibiotics for 24 hours. However, respiratory symptoms persisted and the child remained febrile with subsequent hypothermia and some lethargy. Because of concern for sepsis or meningitis, the child was transferred to an academic medical center children's hospital. A chest radiograph on admission demonstrated dense bulging right upper lobe consolidation with a medial area of cavitation or pneumatocele formation as well as a diffuse macronodular and micronodular pattern elsewhere throughout both lungs (Fig. 18.1a). There also appeared to be prominent paratracheal as well as subcarinal adenopathy with mild mass effect on the airway (Fig. 18.1a). The radiographic appearance raised concern for an unusual infection including tuberculosis (TB) or fungal disease such as *Cocidioidiomycosis* or *Cryptococcus*, less likely an unusual viral or pyogenic bacterial infection. A lumbar puncture demonstrated findings of subacute meningitis (lymphocytic predominance of cells).

A contrast-enhanced CT scan was obtained, demonstrating diffuse consolidation in the right upper lobe with several medial air-containing areas of irregular cavitation (Fig. 18.1b, c). There were diffuse tiny (miliary) and larger nodules as well as confluent patchy areas of opacity in both lungs and peripheral tree-in-bud opacities (Fig. 18.1d). There were large low-density mediastinal, right hilar, and subcarinal nodes. In addition, small hypodense lesions were noted in the spleen (not shown). MR imaging revealed multiple ring-enhancing lesions in the brain (Fig. 18.1e). Although a purified protein derivative (PPD) and cerebrospinal fluid (CSF) polymerase chain reaction (PCR) for TB were negative, subsequent bronchoalveolar lavage and gastric washings were positive. A close family relative was subsequently found to have active TB.

Importance

There is considerable overlap in the radiographic appearance of pneumonias in childhood and imaging is usually relatively poor at predicting viral, bacterial, or other causes. Bacterial pneumonias predominate in the newborn period and are often acquired during labor and delivery. Viral pneumonias are relatively infrequent in the first few months of life due to protection from maternally acquired antibodies. Viral respiratory infections predominate from two months to two years of age, with bacterial infections relatively more common between 2 and 18 years of age.

Acute and subacute pneumonias in children can be divided into several major etiologic categories. These include:

1. acute bronchiolitis–<two years, fever, wheezing, hyperinflation, diffuse peribronchial thickening, and patchy atelectasis–most often due to respiratory syncitial virus, a similar appearance is seen in bronchitis in older children.
2. acute focal pneumonia–high fever, focal lobar or segmental peripheral consolidation, most often bacterial due to *Streptococcus* pneumonia (Fig. 18.2).
3. acute/subacute atypical pneumonia–atypical features include extrapulmonary symptoms, subacute presentation, lack of response to antibiotics, variable radiographic pattern including a streaky reticular pattern, patchy or confluent foci of consolidation. The most common causes are viruses and mycoplasma (Fig. 18.3). TB is a consideration with acute or subacute dense confluent opacity (Fig. 18.1).
4. acute/subacute miliary or nodular pneumonia–most often due to tuberculous or fungal disease but also seen with septic emboli, viral pneumonia, unusual bacterial disease, and lymphocytic interstitial pneumonia.
5. acute/subacute aspiration pneumonia including aspiration of swallowed materials, gastric contents, hydrocarbon ingestion, and near drowning, perihilar and posterior confluent opacity most common.

In most cases chest radiographs are the only imaging study needed to help guide management of acute or subacute pneumonia. Ultrasound (US) may be indicated to evaluate the presence, nature, and extent of pleural fluid, especially when diagnostic or therapeutic drainage is contemplated. While consolidation and even cavitation can be visualized on US, CT provides more detailed evaluation and is useful when plain films are confusing, an unusual organism or mass is suspected, the clinical situation is complex (e.g. immunocompromised child), or complications are of concern.

Acute suppurative lung parenchymal complications include cavitary necrosis, lung abscess, pneumatocele, and bronchopleural fistula. Since young children have little natural tissue contrast, CT along with dynamic intravenous contrast is particularly useful in sorting out fluid from lung or mass or adenopathy, and atelectatic from consolidated lung (Fig. 18.2). Adenopathy is common in association with pneumonia in children. However, there are a few infections in which adenopathy tends to be particularly prominent, especially tuberculosis and atypical mycobacteria (Fig. 18.3) but also fungal and adenovirus infection. The nodes in TB are characteristically low density on contrast-enhanced CT imaging (Fig. 18.1) and the nodes as well as parenchymal lung disease in both TB and other granulomatous conditions may calcify. A large nodal mass may compress adjacent bronchi producing distal air trapping or atelectasis (Fig. 18.4); this most commonly affects the right middle lobe bronchus, hence the term right middle lobe syndrome.

Typical clinical scenario

Similar to adult TB exposures, most newly infected older children have completely asymptomatic infection. A small number form a primary (Ranke's) complex consisting of a relatively small primary lung parenchymal lesion, draining lymphatic vessels, and regional lymph nodes. This primary complex may resolve completely or become fibrotic and calcify (Ghon complex) with the possibility of future reactivation. Unlike older children and adults, 40–50% of infants exposed to TB become symptomatic and have progressive radiographic abnormalities. Tuberculous pulmonary infection most often presents clinically as a subacute or chronic respiratory infection, although an acute or fulminating presentation does occur, as in this case example.

The primary lung parenchymal lesion may enlarge and become necrotic with liquefaction of the caseous material produced. The bacilli from the primary lesion and adjacent caseating nodes can then spread by direct extension to form secondary nodular and coalescent patchy lung opacities, endobronchial spread, pleuritis or pericarditis (unusual in young children), or even direct spread to the chest wall. Hematogenous seeding may occur to remote organs or produce miliary disease in the lungs. The organs most commonly involved are the lungs, liver, spleen, meninges, brain, peritoneum, lymph nodes, pleura, and bones (Fig. 18.1e).

Both TB and atypical mycobacteria are important causes of pulmonary disease in immunosuppressed patients. Atypical mycobacterial infection may present with bulky neck or mediastinal adenopathy as the major finding (Fig. 18.4). Parenchymal lung changes tend to be reticular, reticulonodular, or patchy rather than confluent and bronchiolar involvement with a tree-in-bud appearance is common; miliary disease may also occur.

Differential diagnosis

Since the lungs can respond to diverse disease processes in only a limited number of ways, it is common for the radiographic features of acute infectious pneumonia to overlap considerably with many non-infectious lung diseases. These include alveolar hemorrhage, pulmonary edema, pulmonary embolism and infarction, drug reaction, hypersensitivity pneumonitis, lymphoid interstitial pneumonitis, benign and malignant lymphoproliferative disorders, bronchiolitis obliterans with organizing pneumonia, collagen vascular diseases, toxic inhalation, lipoid pneumonia, alveolar proteinosis, and confluent neoplasms. Anomalies of the lung, mediastinum, and diaphragm that may mimic an acute or chronic pneumonia pattern include atypical thymus, diaphragmatic eventration and hernia, tracheal bronchus, lung hypoplasia, and congenital bronchopulmonary malformations. Both congenital lung malformations and pulmonary neoplasms may become infected or hemorrhage and present as an acute pneumonia-like illness.

A miliary pattern in the lungs can be seen in some non-infectious entities, including pulmonary edema and inhalation of toxic chemicals, gases, fumes, and vapors. A nodular pattern may be seen with Wegener's granulomatosis, recurrent aspiration, and pulmonary metastases while a reticular or reticulonodular pattern may be seen in conditions such as Langerhans cell histiocytosis, hypersensitivity pneumonitis, and lipoid pneumonia.

Careful attention to the clinical history, symptoms, and course as well as the radiographic features can often produce a short list of the most likely possibilities. The specific diagnosis may then be reached by more directed diagnostic tests that may include blood tests, bronchoscopy, CT, lung scintigraphy, and lavage or biopsy as needed.

Teaching point

Knowledge of the spectrum of causes and presentations of childhood pneumonias and useful differentiating features on plain film and CT may help in evaluating possible complications of pneumonia as well as prompt recognition of unusual infections. Acute or subacute tuberculous infection with local and miliary spread is most likely to occur in young infants. Prominent low-density and/or calcified adenopathy with or without impingement on adjacent bronchi along with variable parenchymal lung disease should raise the possibility of tuberculosis.

REFERENCES

1. Eslamy HK, Newman B. Pneumonia in normal and immunocompromised children: an overview and update. *Radiol Clin North Am* 2011;**49**(5):895–920.

2. Marais BJ, Gie RP, Schaaf HS, *et al*. The natural history of childhood intrathoracic tuberculosis: a critical review of literature from the pre-chemotherapy era. *Int J Tuberc Lung Dis* 2004;**8**(4):392–402.

3. Powell DA, Hunt WG. Tuberculosis in children: an update. *Adv Pediatr* 2006;**53**:279–322.

4. Virkki R, Juven T, Rikalainen H, *et al*. Differentiation of bacterial and viral pneumonia in children. *Thorax* 2002;**57**(5):438–41.

5. Westra SJ, Choy G. What imaging should we perform for the diagnosis and management of pulmonary infections? *Pediatr Radiol* 2009;**39**(Suppl 2):S178–83.

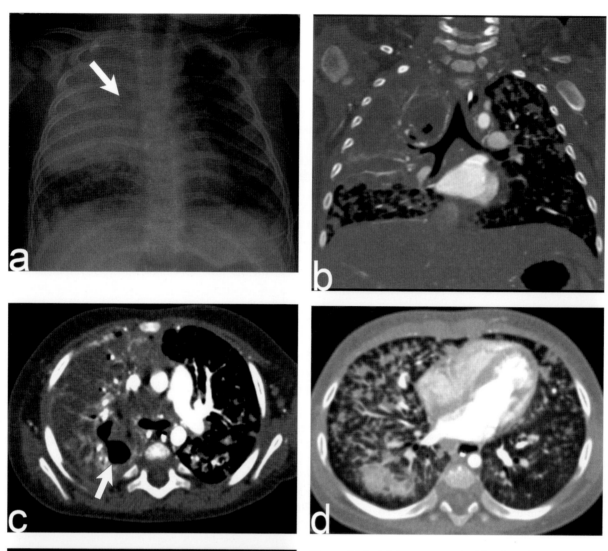

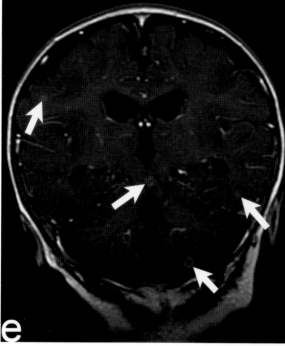

Figure 18.1. (a) A seven-month-old male with acute tuberculous pneumonia. Frontal chest radiograph demonstrates a bulging dense consolidation in the right upper lobe with a suggestion of an irregular cavity medially (arrow). In addition there are multiple large and small nodular opacities in the remainder of the lungs. The trachea appears slightly displaced to the left and the carina is splayed, suggesting the presence of moderate mediastinal adenopathy. **(b, c)** Contrast-enhanced CT scan [coronal, (b) and axial, (c)] demonstrates heterogeneous largely low-density consolidation of the right upper lobe with irregular air-filled cavities medially [arrow in (c)]. The parenchymal abnormality is suggestive of a necrotizing pneumonia; the addition of large low-density mediastinal and hilar adenopathy raises concern for TB. The presence of extensive small and large nodules in the remainder of the lungs suggests both endobronchial spread and hematogenous miliary disease. **(d)** CT–lung window demonstrates large and small pulmonary nodules, confluent opacities, and peripheral tree-in-bud opacity consistent with both endobronchial/bronchiolar disease as well as miliary disease. **(e)** Brain MR (coronal postcontrast image) demonstrates multiple supra- and infratentorial nodular and ring-enhancing lesions (arrows) consistent with cerebral seeding of TB.

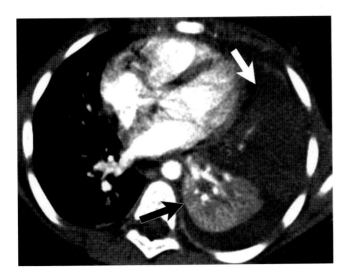

Figure 18.2. A three-year-old with acute pneumococcal pneumonia. There was complete opacification of the left lung on the chest radiograph (not shown). This axial slice from a contrast-enhanced CT scan demonstrates the value of contrast in differentiating consolidated poorly enhancing left upper lobe (white arrow) from densely enhancing atelectatic left lower lobe (black arrow) and adjacent left pleural effusion.

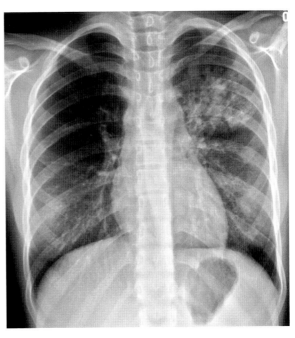

Figure 18.3. An 11-year-old girl with a one-week history of cough and fever. The frontal chest radiograph shows a diffuse mild bilateral reticular appearance with more patchy confluent opacity in the left upper lobe. Both the clinical and radiographic findings suggest an atypical pneumonia. *Mycoplasma pneumoniae* PCR was positive.

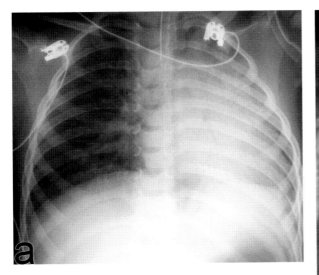

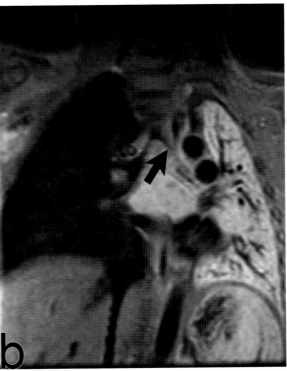

Figure 18.4. *Mycobacterium avium-intracellulare* infection in a two and a half-year-old boy with low grade fever and acute respiratory distress (requiring intubation). **(a)** On the frontal chest radiograph there is complete opacification of the left hemithorax with ipsilateral cardiomediastinal shift, suggesting that left lung atelectasis is the predominant abnormality. Bronchoscopy, obtained to rule out a left endobronchial lesion, demonstrated compression of the carina and left bronchus by an extrinsic mass. **(b)** Chest MR was obtained for further evaluation. This coronal postcontrast image demonstrated splaying of the carina and marked narrowing of the left bronchus by a large enhancing subcarinal solid mass, likely nodes. The left lung was airless but enhanced brightly and homogeneously, suggesting atelectasis rather than consolidated lung. Both inflammatory and neoplastic adenopathy were considered with confirmation of atypical mycobacterial infection on biopsy.

Thymus: normal variations

Beverley Newman

Imaging description

An asymptomatic three-week-old male infant with congenital heart disease (small atrial septal defect [ASD] and ventricular septal defect [VSD]), hypotonia, and dysmorphic facial features was admitted to the neonatal ICU for further evaluation. A portable frontal chest radiograph was obtained, which demonstrated a very prominent mediastinal shadow (Fig. 19.1a). On the left there was a clear thymic wave sign (Fig. 19.1a) but there was concern as to whether the right side was also thymus or if there was a mediastinal mass. A CT scan was ordered. The pediatric radiologist protocolling the CT reviewed the chest radiograph and suggested that this was likely normal thymus and recommended a lateral chest radiograph (Fig. 19.1b) and if necessary an ultrasound (US) study (Fig. 19.1c, d) as the more appropriate examinations to address the clinical concerns. The US examination (Fig. 19.1c, d) was still requested in spite of the reassuring appearance of the lateral chest radiograph showing that all the soft tissue prominence was anterior. The US clearly identified prominent normal thymic tissue, larger on the right than the left, extending from the thoracic inlet to the diaphragm.

Importance

The thymus is an important organ that is responsible for several immunologic functions including the processing and maturation of T lymphocytes. It contributes to normal immunologic function and prevention of autoimmune disease.

Normal variations of the thymus in children include bilateral or unilateral prominence (more common on the right) (Figs. 19.1 and 19.2), thymic hyperplasia or rebound (Fig. 19.3) as well as ectopic thymic tissue (Fig. 19.4). These variations are common reasons for concern being raised about a possible mediastinal or neck mass on a chest radiograph (or even on cross-sectional imaging). The concern can frequently be allayed and additional studies avoided simply by having an experienced pediatric radiologist review the chest radiographs. Both frontal and lateral radiographs are helpful (Fig. 19.1a, b).

The absence of intervening air-filled lung between the US transducer and anterior mediastinum renders the thymus readily available for interrogation by US. Therefore, when concern persists as to whether findings represent a variation of normal or a mass, directed US examination by an experienced pediatric imager is usually effective in identifying normal uniform hypoechoic thymic tissue containing small punctate and linear echogenic areas (Fig. 19.1c, d) from a mass in or adjacent to the thymus. Thymus also has a characteristic appearance on CT (hypodense, mild homogeneous enhancement) (Fig. 19.3) and MR (dark T1, bright T2, homogeneous mild enhancement) (Fig. 19.4) without mass effect on adjacent structures. Although CT and MR can also typically differentiate normal thymic tissue from pathology, it is usually unnecessary to subject the child to the radiation, sedation, and expense that these examinations may entail.

Typical clinical scenario

The thymus is the most common cause of an unusual upper mediastinal contour in children. In young infants the thymus tends to be quadrilateral in shape (more triangular in adolescents) with progressive fatty infiltration. The thymus is largest in small infants and can extend from the superior mediastinum to the diaphragm (Fig. 19.1). Common imaging variations include the thymic wave sign (soft thymic tissue indented by the anterior ribs) (Fig. 19.1) and the thymic sail sign (thymus extending outward overlying the lung, usually on the right and with a sharp inferior border along the minor fissure) (Fig. 19.2). Ectopic normal thymic tissue commonly extends into the neck (most often left sided) (Fig. 19.4) (see Case 7, Fig. 7.1) or behind the superior vena cava. Ectopic or atypical thymus is similar in appearance and enhancement and usually directly contiguous with the normal intrathoracic thymus (Fig. 19.4). Thymic cysts are common, especially in ectopic thymus in the neck (see Case 7, Fig. 7.2).

The thymus is typically more prominent on an expiratory radiograph and is readily compressed by the expanded lungs on inspiration so that a repeat better inspiratory radiograph or fluoroscopic visualization may also be options for separating normal thymus from pathology (Fig. 19.2). A prominent thymus is a sign of robust health in an infant; with stress the thymus may rapidly atrophy, within 24–48 hours. With resolution of the illness, the thymus tends to rebound and may become even more prominent than it was before (Fig. 19.3).

On occasion the thymus may be congenitally absent or hypoplastic. This is seen most commonly in Di George syndrome with resultant T-cell immunodeficiency.

Differential diagnosis

The thymus is not uncommonly the site of origin or directly infiltrated by anterior mediastinal neoplastic lesions, both benign and malignant. These include lymphangioma (Fig. 19.4), hemangioma, Langerhans cell histiocytosis, thymolipoma (Fig. 19.5), teratoma/germ cell tumor (Fig. 19.6), lymphoma (Fig. 19.7), thymoma, and thymic carcinoma.

Other causes of superior mediastinal widening include mediastinal inflammation, abscess or hematoma, middle and posterior mediastinal masses such as foregut duplication cyst, adenopathy, and neuroblastoma, as well as abnormal vessels such as the snowman sign seen in supracardiac anomalous pulmonary venous drainage (Fig. 19.8).

REFERENCES

1. Ben-Ami TE, O'Donovan JC, Yousefzadeh DK. Sonography of the chest in children. *Radiol Clin North Am* 1993;31(3):517–31.

2. Binkovitz LA, Binkovitz I, Kuhn JP. The mediastinum. In: Slovis T, ed. *Caffey's Pediatric Diagnostic Imaging*, vol. 1. 11th edition. Philadelphia: Mosby Elsevier, 2008; 1324–88.

3. Newman B. Thoracic neoplasms in children. *Radiol Clin North Am* 2011;49(4):633–64.

4. Newman B. Ultrasound body applications in children. *Pediatr Radiol* 2011;41(Suppl 2):555–61.

5. Siegel MJ. Chest. In: Siegel MJ, ed. *Pediatric Sonography*, 3rd edition. Philadelphia: Lippincott Williams & Wilkins, 2002;167–72.

Teaching point

Many suspected anterior mediastinal masses and some neck masses in children are due to normal thymic variations.

It is important to recognize these on imaging and use US as the primary problem-solving tool in children.

Many anterior mediastinal lesions, both benign and malignant, originate in or involve the thymus.

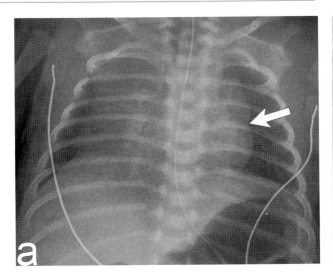

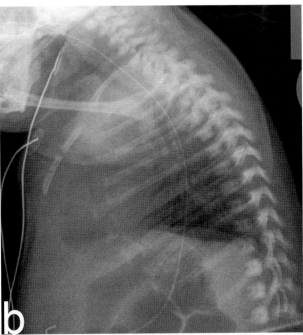

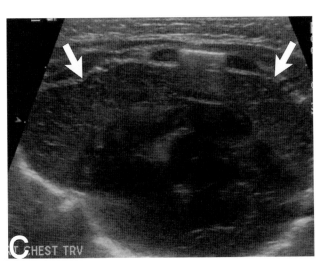

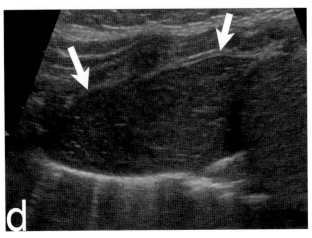

Figure 19.1. Prominent normal thymus in a three-week-old boy with dysmorphic features, hypotonia, and small ASD, VSD. **(a)** Frontal chest radiograph with prominent right mediastinal soft tissue extending to the diaphragm, thought to probably represent normal asymmetric prominence of the thymus. A normal thymic wave sign (indentation of the margin of the thymus by the adjacent ribs) is seen on the left (arrow) but not the right. **(b)** Later lateral chest radiograph confirms impression that the soft tissue is all anterior and likely normal thymus. **(c)** Transverse US and **(d)** right sagittal US images demonstrate the normal sonographic appearance of the anterior thymus (arrows), hypoechoic with small punctate and linear areas of echogenicity, with asymmetric prominence of the right lobe **(c)** extending down to the right hemidiaphragm **(d)**. (Figures 19.1a, c, d: Reprinted from Newman B, Thoracic neoplasms in children. *Radiol Clin North Am* 2011;**49**(4):633–64, Copyright 2011, with permission from Elsevier.)

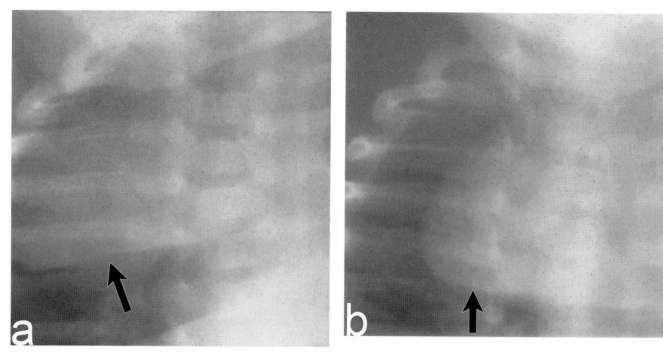

Figure 19.2. A 16-month-old with respiratory distress and upper respiratory infection, normal thymus. **(a)** This expiratory coned down view of the right upper chest demonstrates a large thymus overlying the right upper lobe, simulating a mass or consolidation. Note the sharp inferior border (arrow). This appearance constitutes the thymic sail sign. **(b)** Inspiratory image still demonstrates a right thymic sail sign (arrow); however, the thymus is much smaller, compressed medially, uncovering the normal right upper lobe.

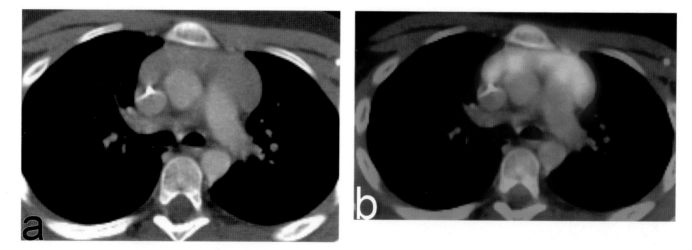

Figure 19.3. Thymic rebound in an 11-year-old previously treated for lymphoma who now has new enlargement of the superior mediastinum. On the contrast-enhanced axial CT **(a)** and axial fused PET/CT image **(b)**, the tissue in the anterior mediastinum has the typical shape, homogeneity, mild enhancement, and diffuse increased metabolic activity typical of normal thymus. (Figure 19.3b: Reprinted from Newman B, Thoracic neoplasms in children. *Radiol Clin North Am* 2011;**49**(4):633–64, Copyright 2011, with permission from Elsevier.)

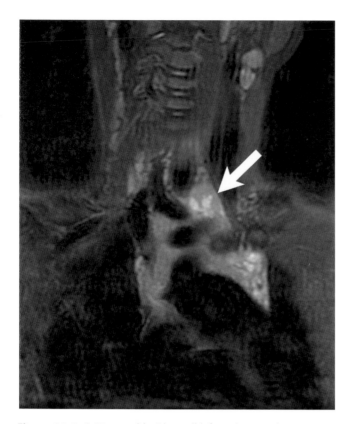

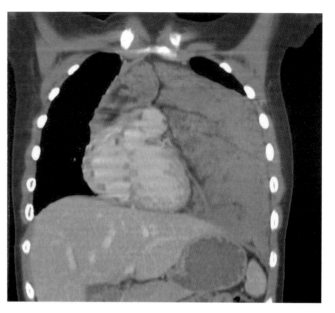

Figure 19.4. A 10-year-old with small left neck mass: thymic lymphangioma with ectopic thymus extending into the neck. T2-weighted coronal MR image demonstrates T2 bright superior mediastinal thymic tissue contiguous with ectopic thymus in the left neck (arrow). Within the thymus there are multiple small brighter cysts on the left, including in the ectopic thymus, which proved to be a small cystic lymphangioma.

Figure 19.5. A 10-year-old asymptomatic boy with incidental discovery of a chest mass, histology consistent with thymolipoma. This coronal CT reconstruction demonstrates a large mass replacing the thymus and extending to the left inferiorly to the diaphragm. The mass consists of large septated lobulations with patchy low attenuation areas with negative Houndsfield numbers consistent with fat. The CT appearance is strongly suggestive of thymolipoma, a benign thymic neoplasm.

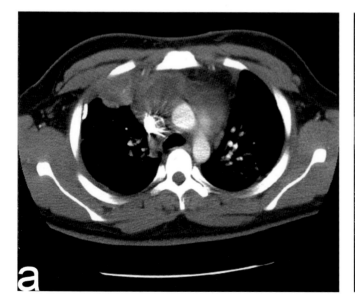

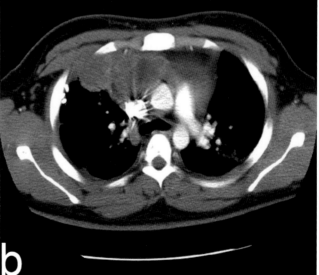

Figure 19.6. Teenage male with a mediastinal non-seminomatous germ cell tumor. Serial axial contrasted CT images extending from superior to inferior demonstrate normal thymic tissue on the left and an irregular hypodense lobulated tumor involving the remainder of the thymus and extending anterolaterally. This tumor has a worse prognosis than mediastinal seminoma and is associated with Klinefelter's syndrome and hematologic disorders. Most patients have elevated beta-HCG (human chorionic gonadotropin) or alpha-fetoprotein levels.

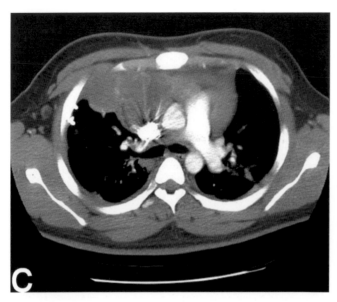
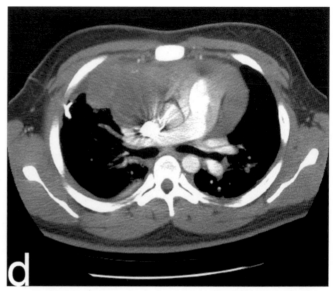

Figure 19.6. (cont.)

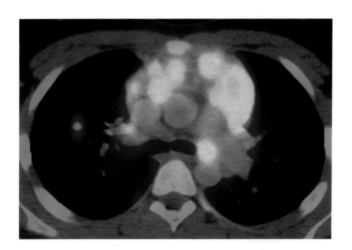

Figure 19.7. A 14-year-old with newly diagnosed Hodgkin's disease. In contrast to the appearance of normal thymic tissue in Fig. 19.3, this axial PET/CT image shows nodularity and irregular metabolic activity in the thymus infiltrated by lymphoma. There are also several other "hot" mediastinal nodes as well as lung nodules. (Reprinted from Newman B, Thoracic neoplasms in children. *Radiol Clin North Am* 2011;**49**(4):633–64, Copyright 2011, with permission from Elsevier.)

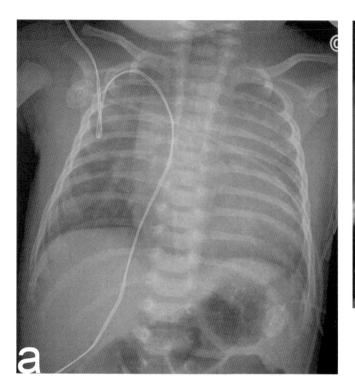

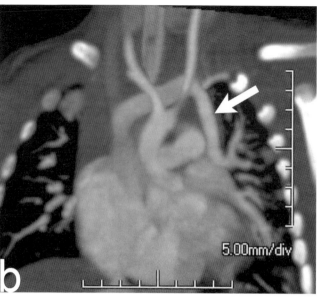

Figure 19.8. A one-month-old boy with respiratory distress and a heart murmur. **(a)** Frontal chest radiograph. There is probable cardiomegaly and a prominent superior mediastinal shadow. **(b)** Coronal MIP reconstruction from a CTA obtained after a cardiac echo that raised concern for anomalous pulmonary venous drainage. Both the normal thymus as well as abnormal enlarged mediastinal veins (snowman sign) contribute to the enlargement of the superior mediastinum. There is partial anomalous venous drainage, with the left upper lobe veins draining to an enlarged left-sided vertical vein (arrow), which joins the left innominate vein to the superior vena cava and right atrium. The other pulmonary veins drained normally to the left atrium (not shown).

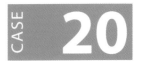

20 Airleak in the neonate

Beverley Newman

Imaging description

A premature newborn infant with respiratory distress was intubated at birth. A frontal chest radiograph (Fig. 20.1a) was obtained which demonstrated an endotracheal tube and nasogastric tube in place. The lungs were mildly underinflated with diffuse symmetric bilateral hazy (ground glass) opacity of the lungs. The appearance was thought to be most consistent with surfactant deficiency although at this early stage there could be some contributory element of residual fetal lung fluid. While neonatal pneumonia, especially infection with group B *Streptococcus*, could have this appearance, there was no clinical history or other findings to suggest infection. There was an unusual central air collection extending from just above the heart to the diaphragm and posterior in location on the lateral view most suggestive of a posterior retrocardiac pneumomediastinum. There was no history of a traumatic tube placement and the air collection dissipated without any specific treatment.

Importance

Retrocardiac pneumomediastinum has been variously thought to be loculated air in the infra-azygos space or air in the pulmonary ligament. In general, pulmonary ligament air tends to adopt a slightly more parasagittal location consistent with the anatomic location of the pulmonary ligament, whereas air in the infra-azygos mediastinum is more midline in position, as in this case. Extension of air from this space superiorly is usually prevented by fascia reflected from the underside of the carina to the fibrous layer of the parietal pericardium. However, the air collection in this case does seem to be present more superiorly than an infra-azygos location.

Similar to other airleak phenomena in babies, retrocardiac pneumomediastinum most often results from the barotrauma of positive pressure ventilation. This first causes alveolar rupture with dissection of air into the interstitium that may then break through into the mediastinal, pleural, or pericardial spaces. In the case of posterior pneumomediastinum, there is also an association with iatrogenic airleak typically related to a surgical mishap (Fig. 20.2) or perforation of the airway or esophagus associated with intubation, nasogastric tube placement, or suction. There may not be clinical recognition of a traumatic tube placement; the presence of new or increasing respiratory distress following tube placement, malposition of the tube radiographically, ongoing airleak, hemorrhage, or effusion should raise suspicion of an iatrogenic perforation. Further imaging investigations such as an esophagram or CT scan may be warranted. Pneumomediastinal collections generally do not require specific treatment; occasionally very large

collections may compress the heart and great vessels and compromise venous return, necessitating drainage.

Typical clinical scenario

Pneumomediastinum or pneumothorax may occur spontaneously at birth (Fig. 20.3) and are thought to be related to precipitous delivery with an abrupt change in intrapulmonary pressure.

Mechanical ventilation of young infants, especially small premature babies, carries a risk of airleak including pulmonary interstitial air, pneumomediastinum, pneumothorax, pneumopericardium, and even intravascular air embolism. Mediastinal air may also dissect into the neck and superficial soft tissues (uncommon in infants) as well as inferiorly into the retroperitoneal and intraperitoneal compartments. Mediastinal airleak in infants is most often located anteriorly and typically elevates the thymus away from the heart, producing an angel's wings appearance (Fig. 20.3). Anterior mediastinal air can extend all the way to the diaphragm (Fig. 20.3) and even dissect along the diaphragm, mimicking a pneumothorax or pneumopericardium. Early treatment with surfactant and use of high-frequency oscillating ventilators has greatly reduced the frequency and severity of airleak in newborns.

Airleak phenomena are particularly prevalent in a variety of underlying conditions and can occur even in the absence of mechanical ventilation. These include meconium aspiration (Fig. 20.4), pulmonary hypoplasia (Fig. 20.5), and neonatal pneumonia.

Differential diagnosis

Pulmonary interstitial emphysema (PIE) appears on imaging most often as multiple linear lucencies radiating from the pulmonary hilum (Fig. 4). The linear areas may coalesce to form small and larger cystic air collections. On CT imaging the air is located immediately adjacent to the vessels; on histology most of the interstitial air is intralymphatic. In general, PIE is not specifically treated and will mostly regress spontaneously. Troublesome persistence has been treated by decubitus positioning (affected side down) and brief administration of 100% oxygen. Occasionally, focal PIE or large peripheral blebs may require surgical resection.

Pneumothorax is characterized by airleak into the pleural space (Figs. 20.4, 20.5), most often from breakthrough of interstitial air. Frequently the lung is abnormal due to underlying pathology such as surfactant deficiency or pneumonia plus/minus PIE so that the lung does not collapse much even with a tension pneumothorax (Fig. 20.4). The free pleural air tends to collect anteromedially in a supine infant and may only be recognized by hyperlucency of the affected hemithorax radiographically or a medial air collection adjacent to the heart

(Fig. 20.6). This can simulate a pneumomediastinum but without elevation of the thymus. Decubitus views may be helpful in moving the free air adjacent to the outer edge of the non-dependent lung when that side is up, facilitating recognition. A pneumothorax under tension (common in a ventilated neonate) is often recognized by mediastinal shift or diaphragmatic inversion (Figs. 20.4, 20.5). A small pneumothorax may be treated conservatively; however, the majority require chest tube drainage, especially if there are new clinical symptoms or signs of a tension pneumothorax.

Pneumopericardium is recognized as being located in the pericardial rather than mediastinal space by the presence of air extending all the way around the cardiac apex (Fig. 20.7). Pericardial air can compress the heart and compromise venous return and is usually drained. Pneumopericardium in postoperative cardiac patients will usually drain spontaneously as the pericardium has been opened surgically.

Air may dissect into the subcutaneous soft tissues as well as the peritoneal cavity, especially with an ongoing source of airleak. Secondary pneumoperitoneum is invariably accompanied by airleak in the chest, the abdomen is usually not tender or symptomatic, and other features of abdominal pathology such as obstruction or pneumatosis and peritoneal fluid are absent.

Large intravascular air embolization is a rare and usually fatal complication; intracardiac and great vessel air may be seen radiographically.

A normal thymic sail sign may be mistaken for an elevated thymus due to pneumomediastinum. Neonatal atypical peripheral atelectasis (NAPA–usually right upper lobe) may also be mistaken for a displaced thymus, apical pleural fluid, or mass (Fig. 20.8). NAPA is a form of unusual atelectasis that is usually a rounded, pleural-based smooth-surfaced lesion that can be located at both apices. Usually this appearance is transient with a more typical appearance of upper lobe atelectasis supervening.

Congenital lobar emphysema with hyperlucent airtrapped lung and sparse vessels may simulate a pneumothorax; careful observation will usually suffice to differentiate although occasionally CT scan may be needed (Fig. 20.9).

Other entities that may be mistaken for airleak phenomena include: air in the esophagus itself, a dilated obstructed esophageal pouch in esophageal atresia; a hiatal, diaphragmatic or paraesophageal hernia; and an air-containing lung cyst or bronchopulmonary malformation. Occasionally, extrinsic artifacts such as a skinfold or overlying equipment may simulate pneumothorax or pneumomediastinum.

Teaching point

Airleak phenomena are common in newborn ventilated infants as well as in association with a variety of underlying conditions. PIE may be the harbinger of other more serious airleak phenomena.

Careful perusal of plain films will often differentiate the location of air collections, although multiple sites of airleak may be present simultaneously. Occasionally CT may be needed to evaluate airleak and differentiate it from other lesions.

The presence of a posterior pneumomediastinum can be spontaneous but should raise the question of iatrogenic tracheal or esophageal perforation, especially if accompanied by an acute clinical deterioration.

REFERENCES

1. Newman B, Oh KS. Iatrogenic tracheobronchial perforation in infants. *J Thorac Imaging* 1994;**4**:269–72.
2. Newman B, Varich L. Neonatal imaging. In: Daldrup-Link H, Gooding C, eds. *Essentials of Pediatric Radiology. A Multimodality Approach.* New York: Cambridge University Press, 2010; 19–30.
3. Swischuk LE. *Respiratory System. Imaging of the Newborn, Infant and Young Child*, 4th edition. Baltimore: Williams and Wilkins, 1997; 74–84.
4. Tamaki Y, Pandit R, Gooding CA. Neonatal atypical peripheral atelectasis. *Pediatr Radiol* 1994;**24**:589–91.

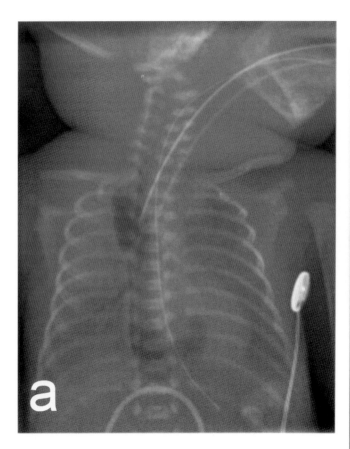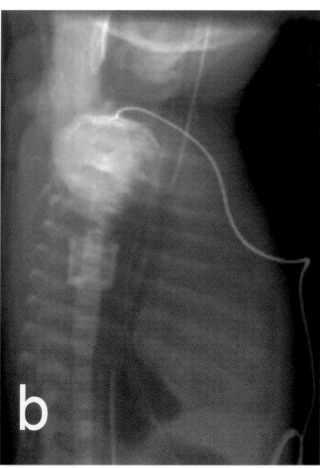

Figure 20.1. Newborn premature infant with respiratory distress due to surfactant deficiency, developed posterior pneumomediastinum. Frontal **(a)** and lateral **(b)** chest radiographs demonstrate diffuse hazy opacification of the lungs (ground glass) with some air bronchograms visible and slightly decreased lung volume. An endotracheal tube and nasogastric tube are in place. There is an unusual central air collection extending from just above the heart to the diaphragm and posterior in location on the lateral view most suggestive of a posterior retrocardiac pneumomediastinum.

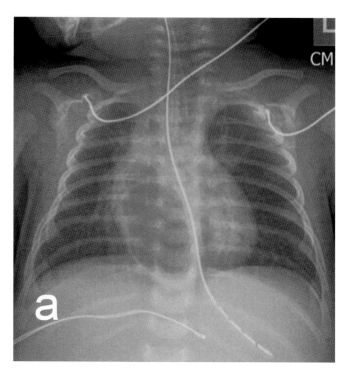

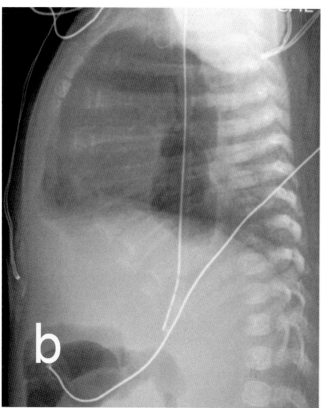

Figure 20.2. A five-week-old infant post repair of H-type fistula with postoperative development of posterior pneumomediastinum related to breakdown of the repair. The frontal **(a)** and lateral **(b)** chest radiographs demonstrate a prominent midline, inferior and posterior air collection consistent with an infra-azygos posterior pneumomediastinum.

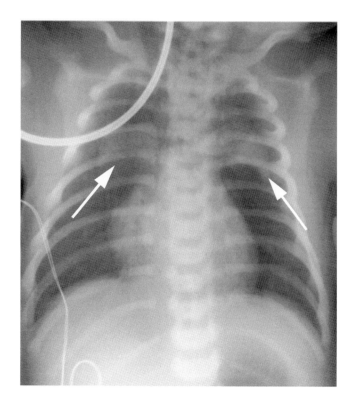

Figure 20.3. Term newborn infant with spontaneous pneumomediastinum. Frontal chest radiograph demonstrates the mediastinal air to be located anteriorly with the typical elevation of the thymus off the heart (arrows) (angel's wings). Note that on the left the mediastinal air extends all the way to the diaphragm. Image courtesy of Laura Varich. (Previously published as Fig 2.17A in Newman B, Varich L. Neonatal imaging. In: Daldrup-Link H, Gooding C, eds. *Essentials of Pediatric Radiology. A Multimodality Approach.* New York: Cambridge University Press, 2010; 19–30.)

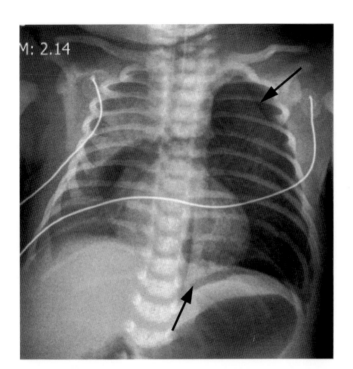

Figure 20.4. A 37-week gestation infant with meconium aspiration. The baby is intubated and on mechanical ventilation. This frontal radiograph demonstrates right-sided pneumomediastinum with typical elevation of the thymus. The left lung is hyperlucent with multiple streaky linear lucencies extending peripherally from the hilum consistent with pulmonary interstitial emphysema (PIE). In addition there is a left pneumothorax with the displaced lung edge best seen superolaterally and inferomedially (arrows). Note that the affected lung collapses poorly due to the PIE. There is some tension component to this pneumothorax (expected with positive pressure ventilation), manifested by mild mediastinal rightward shift and right lung deaeration.

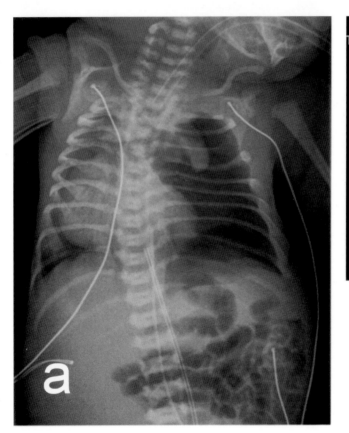

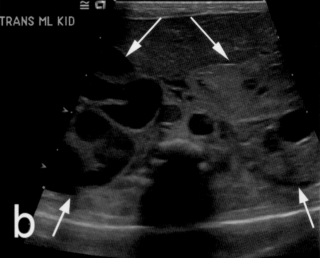

Figure 20.5. Posterior urethral valves with obstructive renal dysplasia. Newborn male infant with severe oligohydramnios in utero and immediate respiratory distress at birth. Although Potter's syndrome was originally described as bilateral renal agenesis, bilateral severe renal dysfunction with oligohydramnios is considered part of the spectrum of a Potter-like syndrome. (a) This frontal chest radiograph demonstrates spontaneous left pneumomediastinum and pneumothorax with cardiomediastinal shift to the right. In addition the chest wall is noted to be deformed with wavy ribs related to oligohydramnios in utero and pulmonary hypoplasia. There is fullness in the right side of the abdomen due to an enlarged right kidney. (b) Transverse ultrasound (US) image at birth demonstrates a markedly hydronephrotic right kidney with virtually no parenchyma and very echogenic left kidney with peripheral dysplastic cysts (arrows).

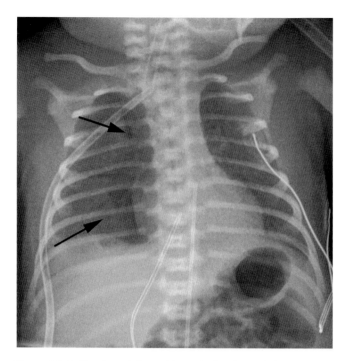

Figure 20.6. Newborn infant with residual right medial pneumothorax. On frontal chest radiograph, this premature infant has granular and mottled changes in the lungs consistent with partially treated surfactant deficiency. There is a right chest tube in place to treat a right pneumothorax. There is residual medial right pneumothorax noted as a band of medial lucency in this supine infant (arrows). Note the absence of thymic elevation.

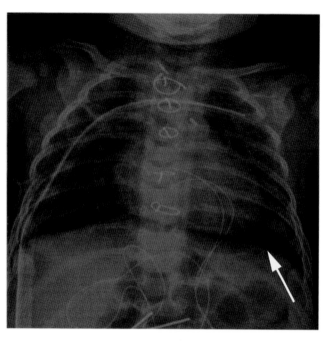

Figure 20.7. Pneumopericardium after ventricular septal defect (VSD) repair. Note the air extending continuously around the cardiac apex, displacing the pericardium from the heart (arrow).

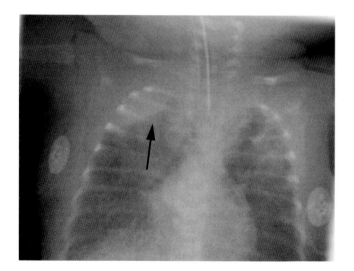

Figure 20.8. Neonatal atypical peripheral atelectasis (NAPA)–four-week-old premature male infant treated for surfactant deficiency now with moderate mottled chronic lung changes. A new right apical density has appeared on the frontal chest radiograph (arrow). Normal thymus appears to be present centrally. This appearance was transient and quickly changed on a repeat radiograph to the more typical appearance of right upper lobe atelectasis.

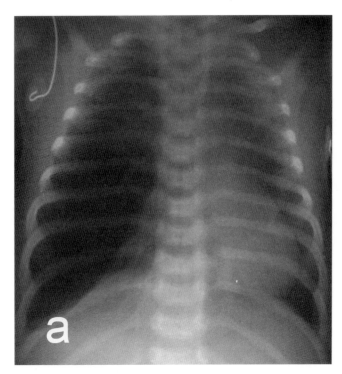
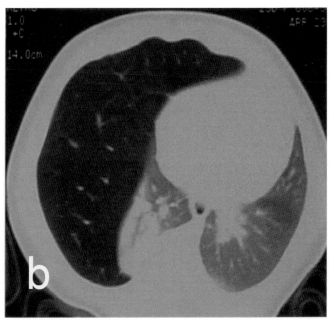

Figure 20.9. Newborn infant with right middle lobe congenital lobar emphysema (CLE). **(a)** Frontal chest radiograph. At first glance the hyperlucent right lung with leftward shift may be mistaken for airleak. Recognition that there is complete right lower lobe atelectasis inferiorly and partial right upper lobe atelectasis superiorly facilitates recognition of the emphysematous right middle lobe. **(b)** The axial CT slice confirms the hyperlucent emphysematous right middle lobe with sparse vessels and adjacent medial atelectatic right lower lobe with cardiomediastinal shift to the left.

Bronchopulmonary malformation: hybrid lesions

Beverley Newman

Imaging description

A chest radiograph (Fig. 21.1a) was obtained on an asymptomatic newborn infant because of a history of a right lower lobe abnormality discovered in utero. The newborn chest radiograph showed only subtle increased markings at the right lung base (Fig. 21.1a). Prenatal imaging had included ultrasound (US) and MRI at 29 weeks (Fig. 21.1b). Both studies had shown a large somewhat heterogeneous complex lesion, mostly solid with some cystic components, occupying most of the right lung posteriorly and with some midline mass effect (Fig. 21.1b). There was also a linear low signal branching structure noted inferiorly suggesting a systemic vascular supply to the lesion from below the diaphragm (Fig. 21.1b). The findings were consistent with a bronchopulmonary malformation (BPM), with hybrid feature of pulmonary sequestration (systemic arterial supply) and cystic pulmonary airway malformation (CPAM) (cysts). Serial ultrasound studies demonstrated moderate progressive decrease in the size of the lesion in the third trimester of pregnancy.

The child remained asymptomatic and thrived. A CTA was obtained at 10 months of age to determine the size, extent, and detailed anatomy of the residual lesion, and provide guidance on appropriate management. This demonstrated a moderate-sized residual lesion in the right lower lobe, with hybrid features including cystic and solid non-aerated components, similar to those seen prenatally. There was a large systemic artery supplying the lesion that arose from the celiac axis with pulmonary venous drainage to the right inferior pulmonary vein and left atrium. The mass was resected thoracoscopically with pathologic confirmation of a BPM with histologic hybrid features of pulmonary sequestration and CPAM.

Importance

The major lesions incorporated under the umbrella of the congenital BPMs include bronchogenic cyst, bronchial atresia, congenital lobar/segmental overinflation, CPAM, and pulmonary sequestration. An increasing number of these lesions are being recognized as having considerable overlap (>50%) in features both at imaging and pathology. This has been explained by suggesting that they share a common underlying etiology of in utero airway obstruction and that the timing and degree of obstruction determines the anatomic and pathologic features that predominate. Histologic changes of lung malformation including pulmonary hyperplasia and cystic dysplasia are common overlapping features in these lesions. Several careful specimen studies have shown that ~80% of these anomalies have underlying associated atresia of the supplying bronchus.

Imaging studies provide some confirmation of this obstruction malformation concept in that features associated with airway obstruction are common in these lesions and cystic dysplastic changes correlate well with pathology. Features of airway obstruction on imaging include complete lack of air in some lesions as well as slow clearing of fetal lung fluid from the cystic or complex lesions that become aerated, with subsequent overaeration/hyperlucency, consistent with partial airway obstruction and/or collateral ventilation. Another common feature that can be seen in both prenatal as well as postnatal imaging studies is the presence of dilated airways with mucoid impaction, a typical finding in the airways distal to focal bronchial atresia. This finding may be subtle, especially early in life. Cystic changes of varying size, either fluid or air filled, are common and are considered to be secondary dysplastic changes (typical findings in bronchogenic cyst and large or small cyst CPAM).

The current imaging approach to the BPM lesions has changed considerably with their common discovery and detailed imaging in utero. The early imaging and management will depend on the presence of symptoms at birth. The most commonly symptomatic lesions at birth are large cyst CPAM or congenital lobar overinflation. A chest radiograph followed by an early CT scan is typical if emergent surgical removal of the affected lobe is likely. When the child is asymptomatic a chest radiograph is often the only study obtained at birth. Early postnatal US may be useful, especially if the lesion is non- or only partially aerated (Fig. 21.2). An interval CT is often delayed until six to 12 months, when surgical removal is being contemplated. CT angiography, including the upper abdomen, is indicated to fully define the detailed arterial and venous anatomy and ensure that small systemic arteries are not overlooked. High-quality studies can be obtained with low radiation dose, particularly by using lower kVp and thereby taking advantage of the increased contrast resolution afforded by the concomitant use of intravenous iodine. Multiplanar, volumetric, and maximum and minimum intensity projection reconstructions are indispensable in elucidating the anatomy. Postnatal MRI has a limited role in evaluating the BPMs. While the vascular supply can be defined on MRA similar to CTA, the detailed pulmonary anatomy is less well delineated by MR. Fluid-filled cysts and mucoid impaction in dilated bronchi, denoting bronchial atresia, associated with the lesion are well seen on T2-weighted MRI (Fig. 21.3) and it is possible to follow some of the lesions that are not removed surgically by MR when plain film radiographs are insufficient.

Typical clinical scenario

Many BPMs are found by US in the second trimester of pregnancy. A small number of these lesions progressively enlarge and produce marked mass effect in utero with compression of the esophagus and compromise of systemic venous return to the heart resulting in polyhydramnios and hydrops fetalis with significant fetal morbidity and mortality. Fetal interventions such as in utero drainage, fetal surgical resection, or emergent early delivery may be required. However, most of the lesions reach their largest size in the second trimester and then remain stable or decrease in size during the third trimester. Many lesions that were known to be present in utero are not symptomatic at birth and show no or only subtle findings on chest radiographs (Figs. 21.1, 21.4). However, a residual lesion is almost always present on CT imaging (Figs. 21.1, 21.4).

Some BPMs are symptomatic at birth with respiratory distress due to their size and mass effect on the remainder of the lung. Others become clinically manifest later in life due to superimposed infection, large shunting (Fig. 21.4), or even torsion (Fig. 21.5a, b) while others may be discovered incidentally (Figs. 21.3 and 21.5c). Associated anomalies such as cardiovascular or diaphragmatic abnormalities might be more clinically significant and overshadow the BPM. Still other BPMs may occur as a mass in an extrapulmonary or frankly ectopic location; the most frequent are a middle mediastinal mass or hybrid CPAM/sequestration in the left suprarenal area (Figs. 21.5c, 21.6). There have been suggestions in the past that extrapulmonary sequestrations (non-aerated with separate pleural investment, drain to systemic veins) are congenital lesions and intrapulmonary sequestrations (tend to be at least partially aerated, drain to pulmonary veins) are acquired postnatally, secondary to chronic infection. This and the myth that pulmonary sequestrations are all airless at birth and only become aerated after an infection have been debunked by widespread prenatal and early postnatal imaging (Fig. 21.4). There is quite a lot of overlap between intra- and extrapulmonary sequestration, especially with regard to pulmonary venous drainage, which may be mixed, and generally the distinction is not clinically very important. Extralobar sequestrations have a higher association with other systemic malformations and by definition an ectopic lesion is extralobar (Fig. 21.6). Both intra- and extralobar sequestrations may occur in concert with other BPMs (Fig. 21.5) and both occasionally have a connection with the gastrointestinal tract (usually esophageal) that tends to be overlooked for a prolonged time period.

There are two major postnatal concerns regarding asymptomatic BPMs. These are the risk of superimposed infection and the possibility of malignancy. Infection is uncommon in early infancy and is thought to occur later in ~10–30% of lesions, most prevalent in larger lesions with macroscopic cysts. Prior infection/scarring may render surgical resection more difficult.

There have been multiple case reports of malignant tumors occurring in pre-existing cystic congenital lung lesions. Recent pathology literature has suggested that most, if not all, of these lesions were de novo pleuropulmonary blastomas (PPB) that had been mistaken for congenital lung lesions. There appear to be a very small number of bronchoalveolar carcinomas in children and adults that have been associated with pre-existing BPMs, not only within the lesion but also in some cases in lung tissue adjacent to the site of a previously resected lesion.

There is considerable controversy regarding the surgical versus conservative management of BPMs. Those that have significant clinical symptoms or large systemic arterial supply are obvious surgical candidates (Fig. 21.4). The asymptomatic lesions are more problematic, indeed many of them may not have been detected postnatally had there not been in utero US. There is an increasing tendency to leave some of the asymptomatic lesions alone and follow them clinically. The nature, timing, and length of the follow-up needed are not certain. The asymptomatic lesions most likely to be managed conservatively are lobar and segmental overinflation as well as other lesions with clearly defined bronchial atresia. Small pulmonary sequestrations with minimal systemic supply may also be left alone. Another possible option for managing pulmonary sequestration lesions is interventional vascular embolization. Asymptomatic lesions with macroscopic cysts are more likely to be removed surgically; complete lobectomy is typically performed. It is therefore important to carefully describe the anatomy, location, extent, and specific features, including presence of macroscopic cysts, mucoid impaction, lung overinflation, and systemic arterial supply.

Differential diagnosis

BPMs tend to be quite distinct and identifiable on imaging. Other uncommon prenatal intrapulmonary masses include congenital peribronchial myofibroblastic tumor thought to possibly be a low grade fibrosarcoma, characterized by its large size but benign behavior; fetal lung interstitial tumor, a recently described solid entity resembling normal lung with arrested development; PPB, synovial sarcoma, and rhabdomyosarcoma. Only a small number of pulmonary neoplasms have been described in utero, usually not before the third trimester, and they tend to progressively increase in size, unlike the BPMs. Postnatally the most troublesome distinction is between cystic PPB and CPAM. PPB is less likely to be found prenatally or at birth, tends to be more peripheral, presents more frequently with pneumothorax or multiple lesions, and may contain solid nodular components. CPAM may be distinguished by its tendency to be found early and often regress in utero as well as a common association with hybrid features of BPMs including mucoid impaction and systemic arterial supply.

While BPMs may become secondarily infected and be a source for chronic or recurrent infection, the radiographic presence of a partially or non-aerated lesion (most common in medial left lower lobe) may be mistaken for recurrent pneumonia in a child with only repeated upper respiratory infections. In addition, cystic changes such as pneumatocele formation in pneumonia may sometimes be difficult to differentiate from an underlying infected BPM. Chest radiographs should be carefully reviewed for changes in appearance or resolution when the child is well. Detailed CT imaging may also be helpful in the distinction. Chronic lower lobe pneumonia may occasionally acquire a secondary blood supply from phrenic vessels somewhat simulating a sequestration.

BPMs located in the mediastinum include bronchogenic cyst (Fig. 21.5c) (most common at the carina), esophageal duplication cyst, and neurenteric cyst. Bronchogenic cysts, in particular, may cause extrinsic airway compression with distal lung overinflation or atelectasis. Differential considerations for these lesions include other middle mediastinal masses such as infectious or neoplastic adenopathy, pericardial cyst or neoplasm, and vascular lesions such as rings or aneurysm.

Abdominal BPMs, specifically a cystic/solid mass in the left suprarenal area, are a major differential consideration for neonatal adrenal masses, including adrenal hemorrhage and neuroblastoma. Features favoring a hybrid BPM lesion include early presence in utero, location adjacent to rather than in the adrenal, visible systemic arterial supply, lack of growth over time, and adjacent diaphragmatic abnormality such as eventration (Fig. 21.6).

Teaching point

There is a broad spectrum of presentation and appearance of congenital BPMs. Both prenatal and postnatal imaging should carefully evaluate the anomalous airway, vascular, foregut, and pulmonary parenchymal components of these lesions as well as possible other associated lesions. Recognition of the considerable clinical, histologic, and imaging overlap of BPMs as part of an obstruction malformation complex is helpful in understanding and recognizing the imaging features.

REFERENCES

1. Epelman M, Kreiger PA, Servaes S, Victoria T, Hellinger JC. Current imaging of prenatally diagnosed congenital lung lesions. *Semin Ultrasound CT MR* 2010;**31**:141–57.

2. Kunisaki SM, Fauza DO, Nemes LP, *et al.* Bronchial atresia: the hidden pathology within a spectrum of prenatally diagnosed lung masses. *J Pediatr Surg* 2006;**41**(1):61–5.

3. Laberge JM, Puligandla P, Flageole H. Asymptomatic congenital lung malformations. *Semin Pediatr Surg* 2005;**14**:16–33.

4. Langston C. New concepts in the pathology of congenital lung malformations. *Semin Pediatr Surg* 2003;**12**:17–37.

5. Newman B. Congenital bronchopulmonary foregut malformations: concepts and controversies. *Pediatr Radiol* 2006;**36**:773–91.

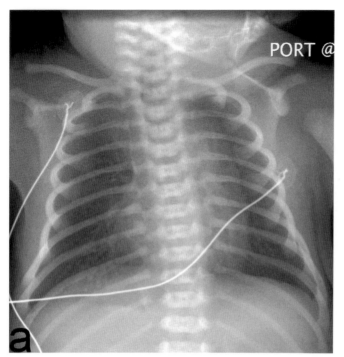

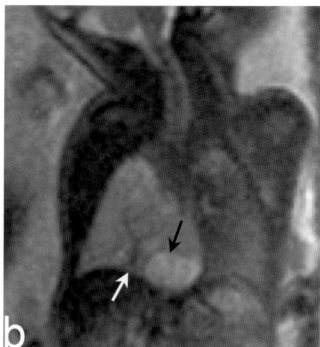

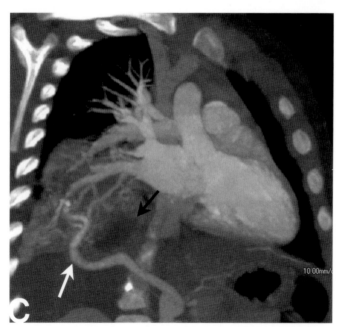

Figure 21.1. Bronchopulmonary malformation–hybrid pulmonary sequestration/CPAM. **(a)** Chest radiograph at birth shows only subtle right lower lobe streaky opacity. **(b)** Prenatal T2-weighted coronal MRI at 29 weeks with a large increased signal lesion affecting most of the right lung with some normal lung seen superiorly. There is mass effect with some leftward mediastinal shift. The lesion is heterogeneous with some cystic components (black arrow). A branching low-density feeding vessel is seen extending into the lesion from inferiorly (white arrow). **(c)** CTA at 10 months of age. Coronal MIP reconstructed image demonstrates an airless right lower lobe lesion containing several fluid-filled cysts (black arrow). There is a large systemic artery from the abdominal aorta supplying the lesion (white arrow), with drainage to the right pulmonary veins. The airless nature of the lesion suggests an extralobar sequestration in spite of the venous drainage. The features of the lesion correspond very well to the prenatal MR, although it is smaller, occupying less of the right lung than previously, and midline mass effect is no longer present.

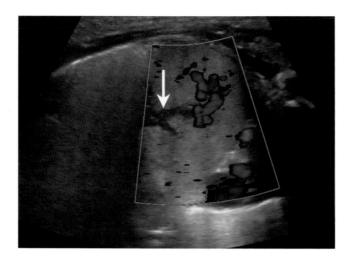

Figure 21.2. Pulmonary sequestration, newborn infant. Oblique transverse US of the medial left lower lobe, seen here adjacent to the liver. The lesion was airless and homogeneous with a large systemic artery and draining vein partially visualized within the lesion. A medial fluid-filled branching structure close to the vessels (arrow) represents a dilated mucoid impacted bronchus indicative of proximal bronchial atresia.

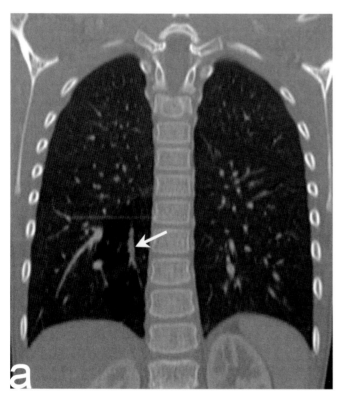

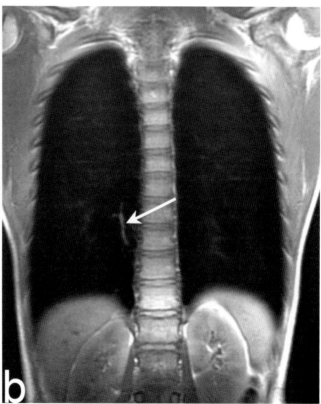

Figure 21.3. An eight-year-old boy, incidental finding of asymptomatic BPM–segmental overinflation with bronchial atresia on CT obtained for appendicitis. **(a)** Coronal reconstruction from CT demonstrates a small area of focal medial and basilar hyperinflated lung containing a non-vascular medial linear dense branching structure consistent with mucoid impaction in a dilated bronchus (arrow). Findings indicative of segmental bronchial atresia with distal mucoid impaction and overinflated adjacent lung aerated through collateral channels. **(b)** Follow-up coronal T2-weighted MR 1 year later demonstrates the same findings of hyperlucent lung and bronchial mucoid impaction. Although lung parenchymal detail on MR is less distinct compared with CT, the mucoid impaction is particularly easy to see and distinguish from vessels on MR.

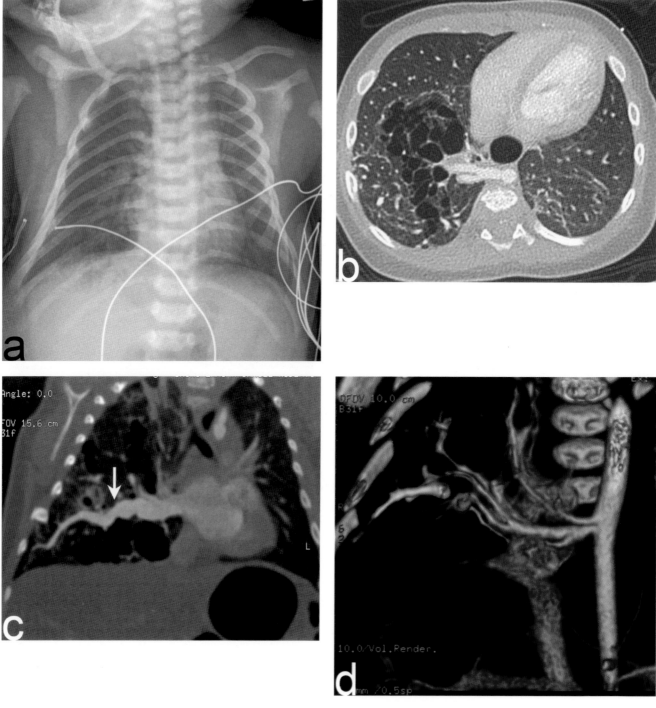

Figure 21.4. CPAM/sequestration hybrid lesion. **(a)** Chest radiograph at birth in a one-day-old child with known large right-sided cystic lung lesion in utero, with progressive decrease in size in the third trimester (not shown). Small ill-defined aerated cysts are seen in the inferomedial right lower lobe. **(b)** CTA at age four months–axial slice, lung window. The right lower lobe lesion consists of small aerated cysts with large systemic arterial supply from the aorta. **(c)** CTA–coronal MINIP reconstruction. The right lower lobe lesion with multiple small cysts is interspersed with the normal right lower lung, consistent with absence of a separate pleural investment, i.e. intralobar. The enlarged pulmonary vein (arrow) draining the lesion to the left atrium indicates a large shunt. **(d)** CTA–coronal volumetric reconstruction showing several large arteries from the subdiaphragmatic aorta supplying the right lower lobe.

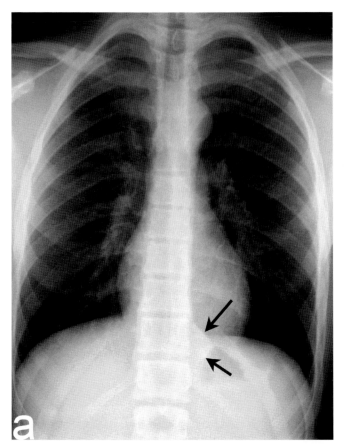

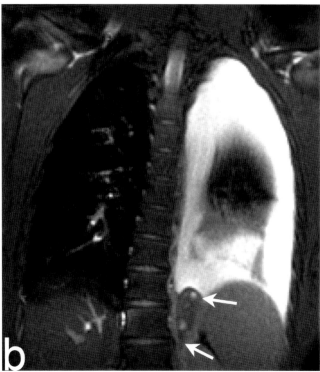

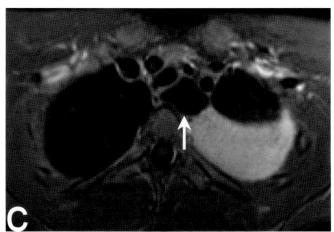

Figure 21.5. Torsion of an extralobar sequestration – six-year-old boy with acute left chest pain. **(a)** The frontal chest radiograph appeared normal except for a small left inferomedial paraspinal density (arrows). **(b)** Coronal T2-weighted MR image 24 hours after the chest radiograph demonstrates development of a large left pleural effusion. The arrows point to the small low signal left paraspinal mass at the medial left lung base containing small cysts. This lesion did not enhance postcontrast. **(c)** Postcontrast T1-weighted axial image of the upper chest demonstrates an additional small mediastinal cyst (arrow). Note that the pleural fluid is bright on both T1- and T2-weighted images, suggesting it is likely blood. The radiologic diagnoses of a torsed infarcted extralobar sequestration with hemorrhage and separate upper mediastinal bronchogenic cyst were confirmed at surgery.

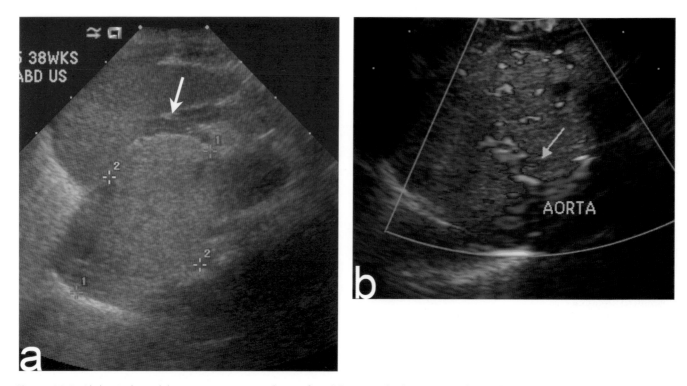

Figure 21.6. Abdominal extralobar sequestration–newborn infant. **(a)** Longitudinal sonogram of the left upper abdomen shows a rounded mostly solid suprarenal mass with some cystic components, located medial to and separate from the spleen and adrenal gland (arrow). Note also focal eventration of the left posteromedial hemidiaphragm superior to the mass. **(b)** Longitudinal color Doppler image shows a large arterial feeder (arrow) from the aorta to the sequestration mass in the left upper abdomen.

Lymphatic abnormality in the pediatric chest

Beverley Newman

Imaging description

A previously healthy 10-year-old girl presented with shortness of breath for 10 days. A frontal chest radiograph (Fig. 22.1a) demonstrated complete opacification of the left hemithorax with cardiomediastinal shift to the right, raising concerns of a left-sided mass versus large effusion. She was afebrile. A contrast-enhanced CT scan (Fig. 22.1b) revealed low-density material, thought to be fluid, filling the left pleural space; the left lung was completely atelectatic. A subtle finding on the CT was lytic expansion of two lower left ribs (Fig. 22.1b). Concern was raised for an underlying neoplasm such as Ewing's sarcoma or leukemia/lymphoma and a chest MR was obtained (Fig. 22.1c). This demonstrated bright T2-weighted signal in the pleura, mediastinum, lower ribs, and adjacent chest wall with large complex organizing pleural fluid. In addition, multiple splenic cysts were noted. No discrete mass and no abnormal enhancement was seen postcontrast. The diagnosis of lymphatic abnormality, likely lymphangiomatosis, with pleural, bone, and splenic involvement was suggested by the interpreting radiologist. On ultrasound (US), the fluid was also shown to be complex and septated consistent with proteinaceous fluid (Fig. 22.1d). The pleural fluid was drained and found to be chylous; pleural biopsy showed dilated lymphatics without definite proliferative findings.

The child initially did well with pleural drainage with re-expansion of the left lung. However, she returned 10 months later with recurrent left pleural fluid accumulation and increased left lower rib lytic changes (not shown).

Importance

Chylothorax is an important and frequently overlooked cause of pleural effusion in children. It is the most common cause of a large pleural effusion in the newborn; the etiology is frequently not ascertained (idiopathic).

There are extensive lymphatic channels throughout the body that grow along with the venous system. The lower extremity and abdominal lymphatics drain into the thoracic duct, which connects into the left innominate vein. In the chest, in addition to the thoracic duct, there are bilateral internal mammary lymphatic chains as well as bilateral pleural and lung to bronchomediastinal lymphatic pathways that usually drain into ipsilateral innominate veins. Absence, malformation, disruption, obstruction, or lack of normal venous drainage of the lymphatics may result in abnormal dilated lymphatic channels with diffuse or focal lymphatic malformation masses or free lymphatic fluid including lymphedema, chylothorax, chylopericardium, and chylous ascites. Abnormal intra- or extralymphatic chylous fluid collections may disrupt the function of the organ in which they reside; for example, intestinal lymphangiectasia is associated with malabsorption and protein-losing enteropathy, and pulmonary lymphangiectasia may disrupt

normal alveolar gas exchange. Lymphangiomas can compress adjacent structures such as vessels and airways and free chylous fluid can produce mass effect and compression of adjacent organs such as the lungs.

Clinical scenario

Acquired intrathoracic lymphatic abnormalities include birth trauma (disruption of the thoracic duct), surgical disruption/obstruction of lymphatics, lymphatic obstruction by superior vena cava (SVC) or innominate vein thrombosis (usually bilateral but occasionally unilateral left sided) (Fig. 22.2), pulmonary venous obstruction (Fig. 22.3), and lymphatic obstruction by a neoplasm.

Congenital lymphatic abnormalities include absent, malformed, or obstructed lymphatics, which result in focal or diffusely dilated lymphatic channels (lymphangiectasia, lymphatic malformation, and lymphatic dysplasia); these anomalies are especially associated with Turner's, Noonan's, and Down syndromes.

Lymphatic dysplasia syndrome is the term used to describe focal or diffuse soft tissue lymphedema due to malformation of major lymphatic channels. This is frequently associated with chylothorax at birth. Recurrent sinopulmonary infection and bronchiectasis occur due to associated IgG deficiency.

Lymphangiectasia refers to non-proliferative linear or cystic lymphatic dilatation that may be primary and present at birth or secondary, often accompanying lymphatic obstruction. Primary lymphangiectasia in the lungs is most often idiopathic and thought to be due to lack of normal pulmonary lymphatic regression prenatally. However, lymphangiectasia is associated with left-sided cardiac obstructive lesions such as hypoplastic left heart or obstructed pulmonary veins in approximately one-third of cases (Fig. 22.3). After correction of the cardiac obstructive lesion, lymphangiectasia may not resolve and can be a cause of ongoing respiratory symptoms. Mild or severe respiratory distress and chylous pleural effusion may accompany pulmonary lymphangiectasia, with exacerbation of symptoms in association with superimposed respiratory infection. Dilated mediastinal and perihilar lymphatic channels may simulate a mediastinal mass (Fig. 22.3).

A lymphatic malformation (aka lymphangioma) is thought to be due to focal malformation or obstruction of lymphatics with lymphatic proliferation and lymph accumulation. The lesion may be macrocystic (cystic hygroma) (Fig. 22.4) or cavernous (Fig. 22.5) depending on the density of the tissue involved. They may occur throughout the body. In the chest the most common locations are the neck, chest wall, axilla, and less commonly mediastinum and lung (Figs. 22.4, 22.5). Lymphangiomas may be present at birth or only be appreciated later and can progressively enlarge, especially with superimposed infection or hemorrhage.

Lymphangiomatosis is the term used when there are multi-focal lymphangiomas involving multiple sites and organs. Common locations are the lung, pleura, pericardium, spleen, and bone (Fig. 22.1). The combination of a soft tissue mass and/or chylothorax with bone and splenic cystic changes is very suggestive of lymphangiomatosis on imaging. Pathologically lymphangioma and lymphangiomatosis are defined as benign neoplasms with proliferating lymphatics.

Lymphangioleiomyomatosis is a benign smooth muscle proliferation obstructing veins, lymphatics, and bronchioles, seen in conjunction with tuberous sclerosis, mostly found in young adult women, with innumerable tiny thin-walled cysts within the lungs. Pneumothorax and/or pleural effusion are common features.

Respiratory distress, prominent interstitial markings (Figs. 22.2 and 22.3), complex effusion (Figs. 22.1 and 22.2), microcystic (Fig. 22.5) or macrocystic mass (Fig. 22.4), and multiorgan involvement (Fig. 22.1) are the modes of presentation of lymphatic abnormality in the chest in children.

Contrast-enhanced CT, CTA, and high-resolution thin-cut chest CT are useful in evaluating suspected pulmonary lymphatic abnormality. Lymphatic congestion or obstruction of pulmonary lymphatic drainage e.g. by a central mass is visualized on high-resolution CT (HRCT) as smoothly dilated interlobular septal lymphatics (Figs. 22.2 and 22.3) whereas spread of tumor along the lymphatics, lymphangitic carcinomatosis, produces irregular or nodular interlobular septal thickening. Chest wall, intrapulmonary, and mediastinal lymphangiomas can be seen on CT but may be difficult to differentiate from other masses. Contrast is necessary to sort out fluid versus mass versus atelectatic lung and hemangioma from lymphangioma. MR (usually including contrast enhancement) is superior in defining the location, extent, and nature of lymphatic masses, particularly with soft tissue lesions (Fig. 22.4). Both MR and US are better than CT imaging at differentiating simple from complex fluid (Fig. 22.1) and a cystic from a solid lesion although very complex organizing fluid may be quite difficult to differentiate from a cystic mass on all modalities. Since lymphatic fluid is proteinaceous, it may be echogenic on US (Fig. 22.1), dense on CT, and bright on both T1- and T2-weighted MR images, simulating blood or a solid lesion. Lymphatic lesions do not usually enhance after intravenous contrast except for the septations of macrocystic lesions or when they occur in conjunction with a vascular malformation.

Lymphangiography following webspace injection of dye followed by cannulation of a lymphatic channel and injection of Lipiodol to opacify the lymphatics has been performed for many years but is technically challenging, especially in children. There has been recent description of improved visualization of the lymphatics and thoracic duct using an US-guided technique with injection of Lipiodol into inguinal nodes. Once the thoracic duct is opacified it can be cannulated percutaneously and contrast or other agents injected into the lymphatic system for diagnostic or therapeutic purposes. Nuclear lymphoscintigraphy has been helpful in some select instances of congenital or acquired lymphatic abnormality. The agent technetium 99m albumin is injected subcutaneously, usually in several webspaces of the feet and/or hands, with serial imaging attempting to trace lymphatic drainage pathways. Anatomic definition is somewhat poor using this technique especially as the agent dissipates higher up in the abdomen or chest. There have been some recent descriptions of good anatomic definition of lymphatic channels in the legs and lower abdomen with MR imaging following webspace injection of gadolinium agents.

Management of chest lymphatic lesions varies. Frequently the exact underlying abnormality is unknown. Traumatic or iatrogenic entities, idiopathic chylothorax, and lymphangiectasia are often treated conservatively with hyperalimentation and/or a low fat, high protein, medium chain triglyceride diet to decrease lymph flow. More insidious or prolonged chylothorax may be managed by surgical, or more recently percutaneous ligation or ablation of the thoracic duct or other lymphatic ducts.

If a discrete malformation is present, management may consist of percutaneous sclerosis (for superficial lesions) or surgical removal. There is a relatively high incidence of recurrence at the same site or close by. More extensive lesions or those in critical locations may not be able to be surgically removed or sclerosed and may be treated by a variety of palliative methods including various drugs, pleurodesis, and percutaneous ablation to prevent reaccumulation of chylothorax. The more extensive or complex lesions have a tendency to gradually worsen with high long-term morbidity and mortality.

Differential diagnosis

The differential diagnosis of an opacified hemithorax is quite broad including lung consolidation or atelectasis; pleural effusion; pulmonary, pleural, or even mediastinal mass. The presence of contralateral mediastinal shift implies a space-occupying lesion such as a large pleural effusion or an underlying mass or both.

Pleural fluid may be simple and transudative (congestive heart failure, accompanying some infections, sympathetic effusion, e.g. abdominal pathology such as pancreatitis) or complex and exudative (proteinaceous fluid such as pus [empyema], blood [trauma, post-surgical] or lymph). Complex effusions tend to septate and loculate (Fig. 22.1) whereas simple effusions often remain clear and free flowing. After plain chest radiographs, US imaging is often useful to evaluate the presence, quantity, and nature of pleural fluid and rule out an underlying mass. Decubitus radiographs are not useful when there is marked or complete opacification of a hemithorax since the movement of fluid and visualization of the adjacent lung cannot be seen. CT and/or MR imaging may be used to further define the anatomy in complex cases.

Multiorgan involvement with cystic/lytic lesions and pleural effusion raises other differential diagnostic possibilities including Langerhans cell histiocytosis, hemangiomatosis, and malignancy such as lymphoma, neuroblastoma, or Ewing's sarcoma. The combination of clinical information and multi-modality imaging may be needed to help evaluate the most likely diagnostic possibilities. Imaging is often useful in defining appropriate locations for biopsy.

Teaching point

Lymphatic abnormality in the chest can present in a wide variety of ways, mimicking multiple other pathologic entities including infection, interstitial lung disease and intrapulmonary, mediastinal, pleural, or chest wall neoplasms. Lymphatic abnormalities of the chest in children include lymphatic dysplasia, lymphangiectasia, lymphatic malformation (lymphangioma), and lymphangiomatosis; these entities overlap. While these abnormalities are rare, their recognition and differentiation from other pathologic entities is important. The observant, knowledgeable radiologist may be the first person to consider lymphatic abnormality as the underlying diagnosis. As the chest, abdomen, soft tissues, and many different organs (especially spleen and bone) may be involved, careful and comprehensive evaluation is required.

REFERENCES

1. Faul JL, Berry GJ, Colby TV, *et al.* Thoracic lymphangiomas, lymphangiectasis, lymphangiomatosis, and lymphatic dysplasia syndrome. *Am J Respir Crit Care Med* 2000;**161**(3 Pt 1):1037–46.

2. Itkin M, Krishnamurthy G, Naim MY, *et al.* Percutaneous thoracic duct embolization as a treatment for intrathoracic chyle leaks in infants. *Pediatrics* 2011;**128**(1):e237–41.

3. Lohrmann C, Foeldi E, Langer M. Diffuse lymphangiomatosis with genital involvement: evaluation with magnetic resonance lymphangiography. *Urol Oncol* 2011;**29**(5):515–22.

4. Nadolski GJ, Itkin M. Feasibility of ultrasound-guided intranodal lymphangiogram for thoracic duct embolization. *J Vasc Interv Radiol* 2012;**23**(5):613–16.

5. Raman SP, Pipavath SN, Raghu G, *et al.* Imaging of thoracic lymphatic diseases. *AJR Am J Roentgenol* 2009;**193**(6):1504–13.

6. Wadsworth DT, Newman B, Abramson S, *et al.* Splenic lymphangiomatosis in children. *Radiology* 1997;**202**(1):173–6.

7. Yang DH, Goo HW. Generalized lymphangiomatosis: radiologic findings in three pediatric patients. *Korean J Radiol* 2006;**7**(4):287–91.

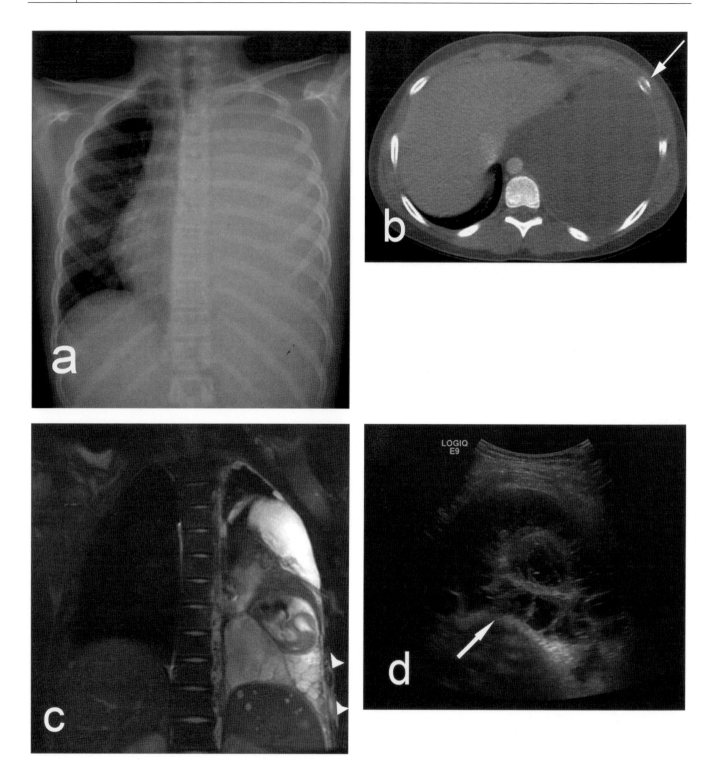

Figure 22.1. Chylothorax–10-year-old with shortness of breath. **(a)** Frontal chest radiograph with complete opacification of the left hemithorax with moderate cardiomediastinal shift to the right. **(b)** Axial slice from contrast-enhanced CT demonstrates uniform fluid density in the left lower chest as well as a subtle expansile lesion of two anterior left lower ribs (one shown – arrow). **(c)** Coronal T2-weighted MR demonstrates complex organizing fluid in the left chest, thickened pleura, multiple cysts in the spleen, and bright T2 signal in two lower left ribs (arrowheads) with surrounding increased soft tissue signal. **(d)** Transverse US of the lower left chest post partial drainage demonstrates heavily septated complex organizing fluid. A small piece of echogenic partially atelectatic lung is seen in the center (arrow).

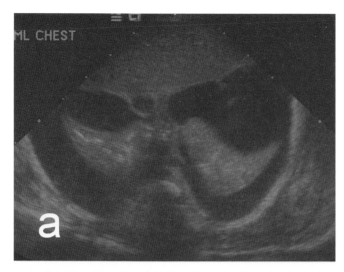

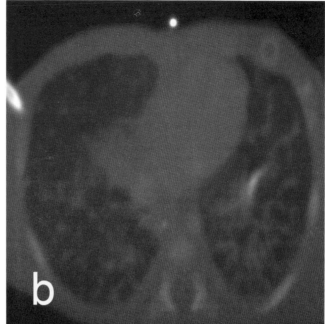

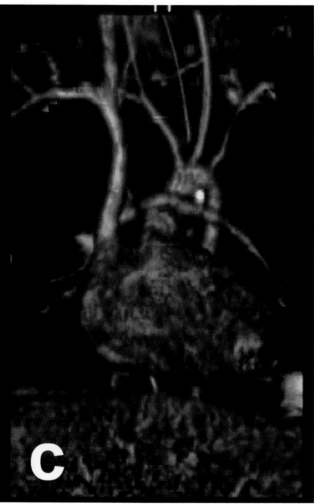

Figure 22.2. Iatrogenic lymphatic obstruction. Ex 1200 g 28 weeks' gestation infant with transposition of the great arteries post successful arterial switch at 10 days of age. Respiratory distress at 3 weeks of age with bilateral chylous pleural effusions. Normal cardiac echo. **(a)** Transverse US of lower chest demonstrates bilateral atelectatic lower lobes surrounded by prominent bilateral pleural effusions containing some echogenic debris. **(b)** Axial chest CT lung window demonstrates mediastinal widening (lymphedema) and increased bilateral pulmonary interstitial markings and interlobular septal thickening (intrapulmonary lymphangiectasia). Pleural fluid has been drained. **(c)** Volume rendered coronal reconstruction of CTA demonstrates intact right-sided upper extremity veins but complete thrombosis of the left subclavian and innominate veins related to a prior PICC line that had been located in the left innominate vein.

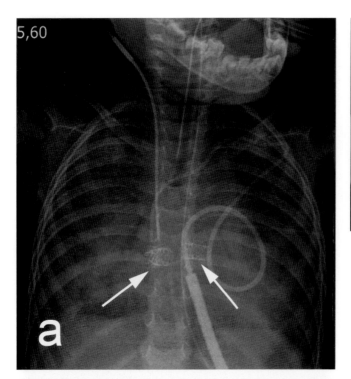

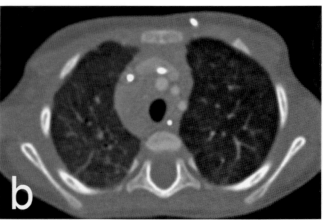

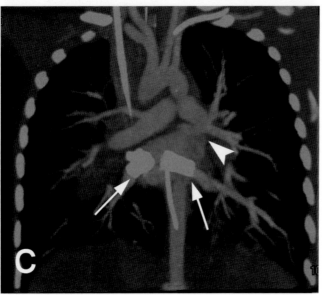

Figure 22.3. Pulmonary vein stenosis and lymphangiectasis. A two-year-old girl with congenital pulmonary venous stenosis with continued shortness of breath post multiple pulmonary vein stents. **(a)** Frontal chest radiograph demonstrates bilateral lower pulmonary vein stents (arrows). There is marked diffuse pulmonary venous congestion. **(b)** Axial CT slice demonstrates marked pulmonary ground glass opacification with some interlobular septal thickening consistent with alveolar edema and lymphatic congestion. There was unusual mediastinal widening with diffuse low-density signal. **(c)** CT coronal MIP reconstruction demonstrates diffuse mediastinal and perihilar low signal soft tissue (pathologically proven mediastinal lymphangiectasia). The lower pulmonary veins appear patent with central stents (arrows). The left upper pulmonary vein was stenotic centrally (arrowhead) and the right upper vein completely thrombosed.

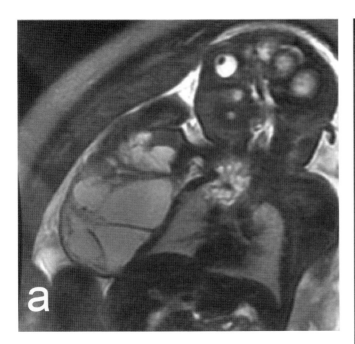
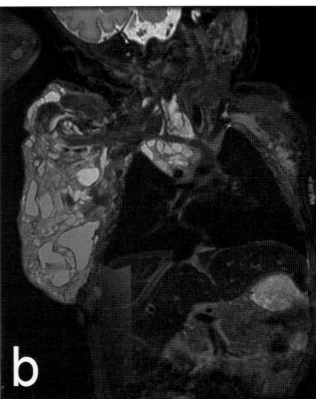

Figure 22.4. Lymphangioma chest 30 weeks' gestation prenatal coronal T2-weighted image **(a)**. Coronal T2 image at 10 days old **(b)**. Both studies show a large right multicystic chest wall mass extending into the right neck, upper pleura, and mediastinum. (Reprinted from *Radiologic Clinics of North America*, Vol. **49**(4), Newman B, Thoracic neoplasms in children, Pages 633–64, Copyright 2011, with permission from Elsevier; Figures 34a–b.)

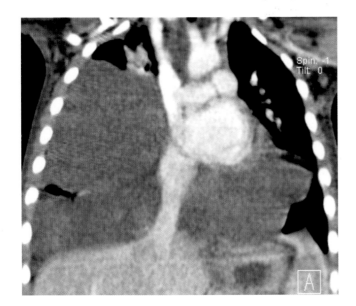

Figure 22.5. Pulmonary/mediastinal lymphangioma in a two-year-old boy. CT–coronal reconstruction demonstrates a diffuse low-density mass infiltrating the right lung and mediastinum.

Tetralogy of Fallot with pulmonary atresia

Beverley Newman

Imaging description

A routine prenatal ultrasound (US) demonstrated cardiac abnormality later determined at dedicated prenatal cardiac echo to be suggestive of tetralogy of Fallot (TOF) with severe pulmonary stenosis or atresia and a large patent ductus arteriosus (PDA). Arrangements were therefore made for delivery at a major medical center. The baby was born by normal vaginal delivery at 39 weeks' gestation and was noted to be mildly cyanotic with a soft systolic ejection murmur at the left sternal border. A frontal chest radiograph demonstrated mild cardiomegaly with a concave main pulmonary artery (PA) segment and uplifted cardiac apex (Fig. 23.1a) consistent with TOF. Pulmonary vascularity appeared normal. TOF with pulmonary valve atresia and large PDA were confirmed on postnatal echocardiography. Prostaglandin therapy to maintain patency of the ductus arteriosus had been initiated in the delivery room because of the prenatal echo findings.

A gated CT angiogram (80kVp, mean mAs 102, DLP 30, approximate effective dose 2.4mSv) was obtained at 4 days of age to further define the size and appearance of the native pulmonary vessels and systemic collateral arterial supply to the lungs. CT images including multiplanar, maximum intensity projection (MIP) and 3D volumetric reconstructions demonstrated the typical cardiac anatomy of TOF (large outlet ventricular septal defect (VSD), overriding aorta, right ventricular hypertrophy, and right ventricular outflow stenosis, in this case atresia) (Fig. 23.1b). A large tortuous PDA (5mm) was seen extending from the distal aortic arch to the proximal left PA (Fig. 23.1c). This was the only systemic arterial supply to the lungs, no additional aorticopulmonary or other collaterals were identified. The distal main PA and right and left branch PAs were normally patent (approximately 3–4mm) without stenoses (Fig. 23.1d). There was mild kinking of the proximal left PA proximal to the PDA. There was mild anomalous branching of the left-sided aortic arch with a common origin of the right brachiocephalic and left common carotid arteries and separate left subclavian artery (Fig. 23.1c). The coronary arteries appeared normal. There was moderate left upper lobe and lingular atelectasis with partial compression of the left bronchus by the PDA (not shown).

Importance

This case illustrates the important advances that have been made in pre- and perinatal care with early identification of fetal anomalies by means of screening fetal US. Once an abnormality has been identified it can be further characterized with additional prenatal imaging (US and/or MRI). This allows for counseling and preparation of the parents as well as formulation of appropriate prenatal, delivery, and postnatal care plans.

Plain chest radiographs are still usually the first imaging studies obtained postnatally in infants with suspected or known congenital heart disease, albeit followed quickly by cardiac echocardiography. While chest radiographs can be entirely normal in infants with significant congenital heart disease or depict only non-specific abnormality, there are some radiographic findings that suggest the presence and nature of the underlying cardiac anomaly. The *coeur en sabot* or boot-shaped heart typical of TOF consists of mild cardiomegaly, an uplifted cardiac apex (right ventricular hypertrophy), and concave major pulmonary artery (MPA) (obstructed pulmonary outflow). A right-sided aortic arch is also quite common, occurring in 25–30% of cases. Normal to decreased pulmonary vascularity typically accompanies TOF depending on the degree of pulmonary obstruction. Right-sided cardiac outlet obstruction is the most variable component of TOF, ranging from mild (pink TOF) to severe (blue TOF) to complete pulmonary atresia. There may be obstruction at multiple levels including the right ventricular outflow tract, pulmonary valve, main and central PAs, and peripheral PA stenoses. When pulmonary atresia is present pulmonary blood supply relies on systemic arterial collateral vessels known as major aorticopulmonary collaterals (MAPCAs) (Fig. 23.2). These most often arise from the descending aorta and are frequently multiple, irregular, or stenotic vessels that may connect with the native PAs in the lungs. They may also arise from the upper extremity arteries, aorta below the diaphragm, ductus arteriosus, or coronary artery. When systemic collaterals provide blood supply to the lungs, the appearance of the pulmonary vasculature tends to be atypical on imaging studies. There may be increased or asymmetric rather than decreased pulmonary vascularity depending on the source and size of the MAPCAs.

Echocardiography provides highly sophisticated and detailed imaging evaluation of intracardiac anatomy but may have some difficulty depicting broad details of the extracardiac vasculature including the aortic arch, MAPCAs, coronary and pulmonary arteries, as well as airways and lungs. Depending on the information required, CT, MR, or cardiac catheterization may be utilized for further evaluation. Because of relatively poor renal function in the first week of postnatal life, contrast administration is generally avoided unless absolutely necessary. As with all other imaging studies in children, attention should be paid to obtaining a diagnostically useful study at the lowest possible dose. In this case, for example, a gated cardiac study was done in order to clearly identify the detailed anatomy, course, and caliber of potentially small tortuous MAPCAs and native PAs. This CTA examination was done at 80kVp to take advantage of the known greater contrast resolution present in enhanced studies at lower kVp.

Typical clinical scenario

TOF is a conotruncal developmental anomaly in which anterior malposition of the conal septum produces uneven separation of the aorta and MPA and results in the four cardinal features: overriding aorta, pulmonary outflow obstruction, ventricular septal defect, and right ventricular hypertrophy. Additional associated anomalies may include atrial septal defect and common atrioventricular canal (especially in Down syndrome). TOF is often associated with other anomalies, including chromosomal disorders such as Down and DiGeorge syndromes. Cyanosis and early symptoms in TOF (heart murmur, dyspnea) are typically related to more severe pulmonary outflow obstruction, often accompanied by decreased pulmonary flow and right to left shunting. Milder forms of TOF may be completely asymptomatic and only discovered at a later age, because of a heart murmur or symptoms with exertion. Tetralogy of Fallot with pulmonary atresia may also be asymptomatic when pulmonary and systemic blood flows are well balanced. As with many other conditions, congenital heart lesions may be discovered by in utero US and investigated immediately after birth even if the infant has no symptoms.

Initial management of symptomatic infants with TOF used to be geared toward increasing pulmonary blood flow (a systemic to pulmonary artery shunt, most often subclavian to PA–Blalock–Taussig shunt), with later complete repair and removal of the shunt. Current management in uncomplicated cases is usually complete repair in infancy.

The surgical repair of TOF consists of VSD closure (ensuring patency of the left ventricle (LV) outflow tract) and pulmonary valvuloplasty and/or patch enlargement of the outflow tract. Patients generally do well postoperatively with the major problems being residual central or peripheral pulmonary stenoses and pulmonary regurgitation that may lead to subsequent right ventricular dysfunction. Reoperation at a later age to place a homograft or other pulmonary valve is frequently required. The timing of this is often monitored by regular echocardiography and MRI studies to evaluate right ventricular size and function and pulmonary anatomy and regurgitation.

The scenario of TOF with pulmonary atresia is often more complex. The timing and type of surgical intervention depends on the nature and source of pulmonary blood supply. When the ductus arteriosus is the major or sole collateral supply to the lungs (duct dependent) the infant may become critically ill when the ductus begins to close and prostaglandin infusion is needed to keep the duct open. This tends to be a precarious situation and early surgical intervention (a central shunt or complete repair) is usually necessary to ensure a reliable pulmonary blood supply. A large collateral from the coronary circulation may be another indication for early surgery to prevent coronary steal and ischemia. If there are adequate collateral vessels, surgical intervention may be postponed until after the immediate neonatal period. The type and timing of surgery depends on the presence and size of the native central PAs and their connections with the MAPCAs. If the native PAs are present but very hypoplastic, the initial surgery may consist of a central aorta to PA shunt to promote growth of the PAs. Ultimate surgical correction may require several steps that include closure of the VSD and unifocalization of the collaterals by ligating them (if they connect with the native PAs) or removing them from the aorta and connecting them centrally to the PAs or central graft material to fashion central PAs that connect to the right ventricle directly or via a conduit.

Differential diagnosis

The *coeur en sabot* appearance is not exclusive to TOF and can occur in other right-sided obstructive heart lesions including tricuspid atresia, pulmonary atresia with intact ventricular septum, and Ebstein's anomaly (usually marked cardiomegaly); these lesions, however, are much less common than TOF. When accompanied by pulmonic stenosis, other congenital lesions including double outlet right ventricle, transposition of the great vessels, and truncus arteriosus may also look similar to TOF. A common pitfall is the false appearance resembling an uplifted cardiac apex in a normal but lordotically positioned chest radiograph.

Another unusual variant of TOF is absence of the pulmonary valve leaflets in which severe in utero and postnatal pulmonary regurgitation produces aneurysmally dilated central PAs that may simulate a large mediastinal mass (Fig. 23.3a). These dilated vessels frequently compress the central bronchi, producing diffuse lung abnormality including areas of atelectasis and overinflation (Fig. 23.3b).

> ## Teaching point
>
> The pulmonary anatomy and blood supply in TOF is widely variable with corresponding variability in imaging appearance and requirements as well as clinical and surgical management. Correlation with other imaging studies, a thorough understanding of the clinical findings, and questions and adherence to ALARA (as low as reasonably achievable) principles should guide imaging decisions.

REFERENCES

1. Frank L, Dillman JR, Parish V, *et al.* Cardiovascular MR imaging of conotruncal anomalies. *Radiographics* 2010;**30**:1069–94.

2. Gaca AM, Jaggers JJ, Dudley LT, Bisset GS, 3rd. Repair of congenital heart disease: a primer – Part 2. *Radiology* 2008;**248**:44–60.

3. Jonas RA, DiNardo JA. *Comprehensive Surgical Management of Congenital Heart Disease*. London, England: Arnold/Oxford University Press, 2004.

4. Yoo S, Macdonald C, Babyn P. *Chest Radiographic Interpretation in Pediatric Cardiac Patients*. New York, NY: Thieme, 2010.

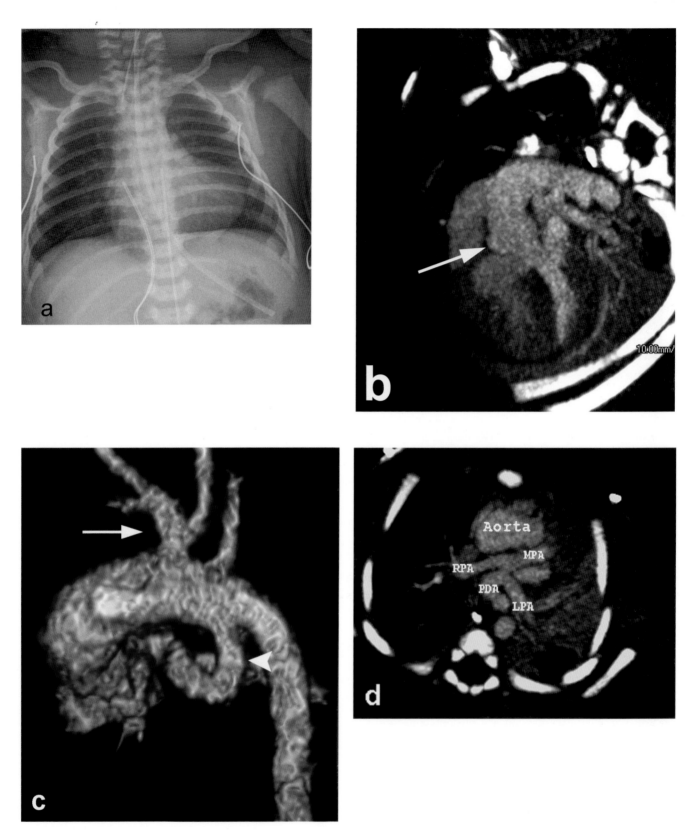

Figure 23.1. Newborn infant with TOF with pulmonary atresia. **(a)** Frontal chest radiograph demonstrates mild cardiomegaly with an uplifted cardiac apex and concave main pulmonary artery, *coeur en sabot* appearance, typical of TOF. Pulmonary vascularity is within normal limits. **(b)** CT angiogram at age four days–oblique axial MIP view of the heart demonstrates the anatomy of TOF including a large outlet VSD and enlarged overriding aorta (arrow). **(c)** CT angiogram–3D volume rendered oblique sagittal image demonstrates the dilated ascending aorta, intact arch with common origin of the right brachiocephalic and left common carotid arteries (arrow) and a large tortuous PDA arising from the distal arch (arrowhead). **(d)** CT angiogram–oblique axial MIP demonstrating the PDA connecting with the proximal left pulmonary artery (LPA). The LPA above the PDA is kinked without focal stenosis. Likewise the MPA and right pulmonary artery (RPA) are patent and normal in size, filling through the PDA. Note moderate left lung atelectasis.

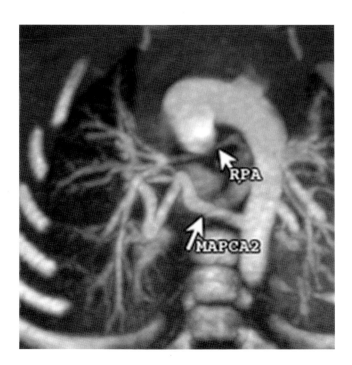

Figure 23.2. CT angiogram–TOF with pulmonary atresia and MAPCAs. Oblique coronal MIP from another newborn infant. There are multiple tortuous descending aorta MAPCAs one of which is shown here. Note the much smaller caliber of the hypoplastic (1–2 mm) native pulmonary arteries (arrow on RPA).

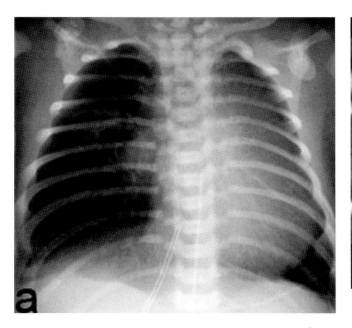

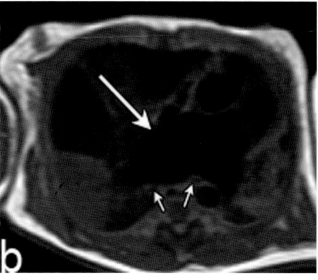

Figure 23.3. **(a)** TOF with absent pulmonary valve. Newborn infant with respiratory distress. There is marked overinflation of the right lung with leftward cardiomediastinal shift and the suggestion of a right perihilar mediastinal mass. **(b)** Axial T1-weighted MR image demonstrates aneurysmally dilated central PAs (arrow) compressing the mainstem bronchi (small arrows). There are multiple areas of atelectasis and overinflation in the lungs.

Left pulmonary artery sling

Beverley Newman

Imaging description

A six-month-old girl was evaluated by her primary care physician for noisy breathing while feeding and failure to thrive. He ordered an upper gastrointestinal study which was normal except for an anterior impression on the mid esophagus (Fig. 24.1a). A chest radiograph (Fig. 24.1b) demonstrated cardiomediastinal shift to the right with a slightly small volume right lung; the lower trachea was poorly visualized. A CT angiogram was then obtained to evaluate for vascular abnormality or mediastinal mass. On the CTA a left pulmonary artery sling (LPAS) was identified as well as a right mid tracheal diverticulum and long segment lower tracheal stenosis with a rounded configuration suggesting complete cartilaginous rings (Fig. 24.1c–e).

Importance

A LPAS occurs when the left postbranchial pulmonary vessels connect with the right instead of the left sixth branchial arch with the aberrant vessel taking a course from right to left between the trachea and esophagus to reach the left hilum (Fig. 24.1c). This course tends to produce an anterior vascular impression on the esophagus (Fig. 24.1a), separating it from the trachea, whereas the anomalous vessels in vascular rings pass posterior to both trachea and esophagus.

LPAS has been classified into two main types. In type 1, the LPAS abuts the distal trachea and right mainstem bronchus, tending to produce malacia, often with right lung air trapping. The trachea is usually normal in type 1 although a right tracheal bronchus may be present (subtype 1B). Type 2 LPAS is characterized by its almost invariable association with major airway abnormalities, including a low obliquely branching carina with the LPAS at this level and long segment tracheal or tracheobronchial stenosis, hence the term ring/sling complex. There may be a right tracheal bronchus or, as in this case, tracheal diverticulum (subtype 2A) at the normal carinal level with long segment tracheal stenosis with complete cartilaginous rings below this level (Fig. 24.1d, e). Bilateral air trapping may therefore accompany type 2 LPAS unless there is associated right lung hypoplasia or agenesis producing a smaller volume right lung (Fig. 24.1b). Precise definition of the anatomy is usually best seen on CTA. Multiplanar 2D and 3D and volumetric reconstructions are often helpful in displaying and understanding the anatomic relationships (Fig. 24.1d, e). Appropriate management addressing both the airway and vascular anomalies is essential for a good outcome.

Typical clinical scenario

LPAS often presents with respiratory symptoms or feeding difficulty in infancy that may be precipitated by acute respiratory infection. The presentation ranges from catastrophic (type 2) to mild (type 1 or 2) or even asymptomatic in older children with type 1 LPAS. In some cases symptoms from associated anomalies may predominate. Other anomalies beyond pulmonary artery, airway, and lung abnormalities are associated with LPAS; the most common are cardiovascular anomalies in 40–60% of cases, ranging from left, superior vena cava (SVC) or coarctation to Scimitar syndrome and complex congenital heart disease. Similar to vascular ring, LPAS is frequently not suspected on initial chest radiographs; careful scrutiny of the airway and lung is the key to suggesting the diagnosis.

Differential diagnosis

Recognition of narrowing, compression, displacement, or poor definition of the airway with or without air trapping on plain chest radiographs raises the question of an underlying lesion. Possibilities include a lesion intrinsic or extrinsic to the airway. Intrinsic lesions include intraluminal and extraluminal causes that encompass airway foreign body, congenital (Fig. 24.2) or acquired stenosis, and benign (papillomatosis, granuloma) or malignant neoplasm (carcinoid). Extrinsic lesions include congenital bronchopulmonary malformations (especially bronchogenic cyst or esophageal duplication cyst), vascular anomalies, esophageal lesions, lymphadenopathy (especially tuberculosis [TB]), and neoplasms (lymphoma, neuroblastoma). The presence of a hypoplastic lung, usually right-sided, brings up the possibility of pulmonary artery or vein anomalies, including absence or hypoplasia and scimitar syndrome, as well as LPAS.

Congenital tracheal stenosis may involve a short or long segment of the airway. Long segment tracheal stenosis is very strongly associated with pulmonary sling but can also occur independently (Fig. 24.2) and is typified by a narrowed, rounded trachea on imaging, suggesting complete cartilaginous rings with absence of the usually flattened posterior membranous portion of the trachea (Figs. 24.1 and 24.2).

A short segment of tracheal stenosis can usually be simply resected surgically. Relatively recent development of tracheoplasty techniques has markedly changed the previously poor prognosis for long segment airway stenosis. Management of LPAS consists of reimplantation of the LPA to the left, alone in symptomatic type 1 LPAS, and both LPA reimplantation and tracheoplasty in type 2 LPAS with associated tracheal stenosis. Other associated lesions are treated as needed on their own merit.

Teaching point

Radiologists, clinicians, and surgeons should appreciate the spectrum of presentation and imaging appearance of LPAS and its strong association with tracheal stenosis. Once the abnormality is suspected, CTA is usually the imaging study of choice to define the vascular, airway, and lung abnormalities so that appropriate management choices can be made.

REFERENCES

1. Berdon WE. Rings, slings, and other things: vascular compression of the infant trachea updated from the midcentury to the millennium – the legacy of Robert E. Gross, MD, and Edward B. D. Neuhauser, MD. *Radiology* 2000;**216**(3):624–32.

2. Chen SJ, Lee WJ, Lin MT, *et al.* Left pulmonary artery sling complex: computed tomography and hypothesis of embryogenesis. *Ann Thorac Surg* 2007;**84**(5):1645–50.

3. Fiore AC, Brown JW, Weber TR, *et al.* Surgical treatment of pulmonary artery sling and tracheal stenosis. *Ann Thorac Surg* 2005; **799**(1):38–46.

4. Loukanov TS, Sebening C, Springer W, *et al.* The evolution of the pulmonary arterial sling syndrome, with particular reference to the need for reoperations because of untreated tracheal stenosis. *Cardiol Young* 2009;**19**(5):446–50.

5. Newman B, Cho YA. Left pulmonary artery sling: anatomy and imaging. *Semin Ultrasound CT MR* 2010;**31**(2):158–70.

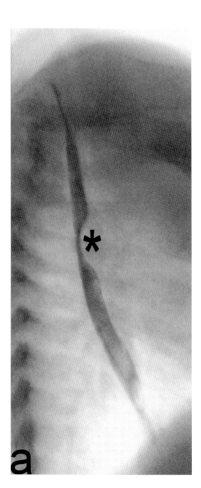
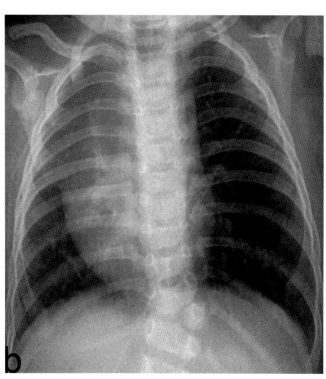

Figure 24.1. Left pulmonary artery sling. A six-month-old girl with noisy breathing with feeding and failure to thrive. **(a)** Lateral view of the esophagus on an upper gastrointestinal study demonstrates an anterior impression on the mid esophageal contrast column (asterisk). **(b)** Frontal chest radiograph with small volume right lung and cardiomediastinal shift to the right. The lower trachea is poorly visualized.

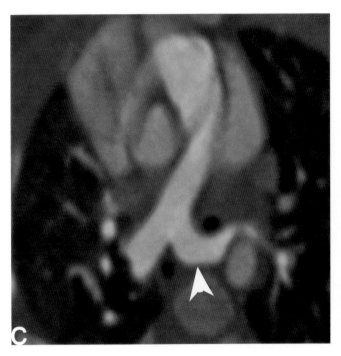

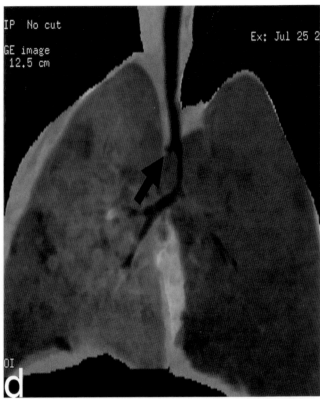

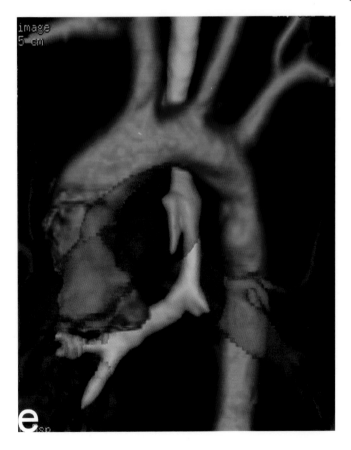

Figure 24.1. (cont.) **(c)** CT angiogram, axial maximum intensity projection (MIP) reconstruction demonstrates anomalous origin of the left pulmonary artery from the right pulmonary artery forming a pulmonary sling (arrowhead) that passes between the trachea anteriorly (note small caliber and rounded configuration) and the esophagus posteriorly to get to the left side. **(d)** CT coronal minimum intensity projection (MINIP) reconstruction of the airway demonstrates a right tracheal diverticulum (abortive tracheal bronchus) at T4 (normal level of the carina) (arrow) with long segment tracheal narrowing from this point to the inferiorly located oblique angled carina. The left bronchus is not well seen due to probable intraluminal mucus. **(e)** CT angiogram oblique sagittal volumetric reconstruction of the great vessels (aorta, red; pulmonary arteries, blue) and airway (white) demonstrates the anatomic relationships, with right tracheal diverticulum and low LPAS passing to the left behind the carina. (Figures 24.1a–d: Reprinted from *Seminars in Ultrasound, CT, and MR*, Vol. **31**(2), Newman B, Cho Ya, Left pulmonary artery sling—anatomy and imaging, Pages 158–70, Copyright 2010, with permission from Elsevier.)

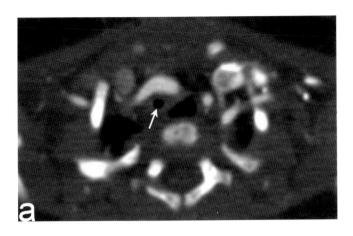

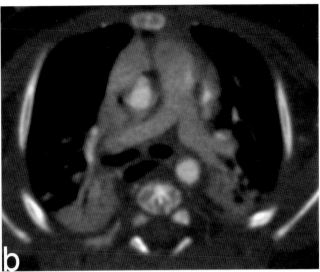

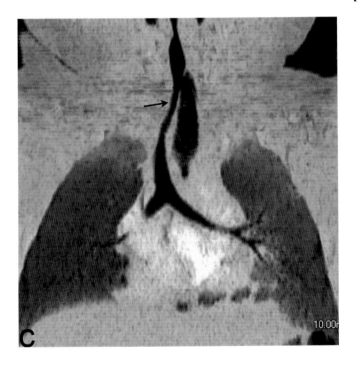

Figure 24.2. A three-month-old with intermittent stridor. Isolated congenital tracheal stenosis. **(a)** CT angiogram axial slice at the thoracic inlet demonstrates a very small rounded trachea (not compressed by the anteriorly crossing innominate artery). The configuration suggests congenital tracheal stenosis with complete cartilagenous rings – this was confirmed at bronchoscopy. **(b)** CT angiogram axial slice, midthoracic demonstrates normal appearance of the right and left pulmonary arteries and no evidence of LPAS. **(c)** CT coronal MINIP reconstruction of the airway demonstrates stenosis of the midtrachea (arrow) with normal upper and lower tracheal caliber.

25 Vascular ring

Beverley Newman

Imaging description

A 16-month-old girl presented to the emergency room with fever and shortness of breath and was wheezing with mild hypoxemia on examination. Her mother offered a history of noisy breathing since birth and repeated episodes of wheezing and respiratory infection. The chest radiographs were interpreted as normal in the emergency room; the infant was admitted to the hospital for probable viral upper respiratory infection. The radiologist called the next morning to report that the chest radiographs demonstrated abnormality of the intrathoracic airway including a right-sided impression on the trachea, possibly representing a right aortic arch (Fig. 25.1a) as well as narrowing and anterior bowing (Fig. 25.1b) of the lower trachea. The appearance raised the question of a vascular ring with tracheal compression.

A CT angiogram was obtained which demonstrated a vascular ring consisting of a double aortic arch variant with atresia of the distal left arch adjacent to a Kommerel diverticulum (Fig. 25.1c–e). The right arch was larger than the left with the descending aorta in the midline. The vascular ring encircled the trachea and esophagus with marked compression of the lower trachea at the site of the vascular abnormality.

Importance

It is essential to include careful evaluation of the airway in the overall assessment of plain chest radiographs. The presence of a right-side aortic arch (often best appreciated by leftward deviation of the airway at the level of the arch) and anterior bowing and narrowing of the lower trachea on the lateral view are the most frequent radiographic clues suggesting the presence of a vascular ring.

Although an esophagram was commonly ordered in the past to assess for the possibility of a vascular ring, it is now infrequently obtained for this indication since the images can suggest the presence of a vascular ring but are non-specific as to the exact anatomy. CT or MR angiography are now the examinations of choice for defining the anatomy when a vascular ring is suspected. The images are typically evaluated in multiple planes with maximum and minimum intensity and 3D volumetric reconstructions common (Figs. 25.1 and 25.2). The major anatomic details that need to be reported can be remembered as an ABCD format as follows: A = Aortic arch location; B = Branching pattern of arch; C = Compression of airway; D = Diverticulum of Kommerell and Descending aorta.

Typical clinical scenario

Underlying vascular abnormalities such as a vascular ring or sling frequently present clinically as repeated episodes of respiratory distress or infection in infancy and are often overlooked on chest radiographs. The presence and severity of symptoms vary with the degree of tracheal compression and a loose ring may be asymptomatic. These vascular anomalies encircle the trachea and esophagus and may occasionally produce dysphagia rather than respiratory symptoms, especially in older children.

The most symptomatic vascular ring in infancy is a double aortic arch (persistence of early fetal anatomy) where the ascending and descending aorta and bilateral arches that give rise to ipsilateral separate carotid and subclavian arteries tightly encircle the airway and esophagus. A fairly common variant of double aortic arch is a double arch with left coarctation or atresia of the distal left arch (Fig. 25.1). In this situation there is a short residual ligamentous connection between the patent left arch and the diverticular remnant of the distal left arch (Kommerell diverticulum) connected to the descending aorta. There is usually a ductal ligament present also.

Right aortic arch with aberrant left subclavian artery is the most commonly occurring type of vascular ring but tends to be a relatively loose ring and may be asymptomatic. The encircling vessels include the left common carotid artery anteriorly, aortic arch to the right and sometimes posteriorly when there is a circumflex posterior arch that sweeps from right to left (Fig. 25.2), the diverticulum of Kommerell posteriorly (remnant of dorsal left arch) extending to the left and giving rise to the aberrant left subclavian artery as well as the ligamentum arteriosum which complete the left side of the ring (Fig. 25.2). There are other rings that occur uncommonly including left arch with aberrant right subclavian and right Kommerell diverticulum and ductal ligament as well as occasional vascular rings associated with a mirror image right arch, left Kommerell diverticulum, and ductal ligament. Much more commonly a mirror image right arch is associated with congenital heart diseases such as tetralogy of Fallot and truncus arteriosus without a ring. Vascular rings infrequently occur in association with other congenital abnormalities, including aortic coarctation (Fig. 25.2), congenital heart disease, and pulmonary abnormalities such as hypoplasia or agenesis.

The surgical approach to vascular rings varies with the exact anatomy and is generally intended to break the encircling ring of vessels and relieve tracheoesophageal compression. This most often entails a left thoracotomy with division of the smaller left arch and ligamentum arteriosum (double aortic arch) or just the ligamentum (right arch with aberrant left subclavian). When anatomy is more complex, other surgical approaches may be needed. For example in the case illustrated in Fig. 25.2, with a circumflex right arch, coarctation with hypoplastic distal arch, and left descending aorta, surgery consisted of ligating the hypoplastic right arch and forming a left arch from the Kommerell diverticulum and proximal left subclavian artery and reimplanting the left subclavian artery to the left common carotid artery.

Differential diagnosis

Differential considerations include other vascular abnormalities that can compress the airway including pulmonary sling and innominate artery syndrome as well as abnormally positioned or enlarged vessels (such as a malpositioned aortic arch in meso- or dextrocardia and right pulmonary hypoplasia or agenesis as well as an enlarged aorta in congenital anomalies such as tetralogy of Fallot or truncus arteriosus). Middle mediastinal masses such as benign or malignant adenopathy, foregut duplication cyst, and esophageal lesions can also produce chronic airway compressive symptoms. Large anterior or posterior mediastinal masses such as lymphoma or neuroblastoma can also displace and compress the airway. Intrinsic airway abnormalities such as malacia, stenosis, bronchospasm, and endobronchial masses may also enter into the differential diagnosis.

Teaching point

An underlying vascular abnormality such as a vascular ring may be responsible for acute or recurrent respiratory symptoms. Careful scrutiny of plain chest radiographs may suggest a possible underlying abnormality that can be further defined by detailed cross-sectional angiographic studies. The major plain radiographic findings that suggest a possible vascular ring are leftward deviation of the trachea by a right-sided aortic arch on the frontal radiograph and anterior tracheal bowing on the lateral radiograph.

REFERENCES

1. Berdon WE. Rings, slings, and other things: Vascular compression of the infant trachea updated from the mid century to the millennium – the legacy of Robert E. Gross, MD, and Edward B. D. Neuhauser, MD. *Radiology* 2000;**216**(3):624–32.

2. Eichhorn J, Fink C, Delorme S, Ulmer H. Rings, slings and other vascular abnormalities. Ultra fast computed tomography and magnetic resonance angiography in pediatric cardiology. *Z Kardiol* 2004;**93**:201–8.

3. Hernanz-Schulman M. Vascular rings: a practical approach to imaging diagnosis. *Pediatr Radiol* 2005;**35**:961–79.

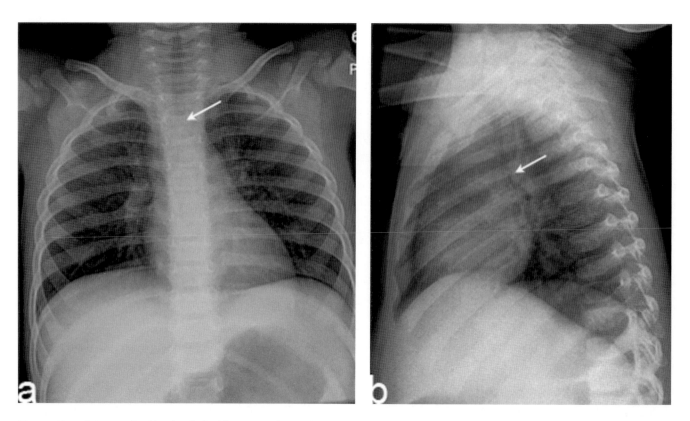

Figure 25.1. A 16-month-old girl with double aortic arch vascular ring and recurrent respiratory distress. **(a)** Frontal chest radiograph with clear, normally aerated lungs. Note the good definition of the upper trachea with loss of definition of the lower trachea. There is a suggestion of tracheal deviation to the left at this level (arrow), suggesting a right-sided aortic arch. **(b)** The lateral chest radiograph demonstrates narrowing and marked anterior bowing of the lower trachea (arrow).

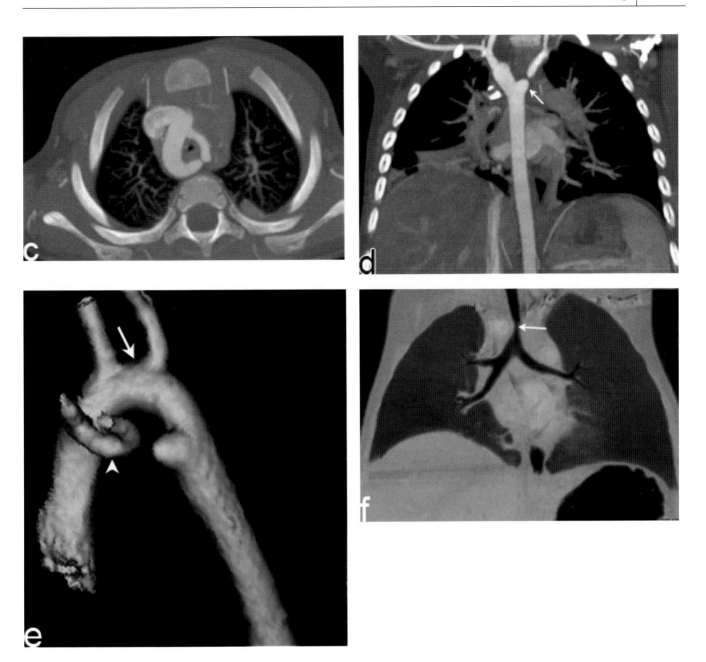

Figure 25.1. (cont.) **(c)** Axial MIP reconstruction from a CT angiogram demonstrating a double aortic arch with distal left arch atresia (ligamentous continuity). The right arch is larger than the left and there is a markedly narrowed and anteriorly displaced airway encircled by the vessels. **(d)** Coronal MIP reconstruction. Note the larger right arch connecting posteriorly to a distal remnant of the dorsal left arch (diverticulum of Kommerell) (arrow). The left arch is atretic posteriorly between the diverticulum and remaining left arch. The descending aorta is midline. **(e)** Oblique sagittal 3D volumetric reconstruction of the aorta demonstrates the larger right (arrow) and smaller left (arrowhead) aortic arches. The branching pattern is typical, with separate ipsilateral carotid and subclavian arteries arising from each arch. Note again the atretic distal left arch. **(f)** Coronal minimum intensity projection (MINIP) of the airway demonstrates marked narrowing of the distal trachea (arrow) (corresponds well with the plain film).

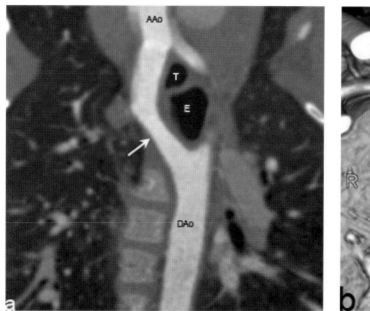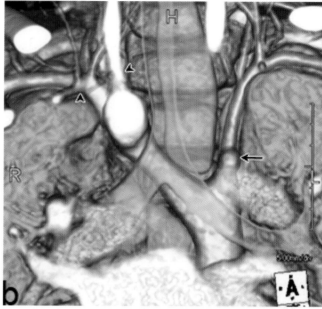

Figure 25.2. A two and a half-year-old girl with a heart murmur and decreased lower extremity pulses. **(a)** CT angiography demonstrated a circumflex right aortic arch with distal arch hypoplasia (arrow) and a vascular ring. This curved planar reconstruction demonstrates the components of the loose vascular ring encircling the trachea (T) and esophagus (E). The left carotid artery forms the anterior vascular component, with the right arch to the right and circumflex posterior and left sweep of the arch and a small Kommerell diverticulum (dorsal left arch remnant) forming the posterior components of the ring. The ring is relatively open on the left side where it is completed by a ligamentum arteriosum (not visible). Note the right-sided ascending (AAo) and left-sided descending aorta (DAo). **(b)** Coronal 3D volumetric slab reconstruction demonstrates the right aortic arch and branching pattern. The first most ventral branch (left carotid artery) is not seen. The subsequent branches off the arch are the right carotid and right subclavian arteries (arrowheads). The aberrant left subclavian artery is the last and most dorsal branch that arises from the left Komerell diverticulum (arrow). The trachea is only mildly narrowed at the level of the right arch.

26 Scimitar syndrome

Rakhee Gawande and Beverley Newman

Imaging description

A full-term neonate developed respiratory distress at birth. There was a history of in utero diagnosis of complex heart disease including hypoplastic left heart as well as a hypoplastic right lung. The chest radiograph at birth (Fig. 26.1a) demonstrated decreased volume of the right lung with dextroposition of the heart. Echocardiography demonstrated a large atrial septal defect (ASD), hypoplastic left heart, and large patent ductus arteriosus (PDA). CT angiography of the chest on day 2 of life demonstrated findings consistent with scimitar syndrome, including abnormal pulmonary venous drainage of the right lung into the inferior vena cava (IVC) via a scimitar vein in the right lower lung (Fig. 26.1b). In addition a small right pulmonary artery was noted with the hypoplastic right lung (Fig. 26.1c). There was also evidence of a right lower lobe horseshoe lung extending posteriorly across the midline behind the IVC to interface with the left lung (Fig. 26.1b). This received arterial supply from an aberrant proximal right pulmonary artery branch (Fig. 26.1c). Venous drainage and airway bronchial branches of this segment were also on the right side (not shown). Dextroposition of the heart was noted along with a hypoplastic left ventricle and large ASD (not shown). Also seen was a large PDA and juxtaductal coarctation of the aorta as well as a left-sided superior vena cava (SVC) draining to the coronary sinus (Fig. 26.1d, e).

Prenatal MR examination had demonstrated right lung hypoplasia, dextroposition of the heart and horseshoe lung (Fig. 26.1f). The vascular anomalies were not defined on the prenatal MR.

Importance

Scimitar syndrome is a rare complex form of partial anomalous pulmonary venous return, in which right-sided pulmonary veins drain to an anomalous vein that descends towards the diaphragm in a vertical crescentic shape (scimitar) and typically drains into the IVC (Figs. 26.1b and 26.2). In two-thirds of the cases the vein provides drainage for the entire right lung and in one-third the lower half of the right lung. The term scimitar syndrome is derived from the curved sword-like shadow created by this anomalous scimitar vein on a chest radiograph (Fig. 26.2a). This typical scimitar sign may not be seen radiographically, especially during infancy. The pathogenesis of this syndrome is unclear, but may be related to a developmental disorder of the lung bud during embryogenesis. Scimitar syndrome rarely presents as an isolated abnormality. The major features of scimitar syndrome are anomalous right pulmonary venous drainage, right lung hypoplasia, dextroposition of the heart, and hypoplastic or absent right pulmonary artery. Other commonly associated features include ASD (40% overall, 80–90% with infantile form) and systemic arterial supply to the right lower lobe from the abdominal aorta (60%) (Fig. 26.2b). Less frequent associations include pulmonary sequestration, pulmonary vein stenosis, hypoplastic or absent bronchi, abnormal lung segmentation, horseshoe lung, eventration of the diaphragm, diaphragmatic hernia, and persistent left SVC. Other associated congenital cardiovascular abnormalities may include ventricular septal defect, coarctation of the aorta, other abnormalities of the aortic arch, and abnormal relationships of pulmonary arteries and bronchi including pulmonary sling. Scimitar syndrome almost always affects the right lung, very occasionally occurring on the left.

Horseshoe lung is a rare congenital malformation, where the posterior basal segments of the lungs fuse behind the pericardial reflection, as seen in this patient. There may be direct lung fusion or separation by a fissure. The arterial and bronchial supply of the ishthmic part is invariably from the hypoplastic lung, also seen in this patient. About 80–85% of horseshoe lungs are associated with scimitar syndrome.

Prenatal ultrasound finding of this syndrome may include dextrocardia with normal situs, polyhydramnios, and narrowing of the pulmonary artery. In the prenatal period abnormal pulmonary veins may be difficult to detect. Scimitar syndrome may be suspected postnatally based on chest radiographs and echocardiography although the anomalous vein may not be appreciated. CT or MR angiography can non-invasively detect the aberrant vascular structures and define the exact anatomy, aiding in medical and surgical decision making and frequently obviating the need for catheter-based angiography (Figs. 26.1 and 26.2).

Typical clinical scenario

The infantile form of scimitar syndrome usually presents within two months of life with tachypnea, recurrent pneumonia, failure to thrive, pulmonary hypertension, and heart failure. This tends to be a more severe form of scimitar syndrome with a poor prognosis associated with major cardiac lesions, large left to right shunt, pulmonary venous obstruction, and pulmonary hypertension. Scimitar syndrome diagnosed later in childhood or even adulthood is often asymptomatic and discovered incidentally although symptoms may be present including recurrent infection, dyspnea, pulmonary hypertension, and hemoptysis.

Management of scimitar syndrome includes surgical correction of intra- and extracardiac anomalies as appropriate. Systemic arterial vessels to the right lung are usually embolized or ligated, especially when they are large. Surgical techniques have improved for redirecting the anomalous pulmonary venous drainage to the left atrium although post-operative pulmonary venous obstruction or occlusion is still problematic.

Differential diagnosis

Lung asymmetry with cardiac dextroposition (not dextrocardia) on a chest radiograph raises several diagnostic possibilities. It is important to evaluate whether the heart is pushed to the right by left-sided pathology such as a pneumothorax, pleural effusion, or mass or pulled across to the right side because of ipsilateral volume loss which might include right lung atelectasis, hypoplasia, or even agenesis. Unilateral pulmonary hypoplasia is most often right-sided and while it can be an isolated finding, it is frequently associated with underlying vascular abnormality, including absent right pulmonary artery or vein, pulmonary sling, and scimitar syndrome.

Teaching point

The presence of respiratory distress, small volume right lung, and dextroposition of the heart should alert the radiologist to the possibility of scimitar syndrome. The scimitar vein may not be visible on plain chest radiographs, especially in infants.

CT or MR angiography can non-invasively detect the complex vascular and lung abnormalities associated with scimitar syndrome and aid in the clinical and surgical management.

REFERENCES

1. Biyyam DR, Chapman T, Ferguson MR, Deutsch G, Dighe MK. Congenital lung abnormalities: embryologic features, prenatal diagnosis, and post-natal radiologic-pathologic correlation. *Radiographics* 2010;**30**(6):1721–38. Review.

2. Korkmaz AA, Yildiz CE, Onan B, *et al.* Scimitar syndrome: a complex form of anomalous pulmonary venous return. *J Card Surg* 2011;**26**:529–34.

3. Midyat L, Demir E, Aşkin M, *et al.* Eponym. Scimitar syndrome. *Eur J Pediatr* 2010;**169**(10):1171–7.

4. Newman B. Congenital bronchopulmonary foregut malformations: concepts and controversies. *Pediatr Radiol* 2006;**36**:773–91.

5. Oguz B, Alan S, Ozcelik U, Haliloglu M. Horseshoe lung associated with left-lung hypoplasia, left pulmonary artery sling and bilateral agenesis of upper lobe bronchi. *Pediatr Radiol* 2009;**39**(9):1002–5.

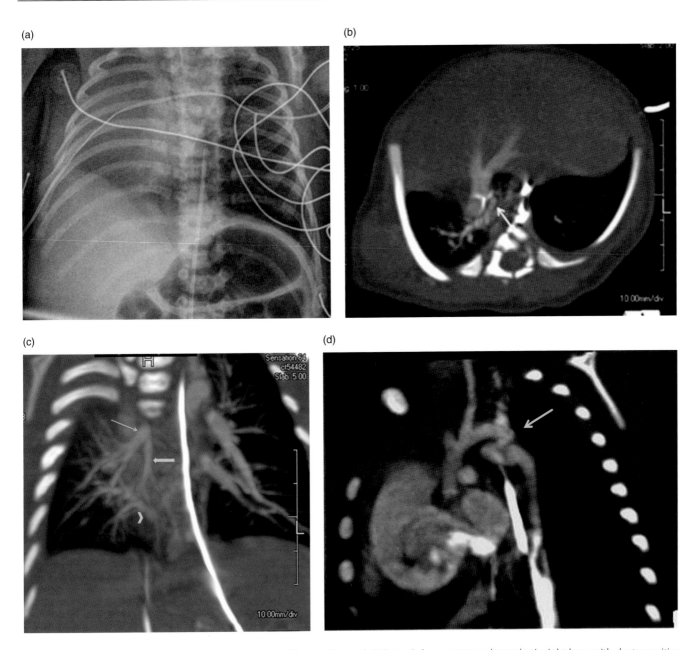

Figure 26.1. **(a)** Newborn infant with scimitar syndrome. Chest radiograph (AP view) demonstrates a hypoplastic right lung with dextroposition of the heart. Note some aerated lung overlying the vertebral column (horseshoe lung). **(b)** CT angiography of the chest (reformatted maximum intensity projection [MIP] axial image) demonstrates an anomalous vessel in the right lower lobe (arrow), draining into the medial IVC above the diaphragm (scimitar vein). Note the horseshoe segment of lung (partially atelectatic) extending behind the IVC and in front of the vertebra to interface with the left lung. **(c)** CT angiography of the chest (coronal MIP reformatted image) demonstrates a small right pulmonary artery (thin arrow) and right lung hypoplasia. A portion of the scimitar vein is visible inferiorly (arrowhead). Note a proximal right pulmonary artery branch extending inferomedially to supply the horseshoe lung (thick arrow). **(d, e)** CT angiography of the chest (oblique sagittal and coronal MIP reformats) demonstrates a large PDA and juxtaductal coarctation (d, arrow) and a left-sided SVC (e, arrow) draining to the coronary sinus. Note that all the dense contrast injected on the left drains to the left SVC, indicating absence of a left bridging innominate vein. **(f)** Fetal MRI (axial single shot fast spin echo [SSFSE]) clearly demonstrates the right lung hypoplasia, dextroposition of the heart, and right posterior horseshoe lung (arrow).

(e)

(f)

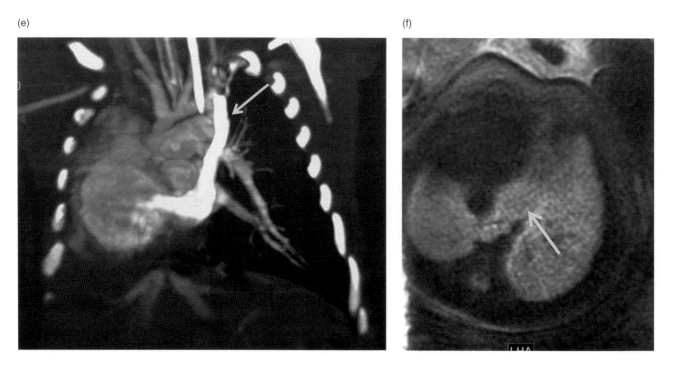

Figure 26.1. (cont.)

(a)

(b)

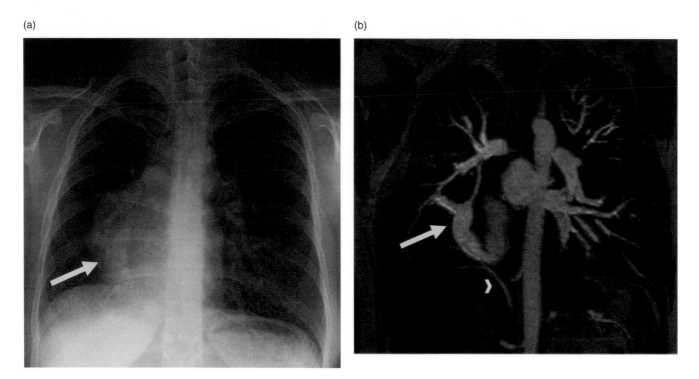

Figure 26.2. (a, b) Radiograph of the chest (PA view, a) of an adolescent with scimitar syndrome demonstrates an abnormal branching curvilinear radio-opacity in the right lower hemithorax [(a) arrow] suggestive of a scimitar vein. The right lung appears hypoplastic with dextroposition of the heart. MR angiogram [coronal reformatted MIP images, (b)] of the same patient demonstrates a small right lung and small right main pulmonary artery with paucity of pulmonary arterial branches on the right. An anomalous pulmonary vein is noted in the inferior right hemithorax, draining to the IVC, suggestive of a scimitar vein [(b) arrow]. In addition, a small systemic artery is noted arising from the subdiaphragmatic aorta (b, arrowhead), supplying the right lower lobe.

Portosystemic shunt and portopulmonary syndrome

Beverley Newman

Imaging description

An 18-month-old girl had persistent shortness of breath and progressive hypoxemia. She had a complicated prior history of liver transplantation at the age of 9 months for biliary atresia accompanying left isomerism with polysplenia. She had had absence of the intrahepatic inferior vena cava (IVC) with azygos continuation, as well as absence of the intrahepatic portal vein. Her current liver function was good; she had undergone prior closure of an atrial septal defect (ASD) but had no other evidence of congenital heart disease.

The frontal chest radiograph (Fig. 27.1a) demonstrated elevation of the right hemidiaphragm (known paralysis), external pacing wires (known heart block), and a nasogatric tube in place (difficulty feeding because of shortness of breath). Sternotomy wires and multiple right upper quadrant clips were present from the prior surgeries. There was no focal abnormality but non-specific prominence of the cardiac silhouette and pulmonary vessels (right side partly obscured by pacemaker), suggestive of shunt vascularity.

A cardiac echo showed no evidence of an intracardiac shunt but a saline bubble study was positive, with appearance of air bubbles after intravenous injection first in the right atrium (normal) and after a few beats in the left atrium (abnormal). The delayed appearance of bubbles in the left atrium suggested intrapulmonary rather than intracardiac shunting.

A CT angiogram of the chest and abdomen was obtained (Fig. 27.1b–d) to evaluate pulmonary and hepatic vessels and assess the possibility of an extracardiac shunt. This demonstrated diffuse prominence of pulmonary vasculature (Fig. 27.1b), polysplenia and large splenic and superior mesenteric veins with a small portal vein (Fig. 27.1c), and a large left splenorenal shunt draining to the hemiazygos vein (Fig. 27.1d). The diagnosis of a congenital extrahepatic portosystemic shunt with portopulmonary syndrome and diffuse intrapulmonary arteriovenous shunting was suggested. The same large left splenorenal shunt in association with polysplenia, absent IVC with azygos and hemiazygos continuation as well as absence of the portal vein (Abernethy malformation type I) and gallbladder (bilary atresia) had been noted on MRI at eight days of age (Fig. 27.1e). The hemiazygos vein joined the azygos in the lower chest (Fig. 27.1e). The splenorenal shunt had not been closed at the time of liver transplantation and was forgotten as a potential source of pulmonary symptoms.

A pulmonary perfusion scan, using technetium macroaggregated albumin, was obtained to verify and quantify intrapulmonary shunting (Fig. 27.1f). This showed moderate abnormal uptake in the brain and abdominal viscera

(Fig. 27.1f). Normally almost all of the particles are trapped in the lungs, unless there is intra- or extracardiac shunting that allows blood to bypass the lung capillaries. Right to left shunt was calculated at 39% (normal = 7%).

The child underwent percutaneous closure of the portosystemic shunt which was followed by a dramatic improvement in oxygen saturation and respiratory symptoms and resolution of cardiomegaly with normalization of pulmonary vasculature on the chest radiograph (Fig. 27.1g). A repeat CTA demonstrated a closure device between the splenic vein and superior mesenteric vein (SMV) with much decreased size of the splenic vein and increased caliber of the portal vein (Fig. 27.1h). Although the splenorenal shunt itself remained, superior mesenteric blood was now directed to the portal vein and liver.

Importance

Recognition of hepatopulmonary or portopulmonary syndrome causing pulmonary arteriovenous shunting, hypoxemia, and pulmonary hypertension is often overlooked, with consequent significant morbidity and even mortality.

Hepatopulmonary syndrome is not uncommon in association with parenchymal liver dysfunction, often but not invariably in association with portal hypertension and the formation of spontaneous, acquired extrahepatic portosystemic shunts that route splenomesenteric flow away from the liver. Portopulmonary syndrome occurs in association with a congenital portosystemic shunt in the absence of liver dysfunction. The exact cause of hepato/portopulmonary syndrome has not been elucidated. However, it appears that when mesenteric blood bypasses the liver some "factor" is missing such that there is an abnormal balance between pulmonary vasodilators and constrictors producing diffuse pulmonary arteriolar/capillary dilatation with arteriovenous shunting and eventually actual small discrete arteriovenous shunts.

This problem is largely reversible with redirection of mesenteric venous blood through the liver before reaching the pulmonary circulation. When it is feasible, and the portal vein and hepatic veins are intact, closure of the shunt either surgically or percutaneously is effective (Fig. 27.1). However, when the portal vein is absent or very small, liver transplantation is the only option for restoring normal mesenteroportal flow. However, liver transplantation alone is not sufficient in the case of a large congenital extrahepatic portosystemic shunt which often will not close spontaneously, unlike the smaller acquired shunts, and will continue to divert flow away from the liver (as in this case) until specifically occluded.

Typical clinical scenario

Portopulmonary syndrome is manifested clinically, in infancy or beyond, by otherwise unexplained respiratory symptoms, progressive hypoxia, and pulmonary hypertension. Congenital portosystemic shunts may be extrahepatic (Abernethy malformation) associated with (type I) or without (type II) absence of the portal vein (Fig. 27.1) or intrahepatic (patent ductus venosus) (Fig. 27.2), other portal to IVC or hepatic vein shunts, or chronic IVC or hepatic vein obstruction with collaterals. There are two major clinical consequences that may follow diversion of mesenteric venous blood away from the liver; these are hepatic encephalopathy (hyperammonemia) and/or hepato/portopulmonary syndrome. They may be present concurrently, or one or the other may predominate in an individual patient.

While a congenital portosystemic shunt may be an isolated phenomenon, there is a propensity for extrahepatic portosystemic shunts (especially splenorenal) to occur in the setting of heterotaxy with left isomerism. Left isomerism is associated with a large variety of cardiovascular and abdominal abnormalities. Cardiovascular anomalies are varied including absent intrahepatic cava with azygos continuation (almost invariably), left atrial and bronchial isomerism, intracardiac shunts and/or complex congenital heart disease, and anomalous pulmonary venous drainage. Abdominal associations include polysplenia, abnormal abdominal situs, biliary atresia, intestinal malrotation, and Abernethy malformation. It is not uncommon for severe or acute cardiac (complex heart disease or large shunt) or abdominal problems (biliary atresia, midgut volvulus) to overshadow less acute problems such as the presence of a portosystemic shunt.

Differential diagnosis

There are many causes of hypoxemia in children. While cardiac and chronic pulmonary conditions are the most common culprits, extrathoracic lesions must also be considered. There are only a few clinical entities that are associated with intrapulmonary arteriovenous shunting. These include hepatopulmonary or portopulmonary syndrome as outlined above, as well as superior cavopulmonary shunts, and pulmonary arteriovenous malformations.

A similar mechanism to hepatopulmonary syndrome is thought to occur in cardiac patients with a single ventricle repair and superior cavopulmonary shunt where a bidirectional Glen anastomosis shunts SVC blood directly to the pulmonary arteries. Lower extremity and mesenteric blood flow are largely excluded from the pulmonary circulation. This results in development of diffuse pulmonary arteriovenous shunting. The problem is correctable by placement of a Fontan conduit (IVC including hepatic veins to pulmonary artery) that restores mesenteric flow via the liver into the pulmonary circulation.

Single or multiple, large or small arteriovenous malformations (AVMs) may be present in the lungs, most often on a congenital basis in association with hereditary hemorrhagic telangiectasia (HHT–Osler–Rendu–Weber syndrome); several genetic mutations have been identified. Although these AVMs are thought to be present at birth, they often do not manifest clinically until they enlarge in late childhood or adulthood. Respiratory-related symptoms include hypoxemia, murmur or bruit, and pulmonary osteoarthropathy. There are frequently AVMs in other organs, including skin, mucous membranes, liver, and gastrointestinal tract. Another entity that can affect multiple organs (especially skin and liver but also lung) and produce arteriovenous shunting is infantile hemangiomatosis (Fig. 27.3). These high flow vascular lesions tend to enlarge in infancy and then spontaneously regress after 1–2 years.

Similar to portopulmonary syndrome, both HHT and pulmonary hemangiomatosis can also demonstrate pulmonary arteriovenous shunting with hypoxemia somewhat responsive to oxygen, a positive ultrasound bubble test, and evidence of right to left shunting on a lung perfusion scan. Large pulmonary AVMs may be visible on a plain chest radiograph but multiple small ones may be invisible or have non-specific findings such as cardiomegaly and shunt vascularity. CTA may be helpful in delineating the discreet pulmonary AVMs that are typical of HHT or hemangiomatosis (Fig. 27.3), versus the diffuse capillary dilatation seen in hepato/porto-pulmonary syndrome (Fig. 27.1), although peripheral pulmonary vessels are better delineated on conventional catheter angiography. Further differentiation is based on the presence of liver disease and/or delineation of portosystemic shunting.

The presence of cardiomegaly and prominent pulmonary vascularity in an infant (with or without features of congestion) conjures up a large differential diagnosis. Possibilities include intracardiac left to right shunts such as ASD, ventricular septal defect (VSD), patent ductus arteriosus (PDA), and common AV canal. These often become clinically symptomatic and radiographically manifest beyond 4–6 weeks of age when pulmonary vascular resistance has dropped and allows increased left to right shunting. The presence of cyanosis adds additional differential diagnostic entities such as admixture lesions including truncus arteriosus, transposition of the great arteries, and partial or total anomalous pulmonary venous return. Other diagnostic considerations include causes of congestive heart failure such as hypoplastic left heart, critical aortic stenosis, interrupted aortic arch, myocarditis, and infantile cardiomyopathies (such as anomalous coronary artery with ischemia and glycogen storage disease). In the absence of an intracardiac anomaly, extracardiac abnormalities should also be considered, including large arteriovenous shunts such as vein of Galen aneurysm and infantile liver hemangioma producing cardiomegaly and congestion.

In addition to pulmonary arteriovenous shunting, other chronic pulmonary conditions should also be considered in the context of hypoxemia and pulmonary hypertension. These include bronchopulmonary dysplasia, chronic interstitial lung disease, cystic fibrosis, bronchiolitis obliterans, lymphangiectasia, and pulmonary venous stenosis or veno-occlusive disease.

Teaching point

Chronic liver disease is increasingly recognized as being associated with hypoxia and pulmonary arteriovenous shunting (hepatopulmonary syndrome). Less well recognized is portopulmonary syndrome, pulmonary arteriovenous shunting in the absence of liver disease related to intra- or extrahepatic congenital portosystemic shunts. Extrahepatic congenital portosystemic shunts or Abernethy malformations have a particular association with heterotaxy with left isomerism and polysplenia. Failure to recognize this entity is associated with delayed or inappropriate therapy of this potentially reversible condition.

REFERENCES

1. Alvarez AE, Ribeiro AF, Hessel G, *et al.* Abernathy malformation: one of the etiologies of hepatopulmonary syndrome. *Pediatr Pulmonol* 2002;**34**(5):391–4.

2. Gupta NA, Abramowsky C, Pillen T, *et al.* Pediatric hepatopulmonary syndrome is seen with polysplenia/interrupted inferior vena cava and without cirrhosis. *Liver Transpl* 2007;**13**(5):680–6.

3. Kinane TB, Westra SJ. Case records of the Massachusetts General Hospital. Weekly clinicopathological exercises. Case 31–2004. A four-year-old boy with hypoxemia. *N Engl J Med* 2004;**351**(16): 1667–75.

4. Newman B, Feinstein JA, Cohen RA, *et al.* Congenital extrahepatic portosystemic shunts associated with heterotaxy and polysplenia. *Pediatr Radiol* 2010;**40**(7):1222–30.

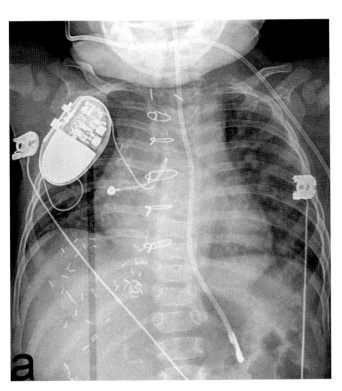

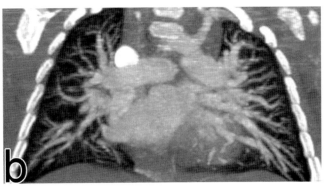

Figure 27.1. An 18-month-old girl with portopulmonary syndrome presented with progressive hypoxemia 1 year post liver transplant for biliary atresia associated with left isomerism. Prior sternotomy for ASD closure. **(a)** The frontal chest radiograph demonstrates elevation of the right hemidiaphragm (known paralysis), external pacing wires (known heart block), and a nasogastric tube in place (difficulty feeding because of shortness of breath). Sternotomy wires and multiple right upper quadrant clips are present from the prior surgeries. There is prominence of the cardiac silhouette and pulmonary vessels (right side partly obscured by pacemaker) with no focal abnormality. **(b, c, d)** CT angiogram [(b, d) coronal MIPs; (c) 3D volumetric coronal slab] demonstrates diffuse peripheral prominence of pulmonary vasculature (b), polysplenia and large splenic (SV) and superior mesenteric (SMV) veins with a small portal vein [(c) arrow], and a large left splenorenal shunt (d, arrow) draining to the hemiazygos vein (d, arrowhead). **(e)** The same large left splenorenal shunt in association with polysplenia, absent IVC with azygos and hemiazygos continuation as well as absence of the portal vein (Abernethy malformation Type I) and gallbladder had been noted on MRI at 8 days of age. This coronal SSSFE MR MIP reconstruction (no contrast) demonstrates the splenorenal shunt draining to the hemiazygos vein (arrow) as well as the azygos continuation of the IVC. The hemiazygos vein joins the azygos in the lower chest (arrowhead). **(f)** Nuclear lung perfusion scan with macroaggregated albumin shows moderate abnormal uptake in the brain and abdominal viscera. Normally almost all the agent is trapped in the lungs. Right to left shunt calculated as 39% (normal = 7%).

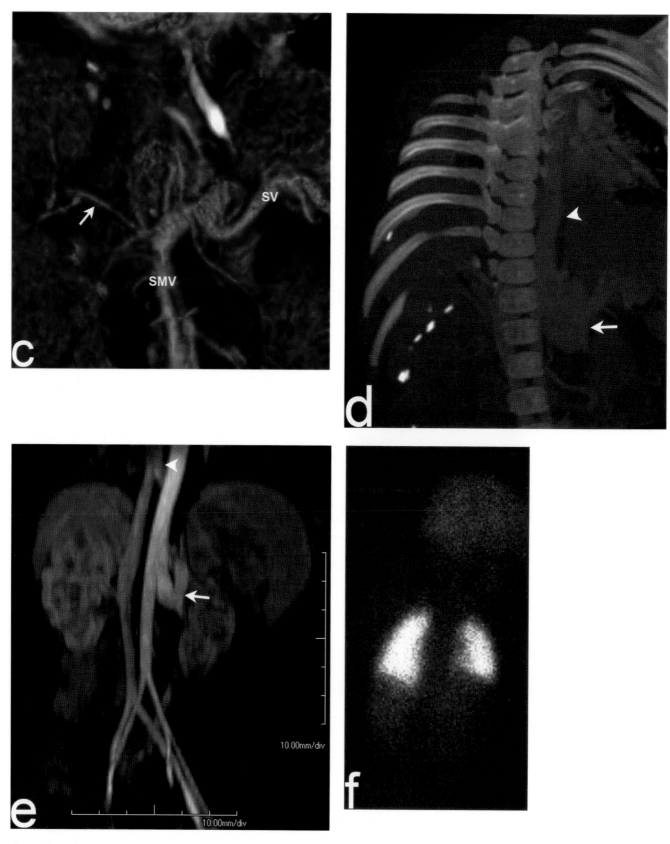

Figure 27.1. (cont.)

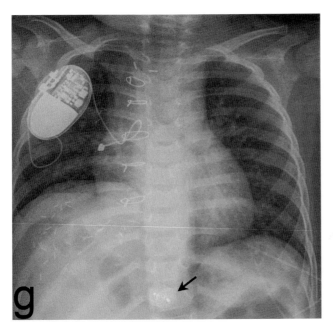
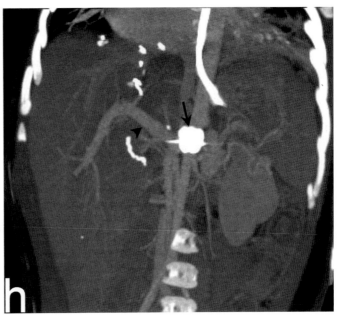

Figure 27.1. (cont.) **(g)** Chest radiograph post shunt closure shows normalization of heart size and pulmonary vasculature (compare with a) that accompanied a dramatic clinical improvement in respiratory symptoms and oxygen saturation. Note shunt closure device in the upper abdomen (arrow). **(h)** CTA angiogram coronal MIP demonstrates a closure device between the splenic vein and SMV (arrow) with much decreased size of the splenic vein and enlargement of the portal vein (arrowhead) [compare with (b)]. Although the splenorenal shunt is actually not completely occluded, superior mesenteric blood is now directed to the portal vein and liver.

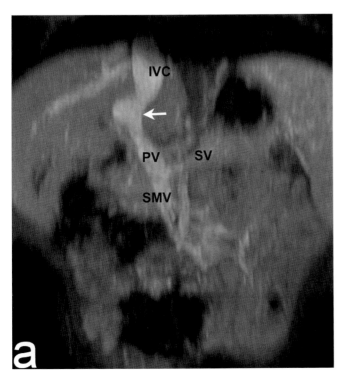
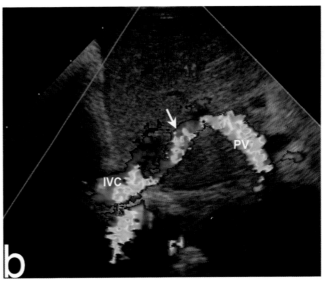

Figure 27.2. Patent ductus venosus and portopulmonary syndrome in a three and a half-year-old with hypoxemia and pulmonary hypertension. **(a)** CT angiogram in the portal venous phase (coronal MIP view) shows an intrahepatic left portal to IVC shunt via a persistent patent ductus venosus (arrow). Note lack of filling of intrahepatic portal venous branches due to predominant flow through the shunt. IVC = inferior vena cava; PV = portal vein; SMV = superior mesenteric vein; SV = splenic vein. **(b)** Oblique sagittal color Doppler ultrasound demonstrates widely patent shunt through a persistent patent ductus venosus (arrow) from left portal vein to hepatic confluence/IVC. IVC = inferior vena cava; PV = portal vein.

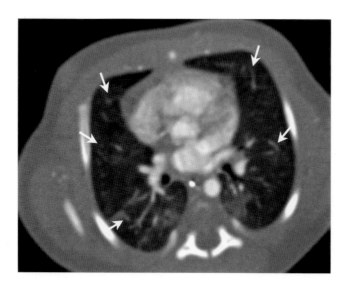

Figure 27.3. A three-day-old girl with multiple skin hemangiomas, hemoptysis, and hypoxemia. Axial CTA image demonstrates multiple abnormal peripheral tangles of vessels in the lung (arrows), some with adjacent ground glass opacity (? hemorrhage). These were thought to represent pulmonary hemangiomatosis. Clinical symptoms resolved spontaneously and the lesions were no longer visible on a follow-up CTA at eight months of age.

Aortic coarctation and interrupted aortic arch

Albert Hsiao and Beverley Newman

Imaging description

A four-year-old girl initially presented with a heart murmur at age 1, which was thought to be benign. On a routine physical examination at three years of age, she was found to have an elevated systolic blood pressure of 125 mmHg. An echocardiogram was performed and coarctation of the aorta was identified. Preoperative MRI of the chest was performed including an MRA (Fig. 28.1a) showing focal narrowing of the distal arch and hypoplasia with some tortuosity of the descending thoracic aorta. 4D flow phase-contrast MRI (Fig. 28.1b, c, d) showed flow acceleration at the site of focal narrowing as well as increased net flow along the course of the aorta, indicating collateral filling through intercostal arteries. Peak velocities exceeded 360 cm/s, corresponding to a pressure gradient over 50 mmHg.

Importance

Aortic coarctation (Fig. 28.1) and interrupted aortic arch (IAA) (Fig. 28.2) lie along a spectrum of congenital abnormalities of the aortic arch. Aortic coarctation is defined by the presence of flow-limiting stenosis in the aortic arch and is generally classified into three types: preductal, ductal, and postductal. There is most commonly focal narrowing in the proximal descending aorta at the site of the ductus arteriosus/ligamentum arteriosum with post-stenotic aortic and sometimes proximal arch and/or great vessel dilatation. The proximal arch may also be involved in the coarctation to a varying extent, most often manifesting as diffuse hypoplasia in the infantile type of coarctation.

At the extreme end of the spectrum is IAA, where blood flow into the descending thoracic aorta is dependent on a patent ductus arteriosus (PDA) (Fig. 28.2). In this latter case, prostaglandin E1 is administered to sustain patency of the PDA until the congenital defect can be surgically repaired. Arch interruption is divided into three types: A: distal to the left subclavian artery; B: between the left common carotid and left subclavian arteries; and C: between the right brachiocephalic and left common carotid arteries.

Early detection and repair of coarctation is critical for prevention of long-term morbidity and mortality, as the mean life expectancy for unrepaired coarctation patients is 34 years. The primary aim of surgical repair is to address the congenital stenosis and reduce cardiac afterload. This may include resection and end-to-end anastomosis for focal lesions or an extended end-to-end repair that also enlarges the hypoplastic arch for the less common diffuse form. Utilization of the proximal left subclavian artery to perform a subclavian flap repair of coarctation is currently less commonly performed. Angioplasty and stent placement has also been attempted, but

its use is generally considered to be more investigative in nature for primary coarctation repair but more commonly utilized in cases of re-coarctation. Unusually long segments of aortic hypoplasia may occasionally require an interposition or jump aortic graft as in the case outlined above.

Despite surgery and intervention, however, many patients continue to have unexplained hypertension either in the immediate postoperative period or at interval clinical follow-up, particularly if repair occurs at an older age. Both of these factors–age of repair and persistent hypertension–appear to be independent predictors of morbidity and early mortality.

Cross-sectional imaging in the form of CT or MRI is often used for routine follow-up of patients after repair of coarctation. These modalities are particularly helpful to survey for late complications that may not be apparent by echocardiography, namely: aneurysm and re-coarctation (Figs. 28.3 and 28.4). Phase-contrast MRI, either in the form of conventional 2D phase-contrast or 4D flow, can help assess the severity of stenosis in re-coarctation. 4D flow has the added advantage of volumetric coverage and increased through-plane resolution over 2D phase-contrast.

Typical clinical scenario

Children and adults with aortic coarctation are often asymptomatic, and much like the case presented above, are incidentally found at an older age on routine physical examination with hypertension, decreased femoral pulses, and differential blood pressure between the upper and lower extremities. In these situations, MRI and CT can help to differentiate this entity from vasculitis, which may also present with a similar constellation of clinical findings.

Patients with more severe coarctation or interrupted aortic arch may alternatively present in infancy with congestive heart failure, where a PDA is required to supply the systemic circulation. Coarctation may also be symptomatic in infancy when it occurs in conjunction with other lesions including ventricular septal defect (VSD) and PDA, known as coarctation syndrome.

Aortic coarctation is associated with other cardiovascular anomalies, especially bicuspid aortic valve (~80%) and associated ascending aortic ectasia. Coarctation is the most common congenital cardiac lesion in Turner's syndrome. Coarctation may also accompany very complex congenital heart lesions, especially those where there is decreased left heart and aortic flow in utero, such as hypoplastic left heart and Shone syndrome (multiple left-sided cardiac obstructive lesions including coarctation and aortic and mitral valve stenosis). Other associations include double aortic arch where the distal aspect of the smaller arch (usually left) may be stenotic, hypoplastic, or interrupted. Coarctation is also associated with remote disease, especially intracranial berry aneurysms.

Focal aortic coarctation may be missed or not manifest in infants in the presence of a PDA. Once the duct closes, distal ductal tissue extending into the aorta may produce the typical posterior shelf appearance of aortic coarctation. On occasion, the coarctation may be more of a membrane with a small central opening; the severity of this form of coarctation is readily missed on anatomic imaging and better appreciated when flow physiology across the narrowing is carefully assessed. This includes velocity (V) and estimated pressure gradient (via the modified Bernoulli equation $\Delta P \approx 4V^2$, where ΔP is the pressure gradient in mmHg and V is the velocity in m/s) across the stenosis on both ultrasound (US) and MR as well as MR assessment of collateral flow.

Interrupted aortic arch types A and B are the most common. While arch interruption may be isolated, it frequently occurs in conjunction with intracardiac anomalies including VSD and PDA and double outlet right ventricle (especially the Taussig–Bing variety with a subpulmonic VSD). Type B arch interruption occurs in association with truncus arteriosus, most often in the context of 22q11 deletion syndromes such as DiGeorge and velocardiofacial syndrome.

Differential diagnosis

The primary differential consideration for a focal stenosis near the ligamentum arteriosum is pseudocoarctation. In pseudocoarctation, the aorta has an irregular contour at the ligamentum arteriosum, but the abnormality does not result in a significant pressure gradient or flow-limiting stenosis, and typically collateral vascular flow is not present. The etiology of pseudocoarctation is unknown, but these lesions are benign, and do not require surgical intervention. Both pseudocoarctation and true coarctation may occur in association with a cervical aortic arch.

Vasculitides, such as Takayasu arteritis, can also result in focal narrowing of medium-sized and large-sized vessels, including the aortic arch. In general, aortic coarctation is more locally confined near the ligamentum arteriosum and although it may involve the arch in the less common diffuse form, it does not typically involve the origins of the arch vessels, as is often seen with Takayasu arteritis. Multiple regions of stenosis and aneurysm, segments of wall thickening, and wall edema are also characteristic features of vasculitis.

Unlike adults, hypertension in childhood is more often associated with an underlying anatomic abnormality. The most common differential considerations include renal artery stenosis (fibromuscular dysplasia, neurofibromatosis, and vasculitis) and aortic coarctation.

The presence of coarctation of the abdominal aorta raises a differential diagnosis that includes vasculitides such as Takayasu arteritis and Kawasaki disease, as well as congenital arteriopathies including neurofibromatosis, tuberous sclerosis, homocystinuria, congenital Rubella, and Williams's syndrome.

Teaching point

- Aortic coarctation can be either symptomatic in infancy or a relatively silent lesion with subtle symptoms. Coarctation should be considered in the differential diagnosis of hypertension in children.
- CT and MRI have supplanted more invasive techniques for detailed evaluation of aortic arch anomalies. In particular MRI and MRA are often employed for anatomic evaluation of aortic coarctation both preoperatively and in assessing postoperative complications.
- Phase-contrast MRI and especially newer 4D phase techniques can quantitatively grade the severity of stenosis in coarctation and evaluate its hemodynamic significance. The degree of collateral circulation can also be assessed.
- Aortic arch interruption is a critical duct-dependent lesion in newborn infants.
- The spectrum of coarctation lesions may be isolated but are often seen in conjunction with other cardiovascular anomalies.

REFERENCES

1. Brierly J, Reddington AN. Aortic coarctation and interrupted aortic arch. In: Anderson RJ, ed. *Pediatric Cardiology*. London: Churchill Livingstone, 2002; 1523–57.
2. Campbell M. Natural history of coarctation of the aorta. *Br Heart J* 1970;**32**(5):633–40.
3. Hom JJ, Ordovas K, Reddy GP. Velocity-encoded cine MR imaging in aortic coarctation: functional assessment of hemodynamic events. *Radiographics* 2008;**28**(2):407–16.
4. Toro-Salazar OH, Steinberger J, Thomas W, *et al.* Long-term follow-up of patients after coarctation of the aorta repair. *Am J Cardiol* 2002;**89**(5):541–7.

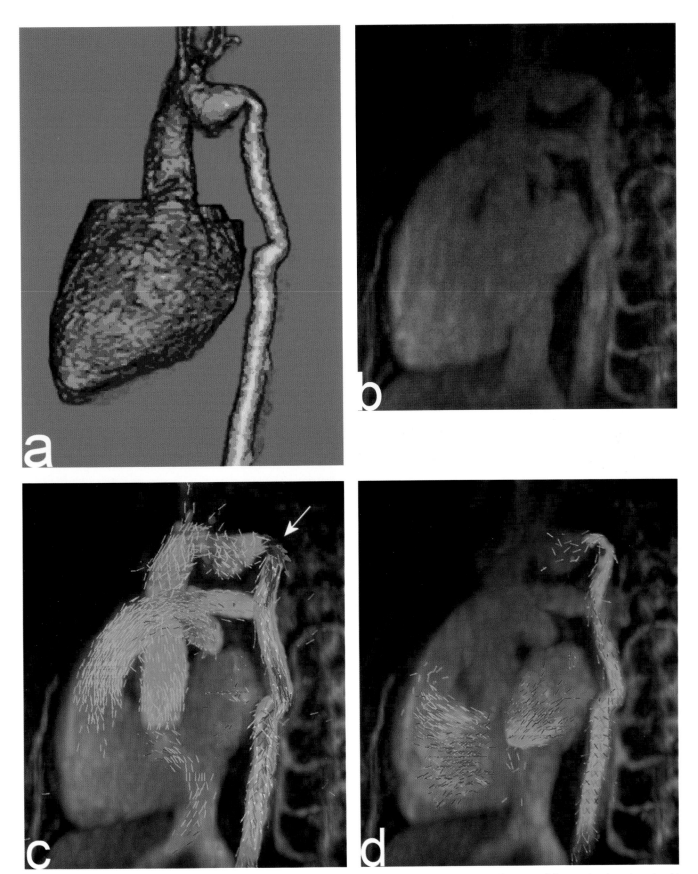

Figure 28.1. **(a)** A four-year-old girl with aortic coarctation. MRA 3D surface rendering demonstrates dilatation of the proximal aortic arch with focal narrowing of the proximal descending aorta and a very unusual tortuous, hypoplastic descending thoracic aorta. No wall thickening or other features were present to suggest vasculitis. **(b–d)** 4D flow 3D volume rendering with superimposed velocity data at (b) end-diastole, (c) early-systole, and (d) early diastole demonstrates flow acceleration just distal to the site of the coarctation (arrow) in early systole and ongoing flow in the distal descending aorta during early diastole. Also note the presence of large posterior collateral intercostal arteries.

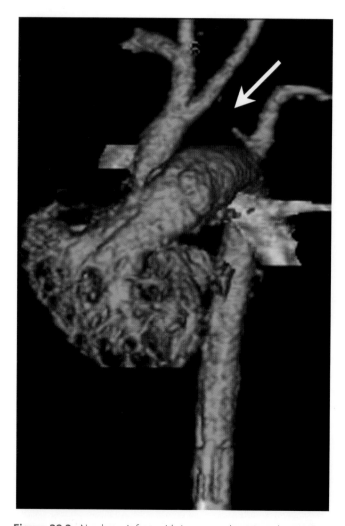

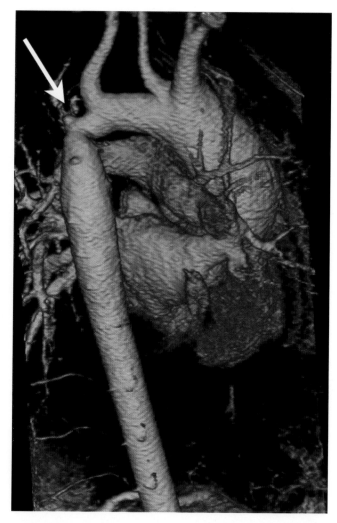

Figure 28.2. Newborn infant with interrupted aortic arch type B. Note the large PDA supplying the descending aorta (arrow). This child also had several other congenital anomalies, including hypoplastic left heart and scimitar syndrome (not shown).

Figure 28.3. MR angiography of the chest (oblique sagittal and coronal 3D surface renderings) demonstrates recurrent narrowing at the site of a previously repaired typical aortic coarctation, just distal to the origin of the left subclavian artery. Phase-contrast imaging did not show a significant pressure gradient. Thus, no immediate surgical intervention was planned.

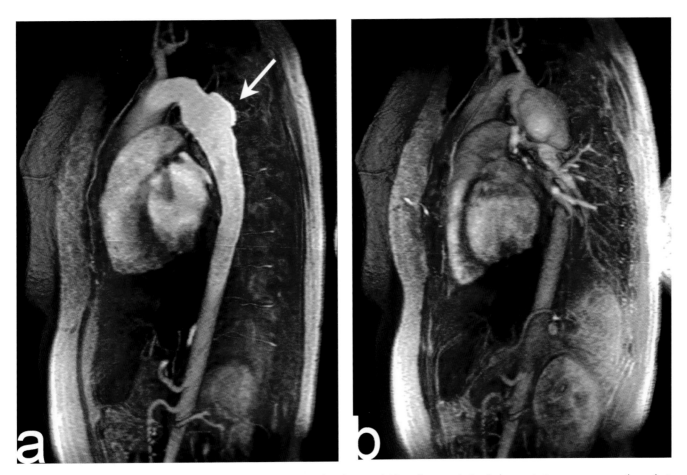

Figure 28.4. (a, b) MR angiography of the chest (oblique sagittal and coronal 3D surface renderings) demonstrates, an aneurysm (arrow) at the site of a previously repaired aortic coarctation in the proximal descending thoracic aorta. This subsequently underwent surgical repair. Note that there are only two vessels off the aortic arch, with an absent proximal left subclavian artery associated with a prior subclavian flap repair. The left subclavian artery in this situation is usually supplied via retrograde flow from the left vertebral artery (not shown).

Ebstein's anomaly

Theo Blake and Beverley Newman

Imaging description

A term infant with trisomy 21 developed cyanosis within the first week of life. A chest radiograph demonstrated a markedly enlarged cardiac silhouette seen in association with normal to diminished pulmonary flow (Fig. 29.1). This "wall-to-wall" or "box-shaped heart" configuration in a newborn is highly suggestive of right atrial enlargement, most often due to Ebstein's anomaly. Cardiac MRI in a different four-month-old infant shows the typical appearance of Ebstein's anomaly including right atrial dilatation (Fig. 29.2a) with apical displacement of the septal and posterior leaflets of the tricuspid valve leading to atrialization of the inflow portion of the right ventricle (Fig. 29.2b, c). MRI also demonstrates marked tricuspid regurgitation (TR) across the dysplastic tricuspid valve (Fig. 29.2d). A secundum atrial septal defect (ASD) is present, a common association.

Importance

Ebstein's anomaly results from embryologic dysgenesis of the tricuspid valve, characterized by incomplete delamination or undermining of the septal and posterior leaflets from the right ventricle. A strong association has been reported between oral lithium therapy during pregnancy and this type of valvular dysgenesis. As a result, affected valve leaflets are apically displaced with atrialization of the inflow portion of the right ventricle. The anterior leaflet may assume a sail-like configuration, and widening of the tricuspid annulus leads to marked tricuspid regurgitation.

If left untreated, up to half the patients with Ebstein's anomaly may die in the first year of life due to right heart failure. If cyanosis is present it is generally most severe in the perinatal period when pulmonary vascular resistance is high. As the lungs mature, vascular resistance drops and the degree of tricuspid regurgitation and right to left shunting decreases. While the majority of cases are diagnosed in childhood, some individuals may remain asymptomatic into adult life. If the shunting is not initially severe, persistent tricuspid regurgitation and elevated right atrial pressure can lead to greater right to left shunting later in life. Pulmonary hypoplasia can also be a cause for morbidity in patients with Ebstein's anomaly and other right heart obstructive lesions such as tricuspid atresia or pulmonary stenosis/atresia due to decreased pulmonary perfusion.

Ebstein's is seen in association with other cardiac anomalies, including a patent foramen ovale or secundum ASD (atrial connection present in 80%), tricuspid stenosis, ventricular septal defect (VSD), patent ductus arteriosus, pulmonary stenosis, pulmonary atresia with intact ventricular septum, tetralogy of Fallot, and transposition of the great arteries.

Typical clinical scenario

Although clinical symptoms vary widely, cases of Ebstein's anomaly that do not present early with congestive heart failure may present later with symptoms of fatigue, dyspnea on exertion, and cyanosis. Exam findings include a holosystolic murmur and a fixed split second heart sound. Right heart conduction abnormalities including Wolf–Parkinson–White syndrome and right bundle branch block are also found in up to 42% of children and adults with Ebstein's.

The management of Ebstein's anomaly is dictated by the severity of the deformity and the symptomatology. Heart failure symptoms are medically managed with ACE inhibitors and diuretics as necessary. Arrhythmias can be addressed with antiarrhythmics or external or transvenous pacemaker placement as needed. Radiofrequency ablation of accessory pathways can be attempted for management of supraventricular tachycardias although the success rates are generally lower than in patients without structural heart disease. Surgical management options generally involve closure of any associated ASD or VSD and either repair of the tricuspid valve if the right ventricle is large enough to attempt a two ventricle repair or a one and a half ventricle repair in instances where it is not. The one and a half ventricle repair connects the superior vena cava (SVC) to the pulmonary artery as a bidirectional cavopulmonary connection (aka bidirectional Glen), thereby unloading a large volume of the systemic return from the right side of the heart.

Differential diagnosis

Other causes of marked cardiomegaly in infancy are typically associated with a very large right atrium, often due to marked tricuspid regurgitation. Those most closely resembling Ebstein's anomaly that also tend to be cyanotic and have decreased pulmonary vascularity include pulmonary atresia with an intact ventricular septum (Fig. 29.3), critical pulmonic stenosis, and occasionally tricuspid atresia (with restrictive ASD). The differential diagnosis of large cardiomegaly,"wall-to-wall heart," in infancy also includes acquired conditions such as pericardial effusion (Fig. 29.4a, b), myocarditis, cardiomyopathy, and occasionally a cardiac neoplasm. Causes of cardiomyopathy in young infants include ischemia–perinatal asphyxia (usually transient TR), anomalous left coronary artery (arising from the pulmonary artery) (see Case 32, Fig. 32.1), and hypoplastic left heart; infectious myocarditis, especially coxsackie virus infection; hypertrophic cardiomyopathy–seen in an infant of a diabetic mother with septal hypertrophy and left ventricle (LV) obstruction (usually transient); LV obstruction with endocardial fibroelastosis (EFE); toxic–drugs, especially steroids, and metabolic–anemia, glycogen storage disease type II (Pompe's) (Fig. 29.5).

Additional differential considerations include other causes of right atrial enlargement such as atrial level left to right shunts (ASD, partial anomalous pulmonary venous return, coronary fistula, and a Gerbode defect (VSD with LV to right atrium [RA] shunt). Shunts can potentially be distinguished based on the presence of increased pulmonary vascularity. However, these shunts even when large rarely produce the degree of cardiomegaly that is typical of Ebstein's anomaly.

An important normal variant in infants that can be difficult to differentiate from marked cardiomegaly is a normally prominent thymus. The thymus can extend from the upper mediastinum down to the diaphragm. On a frontal chest radiograph what is visualized is a composite cardiothymic silhouette (Fig. 29.6a). The lateral view is helpful in enabling visualization of the heart separate from the thymus, which is located anteriorly (Fig. 29.6b). An enlarged heart tends to be globular in infancy, i.e. it will be enlarged on both frontal and lateral views.

Teaching point

When marked cardiomegaly is identified in a cyanotic or acyanotic infant with normal or reduced pulmonary vasculature, an obstructive right heart condition must be considered. Giant cardiomegaly is most often due to a very enlarged right atrium, frequently related to tricuspid regurgitation, most notably Ebstein's anomaly. The detailed anatomy and differential diagnoses can be elucidated by follow-up imaging with echocardiography or MRI.

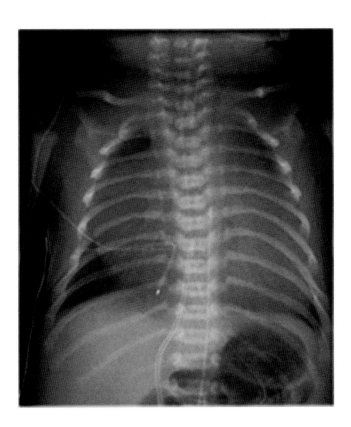

Figure 29.1. Frontal chest radiograph in a neonate showing "wall-to-wall" heart. Cardiomegaly of this size in a newborn suggests right atrial enlargement, most commonly due to Ebstein's anomaly.

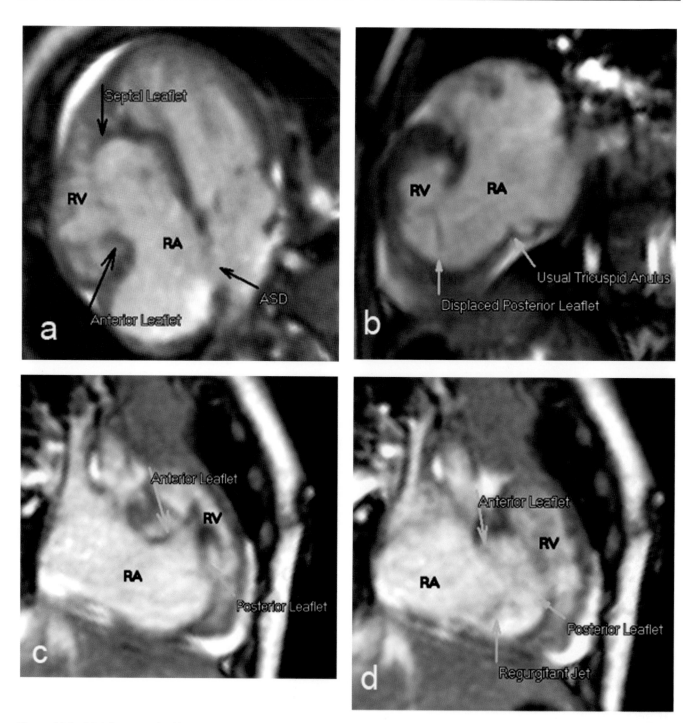

Figure 29.2. (a) A four-month-old girl with Ebstein's anomaly. MRI four-chamber steady state free precession (SSFP) image shows right atrial enlargement resulting from apical displacement of the septal leaflet of the tricuspid valve. A large secundum atrial septal defect (ASD) is also present. RA = right atrium, RV = right ventricle. **(b)** RV two-chamber SSFP image showing apical displacement of the posterior leaflet of the tricuspid valve from its usual site of origin. **(c)** RV three-chamber SSFP image during diastole showing atrialization of the inlet portion of the RV due to a displacement of the posterior leaflet of the tricuspid valve. **(d)** RV three-chamber SSFP image during systole. A jet of tricuspid regurgitation is seen as a result of poor coaptation of the valve leaflets.

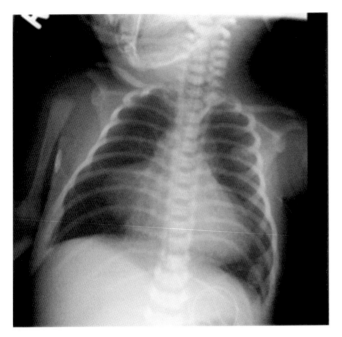

Figure 29.3. Frontal radiograph of a newborn with cyanosis diagnosed on echocardiogram with pulmonary atresia with an intact ventricular septum. There is marked cardiomegaly with a very prominent right atrium and decreased pulmonary vascularity.

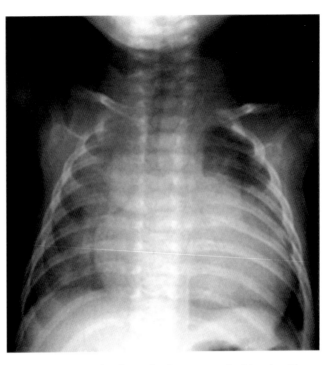

Figure 29.5. Frontal radiograph of a two-month-old male with congestive heart failure and marked cardiomegaly secondary to Pompe disease (glycogen storage disease type II).

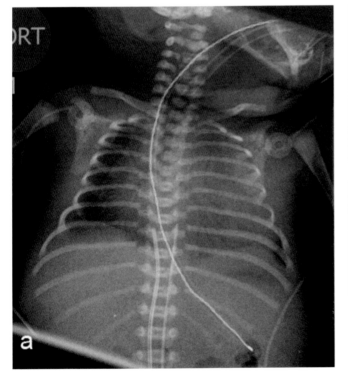

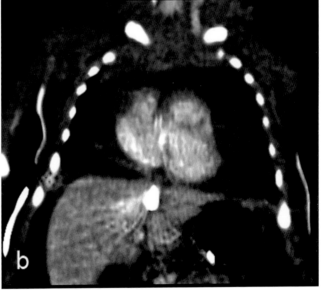

Figure 29.4. (a) Frontal radiograph of a newborn girl with hydrops, ascites, and a large pericardial effusion simulating massive cardiomegaly. **(b)** Coronal CT reconstruction showing low attenuation pericardial fluid filling the thoracic cavity. Note also anasarca and ascites.

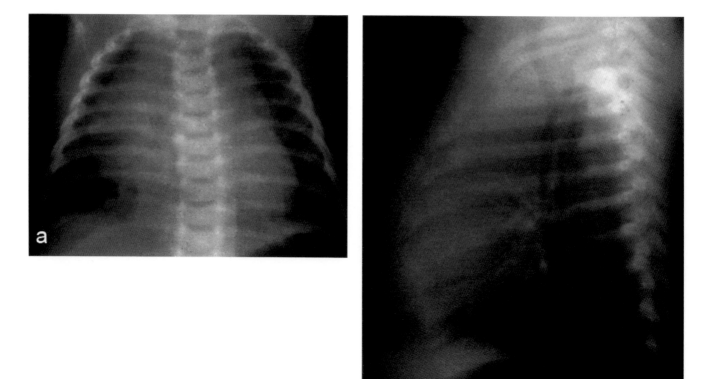

Figure 29.6. **(a)** Frontal radiograph in a two-month-old male delivered following premature rupture of membranes demonstrates a prominent cardiothymic silhouette. **(b)** Lateral radiograph in the same patient reveals that the heart is not enlarged; however, a normally prominent thymus occupies the anterior mediastinum.

Transposition of the great arteries

Beverley Newman

Imaging description

A newborn infant was noted to have moderate tachypnea and cyanosis at birth. A chest radiograph (Fig. 30.1a) demonstrated patchy opacity in the right upper lobe, question atelectasis or pneumonia. There was a slightly narrow mediastinum with an oval-shaped cardiac silhouette ("egg on a string" appearance). Pulmonary vascular markings appeared mildly increased but the main pulmonary artery segment was concave; the possibility of transposition of the great arteries (TGA) was raised and confirmed on cardiac echo. A nonrestrictive secundum atrial septal defect (ASD) was present with no other shunt found. A follow-up chest radiograph at five days of age demonstrated an increase in heart size and prominence of pulmonary vascularity (Fig. 30.1b). An MR examination was obtained to further evaluate anatomy and ventricular size and function. This confirmed transposition of the great arteries (right ventricle connecting to aorta and left ventricle connecting to pulmonary artery) with an anterior and rightward position of the ascending aorta relative to the main pulmonary artery, ASD with no other connection, and normal sized ventricles with good biventricular function (Fig. 30.1c–e). The baby underwent an arterial switch procedure at 10 days of age.

Importance

While chest radiographs are very useful in the initial evaluation of possible congenital heart disease, there are only a few characteristic radiographic findings that suggest a specific diagnosis. More often radiographs help to suggest a category of disease such as left to right shunting (increased vascularity) or a right-sided obstructive lesion (decreased vascularity). The "egg on a string" appearance has been described as characteristic of D-transposition; the narrow appearance of the mediastinum is thought to be related to a combination of the more antero posterior rather than side by side location of the great vessels as well as stress-related thymic atrophy. This appearance is only present in approximately one-third of TGA cases and more commonly, similar to other congenital cardiac conditions, the chest radiographs in TGA may be confusing and are often normal at birth. Cardiomegaly and increased vascularity tend to occur only after a few days when pulmonary vascular resistance drops and increased flow occurs to the pulmonary circuit (Fig. 30.1b).

Typically echocardiography may be the only supplemental imaging required to adequately evaluate congenital heart disease. Depending on complexity, additional imaging such as MRI or cardiac catheterization may be needed. MRI provides excellent anatomic as well as functional evaluation. Catheterization is often deferred or only used when detailed oxygen saturations and pressure measurements are needed or for percutaneous interventions. CTA is most often used when lung parenchymal or airway detail is paramount, or the child is deemed too fragile to tolerate the relatively long MR examination. Gated CTA is used when detailed intracardiac or coronary anatomy is needed, especially in small children.

TGA results in abnormal dual circulations in parallel. Circulatory mixing is essential for survival. There is invariably some form of atrial connection, at least a patent foramen ovale; there may also be a ventricular septal defect (VSD) and/or patent ductus arteriosus. If there is insufficient mixing and marked cyanosis, initial emergency management consists of a Rashkind procedure (enlargement of the interatrial connection), usually achieved in the catheterization laboratory using a regular or cutting balloon.

Typical clinical scenario

TGA is the most common cyanotic congenital cardiac lesion in newborn infants. It is usually symptomatic in the early newborn period with tachypnea and variable cyanosis depending on how much circulatory admixture is present. Pulmonary hypertension tends to occur early in this lesion, especially when a VSD and large pulmonary overcirculation are present. Without surgical intervention, most babies would not survive beyond one year of life.

Currently, corrective surgery is usually performed in the neonatal period and most often consists of an arterial switch procedure (Jatene operation, first performed in 1975) (Fig. 30.2). This surgery includes reanastomosing the coronary arteries as well as the great vessels and has an 88% 15-year survival. The Le Compte maneuver results in draping of the pulmonary arteries anterior to the ascending aorta, producing a very characteristic appearance (Fig. 30.2). A common postoperative complication is asymmetry of the branch pulmonary arteries with narrowing of one or both (Fig. 30.2). Less common problems are anastomotic great artery or coronary stenosis or valvular stenosis/regurgitation.

Prior to the technologic advances that allowed for successful coronary reanastomosis, and also in some circumstances where a switch operation was considered technically challenging or impossible, the surgical procedure performed for TGA was the Mustard or Senning atrial switch operation whereby the atrial septum was removed and surgical baffles placed in the atrium, redirecting pulmonary venous return to the right ventricle and systemic venous return to the left ventricle (Fig. 30.3). This has the advantage of correcting the abnormal circulation but the right ventricle remains as the systemic ventricle. This ultimately results in long-term problems with right ventricular dysfunction, arrhythmia, and eventual failure. The current tendency is to try and use the left ventricle as the systemic ventricle whenever possible and many of these prior atrial switches are being converted to an arterial switch. Unlike in the newborn period, where the left ventricle has seen high in utero vascular resistance as the pulmonary ventricle and is therefore able to function immediately as a systemic ventricle, later switches require "training" of the low resistance pulmonary left ventricle to take over the systemic circulation. This is achieved by banding the pulmonary artery to restrict flow and force the left ventricle to hypertrophy while pumping against increased resistance.

Another variation that may be present in TGA includes pulmonic stenosis (~30% of cases, valvar or subvalvar and typically accompanied by a VSD). If pulmonic stenosis is significant, it may obviate an arterial switch. The approach then is a Rastelli operation with the left ventricle outflow tunneled through the VSD to the aorta and the right ventricle connected to the pulmonary circulation via a pulmonary artery conduit (Fig. 30.4).

Differential diagnosis

The general plain film differential diagnoses for cyanosis with increased vascularity are the "T" lesions, including TGA, truncus arteriosus, total anomalous pulmonary venous return, and occasionally tricuspid atresia. Double outlet right ventricle with a subpulmonic VSD and single ventricle anomalies may also have a similar appearance.

The term D-transposition is used to describe great artery transposition occurring in the context of normal rightward looping of the primitive heart. In this anomaly there is ventriculoarterial discordance (transposition of the great arteries); however, there is atrioventricular concordance.

The term L-transposition or congenitally corrected transposition of the great arteries (CCTGA) describes the situation of cardiac looping to the left in association with great artery transposition (ventriculoarterial discordance) (Fig. 30.5). Because of the aberrant leftward bending of the primitive cardiac tube the position of the ventricles is reversed such that there is additional atrioventricular discordance (right atrium connects with left ventricle and left atrium with right ventricle) (Fig. 30.5). As a result, there is physiologic "correction" of the circulation, with pulmonary venous return directed through the left atrium to the right systemic ventricle and systemic venous return through the left ventricle to the pulmonary circulation. CCTGA is somewhat of a misnomer since there are frequently other associated intracardiac anomalies including pulmonic stenosis, VSD, heartblock, and Ebstein's anomaly (affects the systemic right ventricle) with variable presentation and symptoms. CCTGA may be asymptomatic in childhood and even adulthood. However, similar to the atrial switch procedure, right ventricular dysfunction and failure often supervenes later in life. The current tendency is to do a surgical double switch (atrial baffle as well as arterial switch) in order to have the left ventricle be the systemic ventricle. CCTGA also tends to have a characteristic plain film radiographic appearance with a prominent left superior heart border (with or without dextrocardia) due to the leftward malposition of the ascending aorta relative to the pulmonary artery (Fig. 30.5). On cross-sectional imaging the left-sided and more anterior aorta is readily appreciated as well as an abnormal convex curve to the aortic arch (Figs. 30.5 and 30.6).

Both D- and L-TGA as described above may have some variation in appearance depending on associated cardiac anomalies including ASD, VSD, and patent ductus arteriosus (PDA), pulmonic stenosis, atrioventricular valve abnormalities, and aortic coarctation/interruption. D/L-TGA may also be associated with very complex heart disease including tricuspid atresia and double outlet right ventricle and single ventricle anomalies. Also of note is the fact that coronary anomalies occur commonly in conjunction with transposition as well as other conotruncal anomalies (truncus arteriosus, double outlet right ventricle, and tetralogy of Fallot) (Fig. 30.6).

Teaching point

Plain chest radiographs in TGA are often normal at birth. Specific clues that may be present especially after a few days include "egg on a string" appearance of D-transposition and prominent left superior heart border in L-transposition.

MRI has assumed a primary imaging role in defining cardiac and extracardiac anatomy as well as postoperative complications in complex cardiac lesions such as these.

Current surgical practice is to correct the abnormality, prioritizing the left ventricle as the systemic pump, i.e. switch or double switch whenever possible.

REFERENCES

1. Chan FP. Transposition of the great arteries. In: Ho H, Reddy GP, eds. *Cardiovascular Imaging – Expert Radiology Series*. St. Louis, Missouri: Elsevier, Mosby, Saunders, 2011; Chapter 45.
2. Gaca AM, Jaggers JJ, Dudley LT, Bisset GS, 3rd. Repair of congenital heart disease: a primer – part 1. *Radiology* 2008;**247**:617–31.
3. Gaca AM, Jaggers JJ, Dudley LT, Bisset GS, 3rd. Repair of congenital heart disease: a primer – part 2. *Radiology* 2008;**248**;44–60.
4. Yoo S, Macdonald C, Babyn P. *Chest Radiographic Interpretation in Pediatric Cardiac Patients*. New York: Thieme, 2010.

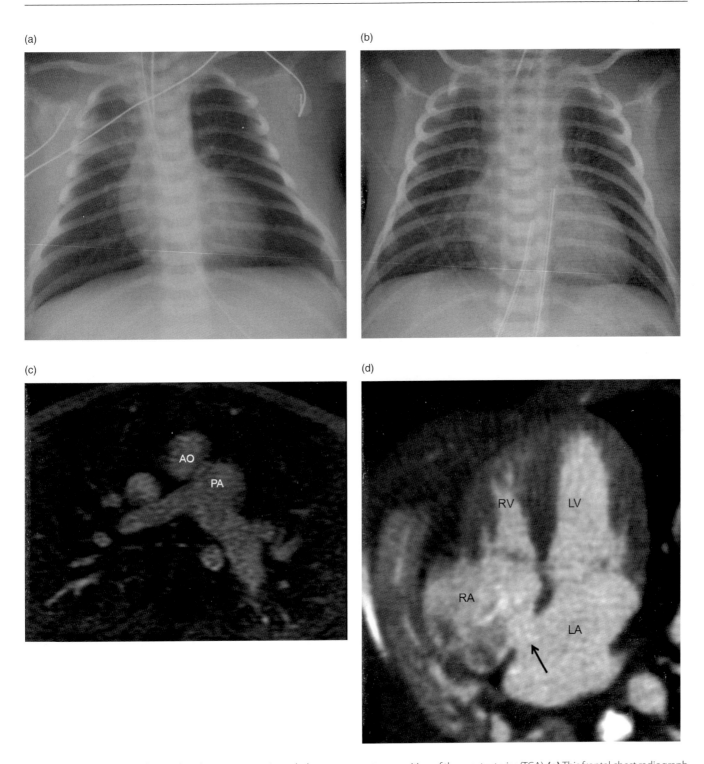

(a)

(b)

(c)

(d)

Figure 30.1. Newborn infant with tachypnea, cyanosis, and a heart murmur; transposition of the great arteries (TGA). **(a)** This frontal chest radiograph just after birth demonstrated an intubated infant with right upper lobe opacity thought to be atelectasis or aspiration. The heart and mediastinum have an "egg on a string" appearance, narrow mediastinum with oval-shaped slightly enlarged heart. Pulmonary vascularity appears mildly prominent. The relatively characteristic cardiomediastinal configuration suggested possible TGA, later confirmed on echocardiography. **(b)** A follow-up frontal chest radiograph at 5 days of age demonstrated increasing cardiomegaly and pulmonary vascularity with mild indistinctness of vascular margins consistent with increased left to right shunting and mild superimposed interstitial pulmonary edema. **(c)** Axial image from an MR angiogram demonstrates the typical aberrant great vessel relationship of D-transposition with the ascending aorta (AO) located to the right and anterior of the main pulmonary artery (PA). The normal configuration is for the PA to be anterior and to the left of the AO. **(d)** MR – four-chamber view: there is atrioventricular concordance with the right atrium (RA) connecting with the right-sided morphologic right ventricle (RV) and the left atrium (LA) connecting with the left-sided morphologic left ventricle (LV). There is a moderate-sized atrial septal defect; no other left/right connection was seen.

(e)

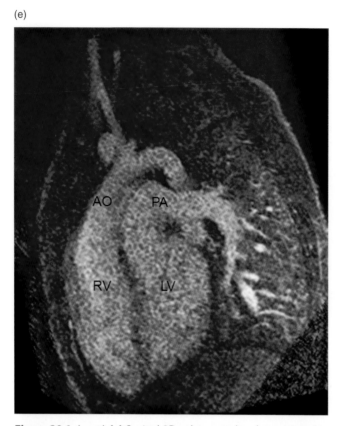

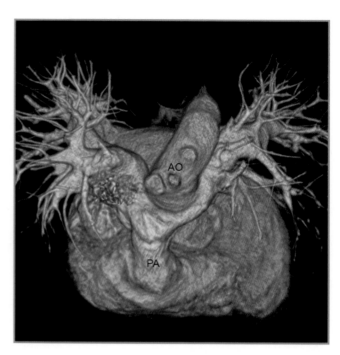

Figure 30.2. TGA post arterial switch operation. This 3D volumetric reconstruction demonstrates the anteriorly reanastomosed pulmonary artery (PA) with the branch PAs draped over the ascending aorta (AO) (Le Compte maneuver). Note some asymmetry of the PAs with mild narrowing of the left side relative to the right PA.

Figure 30.1. (cont.) **(e)** Sagittal 3D volume rendered reconstruction of MRA demonstrating ventriculoarterial discordance (transposition), with the anterior morphologic right ventricle (RV) connecting to the aorta (AO) and the posterior morphologic left ventricle (LV) connecting to the pulmonary artery (PA). Note the parallel rather than crisscrossing orientation of the great arteries, typical of transposition.

(a)

(b)

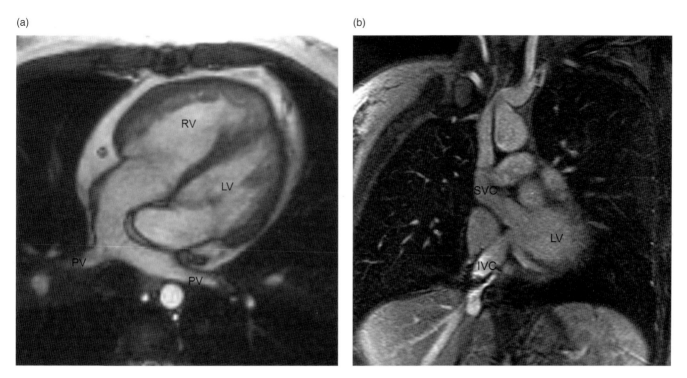

Figure 30.3. TGA post Senning atrial switch repair. **(a)** MRI four-chamber view. Note the atrial baffle that directs pulmonary venous (PV) flow to the systemic hypertrophied right ventricle. **(b)** Coronal reconstruction from MRA demonstrates the systemic veins superior and inferior venae cavae baffled to the left ventricle (pulmonary ventricle).

(a)

(b)

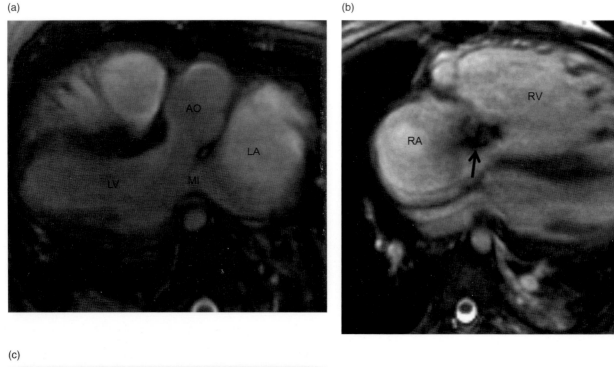

(c)

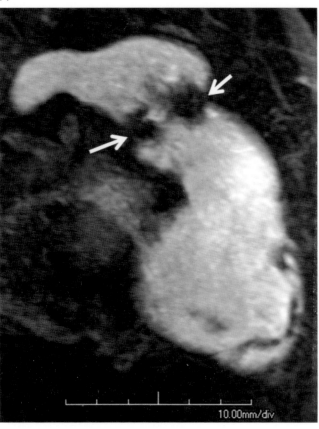

10.00mm/div

Figure 30.4. Rastelli repair for TGA with pulmonic stenosis. **(a)** MR showing LV three-chamber view. The left ventricle (LV) has been tunneled through the prior VSD to the aorta. Note the separation of the mitral (MI) and aortic valves (AO) consistent with prior transposition and a subaortic conus. LA = left atrium. **(b)** Post operative dilatation of RV with conduit valve stenosis and moderate tricuspid regurgitation. MRI four-chamber view demonstrates the dilated RA and RV with a prominent dark jet of tricuspid regurgitation (arrow). **(c)** Thin MIP sagittal reconstruction from the MRA shows a dilated RV connected to the PA via a valved conduit. There is a suggestion of conduit valvar pulmonic stenosis with supravalvar PA dilatation but moderate dark artifact from the prosthetic valve (arrows) makes evaluation difficult. Echocardiography confirmed conduit valve stenosis and moderate tricuspid regurgitation.

(a)

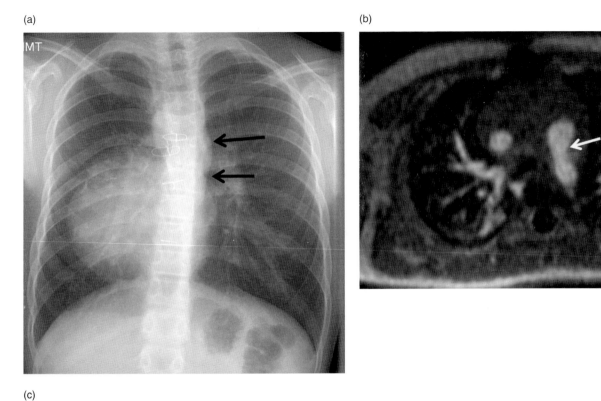

(b)

(c)

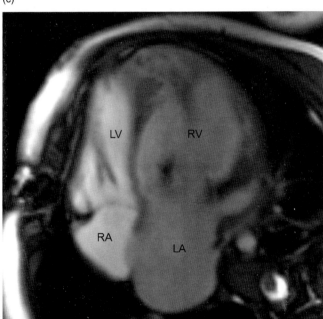

Figure 30.5. CCTGA (L-transposition) post repair of VSD. **(a)** The frontal chest radiograph demonstrates dextrocardia (present in ~25% of CCTGA) and right-sided aortic arch (deviates trachea to left). There is a prominent shadow along the left superior heart border, a characteristic finding in CCTGA, due to the left-sided malposition of the ascending aorta. **(b)** MRA, axial slice demonstrates the characteristic leftward concave shape of the aortic arch (arrow) in L-transposition, where the ascending aorta is malpositioned to the left (as opposed to the normal convex arch when the ascending aorta is to the right of the PA). **(c)** CCTGA (L-transposition) post repair of VSD and placement of pulmonary band – MRI four-chamber view. Note the atrioventricular discordance with the right atrium connecting to the morphologic left ventricle (which is on the right side) and left atrium to the right ventricle (hypertrophied and dilated systemic ventricle on the left side).

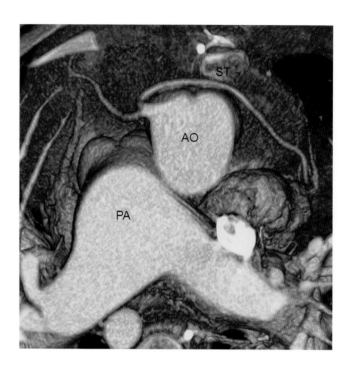

Figure 30.6. CCTGA (L-transposition) with a coronary anomaly. Axial gated CTA 3D slab image demonstrates the aberrant relationship of the anterior and leftward aorta (AO) relative to the PA in CCTGA. There is a single coronary artery arising from the aorta anteriorly and to the right and separating into right and left branches with the left branch coursing anteriorly over the ascending aorta immediately below the sternum (ST). It is important for the surgeon to be aware of this aberrant anatomy so that the coronary artery is not inadvertently injured during a sternotomy incision. (Image courtesy of Frandics Chan, Stanford University.)

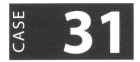

Total anomalous pulmonary venous return

Horacio Murillo, Michael J. Lane, Carlos S. Restrepo, and Beverley Newman

Imaging description

A full-term neonate was noted to be cyanotic and rapidly developed severe respiratory distress requiring endotracheal intubation. A chest radiograph (Fig. 31.1a) showed a diffuse pulmonary edema pattern, but a normal sized cardiac silhouette. Echocardiography demonstrated a large atrial septal defect (ASD) and absence of pulmonary veins entering the left atrium; however, it could not identify the drainage pattern of the pulmonary veins. CT angiography of the chest on the same day showed all pulmonary veins converging into a confluence posterior to the left atrium and draining below the diaphragm (Fig. 31.1b, c), consistent with infracardiac total anomalous pulmonary venous return (TAPVR) with obstruction. Prenatal ultrasound examinations had been reported as within normal limits.

Importance

TAPVR or total anomalous pulmonary venous connection is a rare congenital cardiovascular malformation (2–3% of all congenital cardiovascular anomalies) in which all four pulmonary veins drain into systemic veins or the right atrium with or without pulmonary venous obstruction. More severe obstruction tends to correlate with both earlier clinical presentation and increased severity of symptoms. TAPVR is classified based on the location of pulmonary venous drainage. In all types, the pulmonary veins tend to form a primary confluence, usually behind the left atrium, which then drains ultimately to a systemic vein and the right atrium. Approximately one-third of TAPVR patients have other complex cardiovascular anomalies including asplenia and pulmonary atresia (Fig. 31.2). All types of TAPVR have shunting through the lungs back to the right side of the heart, and require a right to left shunt for survival. An ASD and/or patent foramen ovale (PFO) are essential to allow for the return of blood to the systemic side.

In type I TAPVR, the pulmonary veins drain to supracardiac systemic veins. This is the most common form of total anomalous pulmonary venous drainage pattern (50%). Drainage is most often via a left-sided vertical vein to the left innominate vein and superior vena cava (Fig. 31.3). Less commonly, drainage is to the azygos or hemiazygos veins. Radiographically, the neonatal appearance is unremarkable unless there is pulmonary venous obstruction where type I TAPVR can have a similar appearance to that of type III (Fig. 31.4).

Type II TAPVR is the next most common total anomalous venous drainage pattern (30%), and drains at the cardiac level, most commonly into the coronary sinus or directly into the right atrium (Fig. 31.5). It is less common for this type to present with obstruction. Instead, it commonly presents with right heart failure due to volume overload.

Type III TAPVR (12%) has infracardiac or infradiaphragmatic drainage and almost always exhibits obstruction (Fig. 31.1). The emissary descending pulmonary vein usually extends into the abdomen, anterior to the esophagus, through the esophageal hiatus with drainage into the portal vein, inferior vena cava, or less commonly the ductus venosus or hepatic vein (Figs. 31.1 and 31.2).

Type IV TAPVR has mixed level drainage, which can be any combination of the type I to III drainage levels. The imaging presentation of type IV is variable.

Clinical presentation of all the non-obstructed forms of TAPVR is similar to that of pulmonary shunting with overload of the right heart (Fig. 31.5a, b). Variable cyanosis and congestive heart failure tend to develop soon after birth. Liver congestion is common due to right heart dysfunction or because of the direct drainage of pulmonary veins into the hepatic veins or inferior vena cava (Figs. 31.1 and 31.2).

Typical clinical scenario

In areas of the world where access to medical care during pregnancy and to ultrasound are readily available, anomalies such as TAPVR can be identified prior to birth. Delivery can then be planned at a place where management and care of the newborn can be adequately provided. However, it is not uncommon that even in well cared for pregnancies, prenatal diagnosis can go unnoticed and the presentation at birth is unexpected (Figs. 31.1 and 31.4). The obstructed forms of TAPVR commonly present immediately at birth with respiratory distress and marked cyanosis. Nearly 100% of type III and about 50% of type I TAPVR cases exhibit obstruction near or at the draining site. The obstruction may be due to mechanical compression or because of inherent cellular/connective tissue abnormality, resulting in pulmonary venous dysplasia with irregular enlargement and stricture/stenosis formation.

It is important and often critical to recognize TAPVR promptly. The presentation of TAPVR with obstruction constitutes both a medical and surgical emergency. Prompt diagnosis based on clinical and non-invasive imaging impacts clinical management, surgical planning, and intervention.

Type I (supracardiac) anomalies with a left vertical vein may have the chest radiographic appearance of a "snowman" (Fig. 31.3a). The enlarged vertical vein on the left, the innominate vein superiorly, and the dilated superior vena cava on the right form the head of the snowman. The body of the snowman is formed by an enlarged right atrium and right ventricle. The snowman appearance is often not present or difficult to appreciate early in life because of lack of discernible venous dilatation and obscuration by the thymus. Severe venous obstruction in type I TAPVR may be radiographically indistinguishable from type III, with findings of pulmonary edema and a normal sized cardiac silhouette (Fig. 31.4).

The radiographic appearance of type II (cardiac) TAPVR (Fig. 31.5) is dependent on the timing of presentation. This type tends to manifest slowly over days, weeks, or months and pulmonary venous obstruction is uncommon. An enlarged right cardiac silhouette or frank cardiomegaly and increased pulmonary vascularity are associated with respiratory distress, a variable degree of cyanosis, and increased susceptibility to pneumonia.

Type III TAPVR (infracardiac) has a characteristic radiographic appearance of pulmonary edema and a normal sized cardiac silhouette (Fig. 31.1a). There is usually mechanical obstruction/stenosis at the pulmonary venous drainage site(s) below the diaphragm (Fig. 31.1b, c). In addition, there may be relative obstruction due to passage through the liver with drainage into the portal vein.

The clinical presentation and radiographic appearance of type IV TAPVR is variable, depending on the combination pattern of anomalous connection at two or more levels. As in other types of TAPVR, the presence of obstruction at one or more drainage sites determines the timing, clinical, and imaging manifestations.

Echocardiography and radiography play an essential role in the diagnostic evaluation of patients with TAPVR. However, the patient's body size and the complexity of the anomalous venous morphology and route patterns can be challenging. CT angiography and MR imaging and angiography have become definitive diagnostic imaging modalities, which can provide the three-dimensional anatomic delineation needed for surgical planning and intervention. Multiple post-processing strategies can be used in both CT and MR volumetrically acquired data to aid diagnostic definition, including volume rendering and curved planar reformats (Figs. 31.1 and 31.2). The complex and serpiginous morphology of the anomalous veins may only be appreciated after analysis of multiple imaging post-processing techniques (Figs. 31.1c and 31.3c, d). Because of easier access, faster scanning, and better spatial resolution, CT is most often employed in critically ill infants with obstructed veins. It is imperative to identify all the anomalous veins as well as all the stenotic foci for surgical repair.

In obstructed TAPVR patients, immediate stabilization prior to surgery requires mechanical ventilation, correction of acidosis, inotropic support, and administration of prostaglandin E1 to maintain patency of the ductus arteriosus and or the ductus venosus. Episodic pulmonary hypertension may occur even after repair and requires vasodilators including inhaled nitric oxide.

Prompt surgical repair of obstructed TAPVR is required. The emissary vein or venous confluence behind the left atrium is commonly connected surgically to the posterior left atrium and the ASD or significant PFO closed. Sutures appear to trigger stenosis and strictures of these already dysplastic veins. Evidence supports improved outcomes with the use of a sutureless technique employing pericardium.

The most common postoperative complication after TAPVR repair is pulmonary venous obstruction, which may be progressive. Diagnosis of postoperative complications can be very difficult, with both clinical symptoms and echocardiographic findings being subtle. Postoperative CT and MRI imaging can provide detailed definition of vessels with CT currently having the advantage of greater spatial resolution. However, MR has the added ability to evaluate flow volumes, velocities, and patterns in the pulmonary arteries and veins via phase-contrast imaging.

The surgical repair of non-obstructive TAPVR can be elective. Other associated cardiovascular abnormalities may affect type and timing of surgical intervention.

Differential diagnosis

The radiographic findings of a normal size heart and pulmonary edema should prompt the diagnostic consideration of TAPVR with obstruction. However, other causes of diffuse pulmonary opacification, especially respiratory distress syndrome (typically decreased lung volumes) and neonatal pneumonia may have a similar appearance. The gestational age, timing, and severity of presentation and other clinical data help to differentiate these entities.

Other congenital cardiac lesions can have overlapping clinical and radiographic features with TAPVR, especially the non-obstructive form. These are all characterized by cardiomegaly and increased pulmonary vascularity and/or pulmonary edema. Considerations include left-sided obstructive lesions such as hypoplastic left heart syndrome, congenital mitral stenosis, and critical aortic stenosis. In addition, cyanotic shunt admixture lesions including truncus arteriosus, transposition of the great arteries, and single ventricle can have similar radiographic appearances. If cyanosis is mild or not appreciated and presentation late, left to right shunt lesions such as ASD and/or ventricular septal defect (VSD) also enter into the differential diagnosis.

Teaching point

The presentation of severe cyanosis and respiratory distress at birth and a normal sized heart in a background of pulmonary edema should alert the radiologist to the possibility of TAPVR with obstruction. Non-obstructed forms of TAPVR tend to present later with milder cyanosis, cardiomegaly, and increased pulmonary vascularity. Although neonatal echocardiography is often sufficient for the diagnosis, CT and MR angiography can non-invasively provide comprehensive detailed anatomic delineation of the abnormal venous drainage, which can be used to guide surgical planning and management.

REFERENCES

1. Amplatz K, Moller JH. Radiology of Congenital Heart Disease. St Louis: Mosby-Year Book, 1993; Chapter 46.

2. Chowdhury UK, Airan B, Malhotra A, et al. Mixed total anomalous pulmonary venous connection: anatomic variations, surgical approach, techniques, and results. J Thorac Cardiovasc Surg 2008;**135**(1):106–16, 116.e1–5.

3. Demos TC, Posniak HV, Pierce KL, *et al.* Venous anomalies of the thorax. *AJR Am J Roentgenol* 2004;**182**(5):1139–50.

4. Ferguson EC, Krishnamurthy R, Oldham SA. Classic imaging signs of congenital cardiovascular abnormalities. *Radiographics* 2007;**27**(5):1323–34.

5. Meadows J, Marshall AC, Lock JE, *et al.* A hybrid approach to stabilization and repair of obstructed total anomalous pulmonary venous connection in a critically ill newborn infant. *J Thorac Cardiovasc Surg* 2006;**131**(4):e1–2.

6. Newman B, Grosse-Wortmann L, Charron M, *et al.* A pitfall of radioisotope quantification of the ratio of pulmonary blood flow to systemic blood flow (Qp/Qs) in a patient with severe post-operative pulmonary venous obstruction. *Clin Nucl Med* 2008;**33**(8):521–4.

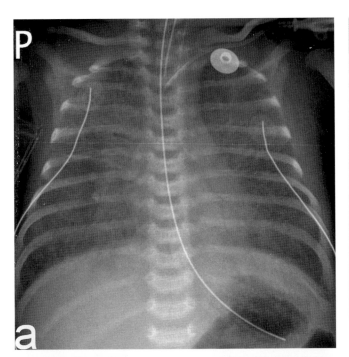

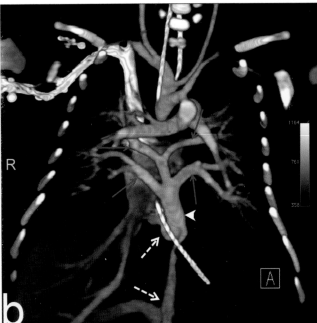

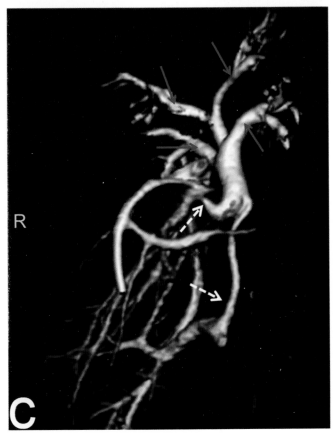

Figure 31.1. Newborn with obstructed infracardiac (type III) total anomalous pulmonary venous return (TAPVR). The patient had severe cyanosis and respiratory distress at birth requiring endotracheal intubation. **(a)** Chest radiograph (AP view) demonstrated diffuse hazy pulmonary opacification and a normal sized cardiac silhouette. This infant was not premature and there were no predisposing factors for sepsis, which led to the diagnostic consideration of obstructed TAPVR. **(b)** CT angiography of the chest. Coronal reformatted thin slab (anterior view) maximum intensity projection demonstrated total anomalous pulmonary veins (blue arrows) converging into a confluent emissary vein (arrowhead) posterior to the left atrium (not seen) and draining inferiorly below the diaphragm. Note two draining sites from the emissary vein into the confluence of the inferior vena cava (IVC) and hepatic veins as well as the portal vein (white arrows). R = right side. **(c)** Subdiaphragmatic venous drainage in type III TAPVR. Post-processed isolation of the TAPVR in the same patient rendered in 3D (right anterior, inferior oblique projection) demonstrated the narrowed connecting vessels to the IVC–hepatic vein confluence and the portal vein (white arrows), which contributed to the obstructing physiology. R = right side.

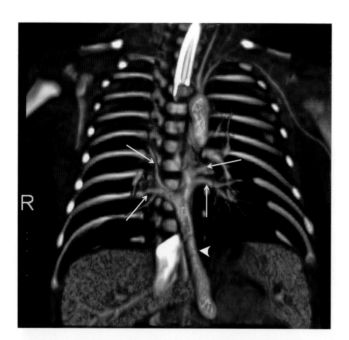

Figure 31.2. Neonate with type III TAPVR associated with complex congenital heart disease and heterotaxia with asplenia. CT angiography, 3D volume rendered reformatting in an anterior projection showing a midline liver and absence of spleen. All pulmonary veins (arrows) converge into an emissary vein (arrowhead), which drains below the diaphragm to the portal vein (not shown). R = right side.

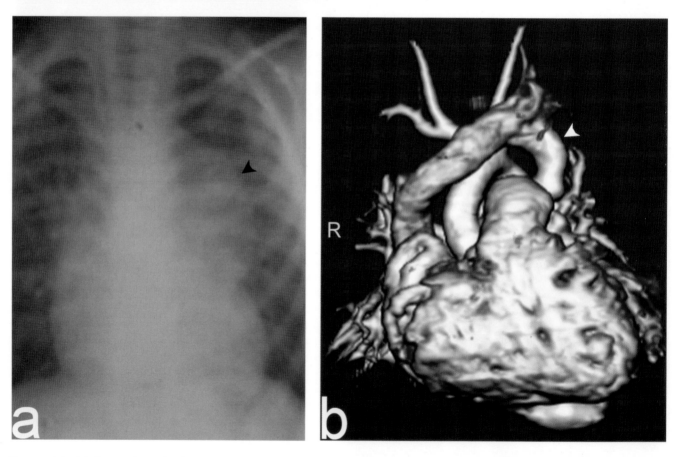

Figure 31.3. **(a)** Chest radiograph of a two-year-old male presenting with pneumonia. PA view demonstrates the "snowman" sign of supracardiac TAPVR (type I), which in this case was unobstructed. Note the large vertical vein silhouette (arrowhead) rising superiorly, over and across the superior mediastinum. **(b)** CT angiography, 3D volume rendered reformatting in an anterior projection showing the vertical vein (arrowhead) rising superiorly, over and across the superior mediastinum, and draining via the left innominate vein into the superior vena cava (SVC). Note the enlarged right ventricle and main pulmonary artery. R = right side.

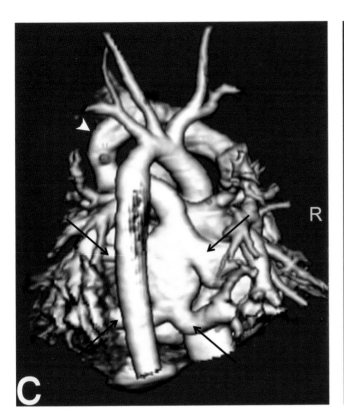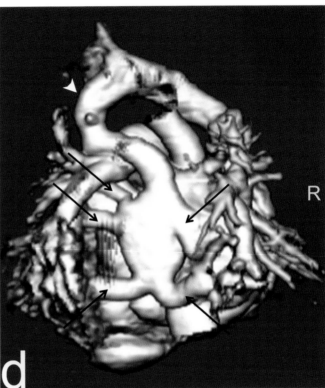

Figure 31.3. (cont.) **(c)** CT angiography, 3D volume rendered reformatting in a posterior projection showing the left vertical vein (arrowhead) rising superiorly, over and across the superior mediastinum, and draining via the left innominate vein to the SVC. Four pulmonary veins (arrows) are discernable from this post-processed view converging into a venous confluence posterior to the left atrium. Note the aortic arch and descending aorta with respect to the pulmonary venous confluence. R = right side. **(d)** CT angiography, 3D-volume rendered reformatting in a posterior projection from the same patient after removal of the aorta from the reformatted image. All five pulmonary veins (arrows) are now visualized draining into the pulmonary venous confluence and from there to the left vertical vein (arrowhead). R = right side.

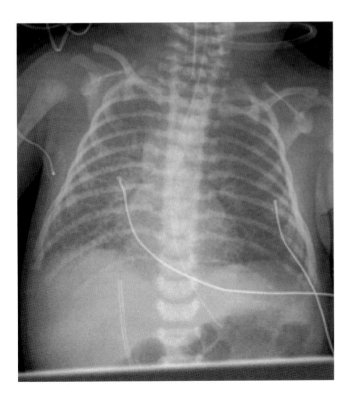

Figure 31.4. Newborn presenting with unexpected severe cyanosis at birth and respiratory distress requiring endotracheal intubation for support. Chest radiograph demonstrates a normal size heart and pulmonary edema with a coarse interstitial pattern. Prenatal care had been uneventful. Cross-sectional imaging demonstrated supracardiac TAPVR with obstruction (not shown).

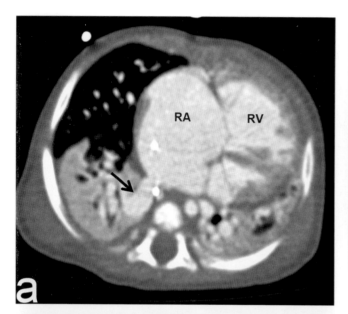

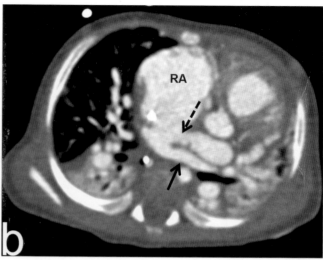

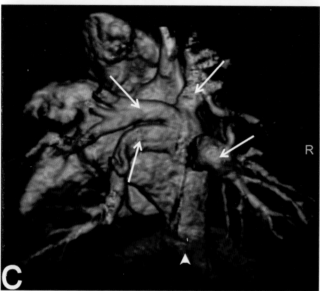

Figure 31.5. CT angiography of a three-month-old boy with cardiac level TAPVR (type II) and unobstructed individual veins draining to the right atrium. Patient had slowly worsening respiratory distress, enlarging cardiac silhouette, and increasing cyanosis. **(a)** Axial CT angiography image at the level of the atria showing right pulmonary vein draining directly (arrow) into the right atrium (RA), which is enlarged. Also note right ventricle (RV) enlargement and relatively small left atrium. **(b)** Axial CT angiography image of the same child showing the left upper lobe pulmonary vein draining directly into the right atrium (solid arrow). An ASD connects the right with the left atrium (dashed arrow). Note anatomic distortion due to enlarged right atrium and its appendage (RA). **(c)** CT angiography, 3D-volume rendered reformatting in a posterior projection. Two right and two left pulmonary veins (arrows) drain all lung lobes directly and unobstructed into the enlarged right atrium. The inferior vena cava is markedly dilated down to the hepatic venous confluence (arrowhead) due to regurgitant flow. R = right side.

Aberrant left coronary artery arising from the pulmonary artery

Beverley Newman

Imaging description

A five-month-old female infant presented with persistent tachypnea and failure to thrive. Frontal and lateral chest radiographs (Fig. 32.1a, b) demonstrated marked cardiomegaly, hyperinflation, and pulmonary venous congestion consistent with cardiogenic pulmonary edema. An echocardiogram was obtained that demonstrated marked left ventricular dilatation with very poor contractility (Fig. 32.1c). No additional abnormality was found. Of note, the coronary origins were thought to be normal on Doppler ultrasound (US), with normal direction of flow (Fig. 32.1d). Additional history, clinical examination, and laboratory investigation failed to reveal an underlying cause for the cardiac dysfunction. A gated CT angiogram was obtained, primarily to confirm that the coronary arteries were indeed normal. The CTA, timed for optimal contrast in the aorta and coronary arteries, demonstrated a single right coronary artery arising from the densely contrast-filled aorta (Fig. 32.1e). The left coronary artery was shown to arise anomalously from the posterior aspect of the pulmonary artery (Fig. 32.1f, g). The relative lack of contrast opacification of the left coronary artery and its branches, similar to the pulmonary artery, confirmed the antegrade flow pattern seen on Doppler. It was hypothesized that chronic hypoxia and pulmonary hypertension resulted in this atypical flow pattern for aberrant left coronary artery arising from the pulmonary artery (ALCAPA). Furthermore, it appeared that the rightward and posterior course of the left circumflex branch close to the aorta produced the appearance mistaken on US for a normal aortic origin of the left coronary artery.

Importance

Early recognition of ALCAPA (aka Bland–White–Garland syndrome) in a young infant with ventricular dysfunction is very important. Unrecognized ALCAPA, along with other congenital coronary anomalies, is an important treatable cause of sudden cardiac death, probably on the basis of ischemia and arrhythmia. Aberrant origin of the right coronary artery (ARCAPA), both coronary arteries, or left anterior descending or circumflex arteries from the pulmonary artery may also occasionally occur (Fig. 32.2).

In utero there is elevated pulmonary vascular resistance and therefore good coronary perfusion irrespective of an aortic or pulmonary coronary origin. Once pulmonary vascular resistance drops, soon after birth, ALCAPA serves as a shunt from the high-pressure systemic circulation to the low-pressure pulmonary circuit via right to left coronary artery connections, tending to bypass the higher resistance coronary capillaries. The result is retrograde flow in the left coronary artery toward the pulmonary artery (Fig. 32.3) and relative cardiac ischemia. If unrecognized or asymptomatic because of adequate coronary supply from the RCA, the coronary arteries become markedly enlarged and tortuous (Fig. 32.3).

Radiographs are usually the first imaging study obtained in a child with cardiac or respiratory symptoms. The presence of cardiomegaly and pulmonary edema suggests an underlying cardiac abnormality. The radiographic features of congestive heart failure in infants and children can be quite subtle. Cardiomegaly is invariable; both frontal and lateral views are helpful to confirm true globular cardiac enlargement versus a normal prominent thymus that can simulate cardiomegaly on an AP view but is anteriorly located on the lateral view (see Case 29, Fig. 29.6). Other helpful features of cardiac congestion in small children include hyperinflation (due to diffuse peribronchial edema and increased secretions causing air trapping), perihilar perivascular indistinctness, and diffuse hazy opacification when alveolar edema is present. Some of the common radiographic findings of congestive heart failure in adults are usually absent or difficult to appreciate in infants, including vascular redistribution, Kerley B lines, and pleural effusion.

Cardiac echocardiography is typically obtained in an infant with a suspected cardiac lesion (Fig. 32.1c, d). This has become a highly sophisticated real-time tool for evaluating detailed cardiac anatomy and function. The thin chest wall and small size of infants creates an ideal acoustic window for the detailed but limited field of view of echocardiography. Visualization of more posterior structures such as the arch and descending aorta and pulmonary arteries and veins may be limited by the adjacent lungs. Even such small vessels as coronary arteries may be visualized on US although US is usually regarded as a screening tool rather than definitive study for coronary evaluation. US visualization of the coronary arteries is less likely to be successful in larger children or adults.

Conventional coronary angiography is still the most definitive method for coronary evaluation but also the most invasive (requires arterial access), with the highest radiation dose. Gated CTA utilizing a modern multidetector (64 slice or greater) CT scanner provides sufficient detail, even in young infants, to evaluate the coronary origins and proximal vessels, with more detailed distal anatomy obtained in cooperative older children and adults (Figs. 32.1, 32.3, 32.4, and 32.5). The disadvantage of CT is exposure to ionizing radiation. Even with careful attention paid to limiting radiation dose, the radiation exposure of a retrospectively gated CTA is approximately four to five times that of a routine chest CT and two to three times that of a non-gated CTA. Newer CT scanners offer prospective gating, differential dose through the cardiac cycle, and ultrafast non-gated CTA techniques that allow for lower dose coronary studies.

MR has the advantage of lack of radiation exposure but affords lower spatial resolution currently, takes much longer, and is seldom adequate for coronary evaluation in young infants. In cooperative older children and adults the coronary origins can be reliably assessed on MR (Fig. 32.2).

Typical clinical scenario

ALCAPA is a rare entity estimated to occur in approximately one in 300 000 births. There are two typical ages of presentation of ALCAPA. Most affected individuals are symptomatic in infancy, often at around two months of age when pulmonary vascular resistance has dropped. Presenting signs and symptoms include congestive heart failure (tachypnea, tachycardia, diaphoresis, irritability, feeding difficulty) and/or a murmur of mitral regurgitation. However, when there is good collateral coronary circulation, ventricular function may be preserved and symptoms may only become manifest later in life with such presentations as chest pain with exercise, syncopal episodes, palpitations, or even sudden death. ALCAPA, along with other coronary anomalies, can occur alone but more commonly coexists with other congenital cardiac lesions (Fig. 32.4), including very complex heart disease.

Without surgical intervention, the mortality rate of ALCAPA is said to be as high as 90%. The early surgical management of ALCAPA consisted of ligation of the left coronary artery at its origin thus preventing the coronary to pulmonary artery steal, with improved cardiac perfusion. Early attempts at coronary reimplantation were typically unsuccessful, usually resulting in left coronary artery occlusion. Modern techniques of coronary reimplantation to the aorta with a vascular plug around the coronary origin have been much more successful. If the left coronary artery is too short to reach the aorta, the Takeuchi aorticopulmonary baffle procedure may be needed.

Differential diagnosis

Other causes of congestive heart failure in infancy include both structural and functional cardiac abnormalities. Structural cardiac lesions that present early in life are most often related to left-sided cardiac obstruction and include hypoplastic left heart, critical aortic stenosis, and critical coarctation or arch interruption. Functional causes of left ventricular failure include myocarditis and congenital or ischemic cardiomyopathies (including perinatal asphyxia, gestational diabetes, and glycogen storage disease), large extracardiac arteriovenous shunts, arrythmias, and metabolic disorders such as anemia, polycythemia, hypoglycemia, or renal dysfunction.

Coronary anomalies can be divided into abnormalities of origin, course, or termination of the coronary vessels. Potentially malignant coronary artery anomalies beyond ALCAPA include aberrant origin of the left (more likely symptomatic) or right coronary artery from the opposite cusp with an interarterial course between the aorta and pulmonary artery (Fig. 32.5), where symptoms are thought to be related to coronary insufficiency and arrhythmia due to a narrowed aberrant coronary orifice and proximal course (often intramural) (Fig. 32.5) as well as increased compression between the great arteries during exercise.

> ## Teaching point
>
> It is important to consider ALCAPA in the context of congestive heart failure in infancy, as well as symptoms of coronary insufficiency later in life. ALCAPA and other coronary anomalies may accompany other structural congenital heart disease. This lesion is eminently treatable by coronary reimplantation, but a severe ischemic cardiac insult may not be reversible and mortality is high without surgical correction. While echocardiographic evaluation is a good screening study for coronary anomalies, it is not foolproof, as in this case. Most cases can be confidently diagnosed by cardiac gated CTA.

REFERENCES

1. Chan FP, El-Helw T. Coronary artery disease in children. In: Slovis T, ed. *Caffey's Pediatric Diagnostic Imaging*, 11th edition. Philadelphia: Mosby Elsevier, 2008; 1648–66.
2. Sahin T, Bozyel S, Acar E, *et al.* A young patient with coronary artery anomaly, whose left anterior descending artery originated from the pulmonary artery, underwent cardiac arrest. *Cardiovasc J Afr* 2012;**23**(8): e15–18.
3. Shriki JE, Shinbane JS, Rashid MA, *et al.* Identifying, characterizing, and classifying congenital anomalies of the coronary arteries. *Radiographics* 2012;**32**(2):453–68.
4. Walsh R, Nielsen JC, Ko HH, *et al.* Imaging of congenital coronary artery anomalies. *Pediatr Radiol* 2011;**41**(12):1526–35.

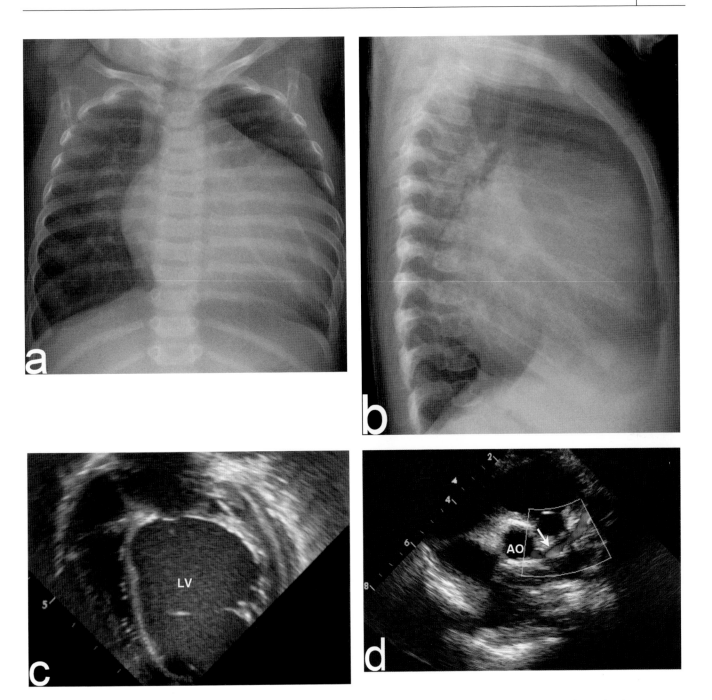

Figure 32.1. A five-month-old girl with failure to thrive and tachypnea (ALCAPA). **(a, b)** Frontal and lateral chest radiographs demonstrate marked cardiomegaly, hyperinflation, and mild pulmonary vascular congestion, indicating cardiogenic pulmonary edema. **(c)** Four-chamber echocardiographic view shows marked dilatation and poor function of the left ventricle (LV). **(d)** Doppler US shows what was thought to be a normal origin of the left coronary artery from the aorta (AO). The normal direction of flow in the left main and anterior descending coronary arteries (arrow) were additional reassuring findings of a normal left coronary artery.

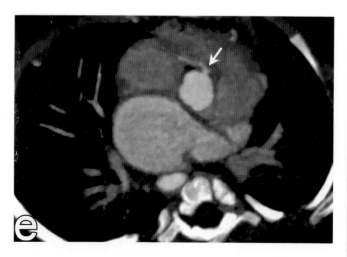

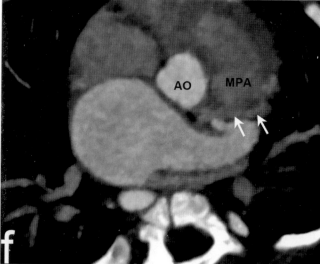

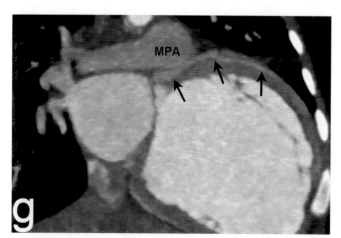

Figure 32.1. (cont.) **(e)** Axial image from a gated coronary CT angiogram demonstrates that only the right coronary artery arises from the AO (arrow). **(f, g)** (f) is a more superior axial image than (e) and the RAO oblique coronal (g) CT angiography images demonstrate the left coronary artery and left anterior descending (LAD) (arrows) arising from the main pulmonary artery (MPA) not the densely contrast-filled AO. Note the lack of contrast in the left coronary similar to the PA indicating forward flow in the left coronary artery as seen on the Doppler US. Typically retrograde flow toward the low-pressure pulmonary system is found in ALCAPA. This unexpected flow pattern was thought to be due to chronic hypoxia and pulmonary hypertension related to congestive heart failure. The left circumflex artery branch extends to the right and posterior (f) close to the AO and was probably responsible for the false US impression of a normal left coronary origin. (Case courtesy of Dr. Gordon Culham, MD, BC Children's Hospital.)

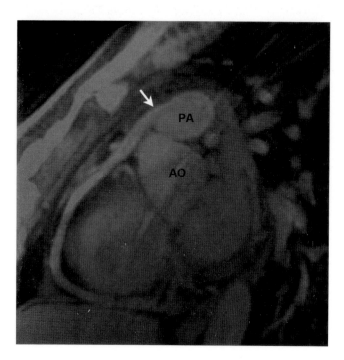

Figure 32.2. A 30-year-old female with palpitations (ARCAPA). Sagittal MIP from a cardiac gated respiratory navigator triggered 3D SSFP MR sequence demonstrates a large right coronary artery (arrow) arising from the PA rather than the AO.

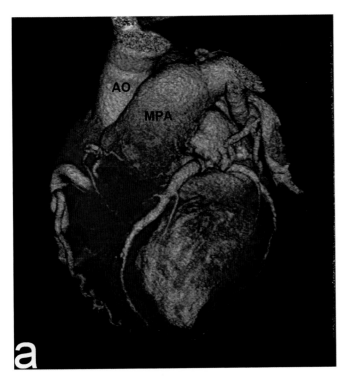
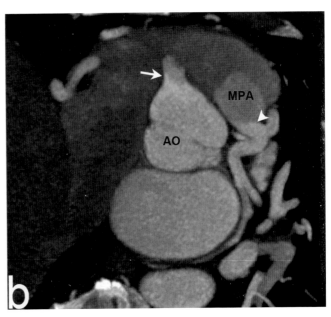

Figure 32.3. A 37-year-old male with chest pain while hiking. **(a, b)** Gated CT angiography volume rendered oblique anterior view (a) and axial reconstructed thin maximum intensity view (b) demonstrate markedly enlarged and tortuous coronary arteries. The right coronary arises normally from the anterior AO (arrow) while the left coronary arises from the posterior MPA (arrowhead). The left to right shunting and flow direction from right to left coronary to PA can be inferred from the large tortuous coronary vessels both containing dense contrast like the AO as opposed to the less densely opacified MPA. Note the bicuspid aortic valve in (b).

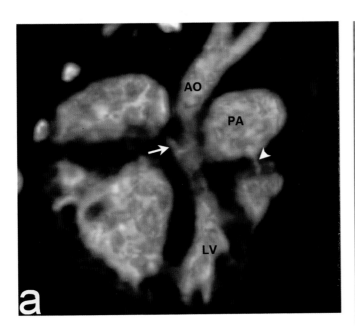
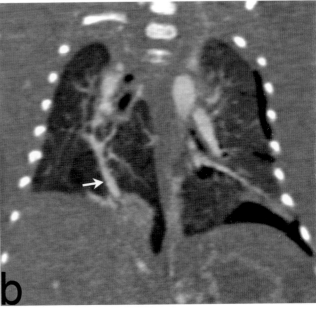

Figure 32.4. Newborn infant with hypoplastic left heart syndrome on cardiac echo and a small right lung on chest radiograph (not shown). Gated CT angiogram obtained for further evaluation also demonstrated scimitar syndrome and ALCAPA. **(a)** Volume rendered oblique coronal reconstruction demonstrates the small left ventricle (LV) and ascending AO. The right coronary artery arises normally from the ascending AO (arrow) while the left coronary arises from the PA (arrowhead). **(b)** Coronal MIP reconstruction demonstrates a small volume right lung with features of scimitar syndrome, including ipsilateral anomalous right pulmonary venous drainage (scimitar vein–arrow) below the diaphragm. There is a small left pneumothorax.

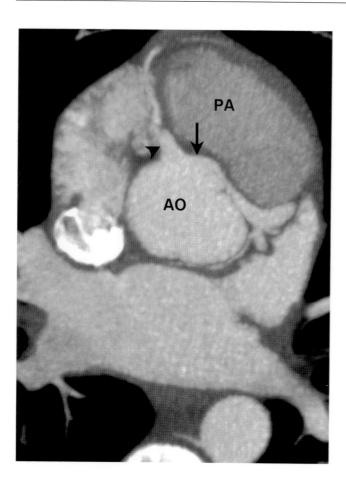

Figure 32.5. A 17-year-old with chest pain on exercise. Aberrant left coronary artery from the right cusp. Gated CTA oblique axial MIP reconstruction demonstrates aberrant origin of the left coronary artery (arrow) from the right anterior aortic cusp adjacent to the right coronary artery (arrowhead). The oblique angle of origin, close apposition of the proximal course to the AO, and mild narrowing proximally suggest an intramural proximal course (in the aortic wall) of the left coronary artery. There is also an interarterial course between the AO and PA. This anatomy allowed for surgical correction by unroofing the intramural left coronary vessel, thus moving the orifice leftward beyond the interarterial pathway, rendering reimplantation unnecessary.

33 Lower extremity ischemia due to homocystinuria

Edward A. Lebowitz

Imaging description

A 19-year-old male presented to the emergency department with gangrene of the right great toe. Figure 33.1 depicts an aortogram and bilateral lower extremity runoff that was obtained the next day. In Figure 33.1a, the nephrograms are abnormal, with atrophy of the right lower pole and contour irregularity in the left mid kidney, which were due to old scarring of uncertain etiology but consistent with either chronic atrophic pyelonephritis, reflux nephropathy, or ischemic infarcts. The aorta and renal, inferior mesenteric, and iliac arteries are normal. Figures 33.1b–d demonstrate occlusion of the right deep femoral artery just distal to its origin, with segmental reconstitution in the mid thigh. Figures 33.1d–i demonstrate occlusion of the right popliteal artery at the adductor canal, with reconstitution of the anterior tibial, posterior tibial, and peroneal arteries distal to the trifurcation. The reconstituted right anterior tibial artery occludes after a short patent segment. The peroneal artery is patent to the ankle where it reconstitutes the anterior tibial artery via the anterior perforating artery. The posterior tibial artery is also patent to the foot, with intact plantar arches to the dorsalis pedis artery. The left lower extremity is normal. Two hundred Units/hour heparin (heparin sodium derived from porcine intestinal mucosa; American Pharmaceutical partners, Los Angeles, CA) was also administered intravenously during this period. No improvement occurred during the infusions, and the patient was brought to the operating room where a right popliteal thrombectomy, saphenous vein patch angioplasty, and proximal popliteal to proximal peroneal artery saphenous vein interposition grafting was performed. Unfortunately, the bypass operation occluded several times over the following four months and cyanosis progressed to include the distal half of the right foot despite multiple tPA infusions and operative revisions. Several months into the patient's course it was recognized that he had a markedly elevated plasma total homocysteine level at 194 μM/L (normal, < 11.4 μM/L), and no cystathionine-β-synthase (CBS) activity in fibroblast tissue (measurement 0.0 nM/h/mg with normal 5.4–18.5). The diagnosis of homocystinuria was made, and vitamins B6, B9, and B12 were added to the aspirin, warfarin, and clopidogrel he was already taking. The plasma homocysteine level fell to 11.1 μM/L within one month of vitamin supplementation. The patient required a forefoot amputation but his bypass graft remained patent for several years.

Importance

Homocystinuria is often unrecognized clinically and therefore untreated. Untreated patients that present with ischemic disease fail to respond to standard pharmacologic, interventional, and operative procedures and instead develop progressive and recurrent arterial occlusion.

Typical clinical scenario

The classic cause of homocystinuria is deficient CBS activity, which is inherited as an autosomal recessive trait and causes homocysteine accumulation in tissues, blood, and urine. When fully expressed, such patients have ectopia lentis, Marfanoid features, osteoporosis, mental retardation, seizures, and psychiatric disease. However, penetrance is variable and patients may, as in this case, display a normal phenotype. Thromboembolism can occur in any vessel at any age and is the most frequent cause of death, which occurs in 25% by 20 years of age and 50% by 30 years of age.

Differential diagnosis

The differential diagnosis of lower extremity ischemia in a young patient includes the following:

1. Emboli from a proximal source.
2. Hypercoagulable state with in situ thrombosis.
3. Buerger disease or other inflammatory arteritis.
4. Fibromuscular dysplasia.
5. Premature atherosclerosis.
6. Drug-induced spasm (ergotism, cocaine, methysergide, vasopressin, catecholamine).
7. Traumatic arterial injury.
8. Spontaneous dissection.
9. Popliteal artery entrapment syndrome.
10. Cystic adventitial disease.
11. Thrombosed popliteal artery aneurysm.

In this patient, traumatic arterial injury, spontaneous dissection, popliteal artery entrapment syndrome, cystic adventitial disease, and thrombosed popliteal artery aneurysm were excluded by the presence of occlusions in the deep as well as the superficial femoral artery distributions. Drug-induced spasm and premature atherosclerosis were excluded by the lack of more general involvement. Angiographic findings of fibromuscular dysplasia and vasculitis were absent, and no proximal source of emboli was identified. Consequently, a hypercoagulable state with in situ thrombosis was the most likely etiology, and homocystinuria was eventually diagnosed and treated.

Teaching point

The biochemical deficiency in homocystinuria is often reversible with relatively inexpensive over-the-counter vitamin supplementation. It should be excluded in any younger patient presenting with a hypercoagulable state, as standard pharmacologic, interventional, and operative treatments are ineffective as long as the hyperhomocysteinemia persists.

REFERENCES

1. Lebowitz EA. SIR 2004 film panel case: gangrene caused by homocystinuria. *J Vasc Interv Radiol* 2004;**15**(9):1013–16.

2. Lobo CA, Millward SF. Homocystinuria: a cause of hypercoagulability that may be unrecognized. *J Vasc Interv Radiol* 1998;**9**(6):971–5.

3. Mudd SH, Levy HL, Kraus JP. Disorders of transsulfuration. In: Scriver CR, Sly WS, Beaudet AL, *et al. The Metabolic and Molecular Bases of Inherited Disease*, vol. 2, 8th edition. New York: McGraw-Hill Medical Publishing Division, 2001; 2007–56.

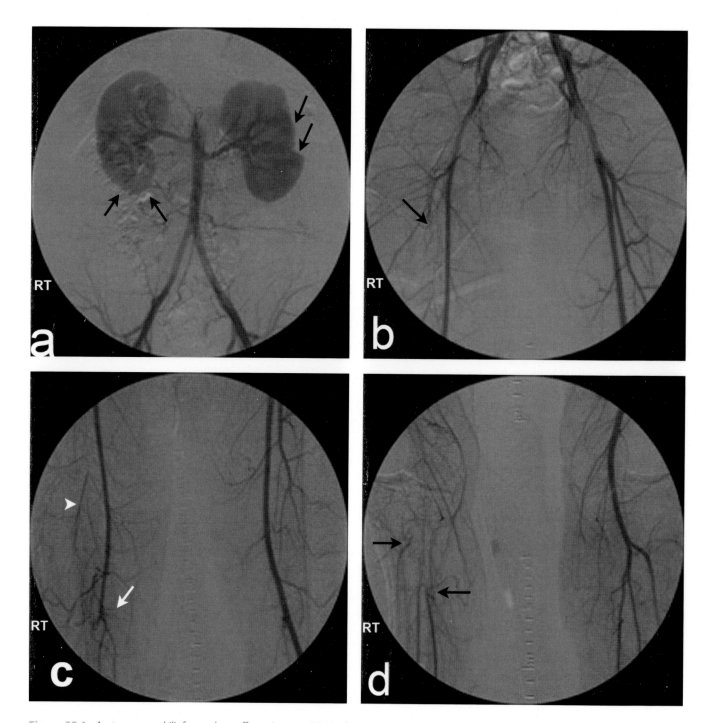

Figure 33.1. Aortogram and iliofemoral runoff arteriogram. (a) Nephrograms indicate atrophy of the right lower pole and contour irregularity in the left mid kidney (arrows) but arteries are normal. (b) Normal origin of the right deep femoral artery (arrow). Occlusion of the right deep femoral artery just distal to its origin (arrow). (c) Segmental reconstitution of the right deep femoral artery (arrowhead) and occlusion of the right popliteal artery at the adductor canal (arrow). (d) Geniculate collateral arteries supply the leg (arrows). Reconstitution of the right anterior tibial artery (lateral arrow), the peroneal artery, and the posterior tibial artery (medial arrow) in the upper calf.

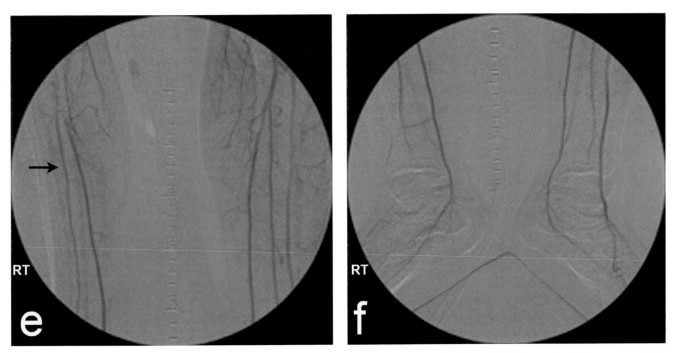

Figure 33.1. (cont.) **(e, f)** Patent right peroneal and posterior tibial arteries the entire length of the calf. Right anterior tibial artery occludes after a short patent segment.

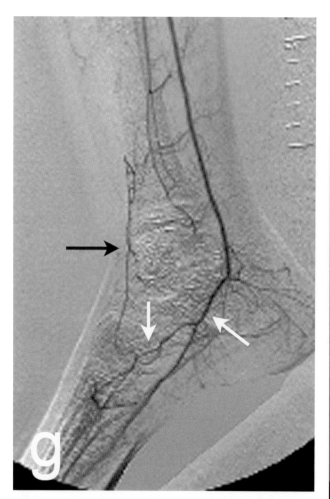

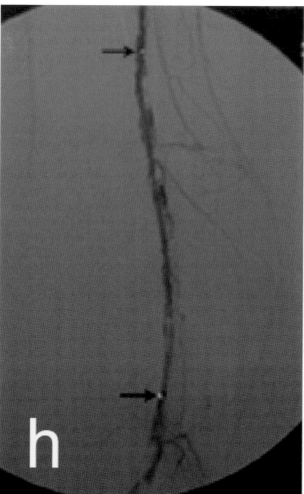

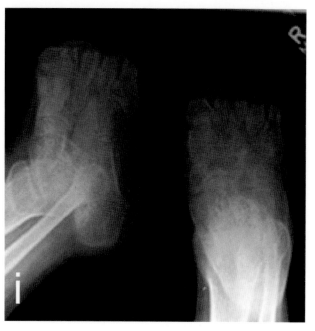

Figure 33.1. (cont.) **(g)** Reconstitution of the distal right anterior tibial artery and dorsalis pedis artery (black arrow) and patent distal posterior tibial artery and plantar arches (white arrows). The left lower extremity runoff is normal in all images. **(h)** Irregular filling defects consistent with thrombus are present throughout the right popliteal artery. Infusion of tissue plasminogen activator (tPA) between the catheter markers (arrows) for approximately 24 hours was without benefit. **(i)** Plain images of right foot status post forefoot amputation. (Reprinted from *Journal of Vascular and Interventional Radiology*, Vol. **15**(9), Lebowitz EA, SIR 2004 film panel case: Gangrene caused by homocystinuria, Pages 1013–6, Copyright 2004, with permission from Elsevier.)

Edward A. Lebowitz

Imaging description

Figures 34.1a and b are chest radiographs obtained following placement of a peripherally inserted central catheter (PICC) by a nurse at the bedside. On the basis of this radiograph, the nurse withdrew the PICC to position its tip at the junction of the superior vena cava and right atrium. Figure 34.1c is a portable abdominal radiograph for nasogastric tube placement obtained 8 days after PICC insertion. Figure 34.1d is an AP portable chest radiograph obtained 9 days after PICC insertion. When this was compared to the earlier chest radiographs, the vertical linear metallic density projecting over the heart was noted. In retrospect, the bottom of this density could be seen at the same location on the abdominal radiograph (Fig. 34.1c). This triggered the AP and cross-table lateral chest radiographs depicted in Figures 34.1e and f, which confirmed the presence of an intrapulmonary foreign body. A CT scan showed that the foreign body was located in a branch of the left pulmonary artery rather than in the left lower lobe bronchus or lung (Fig. 34.1g.) Unbeknownst to the nurse doing the procedure, the guidewire had broken off at the time of PICC insertion and the central guidewire fragment remained in the catheter when the rest of the guidewire was removed, which is noted in retrospect only on close examination of Figures 34.1a and b. At some point between the chest radiograph in Figure 34.1a and the abdominal radiograph 8 days later, the guidewire fragment embolized out of the catheter, through the heart, and into the left lower pulmonary artery branch.

Importance

Catheters of many different types are inserted into hospitalized patients every day, and practitioners may not be aware of complications when they occur. As such, discovery of the complication is often remote from when the procedure was performed and recognizing it is the responsibility of the radiologist reviewing later images (Fig. 34.2). Unfortunately, as in this case, the retained foreign body may look like an artifact and be disregarded. Clinical signs of catheter or guidewire embolization include catheter malfunction, arrhythmia, infraclavicular and shoulder region pain, ipsilateral upper extremity paresthesia, pulmonary symptoms, and sepsis, although about 25–40% are asymptomatic.

Typical clinical scenario

With the rare exception of bullet fragments that enter the vascular system and embolize from their entry point, intravascular foreign bodies are always iatrogenic. The present case, in which the foreign body was recognized remote from the insertion, represents a common clinical scenario. Other common scenarios include the following:

1. A guidewire or catheter may embolize into the patient at the time of insertion (Fig. 34.2).
2. A central venous catheter may pass through the thoracic inlet beside rather than through the subclavian vein with the hard ligaments in the costoclavicular space that surround it, wearing the catheter down until the catheter breaks in a condition known as "pinch off syndrome" (Fig. 34.3). "Pinch off syndrome" sometimes manifests itself with a kink in the catheter where the first rib and clavicle cross each other on the chest radiograph, and, if present, is an indication to remove the catheter before it fractures. Unfortunately, it may still fracture at the time of removal, as in Figure 34.3.
3. A port catheter may disconnect from a port reservoir, which can occur spontaneously (Fig. 34.4) or, more often, at the time of port removal.

In each of these scenarios, the central fragment may either stay in place as in Figure 34.3, or embolize centrally to the heart as in Figure 34.5, or pulmonary arteries as in Figures 34.1 and 34.4.

The interventional radiologist is asked to deal with these patients using endovascular techniques as the alternative may require a major operation. In the retrieval procedure, venous access is obtained, and a wire with a lasso-like snare at the internal end is positioned so the catheter or guidewire fragment passes through the snare loop. The catheter through which the snare-wire is inserted is then cinched down on the snare-wire to grasp the foreign body tightly. The catheter, snare-wire, and foreign body are then pulled together out of the patient's body (Fig. 34.5.) The vein through which access is obtained to perform the procedure depends on the position of the foreign body and is at the discretion of the interventional radiologist. Sometimes the catheter fragment is positioned so that neither end is floating free in which case it needs to be moved with another catheter before it can be ensnared. Also, in the retrieval procedure the foreign body may be dislodged from a stable position by the snare-wire and embolize farther. When that happens, it must be retrieved from the new location.

Differential diagnosis

Artifacts have variable appearances depending on their cause and may be modality specific. They are ubiquitous, and although we strive to eliminate them, this seems to be impossible. Many patients have large numbers of catheters and tubes as well as overlying equipment and it is easy to overlook a subtle finding. In order to avoid false-positive and false-negative interpretations, the radiologist has to carefully scrutinize the images and decide whether an unexpected opacity represents an artifact or pathology. This may require additional imaging with a new cassette, different projection, different technique, removing the patient's clothes, etc. However, in the case of a retained intravascular foreign body, the diagnosis is obvious once you realize that what you are looking at is not an artifact.

Teaching point

Recognition of intravascular foreign bodies is a challenge because they may look like artifacts or parts of medical wires or equipment. Two orthogonal radiographic views are essential to ascertain whether the density is abnormal and whether it is truly located in rather than outside of the patient. Once recognized, intravascular foreign bodies are retrieved using interventional endovascular techniques because surgery is more invasive and because of the potential for future complications even if the patient is asymptomatic at the time of discovery.

REFERENCES

1. Cahill AM, Balla D, Hernandez P, Fontalvo L. Percutaneous retrieval of intravascular foreign bodies in children. *Pediatr Radiol* 2012;**42**:24–31.
2. Hinke DH, Zandt-Stastny DA, Goodman LR, *et al.* Pinch off syndrome: a complication of implantable subclavian venous access devices. *Radiology* 1990;**177**:353–6.
3. Lin CH, Wu HS, Chan DC, *et al.* The mechanisms of failure of totally implantable central venous access system: analysis of 73 cases with fracture of catheter. *Eur J Surg Oncol* 2010;**36**:100–3.
4. Surov A, Wienke A, Carter JM, *et al.* Intravascular embolization of venous catheter – causes, clinical signs, and management: a systematic review. *JPEN J Parenter Enteral Nutr* 2009;**33**:677–85.

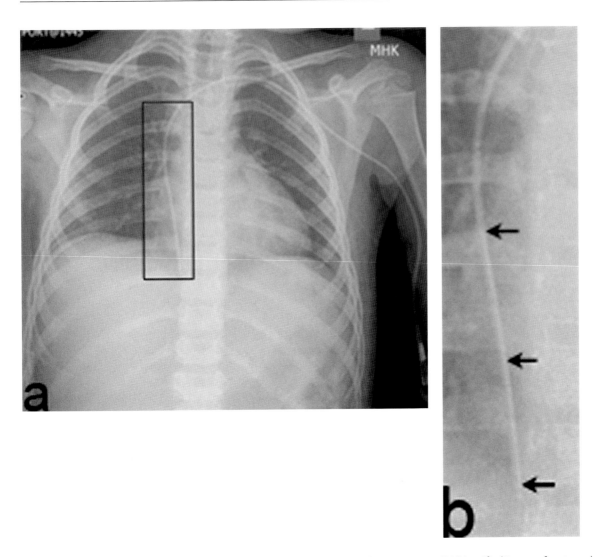

Figure 34.1. **(a)** AP portable chest radiograph following PICC placement for positioning. **(b)** Magnified image of rectangular area in (a). Arrows point to a retained fragment of guidewire within the distal PICC. This was not appreciated at the time.

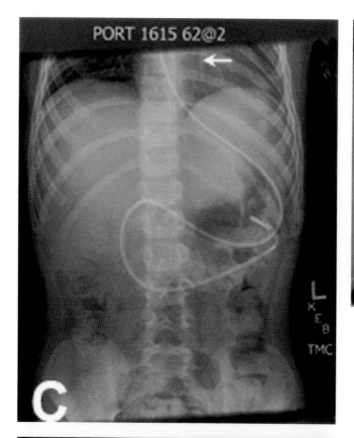

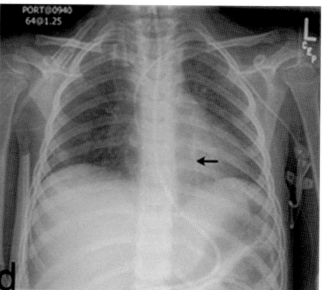

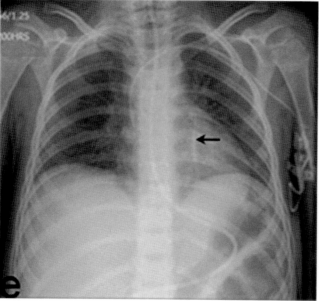

Figure 34.1. (cont.) **(c)** AP portable abdominal radiograph 8 days following prior chest radiograph with the following history: five-year-old male patient. Nasogastric tube placement. History of complicated migraines. Arrow points to embolized guidewire fragment, which was not recognized at the time. **(d)** AP portable chest radiograph obtained 1 day after abdominal radiograph depicted in (c). The history on the requisition was "five-year-old male with probable meningitis." A foreign body (arrow) was suspected, so AP and cross-table lateral chest radiographs were requested. **(e, f)** AP and cross-table lateral portable chest radiographs confirm the presence of a linear metallic foreign body in the left lung (arrows). Note the similarity in appearance of the foreign body with the tip of the metallic guidewire retained in the PICC in parts (a) and (b). **(g)** CT sagittal reconstruction in the plane of the retained guidewire fragment shows the intravascular rather than intrabronchial location.

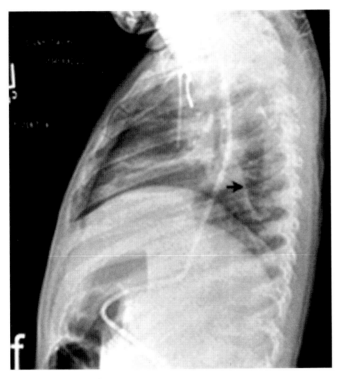

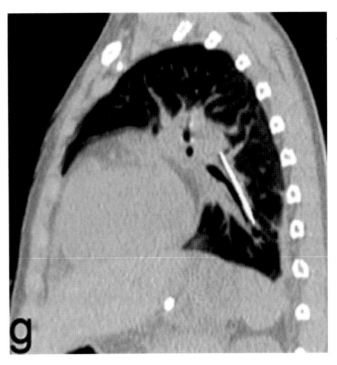

Figure 34.1. (cont.)

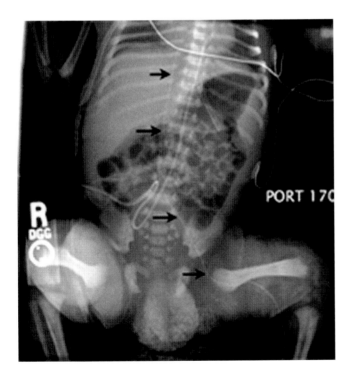

Figure 34.2. PICC placed via left ankle in an eight-day-old neonate inadvertently cut and no longer visible externally.

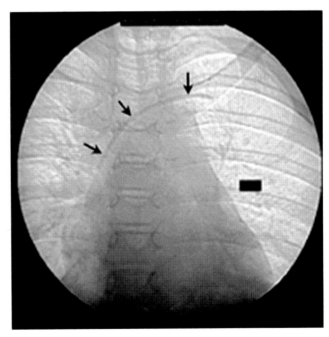

Figure 34.3. Catheter fragment retained after removal of port catheter due to "pinch off syndrome" at thoracic outlet (arrows).

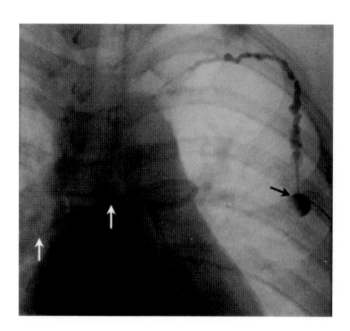

Figure 34.4. Port injection to evaluate patient's complaint of pain with port infusions. Port accessed with Huber needle (black arrow) and injected with contrast medium. Fluoroscopic image shows the tract leading from the port to the left subclavian vein filled with contrast medium. Catheter had detached from port and embolized centrally to straddle the pulmonic valve, with its tip in the right pulmonary artery (white arrows).

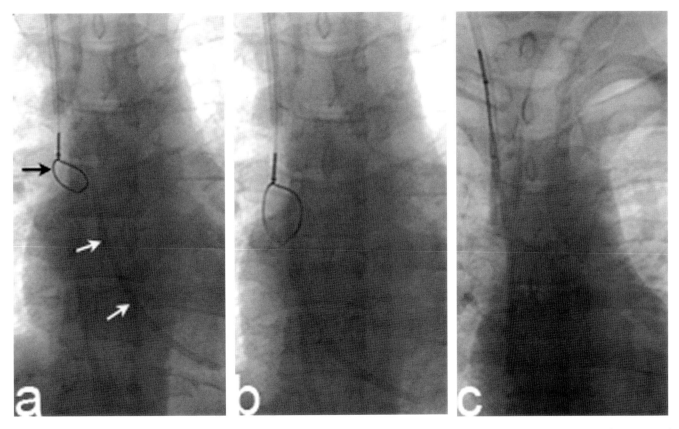

Figure 34.5. Three fluoroscopic images from an endovascular interventional retrieval procedure. (a) Snare (black arrow) approaching retained catheter fragment (white arrows) which straddles the tricuspid valve. (b) Snare engages the upper end of the catheter fragment and is subsequently slid down to surround a point closer to the middle. (c) After cinching the catheter down the snare-wire to grasp the foreign body tightly, everything is pulled out of the patient.

Fibromuscular dysplasia

Edward A. Lebowitz

Imaging description

A 10-year-old boy was discovered to be hypertensive. At ultrasound (US) imaging, as in this child (Fig. 35.1a, b), unilateral renal artery stenosis may demonstrate asymmetry of renal size, with atrophy of the affected and compensatory hypertrophy of the contralateral kidney (Fig. 35.1a, b). Doppler imaging within the kidney typically demonstrates absence of an early systolic velocity peak, a slow systolic upstroke in velocity (long acceleration time), and in consequence a delayed peak systolic velocity with increased diastolic flow, known as the "tardus and parvus" pattern. This finding is seen in the segmental intrarenal vessels downstream from the site of stenosis. The effect on peak systolic flow velocity is variable, depending on where you interrogate; normally peak velocity drops progressively along the course of the renal artery towards the kidney. However, unless flow is critically obstructed, flow velocity is elevated at the stenosis (typically peak velocity in excess of 200 cm/s), and spectral widening due to turbulence is present just distal to the stenosis (Fig. 35.1 c–e). Published criteria for the diagnosis of renal artery stenosis also include elevated peak systolic velocity in the renal artery compared to the adjacent aorta (>3.5 cm/s) and excessive difference in resistive index, which is calculated as (peak systolic velocity–end diastolic velocity)/peak systolic velocity between the two kidneys. The resistive index and resistive index ratio was normal in this patient, reflecting the difficulty in the practical application of this variable. In general, while US is a reasonable screening study for renal artery stenosis, US and Doppler imaging may be normal, especially with milder degrees of stenosis. At CTA (Fig. 35.1f, g) and MRA imaging, which was not obtained in this patient, the location and nature of the arterial stenosis are seen to advantage. Catheter angiography is usually necessary only when interventional/endovascular treatment is going to be attempted. The focal nature of the stenosis, lack of aneurysm formation, and responsiveness to angioplasty (Fig. 35.1) is most consistent with the perimedial fibroplasia type of fibromuscular dysplasia (FMD). Other common angiographic findings of FMD are depicted in a different patient in Figure 35.2.

Importance

Eight to ten percent of hypertensive children have a renovascular etiology as compared to only 1% of hypertensive adults. As in this case, the underlying cause may be amenable to endovascular treatment. Consequently, it is important to recognize the imaging findings.

Typical clinical scenario

Unless one of the important sequelae of hypertension has supervened, most of these patients will be discovered incidentally at either physical examination or clinical evaluation for an unrelated cause.

Differential diagnosis

FMD has been divided by histopathology into five types, which include medial fibroplasia (60–70%), perimedial fibroplasia (15–25%), medial hyperplasia ($<1\%$), intimal fibroplasia ($<10\%$), and adventitial (periarterial) hyperplasia (rare). Each type has a characteristic angiographic appearance, with only medial fibroplasia, the most common, having the classic aneurysmal "string of beads" appearance (Fig. 35.2). FMD may cause unilateral or bilateral main renal artery stenosis or affect only a single segmental renal arterial branch. Other arteries are often affected by FMD as well (Fig. 35.2). Neurofibromatosis is another common cause of renovascular hypertension in children, and since it may have a similar imaging appearance to FMD, other stigmata or genetic markers of neurofibromatosis should be sought. Takayasu disease, another common cause of renovascular hypertension, is a vasculitis that causes thickening of the aortic wall, which may either narrow the entire aorta in midaortic syndrome, or the renal arteries at their origins, either of which may cause renovascular hypertension. Other inflammatory vasculitides may also affect the renal arteries and must be considered in the differential diagnosis. Arterial injury due to trauma, radiation, or anastomotic stenosis of a transplanted renal artery is also in the differential diagnosis, although a specific history would be expected.

Teaching point

Renovascular hypertension is more common in hypertensive children than hypertensive adults. The radiologist should therefore be familiar with the imaging findings, appropriate modalities, and potential for endovascular/interventional treatment.

REFERENCES

1. Bayazit AK, Yalcinkaya F, Cakar N, et al. Reno-vascular hypertension in childhood: a nationwide survey. Pediatric Nephrol 2007;22:1327–33.

2. Foster BJ, Bernard C, Drummond KN. Kawasaki disease complicated by renal artery stenosis. Arch Dis Child 2000;83:253–5.

3. Hughes RJ, Scoble JE, Reidy JF. Renal angioplasty in nonatheromatous renal artery stenosis: technical results and clinical outcome in 43 patients. Cardiovasc Intervent Radiol 2004;27:435–40.

4. Li J, Yan Y, Wei Q, et al. Evaluation of the Tardus-Parvus pattern in patients with atherosclerotic and nonatherosclerotic renal artery stenosis. J Ultrasound Med 2007;26:419–26.

5. Mena E, Bookstein JJ, Holt JF, Fry WJ. Neurofibromatosis and renovascular hypertension in children. AJR Am J Roentgenol 1973;118:39–45.

6. Osborn AG, Anderson RE. Angiographic spectrum of cervical and intracranial fibromuscular dysplasia. Stroke 1977;8:1862–71.

7. Owen CA. *Ultrasound Evaluation of Renal Artery Stenosis.* http://www.gehealthcare.com/usen/ultrasound/education/products/cme_ren_art.html.
8. Slovut DP, Olin JW. Current concepts: fibromuscular dysplasia. *N Engl J Med* 2004;**350**:1862–71.
9. Tublin ME, Bude RO, Platt JF. The resistive index in renal doppler sonography: where do we stand? *AJR Am J Roentgenol* 2003;**180**:885–92.
10. Wiggelinkhuizen J, Cremin BJ. Takayasu arteritis and renovascular hypertension. *Childhood Pediatr* 1978;**62**:209–17.

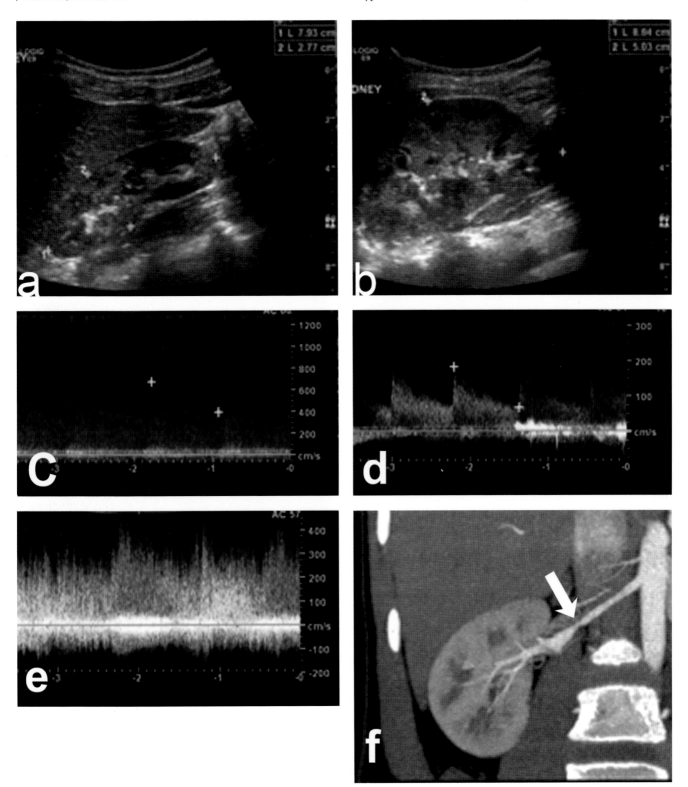

Figure 35.1. Longitudinal US images demonstrate asymmetric renal size, with atrophy of the right (a) and compensatory hypertrophy of the left (b) kidneys. (c–e) Doppler ultrasound images of the abnormal right renal artery (c, e) and the normal left renal artery (d).

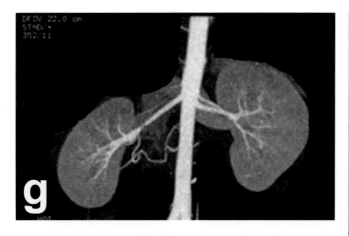
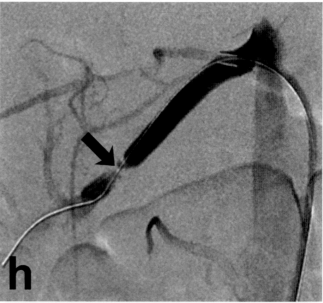
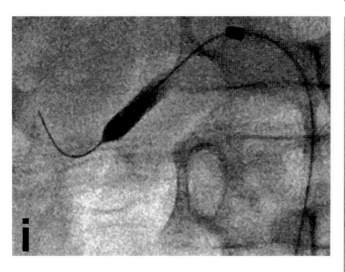
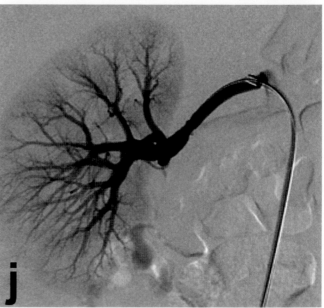

Figure 35.1. (cont.) Note the extremely high velocity, absence of an early systolic peak, and long acceleration time in (c) which was obtained at the level of the stenosis, compared to (d). Note the disorganization of the wave form due to turbulent flow just distal to the stenosis in (e). (f, g) Depicts a coronal CT image (f) in which a tight stenosis (arrow) of the mid-to-distal right renal artery is present. MIP image (g) also demonstrates the discrepant renal sizes and right renal artery stenosis to advantage. The aorta is normal, and there are two left renal arteries, which represents a normal variant. (h) Pre-angioplasty right renal arteriogram with the guidewire across the stenosis (arrow) demonstrates a focal, tight stenosis without aneurysmal dilatation, and although two small "beads" are present it does not qualify as a "string of beads." (i) Angioplasty balloon inflated at stenosis. (j) Post-angioplasty arteriogram demonstrates residual irregular intimal margins, but no residual obstruction and normal flow to the right kidney.

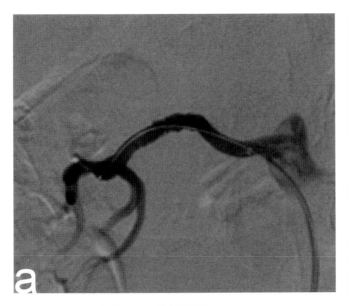

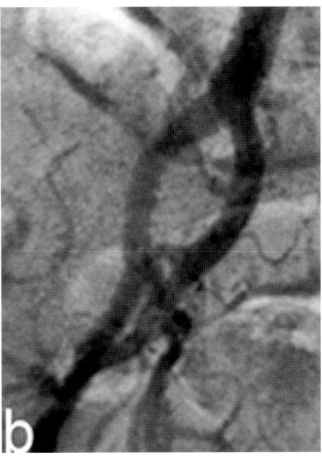

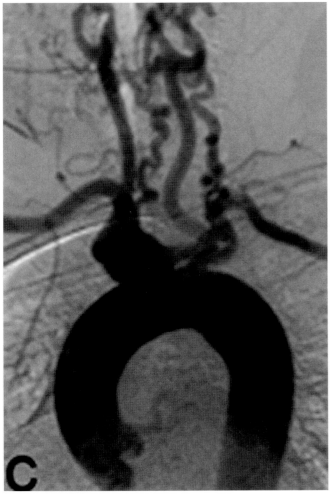

Figure 35.2. Angiographic appearance in a different patient with medial fibroplasia and classic "string of beads" appearance in distal right renal artery (a) and right external iliac artery (b) The same patient also has an aneurysmal innominate artery and extreme tortuosity/redundancy of the vertebral arteries (c).

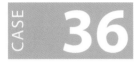

Traumatic vertebral arteriovenous fistulae

Edward A. Lebowitz

Imaging description

A 19-year-old boy was brought to the emergency room following a gunshot wound to the right neck. Figure 36.1a is an axial slice from a CTA at the C2/C3 level that demonstrates bullet fragments along a trajectory from the posterolateral entrance wound through the right facet joint. In addition to subcutaneous emphysema, facet fractures, and bullet fragments, there is a subtle asymmetry of the epidural venous plexus, with enhancement on the right compared to the left. Axial time of flight MRA demonstrated a filling defect (thrombus) in the right vertebral artery in the mid neck (Fig. 36.1b). A diagnosis of traumatic dissection/transection of the right vertebral artery with associated traumatic arteriovenous fistula was suggested. Interventional radiology was consulted for embolization. Figure 36.2 depicts images from the initial pre-embolization brachiocephalic arteriogram that confirm both the right vertebral artery occlusion and arteriovenous fistulae. During the course of metallic coil embolization of the traumatized arteries that fed the arteriovenous fistulae, multiple injections were made into branch arteries. Of note, the occluded right vertebral artery itself did not supply the fistulae (Fig. 36.2d.) However, injections into the right deep cervical, distal right ascending cervical artery, proximal right ascending cervical, right common carotid, right ascending pharyngeal, and right occipital arteries all showed early filling of the epidural venous plexus and each feeding branch was embolized with metallic coils.

Figure 36.2e demonstrates resolution of the early opacification of the epidural venous plexus that had been present prior to coil embolization. Figure 36.3 demonstrates recurrence of the arteriovenous fistulae 10 days later due to partial recanalization of the right vertebral artery, which then fed them. Figure 36.4 demonstrates that the arteriovenous fistulae no longer filled following coil embolization of the right vertebral artery. Figure 36.5 demonstrates that no instability of the cervical spine is present two years following injury. Figure 36.6 depicts findings in a different patient with spontaneous vertebral artery dissection.

Importance

Penetrating trauma in children has reached epidemic proportions, accounting for 10–20% of pediatric trauma admissions in most centers. Spinal cord trauma due to gunshot wounds accounts for approximately 15% of spinal cord injuries overall. Of note, however, in a 2001 review of over 100 admissions for cervical spine injuries in children, none was attributed to a gunshot wound. That gunshot wounds to the spine occur is no surprise and is mentioned in an article detailing the pediatric neurosurgical experience at a United States field hospital in

Iraq in 2007. The etiologies of such injuries may be divided among accidental (often involving children's access to loaded guns in the home environment), intentional (often gang-related), and war zone injuries (host-country civilian children hit by shrapnel or in the line of fire). Rapid transport to specialized trauma centers on the home front and sophisticated field operating rooms in war zones bring many of these patients to medical attention within minutes of injury. As such, early treatment is possible but depends on recognition of treatable complications and availability of interventional and surgical options. Ongoing treatment of the victims occurs over decades, as a quadriplegic injured at 20 years of age has a mean life expectancy of almost 60 years of age.

Typical clinical scenario

With penetrating trauma, the diagnostic problems are not with etiology but with extent of injury. The time from injury to arriving at the hospital is an important variable affecting outcome. Once in the hospital and following a comprehensive trauma evaluation and resuscitation, CT and MRI scans will be obtained. Patients may require emergency operative treatment, as this patient did, from additional gunshot wounds to the chest, but since imaging evaluation can provide important diagnostic information, it is obtained unless the patient is hemodynamically unstable. Patients with severe cervical spine injuries will likely be quadriplegic as this patient was, although his deficit was incomplete and he complained mainly of right upper extremity weakness at discharge several weeks later. A cervical spine series obtained two years later showed no instability or migration of embolization coils (Fig. 36.5).

The arterial supply to the cervical spinal cord is complex, with one anterior and two posterior spinal arteries arising from the vertebral arteries at the base of the skull and descending on the surface of the spinal cord. In addition, one to six radicular arteries enter the cervical intervertebral foramina at multiple levels bilaterally between C2 and T1 and supply the spinal cord through natural anastomoses with the anterior spinal artery. Although 80% of the cervical radicular arteries branch from the vertebral arteries, reported origins also include the deep cervical, superior intercostal, and ascending cervical arteries. However, as numerous anastomoses exist among the cervical, vertebral, and carotid branches, flow will pass from one vascular territory to another under certain conditions.

The selective advantage of a rich network of collateral arteries supplying the spinal cord is obvious; however, in the present case the low-pressure sump of the traumatic arteriovenous fistulae caused them to fill from many sources. The abnormal hemodynamics would be expected to affect the injury in multiple ways. First, the sump effect of the fistulae could affect flow in the spinal arteries themselves, potentially causing an ascending level of deficit by stealing flow from levels above the injury. Second, increased pressure in the epidural venous plexus could cause cord edema and venous stasis with potential thrombosis in stagnant small veins. Third, diversion of flow from the injured bones and soft tissues could interfere with healing. Recognition of the vascular component of injury followed by treatment may therefore forestall clinical deterioration. In this case, the occluded right vertebral artery was obvious on CTA, but the abnormal arteriovenous connections that led to torrential flow through the veins draining the cervical spinal cord required a studied approach by the radiologist on a busy trauma service.

Coil embolization of the arteries that supplied the arteriovenous fistulae could be done safely because of the robust arterial anastomotic network throughout this region. Coils are sized to occlude the arteries and stay in place. Ischemic complications secondary to non-target embolization and arterial occlusion are unlikely as the coils will not migrate from these locations and distal collaterals can supply the vascular territory beyond the coils albeit at a lower pressure. Embolization must extend above and below the origins of the arteries supplying the fistulae. If embolization is limited to the arterial segments proximal to the fisulae, the distal collaterals would continue to fill the fistulae by retrograde flow. Injection of particulate or liquid embolic agents would be riskier than coil embolization because of the potential for ischemic complications due to non-target embolization, especially through dangerous anastomoses between the external and internal carotid artery branches.

Since the left vertebral artery could also have supplied the arteriovenous fistulae through its connection to the distal right vertebral artery, this was assessed by angiography (Fig. 36.3a) and found not to be the case. If this had been present, then a much more dangerous embolization of the distal right vertebral artery by passage of a catheter from the left vertebral artery into the right vertebral artery proximal to the origin of the right posterior inferior cerebellar artery and spinal arteries would have been considered. As left vertebral artery filling was adequate with the left subclavian artery injection (Fig. 36.3a) no catheter had to be placed into the left vertebral artery and thus the likelihood of catheter-induced dissection or spasm that would have been devastating was minimized.

Differential diagnosis

With penetrating neck injury the issue is to evaluate the nature and extent of injuries. Differential diagnosis is usually not relevant although occasionally underlying lesions may confound the evaluation of acute trauma.

Aside from penetrating injuries, vertebral artery injury or dissection may occur from non-penetrating trauma such as seat belt injury or spontaneously. As in this case, as long as the normal anatomy of the right and left vertebral arteries joining

to form the basilar artery is present, flow to the brain is preserved following unilateral vertebral artery dissection. However, ischemia can occur if thrombi formed in the dissected artery embolize distally. For this reason, patients with spontaneous vertebral artery dissection are treated with coagulation inhibitors. An example of this is present in another case (Fig. 36.6) in which the patient presented with occipital headache. MRI (Fig. 36.6a) demonstrated a small left cerebellar infarct due presumably to an embolus into the ipsilateral posterior inferior cerebellar artery, which appeared patent on angiography.

> ## Teaching point
>
> The vascular supply to the cervical spinal cord is complex. Spontaneous or traumatic injuries that affect the supplying arteries and veins to the spine in the neck need to have detailed CT or MR angiographic imaging with careful attention paid to detail to allow for prompt and appropriate management to minimize long-term sequelae. Particularly in the case of penetrating neck injury, multiple arteries and veins may be affected and therapeutic embolization needs to address this.

REFERENCES

1. American Academy of Pediatrics, Committee on Injury and Poison Prevention. Firearm-related injuries affecting the pediatric population. *Pediatrics* 2000;**105**:888–95.

2. Brown RL, Brunn MA. Cervical spine injuries in children: a review of 103 patients treated consecutively at a Level 1 pediatric trauma center. *J Pediatr Surg* 2001;**36**:1107–14.

3. Cotton BA, Nance ML. Penetrating trauma in children. *Semin Pediatr Surg* 2004;**13**:87–97.

4. Hall JR, Reyes HM, Meller JL, Loeff DS, Dembek RG. The new epidemic in children: penetrating injuries. *J Trauma* 1995;**39**:487–91.

5. Hoeft MA, Rathmell JP, Monsey RD, Fonda BJ. Cervical transforaminal injection and the radicular artery: variation in anatomical location within the cervical intervertebral foramina. *Regional Anesth Pain Med* 2006;**31**:270–74.

6. Lasjaunias P, Berenstein A, ter Brugge KG. Craniocervical junction. In: *Surgical Neuroangiography Volume 1: Clinical Vascular Anatomy and Variations*, 2nd edition. Berlin: Springer-Verlag, 2001; 165–260.

7. Li G, Baker SP, DiScala C, *et al.* Factors associated with the intent of firearm-related injuries in pediatric trauma patients. *Arch Pediatr Adolesc Med* 1996;**150**:1160–5.

8. Martin JE, Teff RJ, Spinella PC. Care of pediatric neurosurgical patients in Iraq in 2007: clinical and ethical experience of a field hospital. *J Neurosurg Pediatr* 2010;**6**:250–6.

9. The National SCI Statistical Center, 1717 6th Avenue South, Room 515, Birmingham, AL 35233–7330. *Spinal Cord Injury Facts and Figures at a Glance*. https://www.nscisc.uab.edu. February, 2010.

10. Seshadri R, Goodman D. Prehospital time and outcome in pediatric trauma (Academy of Health Meeting, 2004, San Diego, CA). *Abstr Academy Health Meet* 2004; **21**:abstract no. 1017.

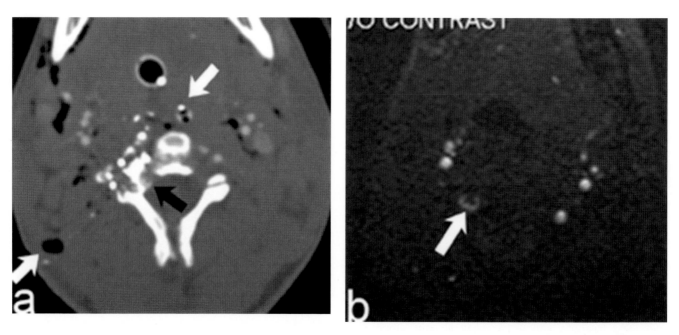

Figure 36.1. (a) Axial contrast-enhanced CT scan through the neck demonstrates bullet and bone fragments along a trajectory through the right-sided cervical facet joint (between white arrows), scattered pockets of air, and asymmetric enhancement of the right epidural venous plexus (black arrow). (b) Axial MRA (time of flight sequence, mid neck) demonstrates a filling defect in the right vertebral artery (white arrow).

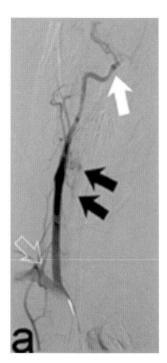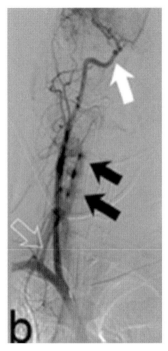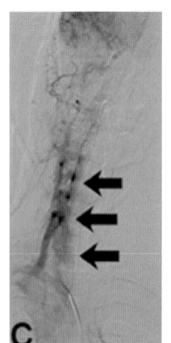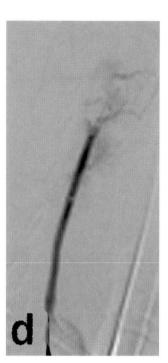

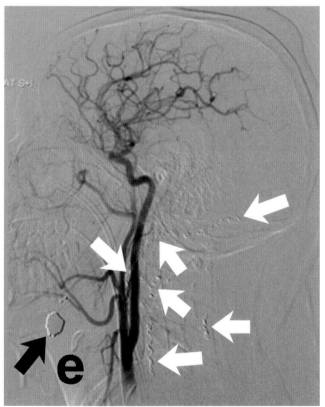

Figure 36.2. Right brachiocephalic arteriogram in early arterial (a), mid arterial (b), and venous (c) phases. Early opacification (black arrows) of the paraspinous venous plexus indicates that acute traumatic arteriovenous fistulae are present. Flow to the brain through the right internal carotid artery is present (white arrows). The proximal right vertebral artery fills, but no opacification of the distal right vertebral artery is present, indicating occlusion due to traumatic dissection and thrombosis (open arrows), better shown with a selective arteriogram of the right vertebral artery (d). Note the occluded vertebral artery does not supply the fistulae at this time. (e) Completion right common carotid arteriogram after embolization of multiple small neck arterial branches supplying the arteriovenous fistulae. There are numerous embolization coils (white arrows) and a bullet fragment (black arrow) but no residual filling of arteriovenous fistulae.

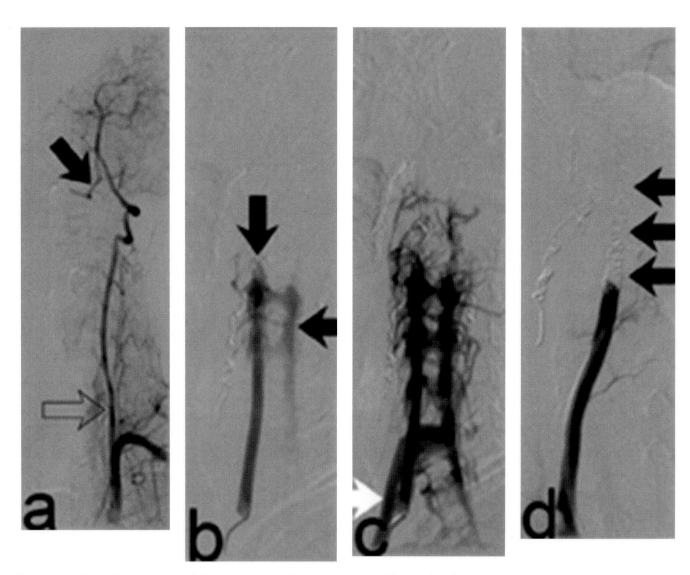

Figure 36.3. **(a)** 10 days later. Left subclavian arteriogram demonstrates normal flow to the left vertebral artery (open arrow), basilar artery, and retrograde filling of distal right vertebral artery (black arrow) with no early venous filling. **(b)** Early arterial phase of right vertebral arteriogram shows rapid filling of epidural venous plexus due to arteriovenous fistulae (black arrows). **(c)** Later phase of right vertebral arteriogram demonstrates intense opacification of the epidural venous plexus and draining vein (white arrow) with lack of flow to the distal right vertebral artery. **(d)** Right vertebral arteriogram post-coil-embolization (arrows) demonstrates no further flow to the arteriovenous fistulae.

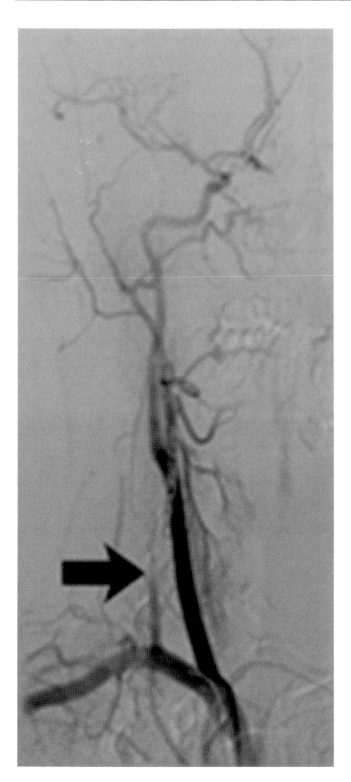

Figure 36.4. Brachiocephalic arteriogram post-embolization demonstrates lack of filling beyond the most proximal segment of the right vertebral artery (arrow) and no further flow to the arteriovenous fistulae, which did not recur. Compare to pre-embolization images in Figure 36.2b.

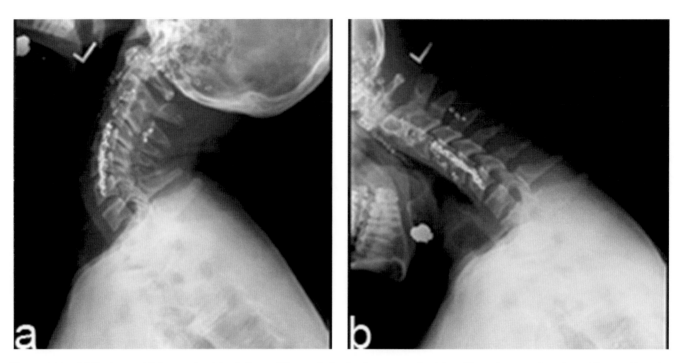

Figure 36.5. **(a)** Flexion and **(b)** extension lateral views of the cervical spine two years after injury. Normal range of motion without subluxation or migration of embolization coils.

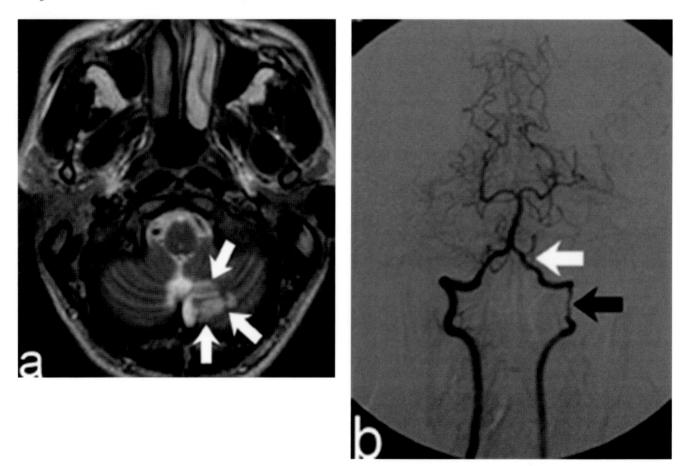

Figure 36.6. **(a)** Axial T2-weighted MRI image through the low posterior fossa in a different patient shows increased signal intensity due to infarction in the inferomedial cerebellum (arrows). **(b)** Narrowing of the left vertebral artery at the V3 segment is typical for spontaneous vertebral artery dissection (black arrow). The ipsilateral posterior inferior cerebellar artery is patent (white arrow).

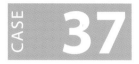

Colonic perforation during intussusception reduction

Edward A. Lebowitz

Imaging description

Figure 37.1 depicts abdominal radiographs obtained in a 14-week-old boy with vomiting and abdominal pain. Figure 37.2 depicts one image from an ultrasound study, which confirmed the diagnosis of intussusception. The patient proceeded immediately to the fluoroscopically guided pneumatic enema reduction shown in Figure 37.3. During the course of this procedure, the diagnosis was confirmed, but just as it appeared that the intussusception was reduced, a popping noise was audible. Insufflation was stopped and the pressure on the sphygmomanometer released based on the appearance at fluoroscopy (Fig. 37.3). On inspection and palpation, the patient's abdomen was massively distended and as hard as a board. A hypodermic needle was inserted into the peritoneal cavity percutaneously, and this was exchanged over a guidewire for a 6 French locking pigtail drainage catheter through which the pneumoperitoneum was aspirated (Fig. 37.4). The patient then went to the operating room where the surgeon noted that the intussusception had been reduced. There were several serosal tears in the small bowel and colon, and there was a 1 cm perforation in the sigmoid colon, which otherwise was normal. As no gross contamination of the peritoneal cavity was present and the patient appeared well, the perforation was repaired and the area irrigated. The patient did well postoperatively.

Importance

Colonic perforation can occur either as part of the natural history of intussusception or as a complication of enema reduction. The incidence of perforation as a procedural complication is reported to be between 1% and 3%. In the present case, the patient developed a tension pneumoperitoneum. Tension pneumoperitoneum is an uncommon but well-recognized complication of gastrointestinal perforation. It results following the rapid accumulation of free air within the peritoneal cavity leading to increased intra-abdominal pressure. Tension pneumoperitoneum is a life-threatening complication that requires emergency treatment. It causes respiratory compromise due to the inability of the diaphragm to move downward, inferior vena caval compression, decreased venous return to the heart, and if pressures exceed systolic arterial pressure can even cause aortic compression. Prompt recognition and treatment are essential to prevent cardiac and respiratory arrest.

Typical clinical scenario

Intussusception occurs when one segment of bowel peristalses telescopically into the segment distal to it. The recipient segment is called the intussuscepiens, and the distally malpositioned bowel is called the intussusceptum. Sometimes there is a polypoid mass such as lymphoma or Meckel diverticulum that serves as lead point, but in typical early childhood ileo-colic intussusception, no obvious pathologic lead point is present other than prominent Peyer's patches in the terminal ileum. There are large numbers of articles written about intussusception, as a query into Pubmed will show. However, the clinically relevant problems can be summarized as: (1) when to suspect it, (2) how to confirm it, and (3) how to treat it.

The problem with diagnosis is the non-specific nature of the presenting findings, which include vomiting, bilious vomiting, abdominal pain and/or tenderness including peritoneal signs, lethargy and/or irritability, palpable abdominal mass, pallor and/or sweating, blood per rectum and/or currant jelly stool, diarrhea, constipation, poor feeding, fever, and abdominal distention. How to sort out who should get advanced imaging to exclude intussusception is important because every pediatric emergency department sees many children with some of these signs and symptoms every day; it is neither cost-effective nor safe to perform a contrast or pneumatic enema reduction on all of them.

Ultrasound scans have proven to be close to 100% sensitive to the diagnosis of intussusception in multiple studies. Such data have led many radiologists to adopt the policy that no enema reduction will be attempted prior to obtaining a positive ultrasound scan. As this reduces the number of unnecessary fluoroscopies, it would seem to be universally acceptable. However, it has been shown that typical clinical findings, such as abdominal pain, lethargy, and vomiting, together with a highly suggestive abdominal radiograph have almost as high a sensitivity as ultrasound, so not everyone agrees on the need for an ultrasound scan in all cases before attempting enema reduction. This controversy may become moot as so-called point-of-care (POC) ultrasound, which is a sonographic imaging procedure by an emergency physician on a patient in the emergency department, becomes more commonplace. One case report documents the diagnosis of intussusception in this manner. The need for a horizontal beam radiograph to exclude a pneumoperitoneum is still necessary as perforation is an absolute contraindication to attempting an enema reduction.

How to treat intussusception is not controversial; enema reduction is the standard. Although some papers have suggested that enema reduction is more or less likely to succeed based on duration of symptoms, presence of small bowel dilatation and air/fluid levels, fluid between layers within the ultrasound target sign, or other imaging signs, in practice most radiologists will attempt an enema reduction in anyone with intussusception that is not dehydrated, hypotensive, septic, or already perforated, which includes the overwhelming majority. The patient, of course, may require fluid resuscitation first.

Barium enema reduction with the rule of threes – three feet high, three minutes, three times–was standard for many years, but air, saline, or isotonic water-soluble iodinated contrast medium are less likely to exacerbate peritonitis if perforation occurs, so barium is no longer used. Whether you use isotonic iodinated contrast medium or air at fluoroscopy or normal saline at ultrasound depends on how comfortable you feel with the techniques. Pneumatic enema reduction is safest with slow rather than abrupt insufflations and pressures below 120 mmHg. Pressures may rise transiently above this level with crying, but these elevations raise pressure on both sides of the bowel wall so do not increase the likelihood of perforation. Straining may even facilitate reduction. Successful enema reductions of idiopathic intussusception are accomplished in approximately 80–90% of cases. Recurrence rates are approximately 4–10%; enema reduction can frequently be achieved a second or occasionally even a third time although consideration might be given to the greater likelihood of an underlying lesion and whether surgery is appropriate.

When perforation occurs during pneumatic enema reduction, the radiologist will likely continue to insufflate the colon before realizing that there is free peritoneal air. Your first reaction may be to suction the enema tube with a catheter tip syringe, or remove the tube when you cannot aspirate the pneumoperitoneum this way. However, the perforation tends to act like a one-way valve, letting the air into the peritoneal space but not back into the colon, so aspirating the enema tube or removing it is insufficient for decompression. The colon can be somewhat decompressed quickly by reversing the three-way stopcock or disconnecting the enema tubing. However, it is more critical to decompress the peritoneal cavity when a tension pneumoperitoneum is present. Such patients should be punctured under fluoroscopic guidance with a hypodermic needle, preferably large gauge, from an anterior approach to avoid the liver and bowel. An angiocatheter or locking pigtail drainage tube is safer, as the plastic catheters will not cause damage to the viscera that a metallic hypodermic needle could. This should all be done as soon as you realize perforation has occurred. Do not send the patient back to the ward, emergency department, clinic, or operating room before decompressing a tension pneumoperitoneum. Obviously, following perforation, operative repair of the colon is urgent even if the intussusception is reduced as in the current patient.

How perforations occur is controversial. In some cases, the enema reduction may uncover a perforation that is already present but tamponaded by the intussusceptum. In the current case, however, the perforation occurred in the sigmoid colon several minutes after this segment had been opened and distended with air. Moreover, the area surrounding the perforation did not appear ischemic or otherwise abnormal on inspection at surgery. As such, one must conclude that the perforation was a direct result of the transmural pressure applied. With injection of air into the body, there is always the potential that the air will go somewhere other than where you intended and the consequences may be dire. For example,

cardiopulmonary arrest during pneumatic reduction of an intussusception was reported in an eight-month-old and was associated with portal venous gas. Although unproved, the arrest may have been due to an air embolus to the heart and pulmonary arteries.

Differential diagnosis

The imaging in this case is very convincing and the next appropriate step is a diagnostic and hopefully therapeutic enema. The imager should not, however, fixate on a single diagnosis and should always consider other possibilities. There are a few entities that can mimic an intussusception on ultrasound imaging and a few important diagnostic pitfalls. A perforated appendix with phlegmon or abscess can quite closely mimic the appearance of an intussusception on ultrasound imaging (see Case 44). The age of the child and clinical symptomatology may help differentiate. Another possible mimic is thick-walled bowel such as may be seen in infectious or inflammatory enterocolitis, where an enema may be contraindicated.

Transient ileoileal intussusception is frequently seen incidentally on CT and may also be found on ultrasound imaging. This entity is usually benign but can be significant when the intussuscepted segment is longer than 2.5 cm and the child is symptomatic. It may be difficult to tell whether an intussusception is in the colon or small bowel on ultrasound. Even when clinically symptomatic this form of intussusception as well as the ileoileal intussusception associated with Henoch–Schonlein purpura may not be amenable to enema reduction.

Idiopathic intussusception is most common in childhood between 3 months and four years of age. Intussusception in older children should not be considered idiopathic and a pathologic lead point should be sought. Enema reduction may not be appropriate if a mass is suspected and exploratory surgery is needed. Similarly, intussusception in a neonate is very uncommon and more likely to be associated with an underlying lesion.

Teaching point

Intussusception reduction is a common procedure in hospitals that treat infants. The radiologist should have a large bore angiocatheter readily available in case of emergency and should know what to do to treat a tension pneumoperitoneum promptly.

Infants undergoing intussusception reduction may be quite ill. It is important that the child has intravenous access in place and it is probably a good idea for an additional trained medical professional to be present to monitor the child during transport as well as the reduction procedure. This is not an appropriate function for the parent and the procedural radiologist's concentration will be on the reduction procedure and fluoroscope. The surgical service should always be aware of an intussusception reduction attempt and be immediately available in the event of a complication.

REFERENCES

1. Applegate KE. Intussusception in children: evidence-based diagnosis and treatment. *Pediatr Radiol* 2009;**39**(Suppl 2):S140–3.

2. Blanch AJM, Perel SB, Acworth JP. Paediatric intussusception: epidemiology and outcome. *Emerg Med Aus* 2007;**19**:45–50.

3. Carey JL, Napoli AM. Tension pneumoperitoneum during routine colonoscopy. *Am J Emerg Med* 2012;**30**(1):261.e1–2.

4. England RJ, Pearse RG, Murthi GV. Tension pneumoperitoneum: bedside management and safe transfer. *Acta Paediatr* 2009;**98**:897–8.

5. Halm BM, Boychuk RB, Franke AA. Diagnosis of intussusception using point-of-care ultrasound in the pediatric ED: a case report. *Am J Emerg Med* 2011;**29**:354.e1–3.

6. Henrikson S, Blane CE, Koujok K, *et al.* The effect of screening sonography on the positive rate of enemas for intussusception. *Pediatr Radiol* 2003;**33**:190–3.

7. Khan MJ, Khan K, Kaleem M, *et al.* Retrospective analysis of clinical presentation of children with diagnosed intussusception. *J Postgrad Med Inst* 2007;**21**:151–3.

8. Maoate K, Beasley SW. Perforation during gas reduction of intussusception. *Pediatr Surg Int* 1998;**14**:168–70.

9. Mendez D, Caviness AC, Ma L, Macias CC. The diagnostic accuracy of an abdominal radiograph with signs and symptoms of intussusception. *Am J Emerg Med* 2012;**30**(3):426–31.

10. Olinde AJ, Maher JM. Tension pneumoperitoneum: a cause of acute aortic occlusion. *Arch Surg* 1983;**118**:1347–50.

11. Ryan ML, Fields JM, Sola JE, Neville HL. Portal venous gas and cardiopulmonary arrest during pneumatic reduction of an ileocolic intussusception. *J Pediatr Surg* 2011;**46**:e5–8.

12. Shiels WE II, Maves CK, Hedlund GL, Kirks DR. Air enema for diagnosis and reduction of intussusception: clinical experience and pressure correlates. *Radiology* 1991;**181**:169–72.

13. Verschelden P, Filiatrault D, Garel L, *et al.* Intussusception in children: reliability of US in diagnosis – a prospective study. *Radiology* 1992;**184**:741–4.

14. Weihmiller SN, Buonomo C, Bachur R. Risk stratification of children being evaluated for intussusception. *Pediatrics* 2011;**127**:e296–303.

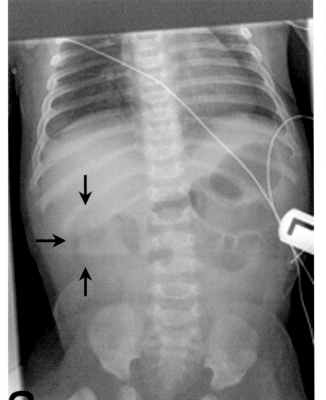

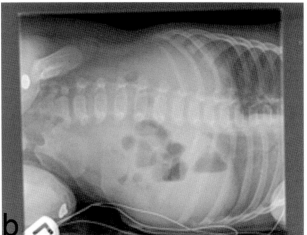

Figure 37.1. Supine (a) and left lateral decubitus abdomen (b) demonstrate gas in the stomach and mildly dilated proximal small bowel in which there are a few air/fluid levels. "Crescent" sign (black arrows), which is caused by a small amount of air in the colon outlining the distal margin of the intussusceptum, is present. No gas is present distally in the colon or rectum, and there is no pneumoperitoneum. The lung bases are clear, and the diaphragm is in normal position.

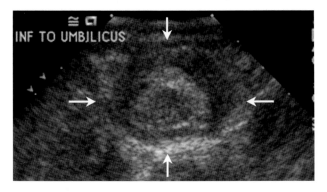

Figure 37.2. Transverse ultrasound image in lower abdomen shows the variously named "pseudokidney," "doughnut," or "target" sign. These designations refer to the oval-shaped mass with concentric layers of contrasting echogenicity demarcated by the white arrows. This confirmed the clinical and radiographic suspicion of intussusception. In the typical ileocolic intussusception, the target comprises from outermost to innermost the uninvaginated colon, called the intussuscipiens, and the invaginated colon, ileum, and attached mesenteric fat, called the intussusceptum.

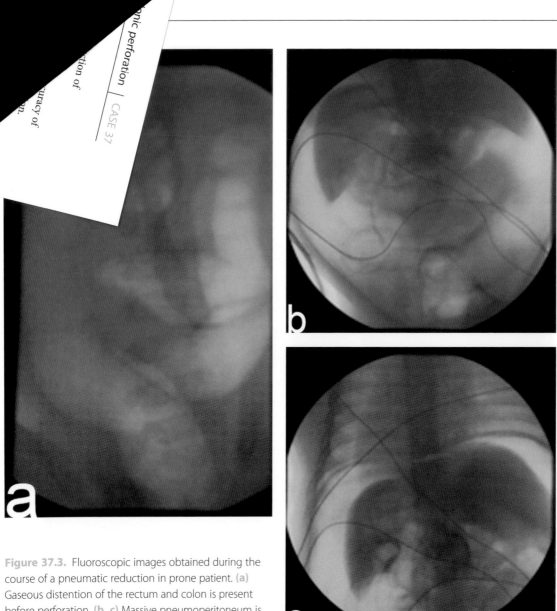

Figure 37.3. Fluoroscopic images obtained during the course of a pneumatic reduction in prone patient. (a) Gaseous distention of the rectum and colon is present before perforation. (b, c) Massive pneumoperitoneum is present.

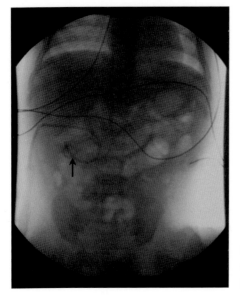

Figure 37.4. Supine fluoroscopic spot image after decompression and complete aspiration of tension pneumoperitoneum. The locking pigtail drainage tube (arrow) was left in place as the patient was transferred to the operating room.

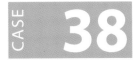
38 Juvenile nasopharyngeal angioma

Edward A. Lebowitz

Imaging description

A 17-year-old boy presented with recurrent prolonged epistaxis. Axial contrast-enhanced CT (Fig. 38.1a) demonstrates an enhancing mass centered at the posterolateral wall of the left nasal cavity and extending in all directions. Bony remodeling is present with posterolateral displacement of the left pterygoid plate, contralateral deviation of the nasal septum, widening of the left sphenopalatine foramen through which the tumor extends into the pterygopalatine and infratemporal fossae, and widening of the posterior nasal aperture through which the tumor extends into the pharynx. Sagittal contrast-enhanced CT (Fig. 38.1b) demonstrates bony destruction of the anterior wall of the sphenoid sinus, filling of the nasopharynx, and extension into the oropharynx. Fluid fills the obstructed left maxillary sinus, but the sphenoid sinus is filled with enhancing tumor. The bony remodeling indicates chronicity, and the bony destruction indicates the locally invasive nature of the tumor. Figure 38.2 demonstrates no tumor opacification on angiographic injection of the left internal carotid artery. A right internal carotid artery injection was similarly negative for tumor enhancement. These injections also demonstrated that the origins of the ophthalmic arteries were from the distal cavernous segments of the internal carotid arteries, which is typical. Figure 38.3a is a pre-embolization left external carotid arteriogram that demonstrates a dense tumor blush. On more selective angiograms, multiple branches of both the left and right external carotid arteries supplied the tumor. Figure 38.3b demonstrates a post-embolization left external carotid arteriogram in which there is abrupt cut-off of embolized arteries and the tumor blush seen in Figure 38.3a is absent. Figure 38.4 demonstrates the resected tumor mass in the same orientation as in the sagittal CT and lateral angiographic images. The demographics, CT, and angiographic appearance are characteristic of a juvenile nasopharyngeal angiofibroma (JNA), and pathology confirmed this diagnosis.

Importance

Epistaxis occurs frequently in children and is usually treated with digital pressure until the bleeding stops. Rarely, bleeding may be recurrent or difficult to stop, and these cases may come to the radiologist's attention for diagnosis and possible treatment. Systemic causes of epistaxis such as coagulopathy will not be diagnosed radiologically, but anatomic causes should be obvious on cross-sectional imaging with CT or MRI.

Typical clinical scenario

Juvenile nasopharyngeal angiofibroma is a benign but locally invasive tumor that almost always occurs in adolescent boys. Presenting symptoms include epistaxis, nasal congestion, pain, snoring, hearing loss, facial deformity, proptosis, and fever from obstructive sinusitis. Intracranial and cavernous sinus extension with cranial nerve compression can also occur. This patient presented to the emergency department for epistaxis that had lasted over 24 hours; however, this was not his first episode of epistaxis, and on questioning and physical examination many of the above signs and symptoms were also present. The mass was obvious on physical examination, which would be expected in such a large lesion. However, smaller lesions could present with epistaxis without being as easy to see on physical exam.

According to the Surgical Pathology Atlas Imaging Database, JNAs are "composed of thin-walled vessels of varying caliber in a mature connective tissue stroma. The vessels typically have a single endothelial cell lining without a muscularis layer, which probably explains the tumors' propensity for hemorrhage." The diagnosis of JNA is not usually confirmed by biopsy prior to definitive surgery because of its hemorrhagic tendency. Instead, preoperative angiography is usually requested. The blood supply of large JNAs by multiple branches of the external carotid arteries bilaterally, as in this case, is common. A dense tumor blush is also characteristic of JNAs, therefore rhabdomyosarcoma, lymphoma, and nasopharyngeal carcinoma should be considered if the angiograms do not show the prominent vascularity present here. Although controversial for smaller JNAs, larger JNAs such as this one usually undergo preoperative embolization in order to minimize blood loss and facilitate operative resection. Embolization may be performed by direct intratumoral injection of embolic materials or by the transarterial route used in this case. Prior to beginning transarterial embolization of the feeding external carotid artery branches, the internal carotid circulation should be evaluated at angiography to exclude true intracranial extension, as this affects resectability, and to avoid blindness due to inadvertent embolization of an ophthalmic artery, which sometimes takes origin from a middle meningeal artery that also supplies the tumor.

To ensure adequate tumor devascularization in the face of the robust collateral network in this region, most interventionalists prefer to embolize with small particles or liquid embolic agents that extend the occlusion to small arteries or arterioles within the tumor tissue rather than simply occluding the larger feeding arteries proximal to the tumor. Although experienced interventionalists can do such procedures safely, particulate or liquid embolic agents increase the risk of non-target embolization, which means that embolic material is deposited into arteries supplying normal structures rather than the targeted vessels. This can occur because of retrograde flow of embolic material that can occur when antegrade flow in the targeted artery slows or stops because of embolic material already deposited, or because the arteries that supply the tumor also supply normal structures or have anastomoses with arteries that do. In the case of JNAs, non-target embolization in the external circulation may cause ischemia or infarction of the tongue, throat, face, orbit, and cranial nerves. Even more importantly, however, embolic materials deposited in the external circulation may flow into the internal circulation through "dangerous" anastomoses that connect branches of the external and internal carotid arteries and thereby cause infarction in the brain.

Differential diagnosis

Solid tumors that affect this region of the head and neck in children include hemangioma, teratoma, nerve sheath tumors, juvenile nasopharyngeal angiofibroma, Langerhans cell histiocytosis, rhabdomyosarcoma, nasopharyngeal carcinoma, lymphoma, and metastatic disease. However, considering the age, sex, symptoms, and imaging appearance in this patient, the diagnosis of JNA is virtually conclusive.

Simple enlargement of the adenoids can be very prominent, however is more common in younger children, tends to have smooth borders and similar enhancement and continuity with the posterior pharyngeal wall. Retropharyngeal cellulitis or abscess is also seen in a younger demographic and usually presents with clinically distinct symptoms, and typically edema/fluid attenuation/signal on CT or MR imaging with or without a discrete abscess.

Teaching point

Juvenile nasopharyngeal angioma should be suspected in the clinical presentation of severe epistaxis in an adolescent boy. Its presence, location, and extent can readily be confirmed on contrast-enhanced CT or MR imaging. Preoperative embolization of this very vascular tumor, especially when large, is often undertaken. There are several pitfalls in this procedure with potentially disastrous consequences including inadvertent occlusion of ophthalmic or internal carotid branches. These are related to atypical vascular supply or anastomoses that require particular knowledge, experience, and care on the part of the interventional radiologist performing the procedure.

REFERENCES

1. Bleier BS, Kennedy DW, Palmer JN, et al. Current management of juvenile nasopharyngeal angiofibroma: a tertiary center experience 1999–2007. Am J Rhinol Allergy 2009;23:328–30.
2. Borghei P, Baradaranfar MH, Borghei SH, Sokhandon F. Transnasal endoscopic resection of juvenile nasopharyngeal angiofibroma without preoperative embolization. ENT J 2006;85:740–3.
3. Gemmete JJ, Ansari SA, McHugh J, Gandhi D. Embolization of vascular tumors of the head and neck. Neuroimaging Clin N Am 2009;19:181–98.
4. Lasjaunias P, Berenstein A, eds. Nasopharyngeal tumors. In: Surgical Neuroangiography 2 – Endovascular Treatment of Craniofacial Lesions. Berlin: Springer-Verlag, 1987; 101–26.
5. Liu Q, Rhoton AL Jr. Middle meningeal origin of the ophthalmic artery. Neurosurgery 2001;49(2):401–7.
6. Robson CD. Imaging of head and neck neoplasms in children. Pediatr Radiol 2010;40:499–509.
7. Surgical Pathology Atlas Imaging Database: http://www.surgicalpathologyatlas.com/glfusion/mediagallery/media.php?f=0&sort=0&s=20091201122528541.
8. Wu AW, Mowry SE, Vinuela F, Abemayor E, Wang MB. Bilateral vascular supply in juvenile nasopharyngeal angiofibromas. Laryngoscope 2011;121(3):639–43. doi: 10.1002/lary.21337.

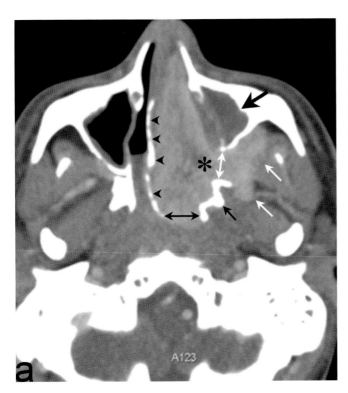
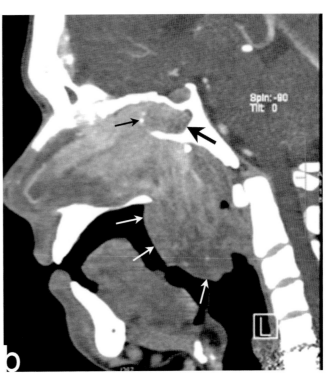

Figure 38.1. Contrast-enhanced CT. (a) Axial. Black asterisk = center of enhancing mass, arrow heads = deviated nasal septum to the right, small black arrow = displaced pterygoid plate, double-headed white arrow = widened sphenopalatine foramen, double-headed black arrow = widened posterior nasal aperture, white arrows = lateral extension of mass through pterygopalatine fossa into infratemporal fossa, large black arrow = fluid filling the left maxillary sinus. (b) Sagittal. Thin black arrow = destruction of anterior wall of sphenoid sinus, white arrows = mass extending downward from nasopharynx into oropharynx, thick black arrow = enhancing mass filling sphenoid sinus.

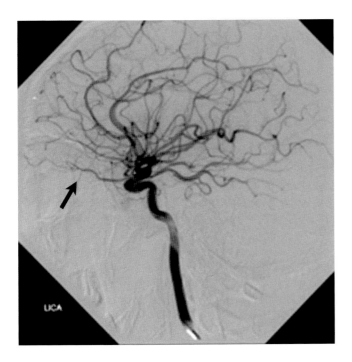

Figure 38.2. Lateral internal carotid arteriogram prior to performing preoperative embolization demonstrates the usual ophthalmic artery origin from the distal cavernous segment of the internal carotid artery (black arrow) and absence of tumor blush, which indicates that the arterial supply to the tumor is entirely from the external carotid circulation.

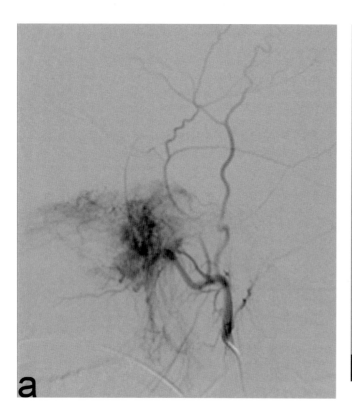
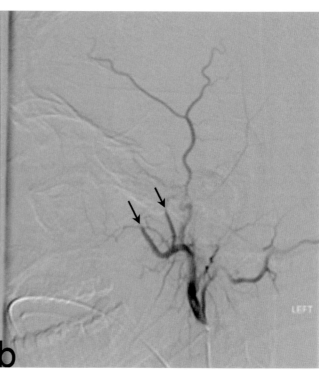

Figure 38.3. Lateral left external carotid digital subtraction arteriograms. (a) Pre-embolization image demonstrates tumor blush. (b) Post-embolization image demonstrates abrupt cut-off of embolized branches (arrows) and no remaining tumor blush.

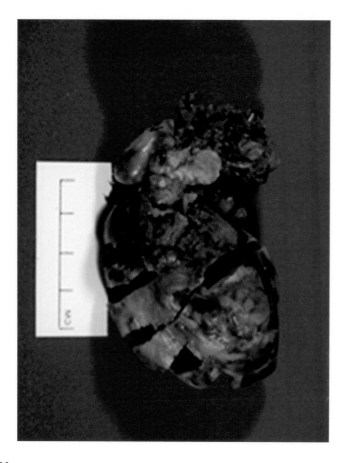

Figure 38.4. Resected tumor mass in same orientation as depicted in sagittal CT and lateral angiograms.

39

Small bowel fistula complicating perforated appendicitis: successful treatment with tissue adhesive

Edward A. Lebowitz

Imaging description

A previously healthy 11-year-old girl presented to interventional radiology with a two-week history of lower abdominal pain and diarrhea without nausea, vomiting, or fever. One week into the course of her present illness, antibiotics were begun empirically when a pediatrician at a neighborhood medical convenience clinic saw the patient. Antibiotics were discontinued two days later when she saw her regular pediatrician. However, as she continued to have pain and subjective fever, the patient's parents sought medical attention four days later. At that time, the patient's temperature was 104.2 °F and her white blood cell count was 21700 with a left shift. An ultrasound scan (Fig. 39.1) demonstrated a large pelvic fluid collection that was drained percutaneously with CT guidance (Fig. 39.2). Following drainage, the patient became afebrile and her leukocytosis resolved. She was discharged from the hospital with instructions on care of her drainage tube. A sinogram/abscessogram was performed two weeks and again five weeks following drainage. Both examinations showed that the abscess cavity had shrunk to the size of the pigtail catheter loop, but a persistent sinus tract leading from the cavity to the terminal ileum was present (Fig. 39.3a). As the patient refused to go to school with the drainage tube in place, it was decided to attempt to close the sinus tract with tissue adhesive (Fig. 39.3b–d). Following treatment, the patient returned to school and resumed other normal activities. However, at six weeks post-treatment, she presented with recurrent abdominal pain, leukocytosis, and fever. CT (Fig. 39.4) demonstrated recurrent appendicitis, and an appendectomy was performed at that time. There have been no problems since.

Importance

Acute appendicitis occurs in 6–8% of the population in Western countries. It is more frequent in males than females and most common in teenagers and young adults. However, it occurs in both sexes in any age group. Abdominal abscess secondary to perforated appendicitis is a common complication, and the surgeons with whom we work prefer to have interventional radiology drain the abscesses prior to appendectomy. An interval appendectomy is usually but not always performed.

Typical clinical scenario

Abscess formation secondary to perforated appendicitis usually occurs in the right lower quadrant or cul-de-sac, as in this patient. Our four criteria for the safe removal of the tube following percutaneous drainage include resolution of fever and leukocytosis, collapse of the abscess cavity around the pigtail catheter, and absence of a patent sinus tract between the bowel and cavity. When these criteria are met, the drainage catheter can be removed without risking recurrent abscess formation. Sinus tracts that connect to bowel usually do so at the site of appendiceal perforation and generally heal following drainage and antibiotics. Although much less common than connection to the appendiceal stump, we have seen other small bowel and even duodenal connections. Since a persistent connection to bowel leaves the patient at risk for abscess recurrence if the pigtail catheter is removed, it is our policy to perform a sinogram/abscessogram to confirm closure prior to removal. The four common causes of a persistent sinus tract to bowel include granulomatous infection or Crohn disease, bowel obstruction downstream, foreign body, or neoplasm at the site of perforation. Systemic corticosteroid therapy is also associated with delayed healing. None of these is likely in an otherwise normal child with perforated acute appendicitis. However, an appendicolith, which was present on this patient's pre-drainage CT scan (Fig. 39.2a), can act like a foreign body and inhibit healing.

In this patient, durable closure of the sinus tract was obtained by application of Bioglue Surgical Adhesive (CryoLife Inc., Kennesaw, GA.) a two-component surgical adhesive composed of bovine serum albumin and glutaraldehyde. Tissue adhesives in general and Bioglue in particular have been used in a variety of clinical settings, including closure of fistulae to bowel. As the Bioglue instructions emphasize the need for a clean dry surface to ensure an optimal result, I flush the tract with copious amounts of normal saline then dry it by injecting carbon dioxide through the 5-French catheter prior to adhesive treatment. I place the Bioglue applicator into the luer hub of the catheter, which is positioned with its tip where the sinus tract connects to bowel. The two are held together as the Bioglue is injected and the catheter withdrawn to the skin surface. Any extra glue that reaches the skin surface is removed. Pediatric applications of Bioglue have been reported, but for neurosurgical applications where sterility is essential results have not been optimistic. The indication in this case appeared to justify the risk. Although the appendicolith disappeared and the sinus tract healed, appendicitis recurred 6 weeks later. This is an accepted risk in appendicitis patients managed non-operatively.

Differential diagnosis

There is little likelihood of any other condition presenting in this manner in a child. The presence of a persistent sinus tract between the abscess cavity and bowel raises concern for the common causes of failure to heal. However, other than the appendicolith, none was found in this patient.

Teaching point

Perforated appendicitis is common in children, frequently managed by percutaneous abscess drainage. There is a small risk of a persistent enteral fistula, most often to the appendiceal stump. An abscessogram is therefore usually performed prior to catheter removal. Tissue adhesives approved for other indications can provide durable closure of enterocutaneous sinus tracts in children.

REFERENCES

1. Addiss DG, Shaffer N, Fowler BS, Tauxe RV. The epidemiology of appendicitis and appendectomy in the United States. *Am J Epidemiol* 1990;**132**:910–25.

2. Aranda-Narváez JM, González-Sánchez AJ, Marín-Camero N, *et al.* Conservative approach versus urgent appendectomy in surgical management of acute appendicitis with abscess or phlegmon. *Rev Esp Enferm Dig* 2010;**102**:648–52.

3. Buckley O, Geoghegan T, Ridgeway P, *et al.* The usefulness of CT-guided drainage of abscesses caused by retained appendicoliths. *Eur J Radiol* 2006;**60**:80–3.

4. Fitzmaurice GJ, McWilliams B, Hurreiz H, Epanomeritakis E. Antibiotics versus appendectomy in the management of acute appendicitis: a review of the current evidence. *Can J Surg* 2011;**54**:307–14.

5. Harbrecht BG, Franklin GA, Miller FB, Smith JW, Richardson JD. Acute appendicitis: not just for the young. *Am J Surg* 2011;**202**:286–90.

6. Hennelly KE, Bachur R. Appendicitis update. *Curr Opin Pediatr* 2011;**23**:281–5.

7. Mason RJ. Surgery for appendicitis: is it necessary? *Surg Infect (Larchmt)* 2008;**9**:481–8.

8. Prytowsky JB, Pugh CM, Nagle AP. Appendicitis. *Curr Probl Surg* 2005;**42**:694–742.

9. Simillis C, Symeonides P, Shorthouse AJ, Tekkis PP. A meta-analysis comparing conservative treatment versus acute appendectomy for complicated appendicitis (abscess or phlegmon). *Surgery* 2010;**147**:818–29.

10. vanSonnenberg E, Wittich GR, Casola G, *et al.* Periappendiceal abscesses: percutaneous drainage. *Radiology* 1987;**163**:23–6.

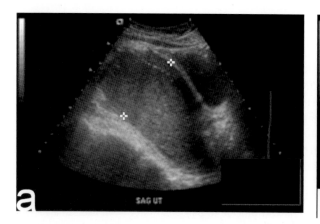 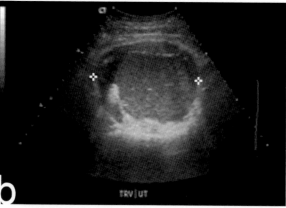

Figure 39.1. Sagittal (a) and axial (b) ultrasound images of the pelvis demonstrate a large echogenic fluid collection in the cul-de-sac.

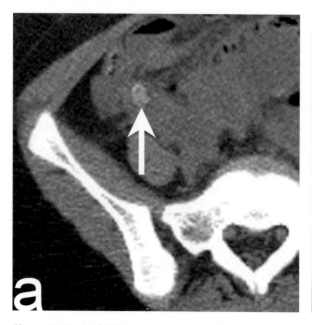 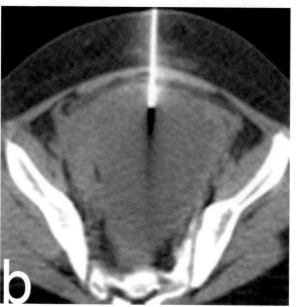

Figure 39.2. Axial CT images show appendicolith (a) entrance of the needle used to drain the abscess (b) and pigtail catheter deep in the cul-de-sac with following aspiration of pus (c).

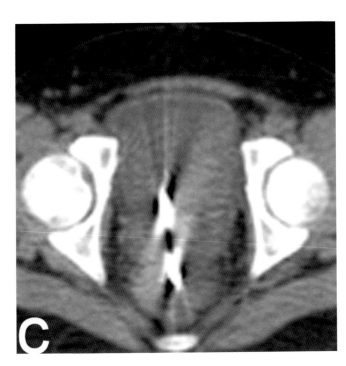

Figure 39.2. (cont.)

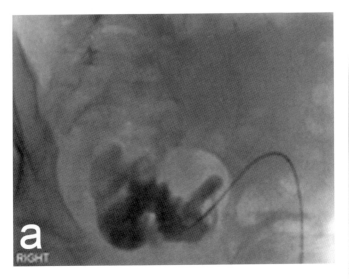

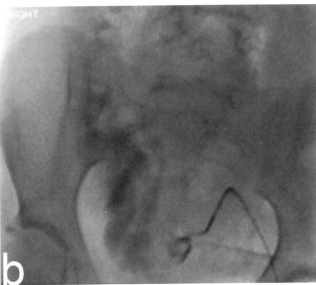

Figure 39.3. Sinogram/abscessogram demonstrates persistent sinus tract connection to small bowel (a). In b, c, and d, a 5-French end-hole catheter was inserted into the tract to the small bowel, and Bioglue Surgical Adhesive (CryoLife Inc., Kennesaw, GA) was infused through the catheter as it was withdrawn.

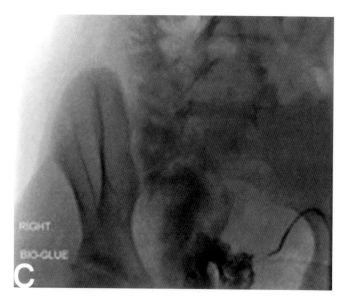
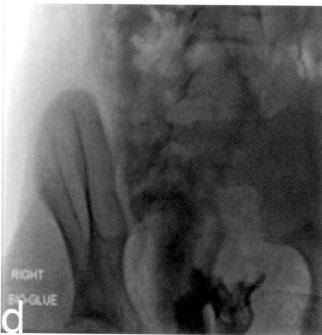

Figure 39.3. (cont.)

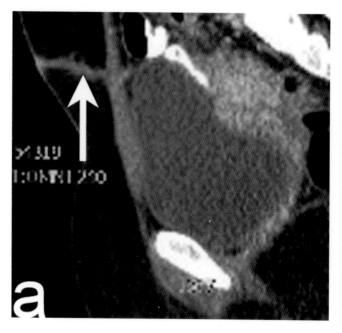
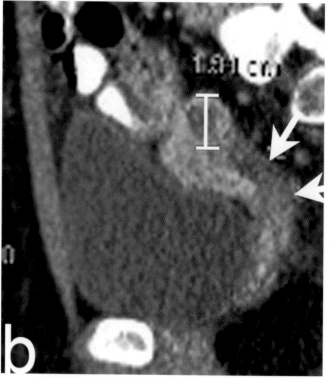

Figure 39.4. CT scan obtained 6 weeks following Bioglue treatment shows a scar corresponding to the closed enterocutaneous sinus tract (a, arrow) and dilated appendix (1.84 cm) with small amount of free fluid (b, arrows) in cul-de-sac consistent with recurrent acute appendicitis with perforation.

Extrahepatic collateral arterial supply to hepatocellular carcinoma

Edward A. Lebowitz

Imaging description

Figure 40.1 depicts an axial MR image obtained in a 17-year-old female with autoimmune hepatitis. On biopsy, the mass in segment 6/7 was consistent with a well-differentiated hepatocellular carcinoma. The patient also had a solitary pulmonary nodule that on resection was consistent with a metastasis from the hepatic primary. Full workup indicated the presence of cirrhosis, portal hypertension, and decreased liver function that precluded operative resection of the tumor. Her metastasis disqualified her from orthotopic liver transplantation. Interventional radiology was consulted to perform transarterial hepatic chemoembolization (TACE) to slow the growth of the primary neoplasm. At angiography, the patient's segment 6/7 tumor was supplied largely by branches of the right hepatic artery that were embolized to stasis with a cisplatin–doxorubicin–Lipiodol mixture. Following each of three TACE procedures over a 12-month period, the patient continued to have a portion of the tumor that failed to accumulate Lipiodol and thus remained untreated (Fig. 40.2). At a fourth TACE procedure, a right inferior phrenic arteriogram was performed (Fig. 40.3). A 2.7-French microcatheter was advanced into the ectatic, tortuous branch of the right inferior phrenic artery shown to supply the tumor, and TACE was performed. A Dyna-CT scan (Siemens Medical Solutions USA, Malvern, PA) performed immediately after TACE treatment demonstrated dense Lipiodol accumulation within the previously untreated portion of the tumor (Fig. 40.4).

Importance

In addition to the usual celiac arterial supply to the liver, 26 named collateral arteries have been described. As TACE and transarterial brachytherapy, so-called radioembolization, have become more common, multiple articles have confirmed clinically important arterial collateral pathways. The need to treat using collateral supply is usually indicated by the presence of untreated portions of tumor following TACE via the usual hepatic arterial branches. TACE via the collateral arteries is essential to obtain complete treatment.

Typical clinical scenario

Hepatocellular carcinoma (HCC) is most often a complication of cirrhosis of the liver. It is the fifth most common cancer worldwide and is usually seen in adults with chronic hepatitis B or C infection or Laennec's cirrhosis due to alcoholic liver disease. In children, liver cancers constitute only 1% of solid organ cancers. About three-quarters of these are hepatoblastoma, which is the most common liver malignancy in children. Fibrolamellar carcinoma also has a younger age demographic than HCC with a peak incidence at approximately 25 years of age. Nevertheless, typical HCC does occur in children, and interventional radiology may be consulted to control its growth or qualify the children for orthotopic liver transplantation. As with adults, liver function and portal hypertension usually preclude operative resection as definitive treatment, and denying liver transplantation in such children is associated with a 100% mortality rate.

The use of TACE is predicated on the fact that HCCs are supplied principally by branches of the hepatic arteries and the surrounding liver parenchyma is supplied principally by the portal venous circulation. As such, arterial embolization seldom causes significant collateral damage if the portal circulation is intact. The exact cocktail of chemotherapeutic agents and embolic material used for TACE varies among institutions. The decision to use TACE when remote metastatic disease is present is predicated on the fact that the majority of patients with advanced HCC die of intrahepatic tumor or hepatic failure rather than from metastatic disease. That said, TACE is still only a palliative treatment and is often combined with other treatments, both local and systemic, in an attempt to prolong patient survival.

Differential diagnosis

In adult patients with typical features of cirrhosis who have focal hepatic masses that display arterial phase enhancement and venous washout, the diagnosis of HCC is made regardless of whether alpha-fetoprotein is elevated, and biopsies are usually not obtained. However, as HCC is rare in children, biopsy is typically obtained.

> ## Teaching point
>
> TACE is a common procedure in most interventional radiology departments that treat adults. TACE is also used in children. To maximize its benefit, the entire tumor should be treated, which, as demonstrated in this patient, can require accessing collateral arterial pathways.

REFERENCES

1. Bulterys M, Goodman MT, Smith MA, et al. Hepatic tumors. In: Reis LAG, Smith MA, Gurney JG, et al., eds. Cancer Incidence and Survival Among Children and Adolescents: United States SEER Program, 1975–1995. Bethesda MD: National Cancer Institute SEER Program. NIH Pub. No. 99–4649, 1999; 91–7.
2. Gupta AA, Gerstle JT, Ng V, et al. Critical review of controversial issues in the management of advanced pediatric liver tumors. Pediatr Blood Cancer 2011;56:1013–18.
3. Malogolowkin MH, Stanley P, Steele DA, Ortega JA. Feasibility and toxicity of chemoembolization for children with liver tumors. J Clin Oncol 2000;18:1279–84.

4. Michels NA. Newer anatomy of the liver and its variant blood supply and collateral circulation. *Am J Surg* 1966;**112**:337–47.

5. Miyayama S, Yamashiro M, Yoshie Y, *et al.* Inferior phrenic arteries: angiographic anatomy, variations, and catheterization techniques for transcatheter arterial chemoembolization. *Jpn J Radiol* 2010;**28**:502–11.

6. Salhab M, Canelo R. An overview of evidence-based management of hepatocellular carcinoma: a meta-analysis. *J Cancer Res Ther* 2011;**7**:463–75.

7. Uka K, Aikata H, Takaki S, *et al.* Clinical features and prognosis of patients with extrahepatic metastases from hepatocellular carcinoma. *World J Gastroenterol* 2007;**13**:414–20.

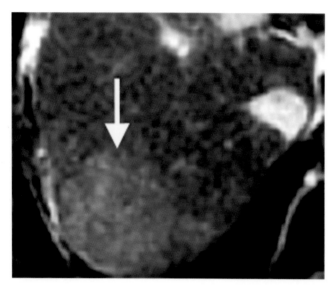

Figure 40.1. T2-weighted axial MR image demonstrates high signal in segment 6/7 corresponding to the biopsy-proven hepatocellular carcinoma (arrow).

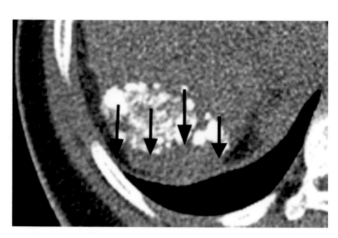

Figure 40.2. Axial CT scan obtained after the third TACE procedure displays excellent accumulation of Lipiodol in the anterior aspect of the tumor (white dots), but no Lipiodol in the tumor mass adjacent to the right hemidiaphragm (black arrows).

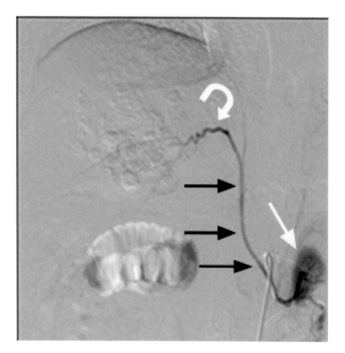

Figure 40.3. Right inferior phrenic arteriogram. The right inferior phrenic artery (black arrows) branched off an artery that originated on the left side of the aorta that also supplied the left adrenal gland, which displays dense parenchymal enhancement (white arrow). A tortuous branch of the right inferior phrenic artery (curved block arrow) supplied the paradiaphragmatic portion of the tumor.

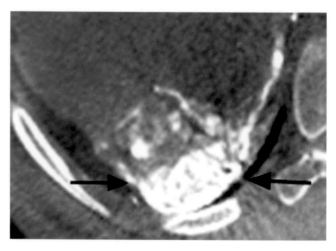

Figure 40.4. Axial Dyna-CT scan obtained following TACE via the tortuous right inferior phrenic artery branch depicted in Figure 40.3. Dense accumulation of Lipiodol (arrows) in the previously untreated paradiaphragmatic portion of the tumor was present.

Use of a curved needle to access an otherwise inaccessible abscess

Edward A. Lebowitz

Clinical course and imaging description

A previously healthy six-year-old boy presented with signs and symptoms of acute appendicitis. Ultrasound (Fig. 41.1a) and CT scan (Fig. 41.1b) were obtained to confirm the diagnosis. The patient had an appendectomy and five days of antibiotics, but due to continued fever and leukocytosis a repeat CT scan (Fig. 41.2) was obtained. This showed a multiloculated abscess that was well above the rectum, making it inaccessible to transrectal drainage, and surrounded by structures that made it seemingly inaccessible without passing through bladder, bowel, or bone. Regardless, the patient was referred to interventional radiology for drainage. Based on reports of successful drainage of such collections using a curved needle, the procedure was approved and the patient transported to the CT scanner, where a non-contrast scan was obtained in the prone position (Fig. 41.3a.) In order to delineate the abscess cavity and right ureter, however, intravenous contrast enhancement was required (Fig. 41.3b.) At this point, a 19-gauge, thin-walled Temno coaxial introducer needle (CareFusion, McGaw Park, IL) was bent to form a curve. Three methods were attempted. One way, without either the stylet or a guidewire through the needle (Fig. 41.4a, d), was unsuccessful because the needle bent at a sharp angle that precluded reinsertion of the stylet (Fig. 41.4b, d.) The second way, with the stylet inside the needle while bending it was stiff and resilient. Although the needle would bend and hold its new shape, the amount of curvature was less than hoped for. The third way was with the stiff segment of an Ultra Stiff Amplatz guidewire (Cook Inc., Bloomington, IN) passed through it (Fig. 41.4c, d). Although this became less curved when the stylet was reinserted, it still gave the most satisfactory result. The curved needle was then inserted through the upper right sacroiliac space aiming slightly laterally. Frequent mid course checks were performed with removal and repositioning required in order to avoid the right ureter. Figure 41.5 depicts the course of the needle from the skin surface to the abscess cavity. After aspirating a small amount of pus for cultures and smears, an Amplatz guidewire was inserted through the Temno needle, and the Temno needle was removed. However, a dilator could not be inserted over the guidewire into the abscess because it was too tight in the sacroiliac space. As such, the 19-gauge guide needle was gently reinserted over the guidewire and the abscess drained through the needle. Dilute Omnipaque was then infused into and aspirated from the abscess to be sure drainage was complete (Fig. 41.6). The needle was then removed. The patient improved and was discharged within 48 hours.

Importance

Pelvic abscess formation following perforated appendicitis is common, and interventional radiology is usually consulted for drainage. Abscesses within the rectovesicle pouch may be drained either percutaneously through the buttocks with CT guidance or transrectally using an endovaginal ultrasound probe, needle guide, and fluoroscopy. In some cases, however, the abscess may be too high to drain transrectally and surrounded by structures that you would prefer not to perforate, especially if you intend to leave a locking pigtail drainage catheter, as in this case. Using a curved needle with careful attention to its course as you insert it will make some of these patients amenable to percutaneous drainage and thereby obviate the need for an open operative procedure.

Typical clinical scenario

Postoperative abscess following appendicitis is discussed elsewhere in this volume (see Case 39).

Differential diagnosis

Postappendectomy fluid collections may be due to hematomas, seromas, or abscesses. In the presence of fever and leukocytosis, there is no credible differential, and an abscess is presumed. CT imaging is helpful in confirming a well-defined fluid collection with enhancing margins and clearly defines the anatomic location and extent. Ultrasound imaging may identify the collection, especially in thin individuals; however, the extent, number, and precise location may be incompletely displayed. More recently, MR imaging has also been utilized effectively to display postoperative fluid collections, including postappendectomy abscesses.

Teaching point

By curving the access needle, the interventional radiologist may be able to drain abscesses that would otherwise require an open operative procedure.

REFERENCES

1. Carrasco CH, Wallace S, Charnsgavej C. Aspiration biopsy: use of a curved needle. *Radiology* 1985;**155**:254.
2. Gupta S, Ahrar K, Wallace MJ, et al. Using coaxial technique with a curved inner needle for CT-guided fine-needle aspiration biopsy. *AJR Am J Roentgenol* 2002;**197**:109–12.
3. Hawkins IF, Caridi JG. Curved stylus for redirection of the fine-needle guide. *Radiology* 1984;**151**:530.
4. Hovsepian DM, Steele JR, Skinner CS, Malden ES. Transrectal versus transvaginal abscess drainage: survey of patient tolerance and effect on activities of daily living. *Radiology* 1999;**212**:159–63.
5. Sze DY. Use of curved needles to perform biopsies and drainages of inaccessible targets. *J Vasc Interv Radiol* 2001;**12**:1441–4.
6. Warnock NG. Curved needle technique for the avoidance of interposed structures in CT-guided percutaneous fine-needle biopsy. *J Comput Assist Tomogr* 1996;**20**:826–8.

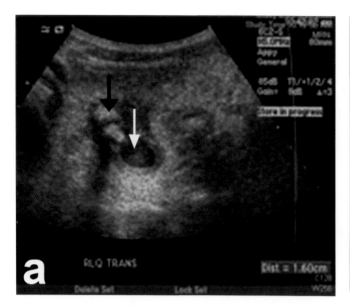
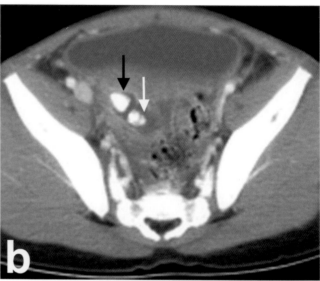

Figure 41.1. Ultrasound (a) and CT (b) scans through the pelvis demonstrate similar findings with dilated appendix (1.6 cm diameter) that contains two appendicoliths (black arrows) and fluid (white arrows).

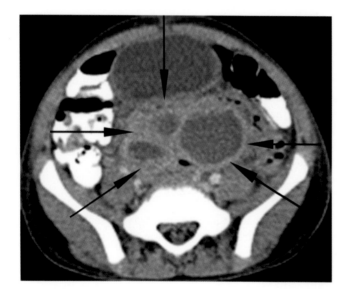

Figure 41.2. CT scan through the pelvis obtained on postoperative day 5 demonstrates a multiloculated abscess (arrows). Note that there is no direct percutaneous drainage route that would not pass through bone, bladder, or bowel.

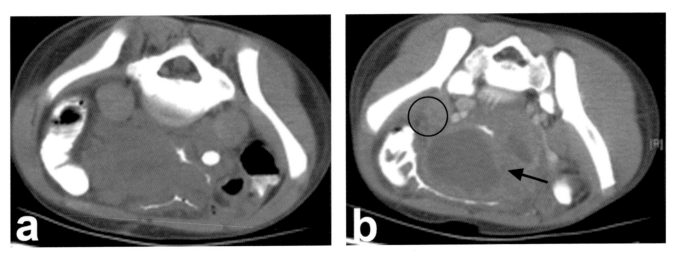

Figure 41.3. Prone CT scans through the pelvis before (a) and immediately after intravenous administration of 2 mL/kg Omnipaque 240 (GE Healthcare Inc., Princeton, NJ) by hand injection. (b) Intravenous contrast medium was administered because satisfactory identification of the abscess cavity (arrow) and right ureter (circle) could not be obtained without it.

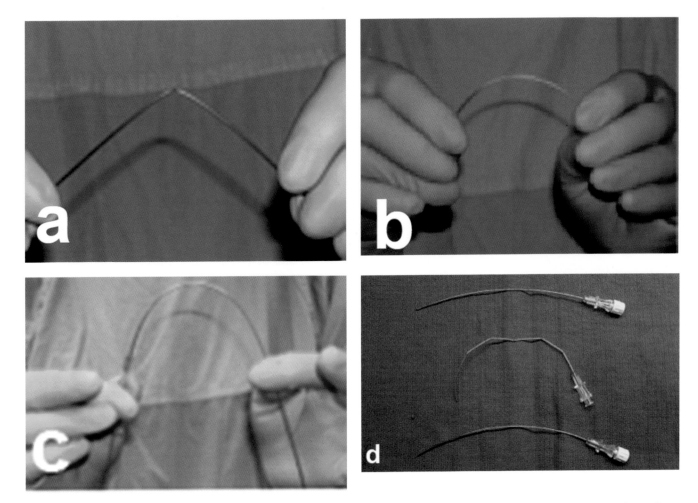

Figure 41.4. Three ways in which bending the needle was attempted, (a) bent without either stylet or guidewire through guide needle, (b) bent with stylet through guide needle, and (c) bent with guidewire through guide needle. (d) The resulting curves after reinsertion of the stylet. Obviously, however, the stylet could not be reinserted into the kinked guide needle.

185

(a)

(b)

(c)

(d)

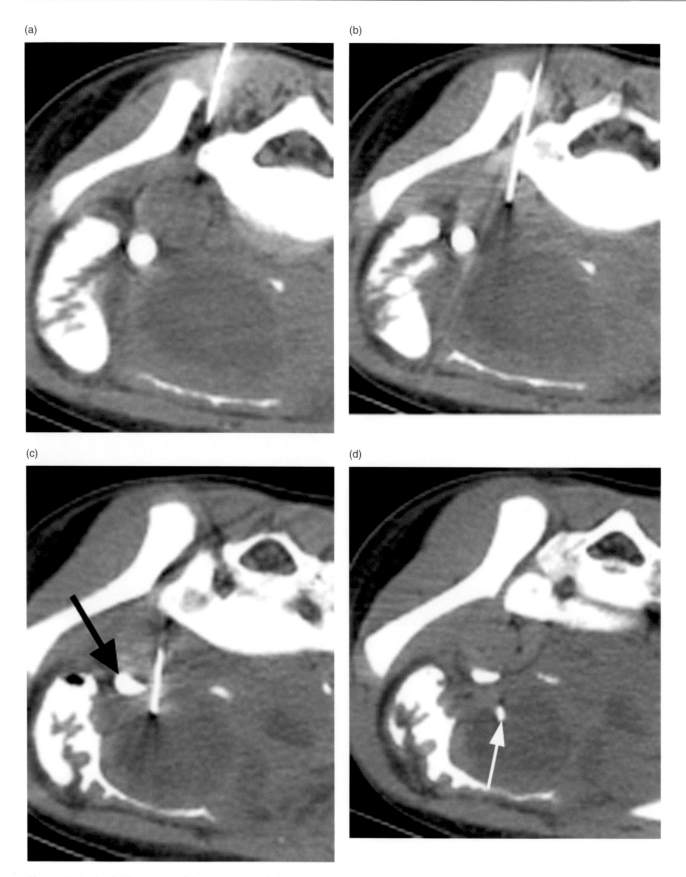

Figure 41.5. (a–d) The course of the Temno needle from the skin surface through the sacroiliac space, psoas muscle, and medial to the right ureter (black arrow), which was densely opacified by the time of needle insertion, to puncture of abscess more caudally (white arrow).

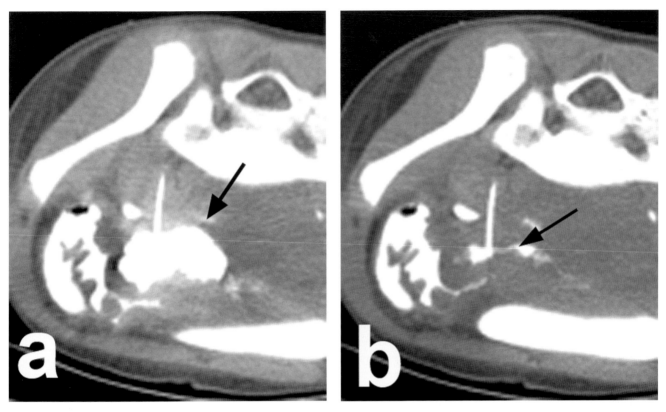

Figure 41.6. (a) The abscess filled with dilute Omnipaque (arrow). (b) The collapsed abscess following aspiration of Omnipaque at the end of the procedure (arrow).

Umbilical venous catheter malposition

Rakhee Gawande and Beverley Newman

Imaging description

A seven-day-old premature neonate presented with elevated liver enzymes and concern for a liver mass. Review of the outside CT scan of the abdomen showed a hypodense non-enhancing lesion in the right lobe of the liver (Fig. 42.1a). The outside ultrasound of the abdomen demonstrated a large thick-walled multilobulated cystic lesion with multiple septations (Fig. 42.1b). Repeat ultrasound (US) after transfer included color Doppler imaging which demonstrated the lesion to be cystic and avascular with mild perilesional hyperemia (Fig. 42.1c). Review of the outside chest radiographs revealed an abnormal anterior course of the umbilical venous line on the lateral view (Fig. 42.1d, e). The pediatric radiologist therefore suggested that rather than a neoplasm the liver "mass" represented a fluid collection/hematoma secondary to malposition of the umbilical venous line into the liver parenchyma with hemorrhage and fluid extravasation. A follow-up US at five months demonstrated complete resolution of the lesion with residual calcification in the liver.

Importance

Umbilical venous catheters (UVC) are one of the most common vascular access routes used in neonatal intensive care units. The umbilical vein extends directly anteriorly from the umbilicus to the liver edge, where it widens into a recess and forms a confluence with the left portal vein. Superiorly the umbilical vein recess connects with the ductus venosus, which then connects to the left hepatic vein/inferior vena cava (IVC). The ideal location of the UVC should be in the IVC, just below its entrance into the right atrium, which usually corresponds to the eighth or nineth thoracic vertebrae on an AP radiograph of the abdomen. To avoid inadvertent instillation of IV fluids into the portal vein, the tip should be advanced at least into the ductus venosus. A lateral radiograph will usually confirm this location, in which the umbilical catheter courses anteriorly in the abdomen, then curves back to the liver with an anterior convexity and then shows a posterior convexity when it has entered the ductus venosus (see Figs. 42.3 and 42.5).

The reported rates of catheter malpositions are 20–37%. A UVC readily enters the left portal vein and can progress to the left (left portal vein), right (left portal vein to right portal vein), or inferiorly (coiled in umbilical vein recess). The catheter can be advanced too far into the right atrium, right ventricle, or even the left atrium via the foramen ovale (Fig. 42.2). The common acute complications of a malpositioned UVC include thrombosis, embolism, vasospasm, vessel perforation, hemorrhage, infection, liver laceration, cardiac arrhythmia, pericardial effusion and tamponade, pulmonary infarction, and lung abscess. Great care is taken to ensure that the UVC is not perfusing the portal vein and the infusion of hypertonic solutions via UVC are restricted as much as possible because of the potential risk of portal vein thrombosis and subsequent presentation years later with portal hypertension and bleeding gastroesophageal varices.

Typical clinical scenario

It may not be clinically apparent when an umbilical venous line has perforated the vessel. Hepatic parenchymal and other injuries associated with a malpositioned UVC carry significant morbidity and mortality and should be suspected if a neonate with a UVC develops abdominal distension. Other signs may include increasing liver size and abnormal liver enzymes. Patients may also have ascites due to hemorrhage and/or extravasation of administered fluids. Careful attention should be paid to the course of the venous catheter on both frontal and lateral views. However, since radiographs may not indicate the exact location of the UVC, US is a useful tool in determining the location of the tip and its relationship to the cardiovascular structures.

When a UVC needs to be replaced and central venous access is still needed, femoral venous percutaneously inserted lines are a common choice (Fig. 42.3). The femoral vein courses posterosuperiorly to the iliac vein, IVC, and right atrium. As with all line placements, iatrogenic misadventures may occur (Fig. 42.4). Optimal position for the tip of a femoral venous line is at the inferior cavoatrial junction but this is less important than with a UVC and location within the IVC is usually considered satisfactory. Important malpositions include placement too high (intracardiac) or in venous branches such as a renal vein or ascending lumbar vein (more common on the left because of the angle between the left iliac vein and lumbar vein) (Fig. 42.5). Lumbar vein malposition should be suggested when the line demonstrates a lateral hump at the L4–5 level on the frontal radiograph or overlies the spine and courses more posteriorly than expected on the lateral view (Fig. 42.5). It is generally a good idea to obtain both frontal and lateral radiographs following placement of a new line; any unusual contour or course should be carefully assessed (Figs. 42.1, 42.3, 42.5) and correlated with clinical concerns.

Differential diagnosis

Malposition of a UVC with extravasation of blood and fluid into the liver is most often confused with a hepatic neoplasm (as in this case) or cyst. Particularly if the catheter has been removed, the possibility of vascular perforation and extravasation may not be considered. It is important to recognize this entity so that additional unnecessary studies including blood work, CT/MR, and biopsy are avoided.

Hepatic neoplasms in the newborn include benign entities such as cystic mesenchymal hamartoma (multicystic with a fibrous stroma), infantile hemangioma (solid hypoechoic hypervascular), and hepatic arteriovenous malformation (vascular tangle). Hepatoblastoma is the most common malignant liver neoplasm in neonates (solid, heterogeneous, and hypervascular, may have areas of necrosis); metastatic tumor is most commonly neuroblastoma in this age group (single, multiple, or diffuse, solid hyperechoic).

Other differential possibilities include hepatic abscess (uncommon in neonates, can result from necrotizing enterocolitis, ascending umbilical or portal venous infection, hematogenous or biliary spread and extravasation associated with UVC or other catheter malposition), bile collection (trauma, biliary atresia, choledochal cyst), or simple hepatic cysts (uncommon in infants and children).

US with Doppler examination should be able to differentiate cysts from solid or vascular masses. The hepatic hematoma/fluid collection related to a misplaced UVC will be avascular although there may be surrounding hyperemia from compressed hepatic parenchyma and reactive inflammatory changes (Fig. 42.1c).

Teaching point

Abdominal distension and a cystic hepatic mass in a neonate with a current or prior UVC should raise the suspicion of erosion of the UVC into the liver. Whenever a line or catheter complication is of concern, two orthogonal radiographic views are helpful in determining abnormality. US is a useful tool in locating the tip of a catheter and investigating the nature and extent of any fluid collection or "mass" that may accompany catheter malpositions.

REFERENCES

1. Michel F, Brevaut-Malaty V, Pasquali R, *et al.* Comparison of ultrasound and X-ray in determining the position of umbilical venous catheters. *Resuscitation* 2012;**83**(6):705–9.

2. Oestreich AE. Umbilical vein catheterization: appropriate and inappropriate placement. *Pediatr Radiol* 2010;**40**(12):1941–9.

3. Ramasethu J. Complications of vascular catheters in the neonatal intensive care unit. *Clin Perinatol* 2008;**35**(1):199–222.

4. Simeunovic E, Arnold M, Sidler D, Moore SW. Liver abscess in neonates. *Pediatr Surg Int* 2009;**25**(2):153–6.

5. Yiğiter M, Arda İS, Hiçsönmez A. Hepatic laceration because of malpositioning of the umbilical vein catheter: case report and literature review. *J Pediatr Surg* 2008;**43**(5):39–41.

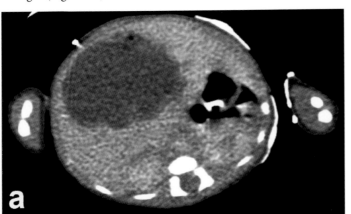

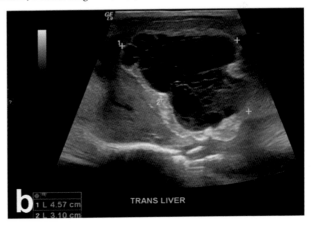

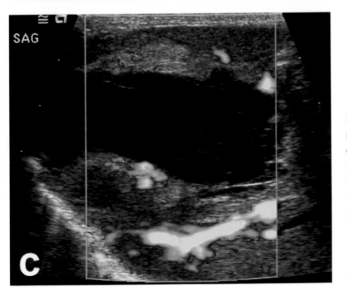

Figure 42.1. A seven-day-old neonate with a liver mass. Iatrogenic UVC perforation with hematoma/fluid extravasation. (a) Outside axial contrast-enhanced computed tomography (CECT) – there is a hypodense non-enhancing rounded anterior right hepatic mass. Note that the umbilical venous line had already been removed. A tiny bubble of air is noted anteriorly. (b) Outside ultrasound (transverse image) of the abdomen performed on the following day shows a large thick-walled multilobulated and multiseptated cystic mass in the right lobe of the liver. (c) Repeat US after transfer. Sagittal power Doppler image shows the mass to be avascular with some perilesional hyperemia, likely reactive or compressed liver parenchyma.

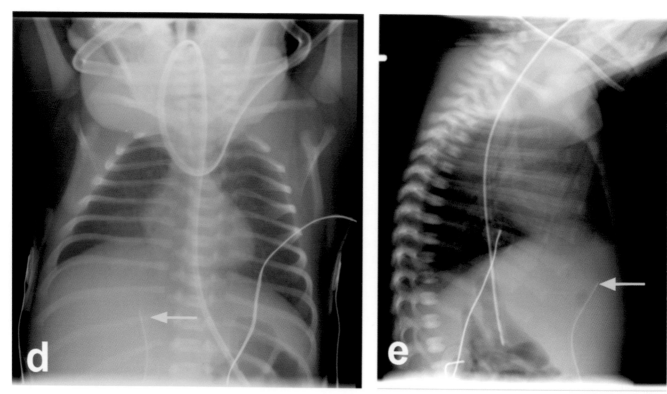

Figure 42.1. (cont.) (d, e) Retrospective review of radiographs of the chest and upper abdomen shows a low umbilical venous catheter with its tip overlying the liver shadow (d, arrow) at the level of T10 vertebra on the frontal view. On the lateral view the umbilical venous catheter was noted to have an abnormal anterior course (e, arrow) with a small amount of air near the tip. The normal course of a UVC through the liver is from anterior to posterior. The findings were therefore suggestive of a hematoma/fluid collection secondary to perforation of the umbilical venous line into the liver parenchyma with hemorrhage and IV fluid extravasation.

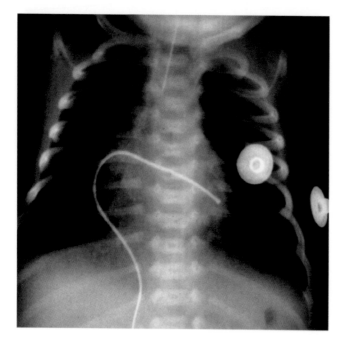

Figure 42.2. Newborn infant. Frontal chest radiograph shows a malpositioned UVC extending into the right atrium and then through a patent foramen ovale into the left atrium.

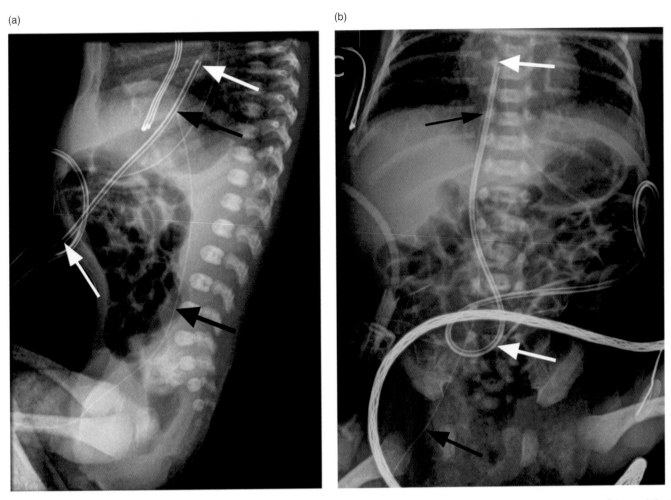

Figure 42.3. Umbilical venous and femoral venous lines. (a) Lateral and (b) frontal abdominal views demonstrate the course of the umbilical venous catheter (white arrows) from the umbilicus directly superiorly and then with a gentle curve posteriorly through the liver with the tip slightly high in the right atrium. Although the course appears relatively straight through the liver, the catheter courses from the umbilical vein to left portal vein, then to the hepatic venous confluence and IVC via the ductus venosus. While the femoral venous (black arrows) and umbilical venous catheters are partially superimposed on the frontal view, the lateral view shows the posterior course of the femoral catheter (femoral vein to iliac vein to IVC with tip at the cavoatrial junction).

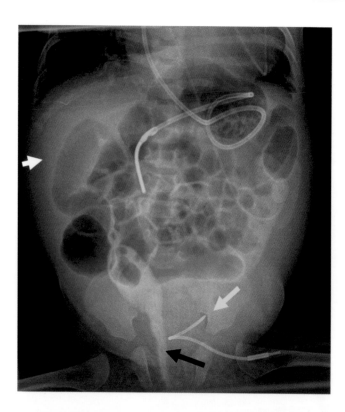

Figure 42.4. Newborn infant with abdominal distention following placement of a left femoral line. Vascular perforation with extravasation and ascites. A frontal abdominal radiograph demonstrates an unusual lateral course (yellow arrow) of the recently placed femoral venous catheter although clinically the catheter was reported to be infusing well. There is mass effect in the pelvis with the rectum displaced to the right (black arrow) (seen well because of residual rectal contrast from recent enema). There is also moderate ascites – the white arrow denotes the dense liver edge with more lucent fluid seen laterally. The findings clearly indicate vascular perforation by the catheter with probable pelvic hematoma and ascites likely consisting of hemorrhage and extravasated IV fluids.

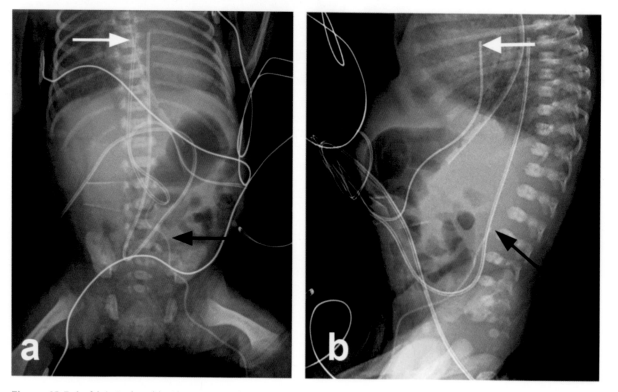

Figure 42.5 (a, b) A six-day-old with respiratory distress syndrome . Malpositioned UVC and left femoral line. Frontal and lateral radiographs of the abdomen demonstrate a well-positioned umbilical arterial line (UAL) at the T6–7 level (optimal position T6–10, away from major branch vessels). The UVC (white arrows) is malpositioned high in the right atrium. A new left femoral line (black arrows) has been placed but could not be further advanced. On the frontal view the femoral line has an unusual wavy buckled appearance with a lateral hump at the L5 level with the tip overlying the spine. On the lateral view, the tip of the catheter extends posteriorly. This appearance is very suggestive of catheter malposition in the left ascending lumbar vein. This line could potentially jeopardize the spinal cord and the catheter was removed promptly and replaced with a right femoral line.

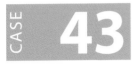
Middle aortic syndrome

Elizabeth Sutton and Heike E. Daldrup-Link

Imaging description

A 12-year-old girl presented with acute abdominal pain. She had undergone chemo and radiation therapy seven years previously for metastatic neuroblastoma. The patient had experienced other, less severe episodes of abdominal pain over the past several months. On clinical examination she had diffuse abdominal pain, hypertension, and non-palpable femoral pulses. A CT scan demonstrated severe narrowing of the infrarenal abdominal aorta as well as occlusions of the celiac trunk, superior mesenteric artery (SMA), left renal artery, and focal narrowing of the proximal right renal artery (Fig. 43.1). The patient underwent a right renal artery angioplasty and right aortorenal bypass surgery.

Importance

Middle aortic syndrome (MAS) is a clinicopathologic term referring to significant, segmental tubular narrowing of the suprarenal, inter-renal, or infrarenal abdominal aorta, frequently associated with concomitant stenoses in the renal and visceral arteries. Ultrasound with Doppler and flow velocity investigations can directly detect the stenosis itself and demonstrate increased flow velocity and mono- or biphasic waveforms of arteries distal to the stenosis (as opposed to the normal triphasic waveforms). CT or MR angiographies can confirm the diagnosis. It is important to consider the possibility of MAS in specific patient populations and in the setting of classical clinical symptoms, described in more detail below. MAS can lead to a series of severe complications, including cerebral hemorrhage, cardiac infarctions, renal insufficiency, and mesenteric ischemia/infarction.

Typical clinical scenario

Depending on the sites of vascular stenosis, patients with middle aortic syndrome may present with uncontrollable hypertension, progressively deteriorating renal function, and/or mesenteric ischemia. A classical clinical finding is hypertension proximal to the aortic stenosis, and relative hypotension distally. Other symptoms may variably include severe headache, nosebleeds, chest pain, cardiac failure, and lower limb claudication. Histologically, the stenotic arteries demonstrate thickening of the intima with dysplastic and/or fibrotic changes. If possible, medical management for MAS is preferred in the pediatric population until the child has ceased growing so as to prevent a second surgery later in life. The treatment of choice for MAS is now either a one-stage reconstructive prosthetic or autologous venous surgical arterial bypass graft.

Differential diagnosis

Other causes of MAS include Takayasu arteritis (Fig. 43.2) (giant cell arteritides), neurofibromatosis, fibromuscular dysplasia (see Case 35), retroperitoneal fibrosis, mucopolysaccharidosis, and Williams syndrome, or other congenital vascular abnormalities of the abdominal aorta and its branches.

Teaching point

As a result of continuing therapeutic advances, children with cancer are surviving longer than in previous decades, rendering long-term follow-up studies essential for optimal treatment and continued care. Radiologists and clinicians should be aware of the possibility of a MAS as a late complication after abdominal irradiation of a malignant abdominal tumor in childhood and a differential consideration for other vasculitides in childhood.

REFERENCES

1. Delis KT, Gloviczki P. Middle aortic syndrome: from presentation to contemporary open surgical and endovascular treatment. *Perspect Vasc Surg Endovasc Ther* 2005;**17**(3):187–203.
2. Lee LC, Broadbent V, Kelsall W. Neuroblastoma in an infant revealing middle aortic syndrome. *Med Pediatr Oncol* 2000;**35**(2):150–2.
3. Lewis VD 3rd, Meranze SG, McLean GK, *et al.* The midaortic syndrome: diagnosis and treatment. *Radiology* 1988;**167**(1):111–13.
4. Sutton EJ, Tong RT, Gillies AM, *et al.* Decreased aortic growth and middle aortic syndrome in patients with neuroblastoma after radiation therapy. *Pediatr Radiol* 2009;**39**(11):1194–202.

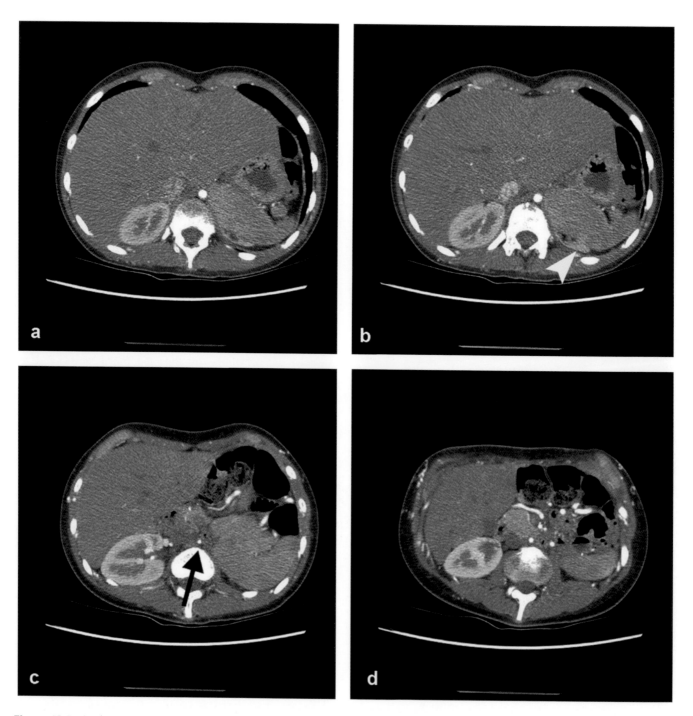

Figure 43.1. Axial contrast-enhanced CT images (a–d) in the arterial phase and a 3D reconstruction of these images (e) show a markedly narrowed infrarenal aorta (arrow). In addition, the celiac trunk, superior mesenteric artery, and left renal artery do not opacify with contrast. The left kidney (arrowhead) is markedly atrophic. The right renal artery demonstrates a mild proximal stenosis. Multiple abdominal collateral vessels are noted. (From *Pediatric Radiology*, Vol. **39**(11), 2009, 1194–202, Decreased aortic growth and middle aortic syndrome in patients with neuroblastoma after radiation therapy, Sutton EJ, Tong RT, Gillis AM, *et al.*, with kind permission from Springer Science and Business Media.)

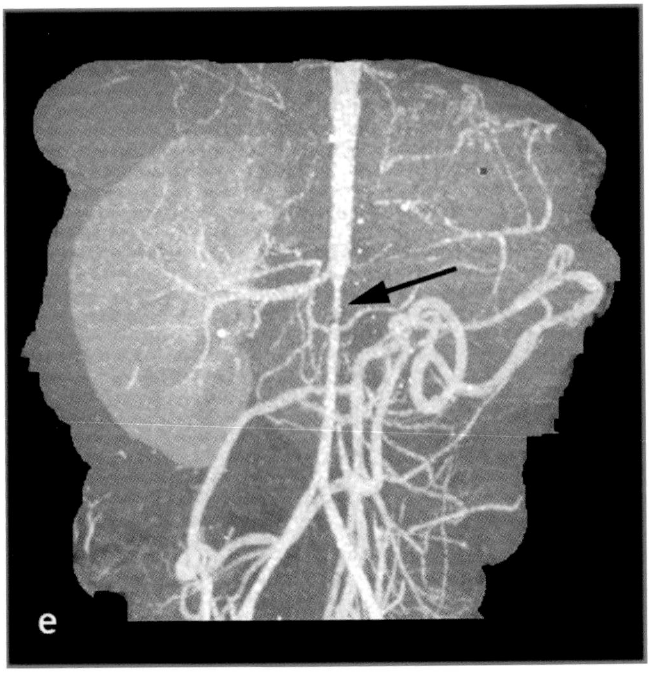

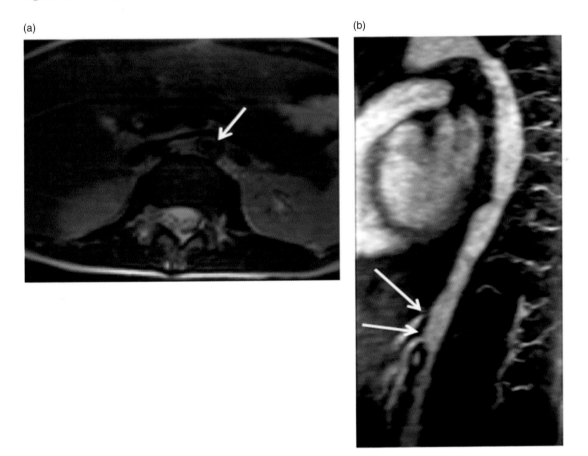

Figure 43.1. (cont.)

Figure 43.2. An 11-year-old girl with Takayasu arteritis. (a) Axial T2-weighted MR scan through the mid abdomen demonstrates thickening and increased signal of the aortic wall, suggesting active inflammation, with decreased luminal diameter of the mid abdominal aorta (arrow). (b) Sagittal MRA MIP reconstruction demonstrates areas of irregular dilatation and narrowing of the descending thoracic and abdominal aorta (arrows). There are stenoses at the origins of the celiac and SMA with narrowing of the abdominal aorta below the SMA.

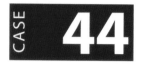

44 Ruptured appendicitis mimicking an intussusception

Rakhee Gawande and Beverley Newman

Imaging description

A six-year-old child presented to the ER with abdominal pain. A ultrasound (US) study (Fig. 44.1a, b) demonstrated a lesion in the right lower quadrant with a pattern of alternating sonolucent and hyperechoic layers, giving an appearance of a bowel loop-within-loop, suggesting intussusception.

A plain radiograph of the abdomen (Fig. 44.1c) revealed blurring of the right flank fat plane, medial displacement of ascending colon gas, and subtle scoliosis of the spine, indicating a right-sided inflammatory process or mass. A contrast enema was obtained to reduce the intussusception diagnosed on US (Fig. 44.1d). The study revealed a possible filling defect at the hepatic flexure which rapidly disappeared (? reduced intussusception) and normal reflux of contrast was noted into the ileum (Fig. 44.1d). The child continued to have abdominal pain, fever, and high white blood cell count. Repeat US the following morning demonstrated a similar, slightly more complex layered pattern and marked surrounding echogenic inflammation was noted (Fig. 44.1e). Taking into account the clinical and laboratory findings as well as the child's age (old for typical idiopathic intussusception), perforated appendicitis with phlegmon/abscess was suggested as a more likely diagnosis. CT examination confirmed ruptured acute appendicitis with an appendicolith and periappendiceal fluid collection/abscess (Fig. 44.1f, g).

Importance

Abdominal pain is a common but potentially serious symptom in children, with acute appendicitis and intussusception high on the list of common differential diagnoses. Appendicitis, especially after perforation, may mimic a variety of other diseases leading to a false-negative diagnosis and vice versa. A misdiagnosis may result in inappropriate or delayed treatment or unnecessary removal of a normal appendix. Both sonography and CT have important roles in the accurate diagnosis of appendicitis and its complications. Subtle radiographic features such as the right lower quadrant inflammation seen in this patient may be helpful diagnostic clues.

Typical clinical scenario

The classic symptoms of acute appendicitis include fever, anorexia, periumbilical pain followed by right lower quadrant pain and vomiting, which can be present in many other causes of acute abdominal pain in children.

Classic symptoms of intussusception include intermittent abdominal pain and irritability, with later diarrhea, bloody stools, and lethargy.

Idiopathic intussusception is most often seen in children between 6 months and 3 years of age and is thought to be related to hypertrophy of bowel lymphoid tissue (Peyer's patches) often triggered by a preceding gastrointestinal illness. Intussusception can occur in older children where it is less likely to be idiopathic and more likely to be associated with a pathologic lead point such as a Meckel's diverticulum, duplication cyst, appendicitis, inspissated meconium (in cystic fibrosis), or a neoplasm such as a polyp or lymphoma. Appendicitis can occur at any age but is relatively uncommon in small infants.

Most idiopathic intussusceptions are ileocolic and therefore are mostly found on the right side of the abdomen. On US transverse sections, an intussusception typically appears as a superficial mass with concentric hypoechoic and echogenic rings representing components of bowel wall and intussuscepted mesenteric fat and lymph nodes, referred to as a target or doughnut sign (Fig. 44.2). On longitudinal scans, the lesion is ovoid in shape with different tissues appearing layered longitudinally, and is often referred to as a sandwich or pseudokidney sign. US is considered a very good imaging study for the detection of intussusception with reported sensitivity of 100% and specificity of 88%.

The classic sonographic signs of appendicitis include a fluid-filled non-compressible hyperemic appendix with diameter exceeding 6mm (Fig. 44.3). The appendix is recognized as a blind-ending tubular structure with bowel wall signature (echogenic mucosa and hypoechoic outer muscular wall) that arises from the base of the cecum. An appendicolith may or may not be present (Fig. 44.3). Sonographic signs of appendiceal perforation include loss of the echogenic mucosa, increased periappendiceal echogenicity due to surrounding inflammation, and a complex mass or focal fluid collection. The appendix itself may be difficult to define from surrounding inflammation, fluid, and gas.

Differential diagnosis

Many acute abdominal conditions can mimic acute appendicitis. Common mimics include mesenteric adenitis, infectious enterocolitis (Fig. 44.4), epiploic appendagitis, omental infarction, Meckel's diverticulitis, Crohn's disease, ileocolic intussusception, pelvic inflammatory disease, hemorrhagic ovarian cyst, ovarian torsion, pyelonephritis, and urolithiasis. Most of these entities can readily be differentiated on imaging.

Teaching point

Several gastrointestinal and genitourinary pathologies can present with similar clinical symptoms and mimic acute appendicitis. Sonography and CT scans are the first line imaging modalities in emergency care. Differential diagnosis of acute appendicitis is broad, but knowledge of specific sonographic and CT appearances and pitfalls will help in accurate diagnosis.

Intussusception has a very characteristic US appearance but there are occasional mimickers. Therefore, in cases in which the age and clinical findings raise questions/discrepancy regarding the appearance on US, radiation exposure concerns should not delay prompt CT imaging.

REFERENCES

1. Shin LK, Jeffrey RB. Sonography and computed tomography of the mimics of appendicitis. *Ultrasound Q* 2010;**26**(4):201–10.
2. Sivit CJ. Diagnosis of acute appendicitis in children: spectrum of sonographic findings. *AJR Am J Roentgenol* 1993;**161**(1):147–52.
3. van Breda Vriesman AC, Puylaert JB. Mimics of appendicitis: alternative nonsurgical diagnoses with sonography and CT. *AJR Am J Roentgenol* 2006;**186**(4):1103–12.
4. Williams H. Imaging and intussusceptions. *Arch Dis Child Educ Pract Ed* 2008;**93**(1):30–6.

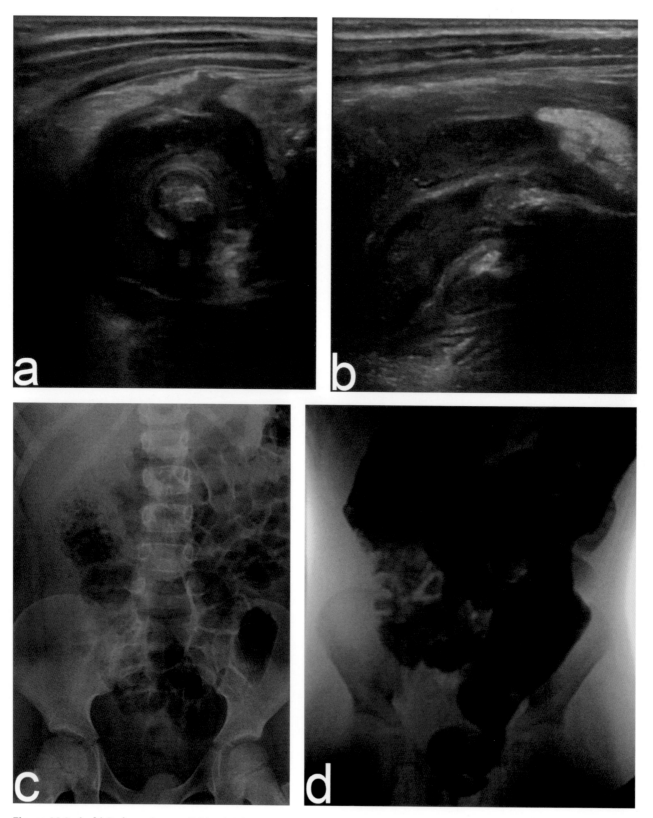

Figure 44.1. (a, b) Perforated appendicitis mimicking intussusception. Transverse (a) and longitudinal (b) US images of the right lower quadrant in this 6-year-old child with abdominal pain reveal a lesion with alternating sonolucent and hyperechoic layers suggestive of an intussusception. **(c)** Supine abdominal radiograph of the same patient demonstrates blurring of the right flank fat plane with medial

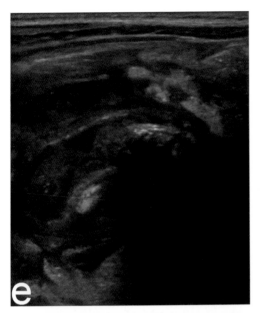

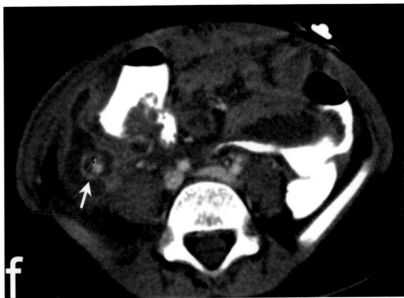

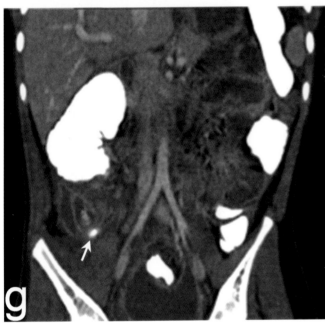

Figure 44.1. (cont.) displacement of the ascending colon and subtle levoscoliosis of the lumbar spine. These findings suggest a right-sided inflammatory process. **(d)** Abdominal AP radiograph of water-soluble contrast enema in the same patient demonstrates opacified colon with reflux of contrast into the small bowel. Mild irregularity/inflammation of the ascending colon is noted. **(e)** Longitudinal US image of the right lower quadrant in the same patient the following day reveals a similar multilayered pattern as on the prior US, somewhat more complex in appearance and with marked surrounding inflammation appreciated, raising concern for a perforated appendix with abscess simulating the appearance of an intussusception. **(f, g)** Axial CT scan of the abdomen (f) with coronal reformat (g) in the same patient reveals a dilated fluid-filled appendix with wall enhancement and periappendiceal fluid collection/abscess, suggestive of acute perforated appendicitis. An appendicolith is noted at the base of the appendix (arrows).

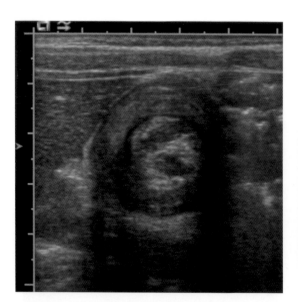

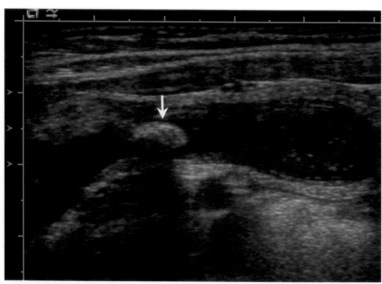

Figure 44.2. Intussusception in a five-month-old. Transverse US image of the right upper quadrant in this child reveals a lesion with concentric rings of sonolucent and hyperechoic bowel walls, consistent with an intussusception. A contrast enema confirmed the diagnosis of ileocolic intussusception, which was partially reduced to the level of the cecum, followed by surgical reduction.

Figure 44.3. Acute appendicitis in a 5-year-old boy with acute right lower quadrant pain. US image of the right lower quadrant demonstrates a dilated (1.2 cm distally), thick-walled, non-compressible blind-ending tubular structure that contains echogenic debris distally and a large shadowing stone proximally (arrow) consistent with acute appendicitis. There was a small amount of free fluid adjacent to the tip but no other signs of perforation.

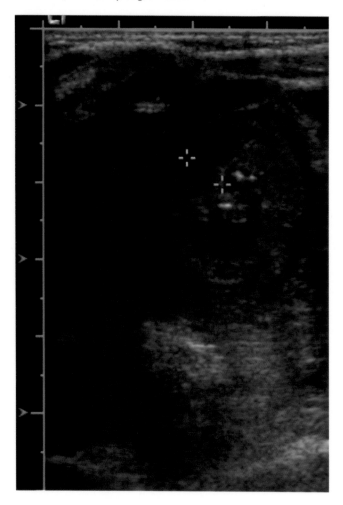

Figure 44.4. Enterocolitis in a three-year-old. Transverse US image of the abdomen demonstrates thickened small bowel in a case of infectious enterocolitis.

Choledochal cyst

Gregory Cheeney and Heike E. Daldrup-Link

Imaging description

A seven-year-old boy presented with nausea, right upper abdominal pain, and jaundice. An initial ultrasound (not shown) demonstrated a cystic lesion in the area of the porta hepatis, separate from the gallbladder. Axial and coronal T2-weighted MR images and 3D MRCP demonstrated fusiform dilatation of the central hepatic ducts and the common bile duct, consistent with a type I choledochal cyst (CC) (Fig. 45.1a–k). The intrahepatic bile ducts appeared normal in caliber. There was no evidence for choledocholithiasis or pancreatitis. An endoscopic retrograde cholangiopancreatography (ERCP) confirmed contrast filling of a fusiform dilated common bile duct without associated dilatation of the intrahepatic bile ducts (Fig. 45.1).

Importance

CCs represent congenital dilatation(s) of the extrahepatic and/or intrahepatic biliary system. The initial diagnostic workup usually entails an abdominal ultrasound, which demonstrates an anechoic cystic structure in the region of the porta hepatis, separate from the gallbladder. Depending on the extent of the cyst, five different types are recognized according to the classification system of Todani (Fig. 45.2). Type I is the most common type, comprising 80–90% of CCs, and representing a fusiform or cystic dilatation of the extrahepatic biliary system. A mild, secondary dilatation of the more proximal intrahepatic biliary system may be visualized; however, the more peripheral intrahepatic bile ducts are typically not dilated.

CCs are often associated with an abnormal high (or proximal) union of the pancreatic duct with the common bile duct (CBD), which results in a long common channel of 1 cm or more. The abnormal proximal insertion of the pancreatic duct into the CBD is thought to lead to pancreatic enzymatic reflux, inflammation, elevated ductal pressures, and cyst formation. Similarly biliary reflux into the pancreatic duct can result in inflammation, stricture, and pancreatitis. Imaging is important in the identification and preoperative planning of CCs, as the operative management depends on the extent of the cyst. The most common surgical approach consists of excision of as much of the abnormal biliary tree as possible and separation of the pancreatic and biliary systems, usually leaving the pancreatic duct draining into the distal CBD/duodenum and draining bile via a choledochojejunostomy. In the pediatric population, MRCP is considered the imaging study of choice for preoperative evaluation. Cholangiography allows for better characterization of CCs, particularly type III choledochocele, and for better identification of aberrant pancreatic duct insertions. Untreated CCs may lead to cholelithiasis or choledocholithiasis, ascending cholangitis, pancreatitis, intrahepatic ductal strictures, hepatic abscesses, and biliary malignancy (malignant transformation rate as high as 15%).

Typical clinical scenario

Patients typically present during childhood (80%), 60% before 10 years of age. Symptoms include nausea, recurrent right upper quadrant pain, jaundice, and a palpable mass. There is an increased incidence in females and Asians.

Differential diagnosis

Differential diagnoses include primary hepatic or pancreatic cysts, gallbladder duplication, or enteric duplication cysts. Duplication cysts are differentiated by their lack of direct connection to the CBD. Other differential considerations in young babies include biliary atresia with associated intrahepatic cyst formation and biliary hamartoma. In older patients, differential considerations may also include secondary biliary duct dilatation due to choledocholithiasis or malignant CBD obstruction. Types IV and V CC, with intrahepatic cystic biliary dilatations, must be distinguished from hepatic cysts, biliary hamartoma, recurrent pyogenic and primary sclerosing cholangitis, and liver abscesses. Identification of CC warrants close examination of the entire biliary system, liver, and pancreas, as other congenital abnormalities such as aberrant ducts and pancreas divisum are seen more commonly.

Teaching point

CC represent the most common congenital anomaly of the biliary system. CC may be distinguished by the presence of focal or diffuse biliary dilatation continuous with the lumen of the CBD. Diagnostic workup with MRCP and/or cholangiography should assess the extent of the cyst, potential intrahepatic abnormalities, presence or absence of chole(docho)lithiasis, relation to the pancreatic duct, and presence or absence of pancreatitis.

REFERENCES

1. Federle MP, Anne VS. Choledochal cyst. In: Federle MP, ed. *Diagnostic Imaging: Abdomen*. Salt Lake City: Amirsys, 2004; II-2-10.
2. Lam WW, Lam TP, Saing H, *et al.* MR cholangiography and CT cholangiography of pediatric patients with choledochal cysts. *AJR Am J Roentgenol* 1999;**173**(2):401–5.
3. Rozel C, Garel L, Rypens F, *et al.* Imaging of biliary disorders in children. *Pediatr Radiol* 2011;**41**(2):208–20.
4. Saito T, Hishiki T, Terui K, *et al.* Use of preoperative, 3-dimensional magnetic resonance cholangiopancreatography in pediatric choledochal cysts. *Surgery* 2011;**149**(4):569–75.
5. Singham J, Yoshida EM, Scudamore CH. Choledochal cysts: part 1 of 3: classification and pathogenesis. *Can J Surg* 2009;**52**(5):434–40.

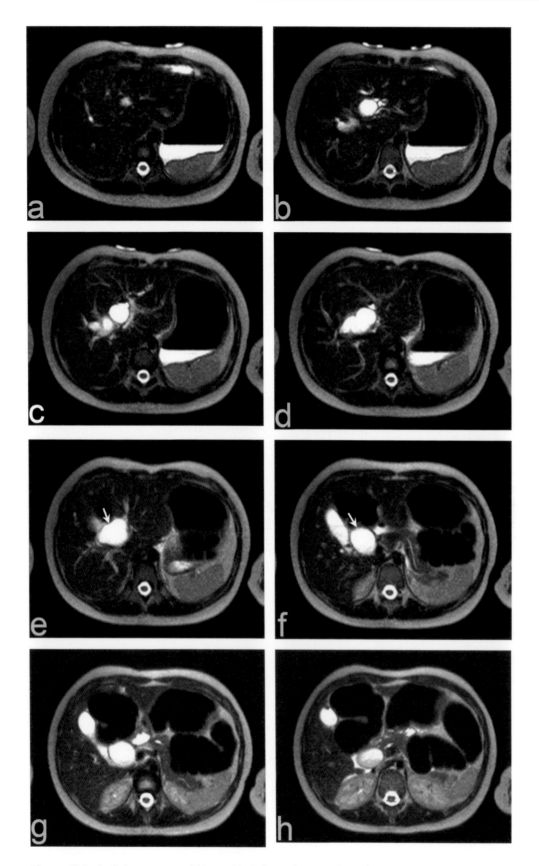

Figure 45.1. (a–i) A seven-year-old boy with abdominal pain and jaundice and Type 1 CC. Axial T2-weighted MR images sequence through the liver demonstrate dilatation of the hyperintense, fluid-filled CBD (arrows), distal common hepatic duct, and central right and left intrahepatic ducts. More peripheral intrahepatic ducts are normal. The gallbladder is seen separately (arrowhead).

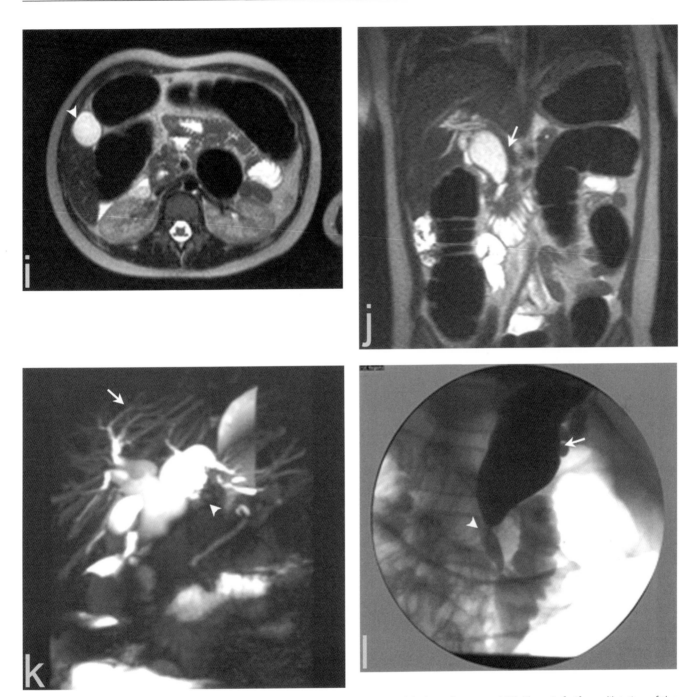

Figure 45.1. (cont.) **(j)** Coronal T2-weighted MR sequence demonstrating typical findings for a type I CC. There is fusiform dilatation of the CBD along most of its course to the duodenum (arrow). **(k)** T2-weighted MRCP image showing normal caliber of peripheral intrahepatic biliary ducts (arrow) and fusiform dilatation of the CBD, consistent with a type I CC. Some dilatation of the adjacent central hepatic ducts may sometimes be seen (arrowheads). **(l)** ERCP showing contrast filling the fusiform markedly dilated upper CBD (arrow) with less dilatation of the distal CBD (arrowhead).

Classification of Choledochal Cysts

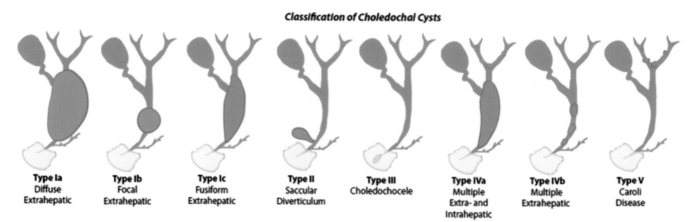

Type Ia	Type Ib	Type Ic	Type II	Type III	Type IVa	Type IVb	Type V
Diffuse Extrahepatic	Focal Extrahepatic	Fusiform Extrahepatic	Saccular Diverticulum	Choledochocele	Multiple Extra- and Intrahepatic	Multiple Extrahepatic	Caroli Disease

Figure 45.2. Classification of choledochal cysts according to Todani. Note the proximal pancreaticobiliary duct junction, one theory as to the etiology of choledochal cysts. Type I cysts are the most common, defined by extrahepatic, luminal dilatation, with subtypes Ia, Ib, and Ic. Type Ia is diffuse dilatation of the CBD that extends distal from the gallbladder. Type Ib is a focal dilatation of the extrahepatic system and type Ic is a fusiform dilatation. Type II represents a saccular diverticulum of the CBD. Type III represents a choledochocele with expansion into the intramural duodenum. Type IV is the second most common type, consisting of type IVa with multiple intra- and extrahepatic dilatations and type IVb with multiple dilatations confined to the extrahepatic system. The intrahepatic cysts of type V or Caroli disease are thought to be due to congenital ductal arrest (art by Tatyana Ter-Grigoryan).

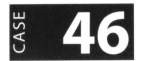

Henoch–Schönlein purpura

Kriengkrai Iemsawatdikul and Heike E. Daldrup-Link

Imaging description

A seven-year-old boy presented with nausea and acute, colicky abdominal pain. The medical history revealed a pharyngitis a few weeks ago and the clinical examination demonstrated multiple small purpura (small areas of hemorrhage) of the skin of the buttocks and upper thighs. An upper gastrointestinal (GI) study demonstrated "thumbprinting" of the duodenum (Fig. 46.1). CT images from another patient after oral contrast media administration demonstrate marked mural thickening of a loop of ileum with narrowing of the lumen and some adjacent free fluid (Fig. 46.2).

Importance

Henoch–Schönlein purpura is a disease of young children (50% are younger than six years of age and 90% are younger than 10 years of age), which typically occurs after an upper respiratory tract infection. The infection leads to formation of complexes of IgA and complement component 3, which accumulate in small vessels and cause a small-vessel vasculitis of the skin, joints, GI tract, and sometimes the kidneys. Acute GI symptoms may precede typical cutaneous lesions in 10–15% of patients and may lead to a laparotomy. It is important to recognize typical clinical and imaging findings of this disease, since it usually resolves spontaneously and does not require invasive interventions.

Typical clinical scenario

The "classic triad" of Henoch–Schönlein purpura is composed of (1) multiple small hemorrhages of the skin (purpura), (2) arthritis, and (3) abdominal pain. The abdominal pain is due to intramural intestinal hematomas in the small bowel, most commonly the duodenum and jejunum; colonic involvement is unusual. Fluoroscopic evaluations of the upper GI tract after administration of oral contrast media demonstrate mucosal fold thickening of the small bowel, "thumbprinting," pseudotumors, and intestinal hypomotility. CT findings comprise multifocal wall thickening of the small bowel, intramural hyperdense (30–80 HU) hemorrhage, mesenteric edema, vascular engorgement, and non-specific lymphadenopathy. A small bowel into small bowel intussusception is a relatively common complication of Henoch-Schönlein purpura. However, false-positive ultrasound diagnoses of intussusception-like target signs have also been described in the past. These false-positive findings are less common with modern high-frequency linear scanners, which can usually differentiate a bowel wall hematoma from the multilayered appearance of a true intussusception. Of note, small bowel into small bowel intussusceptions are not amenable to air or hydrostatic reduction. Henoch–Schönlein purpura usually resolves without complications. However, rarely, secondary vasculitic ischemic insults can lead to bowel perforation or strictures. An accompanying nephritis or nephrotic syndrome may not reveal abnormal findings on ultrasound or CT. However, in some cases, renal enlargement with loss of corticomedullary differentiation due to edema may be observed. Depending on the clinical symptoms, additional imaging studies may include chest x-rays to evaluate for pulmonary hemorrhage, testicular ultrasound to evaluate for testicular hemorrhage or torsion, and brain MRI to evaluate for vasculitis-induced cerebral ischemic lesions.

Differential diagnosis

Differential diagnoses for small bowel wall thickening and hemorrhage include other infectious or inflammatory conditions, trauma, bowel injury by perforating foreign bodies, and tumors, specifically lymphoma. Even though Crohn's disease can cause duodenal fold thickening, isolated lesions of the upper small bowel without involvement of the ileum are rare. Duodenal lymphoma is a possible cause of thickened duodenal mucosal folds, but is usually associated with high blood levels of lactate dehydrogenase (LDH) rather than inflammatory markers.

Teaching point

Henoch–Schönlein purpura is characterized by a classic triad of purpura of the skin, arthritis, and abdominal pain. Acute gastrointestinal symptoms due to wall thickening and hemorrhage of the small bowel may precede typical cutaneous lesions. It is important to recognize typical imaging features in order to initiate adequate conservative management and avoid invasive procedures.

REFERENCES
1. Jeong YK, Ha HK, Yoon CH, et al. Gastrointestinal involvement in Henoch-Schönlein syndrome: CT findings. AJR Am J Roentgenol 1997;**168**(4):965–8.
2. Mills JA, Michel BA, Bloch DA, et al. The American College of Rheumatology 1990 criteria for the classification of Henoch-Schönlein purpura. Arthritis Rheum 1990;**33**(8):1114–21.
3. Shirahama M, Umeno Y, Tomimasu R, et al. The values of colour Doppler ultrasonography for small bowel involvement of adult Henoch-Schönlein purpura. Br J Radiol 1998;**71**(847):788–91.

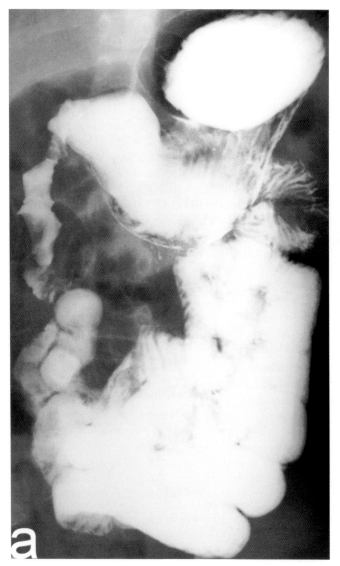

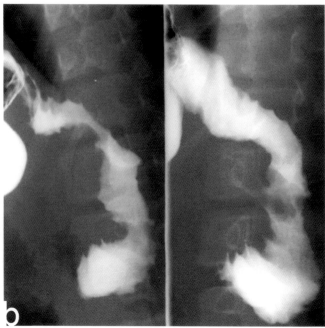

Figure 46.1. Upper GI study after oral administration of thin barium solution demonstrating irregular narrowing of the duodenum with mucosal fold thickening ("thumbprinting").

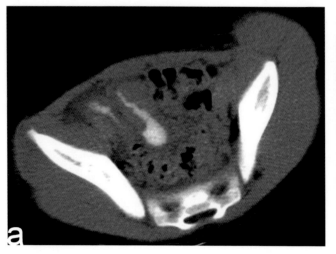

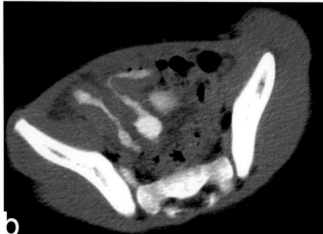

Figure 46.2. CT images from another patient after oral contrast media administration demonstrate marked mural thickening of a loop of ileum with narrowing of the lumen and some adjacent free fluid.

Biliary atresia

Guido Davidzon, Heike E. Daldrup-Link, and Beverley Newman

Imaging description

A three-week-old boy presented with persistent jaundice, dark urine, and light stool. Laboratory evaluation demonstrated hyperbilirubinemia. An ultrasound (US) of the liver showed normal size and echotexture of the liver. The gallbladder was markedly hypoplastic. The common bile duct could not be localized.

A hepatobiliary iminodiacetic acid (HIDA) scan was obtained after intravenous injection of technetium-99 m-HIDA Choletec with dynamic scans over the region of the abdomen in the anterior projection up to 60 minutes as well as static anterior and posterior views at four and 24 hours post injection (Fig. 47.1). Early scans demonstrated rapid uptake of the radiopharmaceutical by the liver, suggesting good hepatocellular function. However, no tracer excretion into the bile ducts or small bowel was seen at 24 hours post injection, suggesting extrahepatic biliary obstruction.

Importance

Congenital biliary atresia occurs with an incidence of 1/10 000 to 1/15 000 live births in the USA. The etiology is unknown, although infection/inflammation and autoimmune reactions may play a significant role. Girls are more commonly affected than boys and the disease is more common in Asian populations. Patients with biliary atresia can be subdivided into two groups: those with isolated biliary atresia (postnatal form), which accounts for 65–90% of cases, and patients with associated situs inversus or polysplenia with or without other congenital anomalies (fetal/embryonic form), comprising 10–35% of cases.

Typical clinical scenario

Patients with biliary atresia present with prolonged jaundice that persists beyond two weeks after birth and is resistant to phototherapy. Laboratory tests show conjugated hyperbilirubinemia. Jaundice and irritability typically worsen during the first month of life as opposed to physiologic jaundice, which usually resolves within two weeks postpartum. Other symptoms may include dark urine, an enlarged spleen, and floating and/or foul-smelling pale or clay-colored stools.

Confirmatory imaging studies include US HIDA scans, and sometimes intraoperative cholangiography. is helpful in both confirming biliary atresia as a likely diagnosis and ruling out other entities associated with neonatal jaundice such as choledochal cyst. It is important to perform US with the infant in a fasting state so as to accurately assess the size of the gallbladder. Sonographic features of biliary atresia include an absent or hypoplastic, typically non-contracting gallbladder (the gallbladder is present in up to 25% of cases, but usually very small and/or in unusual locations) and non-visualization of the common bile duct. An echogenic triangular or tubular area, known as the triangular cord sign, may be visible on US just superior to the portal vein in the liver hilum and is thought to represent the remnant of the common bile duct (Fig. 47.2). Both the triangular cord sign and a more recently described gallbladder ghost triad (length of gallbladder < 1.9 cm, thin or absent mucosa, and irregular gallbladder contour) have high diagnostic sensitivity and specificity for biliary atresia. The diagnosis of biliary atresia is confirmed by a HIDA scan, typically after 4–5 days of pretreatment with pentobarbital, which induces liver enzymes and biliary excretory function: technetium-99 m-labeled bilirubin analog, such as Choletec or Hepatolite, are secreted into the biliary tract. When the biliary system is functioning properly the entire bilirubin pathway from filling of the gallbladder to passage into the common bile duct and duodenum should be visualized. In cases with biliary atresia, there is hepatobiliary uptake of the tracer, but lack of excretion into the biliary tree and intestines. Lack of such excretion on 24-hour delayed scans is highly suggestive of biliary atresia. Of note, the reliability of HIDA scans is diminished at very high conjugated bilirubin levels (> 20 mg/dL). In addition, HIDA scans can be false positive or false negative in about 10% of evaluated cases.

When there is diagnostic uncertainty, especially when a gallbladder is present on US, iodinated, water-soluble contrast agent can be injected directly into the gallbladder in the operating room, prior to a portoenterostomy, and fluoroscopy can confirm the absence of extrahepatic bile ducts (Fig. 47.3). A percutaneous liver biopsy can also help to differentiate between obstructive and hepatocellular causes of cholestasis, with 90% sensitivity and specificity for biliary atresia.

More recently, MR imaging after administration of the hepatobiliary Gd-chelate Gd-DTPA-EOB (Eovist) has been suggested as an alternative to HIDA scans. This application is under investigation at this time and not yet established in clinical practice. Corresponding to HIDA scans, Eovist-enhanced T1-weighted MR scans show vascular and liver parenchymal enhancement in the early phase postcontrast with lack of biliary excretion on delayed postcontrast scans (Fig. 47.4).

The therapy of choice for biliary atresia is a connection of the central bile ducts at the porta hepatis with a Roux-en-Y anastomosis to a 35 cm to 40 cm retrocolic jejunal segment, a "Kasai" procedure. The success of a Kasai portoenterostomy is significantly reduced if the surgery is delayed beyond 60 days of life. Following a Kasai portoenterostomy, symptoms may resolve. However, long-term complications are common and include cholangitis, portal hypertension, and progressive liver cirrhosis. Even in patients with resolution of symptoms after a

Kasai surgery, a considerable number of the patients eventually undergo liver transplantation at variable times after the portoenterostomy.

Differential diagnosis

Differential diagnoses encompass other causes of liver dysfunction and/or extrahepatic biliary obstruction, including idiopathic cholestasis (which should resolve within 2 weeks postpartum), biliary stones, neonatal hepatitis, Alagille syndrome (peculiar facies, ocular abnormalities, biliary hypoplasia, peripheral pulmonary artery stenoses, butterfly vertebrae), Caroli disease, cystic fibrosis, alpha 1 antitrypsin deficiency, choledochal cysts, congenital infections, and neonatal hemochromatosis. The greatest diagnostic uncertainty is in differentiating neonatal hepatitis from biliary atresia. There is considerable clinical and imaging overlap between the two entities and they may actually represent a spectrum of the same fundamental disease process. Normal gallbladder size and contractility, thickened gallbladder wall, and presence of the common bile duct on US along with visualization of biliary excretion on HIDA scans are useful differential findings. However, in some cases, especially with high bilirubin levels and poor liver function, the imaging distinction may be very difficult. In these circumstances liver biopsy or intraoperative cholangiography may be helpful. The fetal form of biliary atresia is particularly associated with heterotaxy with polysplenia in which there are a wide variety of cardiac, vascular, and gastrointestinal anomalies.

Teaching point

Establishing the correct diagnosis in a timely manner is crucial for favorable outcomes. When the diagnosis of biliary atresia is suspected based on clinical and laboratory findings, a combination of US imaging and HIDA scan are often diagnostic. The addition of intraoperative cholangiography or MRI is helpful in equivocal cases.

REFERENCES

1. Schwarz SM. *Medscape. Pediatric Biliary Atresia.* 2011. http://emedicine.medscape.com/article/927029-overview (accessed September 17, 2012).

2. Sleisenger MH, Feldman M, Friedman LS. *Sleisenger and Fordtran's Gastrointestinal and Liver Disease: Pathophysiology, Diagnosis, Management,* 8th edition. Philadelphia: W.B. Saunders, 2006.

3. Slovis T, ed. *Caffey's Pediatric Diagnostic Imaging,* 11th edition. Philadelphia: Mosby Elsevier, 2008.

4. Tan Kendrick AP, Phua KB, Ooi BC, *et al.* Biliary atresia: making the diagnosis by the gallbladder ghost triad. *Pediatr Radiol* 2003;**33**(5):311–15.

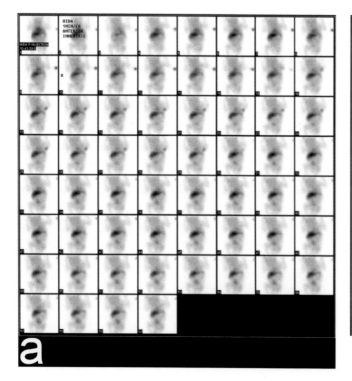
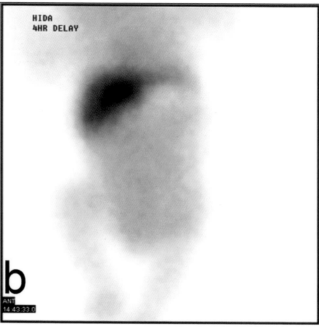

Figure 47.1. A three-week-old with persistent jaundice. **(a)** HIDA scan directly at 1 minute post injection demonstrates tracer uptake by the liver. There is excretion into the urinary bladder. **(b, c)** HIDA scans at four (b) and 24 (c) hours post injection demonstrate tracer retention in the liver with lack of excretion into the duodenum.

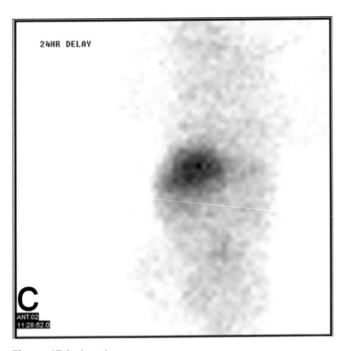

Figure 47.1. (cont.)

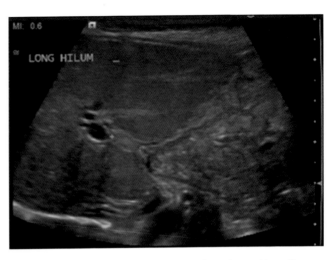

Figure 47.2. A four-week-old patient with prolonged jaundice. Fasting longitudinal US of the region of the liver hilum demonstrates non-visualization of the gallbladder and a tubular echogenic area (calipers) in the liver hilum at the expected location of the common duct. These US findings are strongly suspicious for biliary atresia, later confirmed by both non-visualization of the gallbladder on a nuclear medicine scan and surgical exploration.

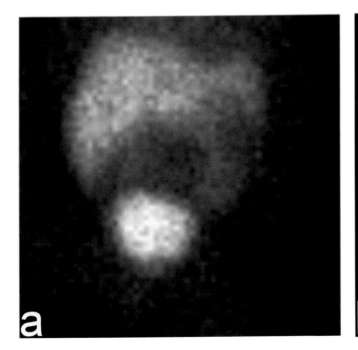

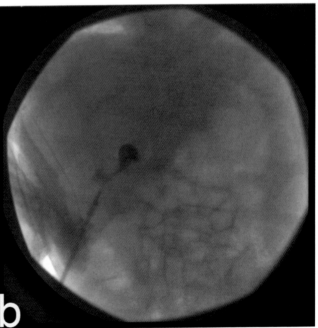

Figure 47.3. Another four-week-old child with severe and prolonged jaundice. **(a)** HIDA scan at 24 hours post injection demonstrates tracer retention in the liver with lack of excretion into the duodenum suggestive of biliary atresia. **(b)** Diagnosis confirmed at intraoperative cholangiogram with direct injection of iodinated contrast agent into a hypoplastic gallbladder showing no evidence for a common bile duct.

(a)

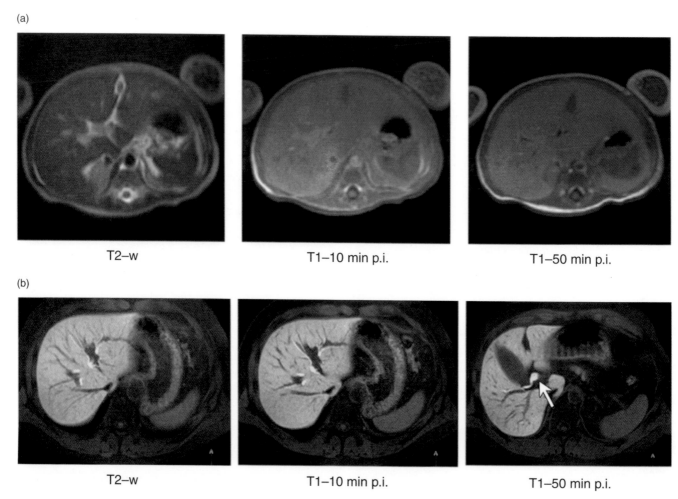

T2–w   T1–10 min p.i.   T1–50 min p.i.

(b)

T2–w   T1–10 min p.i.   T1–50 min p.i.

Figure 47.4. (a) T2-weighted MR scan (a, left) shows no evidence for intrahepatic cholestasis or choledochal cyst. T1-weighted MR scan at 10 minutes after intravenous injection of Gd-DTPA-EOB (Eovist) demonstrates vascular and parenchymal enhancement. T1-weighted MR scan at 50 minutes after intravenous injection of Eovist demonstrates lack of biliary contrast excretion suggestive of biliary atresia. **(b)** A different patient with a comparative normal T1-weighted MR at 50 minutes post injection of Eovist. There is good liver parenchymal enhancement and excretion of contrast agent into intra and extrahepatic bile ducts, with hyperintense delineation of the common bile duct (arrow).

CASE 48

Mesenchymal hamartoma of the liver

Aman Khurana, Fanny Chapelin, and Heike E. Daldrup-Link

Imaging description

An infant who was several weeks old presented with an incidental finding of a palpable abdominal mass on a routine clinical examination. The child did not have fever or any other clinical abnormalities. The liver was palpable 10 cm below the right costal margin. Ultrasound and CT studies demonstrated a large, multiseptated cystic lesion in the right lobe of the liver (Fig. 48.1). This was thought to be most consistent with a mesenchymal cystic hamartoma of the liver.

Importance

Mesenchymal hamartoma is a rare, benign liver neoplasm, typically found in children less than two years of age. The lesion is slightly more common in boys than in girls. It is a developmental cystic liver tumor, composed of proliferations of variably myxomatous mesenchyme and malformed bile ducts. Treatment consists of surgical resection.

Typical clinical scenario

Patients typically present with an asymptomatic abdominal mass. Rarely, complications including ascites, jaundice, and even congestive heart failure can occur. Since mesenchymal hamartomas are congenital malformations, they may be detected prenatally. The size is highly variable. The lesions may grow rapidly in the postnatal period, followed by growth stasis or even some regression. Most lesions are located within the liver parenchyma, although rare cases of pedunculated lesions have been described as well.

On CT scans, a mesenchymal hamartoma typically appears as a multicystic mass with thin septae, which may enhance after contrast media injection. Much more rarely, mesenchymal hamartomas may have predominantly stromal (mesenchymal), solid elements, which enhance after contrast media injection. Hemorrhage occasionally occurs but is not typical. Calcifications are usually not found in mesenchymal hamartomas. The characteristic MRI appearance of mesenchymal hamartoma is that of a multicystic mass. The cystic components of the mass are T2-hyperintense and T1-hypointense compared to liver tissue, with similar signal compared to cerebrospinal fluid (in the spinal canal) as an internal standard. The much more rare predominantly stromal variant appears as a solid mass with multiple cysts of varying size ("swiss cheese" appearance). The stromal components enhance after contrast media injection.

Differential diagnosis

Differential diagnoses in young children include other congenital hepatic cysts (very rare), choledochal cyst or Caroli's disease (irregularly dilated bile ducts), parasitic cysts (such as echinococcal cysts or amebic abscesses), hemorrhage/ hematoma (see Case 42), or pyogenic abscesses (Fig. 48.2). The latter is usually associated with clinical and laboratory signs of inflammation. The presence of high fever and air in a cystic liver mass is very suggestive of a pyogenic liver abscess. Infantile hemangiomas and hemangioendotheliomas can have a somewhat similar appearance on unenhanced scans, but they show peripheral-to-central enhancement after intravenous contrast administration, with contrast pooling on delayed postcontrast scans (Fig. 48.2). Hepatoblastoma is the most common malignant liver neoplasm in infants; this is typically a single or multifocal heterogeneously enhancing solid mass which may have some cystic or necrotic components, particularly after therapy (Fig. 48.3).

In older children, typically teenagers, an embryonal sarcoma of the liver should also be considered in the differential diagnosis of a multicystic hepatic mass. Embryonal sarcomas of the liver present as apparently cystic masses, which contain soft tissue components, that can be delineated on ultrasound, and which show slow, delayed enhancement on delayed postcontrast CT and MR scans (Fig. 48.4). The etiology of these lesions is controversial: while some authors believe that embryonal sarcoma of the liver is a distinct tumor, others postulate that they result from malignant transformation of mesenchymal hamartomas. In accordance with the latter theory, mesenchymal hamartoma and embryonal sarcoma have similar imaging characteristics, although embryonal sarcomas occur in older children and usually have some soft tissue components. Begueret et al. reported a case of a large, cystic hepatic mass in a 17-year-old girl that contained histologic elements of both embryonal sarcoma and mesenchymal hamartoma.

Teaching point

A mesenchymal hamartoma is the most common benign cystic liver mass in a young child and should be the major differential consideration when a multicystic hepatic mass is found in this age group. Embryonal sarcoma has a very similar multicystic appearance but it occurs in older children and contains additional soft tissue components.

REFERENCES

1. Begueret H, Trouette H, Vielh P, et al. Hepatic undifferentiated embryonal sarcoma: malignant evolution of mesenchymal hamartoma? Study of one case with immunohistochemical and flow cytometric emphasis. J Hepatol 2001;34(1):178–9.

2. Buonomo C, Taylor GA, Share JC, et al. Gastrointestinal tract. In: Kirks DR, Griscom NT, eds. Practical Pediatric Imaging: Diagnostic Radiology of Infants and Children, 3rd edition. Philadelphia: Lippincott-Raven, 1998; 963–4.

3. Horton KM, Bluemke DA, Hruban RH, et al. CT and MR imaging of benign hepatic and biliary tumors. Radiographics 1999;19(2):431–51.

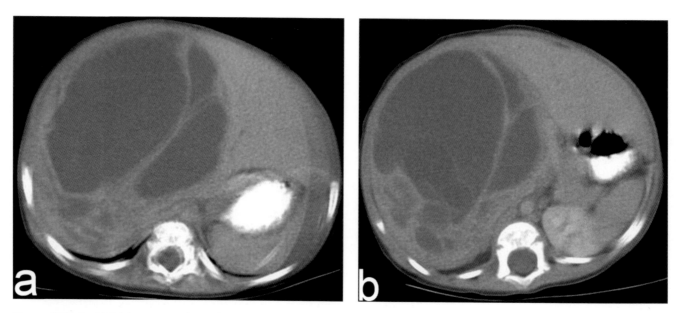

Figure 48.1. (a, b) Axial contrast-enhanced CT scans. Multiseptated, multicystic mass in the right lobe of the liver in an infant, proven to be a mesenchymal hamartoma on histopathology.

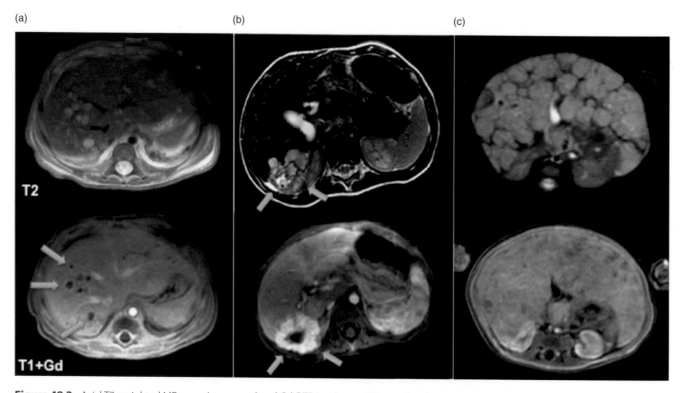

Figure 48.2. Axial T2-weighted MR scans (upper row) and Gd-DTPA-enhanced T1-weighted MR scans (lower row) of multiple hepatic abscesses in a patient with methicillin resistant *Staphylococcus aureus* (MRSA) sepsis **(a)**, a unifocal hemangioendothelioma **(b)**, and a multifocal hemangioendothelioma **(c)**. All lesions show fluid-equivalent signal on T2-weighted sequences, similar to spinal fluid as an internal standard. Solitary hemangioendotheliomas may have a lobulated contour and central inhomogeneities from central calcification, necrosis, or bleeding. Multifocal hemangioendotheliomas can occupy the whole liver parenchyma **(c)**. Liver abscesses show peripheral rim enhancement **(a)**, while hemangioendotheliomas show peripheral-to-central contrast enhancement with contrast pooling on delayed postcontrast scans.

(a)   (b)

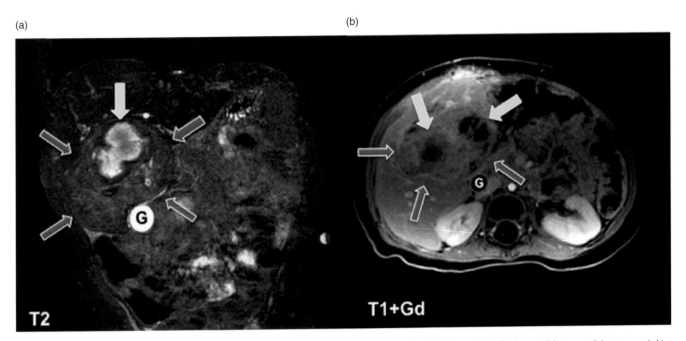

Figure 48.3. Coronal T2-weighted MR scan **(a)** and axial contrast-enhanced T1-weighted MR scan **(b)** of a hepatoblastoma (blue arrows). Note solid tumor component, which shows similar T2 signal and contrast enhancement compared to adjacent liver parenchyma. Areas of central necrosis appear T2-hyperintense and show diminished or no contrast enhancement (yellow arrows).

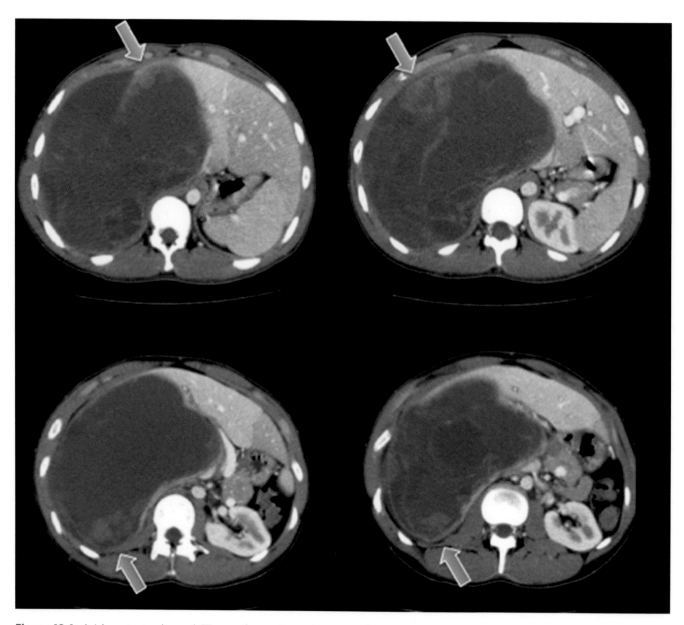

Figure 48.4. Axial, contrast-enhanced CT scan of an embryonal sarcoma of the liver in a teenager. The lesion presents as an apparently cystic mass, which contains inhomogeneous enhancing areas of soft tissue attenuation (arrows). These lesions can be mistaken for a bleed or abscess. However, the patients typically have no clinical or lab signs of blood loss or infection.

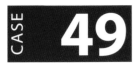

Lymphoid follicular hyperplasia

Heike E. Daldrup-Link

Imaging description

An 11-year-old patient presented with diffuse abdominal pain. The medical history, clinical examination, and laboratory values did not reveal any abnormal findings. A fluoroscopic barium upper gastrointestinal (GI) study with small bowel follow through (SBFT) revealed multiple 2 mm nodules on the mucosal surface of the terminal ileum, deforming the thin barium-filled parallel folds that are seen in the contracted ileum (Fig. 49.1). These mucosal nodules are typical of benign enlarged lymphoid follicles, a frequent finding in children and adolescents. Additional examples are shown in (Figs. 49.2 and 49.3).

Importance

Lymphoid follicular hyperplasia of the intestinal tract represents a benign enlargement of the submucosal lymphoid follicles. It is a common condition in children and adolescents. The lesions may present in two forms, a focal or a diffuse type. In the more common focal type, an aggregate of benign lymphoid nodules is found in an isolated area, usually the terminal ileum. In the less common diffuse form, a multinodular pattern is found throughout much of the GI tract, especially the colon. The diffuse follicular hyperplasia may be seen in children with GI infections and/or bleeding and perhaps represents a lymphoid reaction to an unidentified infection. Especially when found in the colon, benign follicular hyperplasia has been confused with multiple polyposis, leading to unnecessary surgery or endoscopic resections. Follicular lymphoid hyperplasia of the appendix is associated with dilatation and thickening of the mucosa and can be mistaken for appendicitis or other pathology (Fig. 49.3). Absence of wall thickening, hyperemia, and periappendiceal inflammation help in making this distinction.

Typical clinical scenario

Patients usually present with highly variable, often non-specific abdominal complaints, which lead to an imaging evaluation and/or endoscopy of the GI tract and incidental finding of focal or diffuse lymphoid follicular hyperplasia. On upper or lower GI fluoroscopies, the lesions are demonstrated as small radiolucent filling defects, which are of uniform size and typically show a small umbilication within the center. Histologically, discrete polypoid lesions of lymphoid tissue with germinal centers are present. Rarely, the lesions can serve as a lead point for intussusception.

Differential diagnosis

The differential diagnoses of benign, idiopathic lymphoid follicular hyperplasia of the GI tract include (1) inflammatory diseases, such as Crohn's disease, (2) bacterial, parasitic, or viral intestinal infections, such as salmonella, campylobacter, yersinia, and tuberculous gastroenteritis, (3) diffuse nodular lymphoid hyperplasia associated with immunodeficiencies, hypogammaglobulinemias, autoimmune disorders, and allergies (particularly food allergies), and (4) neoplastic conditions such as intestinal polyps, malignant lymphoma, or carcinoma. Bronen and colleagues have reported that the presence of unusually prominent lymphoid follicles in adults may be associated with colonic tumors and should promote a vigorous search for the presence of an underlying colonic tumor.

> ### Teaching point
>
> Benign lymphoid hyperplasia of the GI tract is a common normal variant in children, sometimes associated with intestinal infection and/or immunologic disorders. Characteristic imaging features include typical location, especially in the terminal ileum, uniform small size <3 mm, and central umbilication. Lymphoid hyperplasia of the appendix, either idiopathic or reactive, can accompany generalized lymphoid hyperplasia and should be considered when there is mild non-specific dilatation and mucosal thickening of the appendix without other clinical and imaging signs of inflammation.

REFERENCES

1. Bronen RA, Glick SN, Teplick SK. Diffuse lymphoid follicles of the colon associated with colonic carcinoma. *AJR Am J Roentgenol* 1984;**142**(1):105–9.
2. Iacono G, Ravelli A, Di Prima L, *et al*. Colonic lymphoid nodular hyperplasia in children: relationship to food hypersensitivity. *Clin Gastroenterol Hepatol* 2007;**5**(3):361–6.
3. Lappas JC, Maglinte DDT. The small bowel. In: Putman CE, Rawin CE, eds. *Textbook of Diagnostic Imaging*. Philadelphia: W.B. Saunders Company, 1998; 846–50.
4. Park NH, Oh HE, Park HJ, *et al*. Ultrasonography of normal and abnormal appendix in children. *World J Radiol* 2011;**3**(4):85–91.
5. Parker BR. The abdomen and gastrointestinal tract: the colon. In: Silverman FN, Kuhn JP, eds. *Caffey's Pediatric X-ray Diagnosis: An Integrated Imaging Approach*. St Louis: Mosby, 1992; 1119.

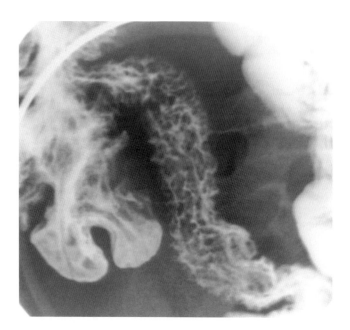

Figure 49.1. Spot view of the terminal ileum on a barium upper GI/SB fluoroscopy, demonstrating a multinodular pattern of the mucosa of the terminal ileum with central small filling defects (umbilication), consistent with lymphoid follicles.

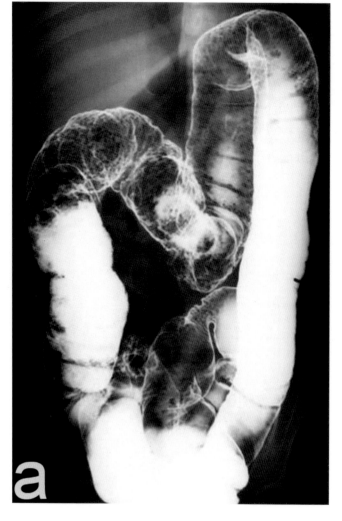

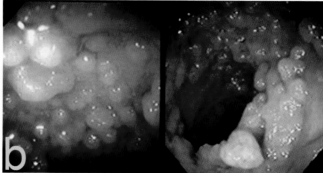

Figure 49.2. (a) Barium enema in another four-year-old patient with lymphoid hyperplasia, demonstrating fairly uniform 1–3 mm nodules diffusely throughout the transverse colon, including the hepatic and splenic flexures. **(b)** Lymphoid hyperplasia shown on endoscopy of the colon and terminal ileum, demonstrating multiple 1–2 mm small mucosal nodules with smooth contour and fairly uniform size.

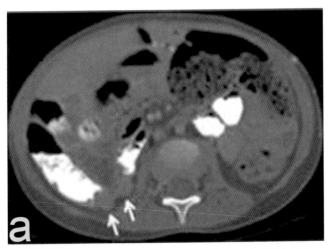

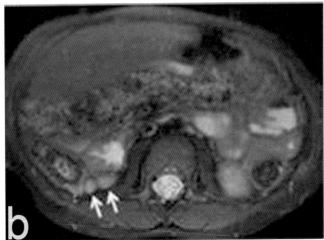

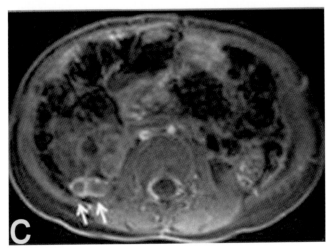

Figure 49.3. Lymphoid hyperplasia including the appendix in a three-year-old asymptomatic male post liver transplant for hepatoblastoma. Routine surveillance contrast-enhanced CT (**a**) and MR scans of the abdomen (**b**: T2-weighted scan, **c**: T1-weighted scan postcontrast) 8 months apart, demonstrate a dilated 8–10 mm appendix (arrows) with wall enhancement and no periappendiceal inflammatory changes or lymphadenopathy. There is mild wall thickening of the terminal ileum and a suggestion of small focal lesions in the proximal colon. Epstein–Barr virus titers were negative. Two colonoscopies with several biopsies demonstrated diffuse lymphoid hyperplasia of the terminal ileum and proximal colon.

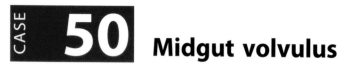

Midgut volvulus

Heike E. Daldrup-Link

Imaging description

A neonate who was a few days old presented with acute bilious vomiting. A radiograph of the abdomen demonstrated a "double bubble" sign with air in the stomach and the duodenum, but no air in more distal loops of bowel. An upper gastrointestinal (GI) fluoroscopy after oral administration of thin barium solution revealed an obstruction of the proximal duodenum and a "corkscrew" appearance of subsequent small bowel loops (Fig. 50.1). These findings are characteristic for malrotation of the small bowel and midgut volvulus around the mesenteric axis (Fig. 50.2).

Importance

Bowel malrotation occurs when there is abnormal rotation of the bowel in utero, resulting in absence of the normal broad mesenteric fixation from the left upper quadrant (proximal jejunum–ligament of Treitz) to the right lower quadrant (cecal fixation). As a result the mesentery and accompanying vessels have a narrow stalk-like configuration. Midgut volvulus is characterized by rotation of the proximal small bowel around the mesenteric stalk with variable compromise of the blood supply to the bowel. Affected bowel may extend from the proximal duodenum to the mid transverse colon. Arterial compromise may lead to mucosal necrosis, pneumatosis, perforation, peritonitis, and death. Thus, immediate and emergent evaluation is warranted in a case of suspected midgut volvulus.

An intermittent volvulus may present with more subacute symptoms, such as intermittent vomiting, alternating constipation and diarrhea, chronic malabsorption, mesenteric cyst formation, and chylous ascites (from venolymphatic congestion).

Typical clinical scenario

Midgut volvulus most often occurs in neonates and young infants. They present with bilious vomiting as well as clinical and radiographic signs of high intestinal obstruction. Associated anomalies include heterotaxy and congenital heart disease, congenital diaphragmatic hernia, omphalocele, gastroschisis, imperforate anus, and biliary atresia. Conventional radiographs typically show a "double bubble" sign with air in a dilated stomach and proximal duodenum, but paucity of gas in more distal loops of bowel. Rarely, an abdominal radiograph can be normal. The additional presence of fixed dilated small bowel loops and/or pneumatosis on plain radiographs indicates possible bowel ischemia/necrosis.

The imaging modality of choice to diagnose a midgut volvulus is an upper GI fluoroscopy. It should demonstrate partial or complete duodenal obstruction, with a "birdbeak"

obstruction of the proximal duodenum and a "corkscrew" appearance of the lower duodenum and proximal jejunum. Malrotation without volvulus is characterized by absence of the normal fixation point of the ligament of Treitz to the left of the spine and superiorly at the level of the pylorus. There may be partial duodenal obstruction without volvulus, most often related to crossing mesenteric Ladd's bands. Continuation of the small bowel series to show abnormally positioned proximal jejunal loops on the right side can be a helpful confirmation of malrotation. Although abnormal position of the cecum is suggestive of malrotation, lower GI studies are not particularly helpful as the cecum can normally be somewhat mobile. In addition, a lower GI study may obscure findings on a subsequent upper GI study.

An ultrasound is rarely performed with a suspected volvulus, but if done for other reasons, it may show an inversion of the position of the superior mesenteric vein and artery (suggestive of bowel malrotation) with a "whirlpool" appearance of these vessels and adjacent bowel (indicative of volvulus). Incidental note of duodenal dilatation and bowel wall thickening due to edema and venous congestion may also support the diagnosis.

Likewise, a CT is not indicated to confirm the diagnosis. However, in children, in whom a contrast-enhanced CT is performed for a different indication, the same abnormal mesenteric vascular relationships (Fig. 50.3), a "hurricane" or "whirlpool" appearance of the mesenteric vessels (Fig. 50.3), and mural edema and hypoperfusion of bowel may be noted.

A midgut volvulus is only possible when there is malrotation of the bowel. Patients at risk for malrotation are screened for this abnormality (Fig. 50.4). An abnormal position of the duodenojejunal junction on upper GI fluoroscopy is the single best sign of small bowel malrotation. Examples are shown in (Fig. 50.4). Other signs of malrotation include absent or incomplete dorsal sweep of the duodenum on a lateral view, as well as an abnormally high position of the cecum, mentioned above.

Malrotation can be suggested by abnormal superior mesenteric vein/artery relationships (normally SMV is located to the right and anterior to the SMA) on abdominal ultrasound, CT (Fig. 50.3), or MR. An attempt can be made on these studies to determine if there is a retroperitoneal course of the duodenum (normal) or not (malrotation). However, an upper GI study is usually required for confirmation and help with determining whether prophylactic surgery (Ladd's procedure with mesenteric fixation) is required to prevent midgut volvulus. Non-rotation of the bowel is an uncommon variation where the small bowel is right-sided and the large bowel all left-sided. In this situation, when the cecum is low, there is broad mesenteric fixation and the child is at very low risk for volvulus.

Differential diagnosis

Differential diagnoses of duodenal obstruction include duodenal atresia, duodenal web, duodenal stenosis, preduodenal portal vein, and annular pancreas. Some authors postulate that the dilatation of the proximal duodenum is more severe in cases with chronic duodenal obstruction as opposed to the usual acute setting of a midgut volvulus. Of note, the above-mentioned diagnoses and malrotation or midgut volvulus can coexist. In cases with complete duodenal obstruction without other typical signs of a midgut volvulus, all of the above differential diagnoses can be considered and a surgical exploration is warranted.

Other differential diagnoses include pathologies that lead to displacement of the duodenojejunal junction, such as abdominal tumor, mesenteric cyst, bowel duplication, or marked splenomegaly.

Some infants demonstrate a redundant duodenum on upper GI studies, which can be difficult to differentiate from malrotation. It is important to localize the duodenojejunal junction in its usual position, to the left of the spine and at the level of the pylorus (Fig. 50.4). A normal position of the cecum in the right lower quadrant can confirm normal bowel rotation.

Teaching point

A suspected midgut volvulus is an emergency warranting immediate evaluation via an upper GI fluoroscopy study. Classic signs of a midgut volvulus include obstruction and "beaking" of the proximal duodenum with abrupt transition to narrowed small bowel loops with a "corkscrew" appearance. Upper GI with small bowel follow through is currently considered the most useful diagnostic study to evaluate possible bowel malrotation without or with obstruction or volvulus.

Malrotation can be suspected, but not confirmed with certainty, on cross-sectional imaging based on an abnormal SMA/SMV relationship. The "whirlpool" sign on cross-sectional imaging is diagnostic of volvulus and should be urgently relayed to the referring clinician.

REFERENCES

1. Applegate KE, Anderson JM, Klatte EC. Intestinal malrotation in children: a problem-solving approach to the upper gastrointestinal series. *Radiographics* 2006;**26**(5):1485–500.

2. Reid JR. *Medscape. Midgut Volvulus Imaging.* 2011 http://emedicine.medscape.com/article/411249-overview#a24 (accessed September 18, 2012).

3. Sizemore AW, Rabbani KZ, Ladd A, *et al.* Diagnostic performance of the upper gastrointestinal series in the evaluation of children with clinically suspected malrotation. *Pediatr Radiol* 2008;**38**(5):518–28.

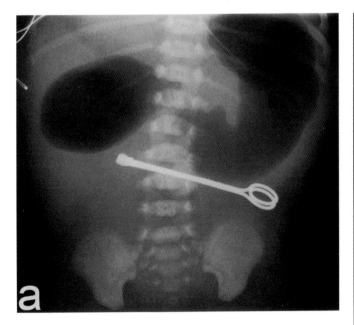
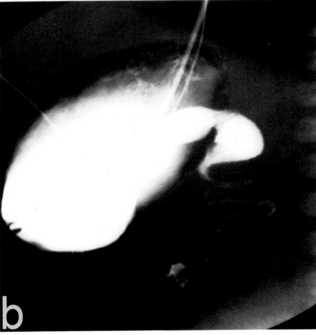

Figure 50.1. (a) A radiograph of the abdomen in a neonate with acute bilious vomiting demonstrates a "double bubble" sign (air in the stomach and proximal duodenum), indicative of a duodenal obstruction. **(b)** An upper GI fluoroscopy after oral administration of thin barium solution demonstrates dilatation of the proximal duodenum with abrupt transition to a narrow lumen of the more distal small bowel loops, revealing a characteristic "corkscrew" appearance, diagnostic of malrotation with a midgut volvulus.

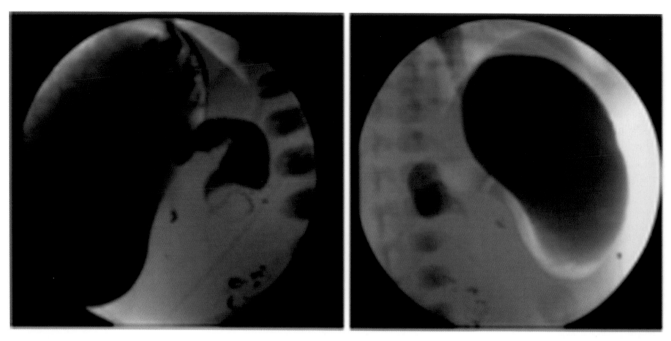

Figure 50.2. An upper GI fluoroscopy study in a different patient also shows the characteristic beaking of the obstructed duodenum and the corkscrew appearance of small bowel volvulus.

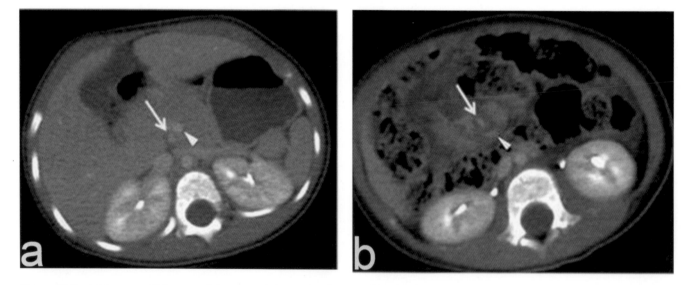

Figure 50.3. Axial contrast CT images of the upper abdomen in a 2.5-year-old girl with acute abdominal pain. **(a)** CT image at level of the renal veins demonstrates an inverted abnormal relationship between the superior mesenteric artery (SMA, arrow) and vein (SMV, anterior and left, arrowhead). Normally the SMV is located anterior and to the right of the SMA. **(b)** Axial CT a few slices lower demonstrates the "whirlpool" or "hurricane" sign of midgut volvulus with the SMV (arrowhead) and adjacent bowel loops twisted around the SMA (arrow).

(b–e) malrotation

(a) normal

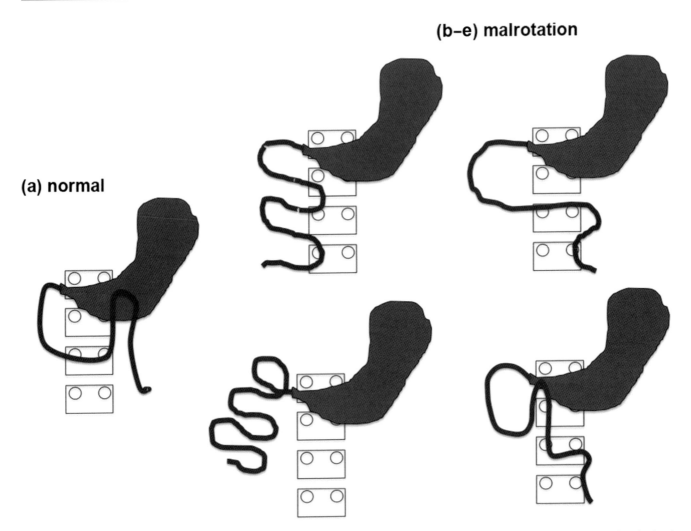

Figure 50.4. (a) Normal rotation of the bowel with normal position of the duodenojejunal junction, to the left of the spine and at the level of the pylorus. **(b–e)** Possible appearances of malrotation on upper GI fluoroscopies. In all of these cases, the duodenojejunal junction is not in its normal position.

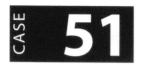

CASE 51

Foveolar hyperplasia: post prostaglandin therapy

Kriengkrai Iemsawatdikul and Heike E. Daldrup-Link

Imaging description

A five-week-old infant presented with projectile vomiting and failure to thrive. There was a prior history of cyanotic congenital heart disease, treated with prostaglandin therapy. On clinical examination, there was no palpable pyloric mass. An ultrasound demonstrated elongation of the pyloric channel without muscular wall thickening, but with markedly prominent hyperechogenic mucosa of the antrum and pylorus (Fig. 51.1a, b). An upper gastrointestinal (GI) fluoroscopy confirmed gastric outlet obstruction with elongation and narrowing of the pyloric channel (Fig. 51.1c, d).

Importance

Prostaglandin therapy can lead to deepening and widening of the gastric fovea (the pits in the mucosa into which gastric glands empty) with hyperplasia and redundancy of the epithelium, especially in the antral and pyloric regions (Figs. 51.1 and 51.2). This "foveolar hyperplasia" can cause obstruction of the gastric outlet, mimicking hypertrophic pyloric stenosis clinically. It is important to differentiate foveolar hyperplasia from hypertrophic pyloric stenosis (Fig. 51.3), since the former is treated conservatively, while the latter is treated with surgical pyloromyotomy.

Typical clinical scenario

Patients are typically neonates and infants with cyanotic heart disease and prostaglandin therapy, who present with projectile vomiting and failure to thrive. The symptoms occur a few weeks to months after start of prostaglandin therapy and reverse completely within two months after stopping prostaglandin.

Differential diagnosis

The main differential diagnosis is pyloric stenosis (Fig. 51.3). In foveolar hyperplasia, the pyloric channel may be elongated (>16mm), but the muscle wall is not thickened (muscle wall thickness <3–4mm). Foveolar hyperplasia can sometimes be focal, then mimicking ectopic pancreas or a gastric neoplasm.

Prostaglandin therapy can lead to other imaging findings that may help confirm the diagnosis, such as periosteal reactions of the long bones, particularly involving the ribs and shafts of the humeri and femura (Fig. 51.2), as well as brown fat calcifications, i.e. dystrophic soft tissue calcifications along the lower neck, axillae, and chest wall. Other differential diagnoses include other causes of gastric outlet obstruction, such as eosinophilic gastroenteritis, duodenal atresia, duodenal web, and annular pancreas.

Teaching point

In patients who present with clinical signs of a gastric outlet obstruction, who also have a history of cyanotic congenital heart disease and prostaglandin therapy, foveolar hyperplasia should be considered. An ultrasound can help to distinguish between muscle thickening in hypertrophic pyloric stenosis and mucosal thickening in foveolar hyperplasia.

REFERENCES

1. Katz ME, Blocker SH, McAlister WH. Focal foveolar hyperplasia presenting as an antral-pyloric mass in a young infant. *Pediatr Radiol* 1985;**15**(2):136–7.
2. McAlister WH, Katz ME, Perlman JM, *et al.* Sonography of focal foveolar hyperplasia causing gastric obstruction in an infant. *Pediatr Radiol* 1988;**18**(1):79–81.
3. Mercado-Deane MG, Burton EM, Brawley AV, *et al.* Prostaglandin-induced foveolar hyperplasia simulating pyloric stenosis in an infant with cyanotic heart disease. *Pediatr Radiol* 1994;**24**(1):45–6.
4. Tytgat GN, Offerhaus GJ, van Minnen AJ, *et al.* Influence of oral 15(R)-15-methyl prostaglandin E2 on human gastric mucosa: a light microscopic, cell kinetic, and ultrastructural study. *Gastroenterology* 1986;**90**(5 Pt 1):1111–20.
5. Voutilainen M, Juhola M, Färkkilä M, *et al.* Foveolar hyperplasia at the gastric cardia: prevalence and associations. *J Clin Pathol* 2002;**55**(5):352–4.

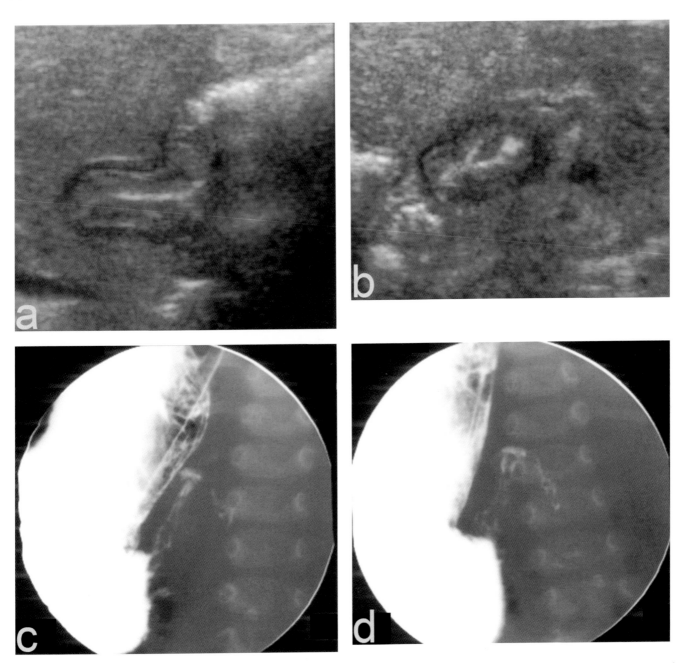

Figure 51.1. Sagittal **(a)** and transverse **(b)** ultrasound scans through the pylorus show normal thickness of the hypoechogenic muscle layer of the pylorus, but thickened hyperechogenic mucosa. **(c, d)** An upper GI fluoroscopy study after oral administration of thin barium solution demonstrates persistent elongation and narrowing of the pyloric channel.

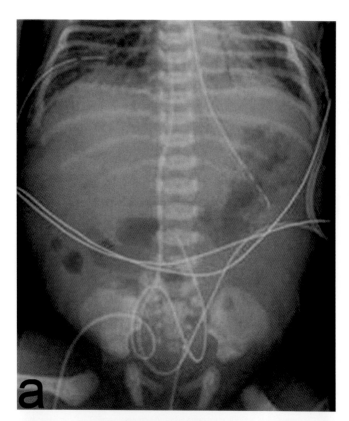

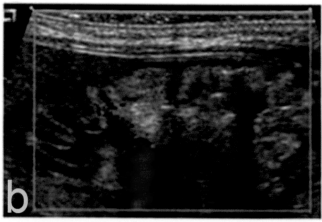

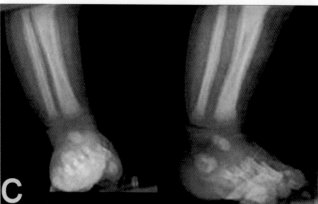

Figure 51.2. Infant with critical aortic coarctation on prostaglandin therapy. Foveolar hyperplasia and bony periosteal thickening. **(a)** Frontal abdominal radiograph at two weeks of age demonstrates thickening of gastric folds. **(b)** Transverse ultrasound image of the stomach demonstrates marked thickening of the gastric/antral wall without hyperemia. **(c)** Frontal and lateral radiographs of the right lower leg at three weeks of age show marked smooth asymptomatic tibial and fibular periosteal cloaking, likely also secondary to prolonged prostaglandin therapy. This was bilateral (not shown).

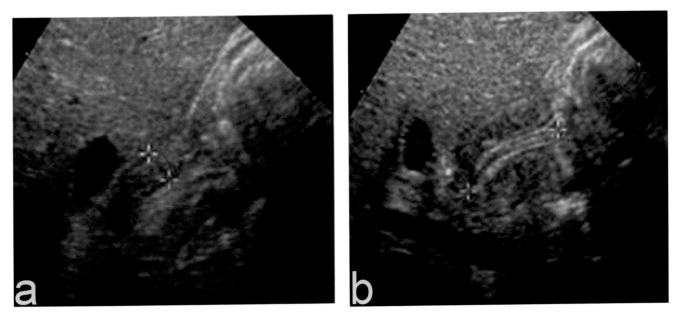

Figure 51.3. Pyloric stenosis. Sagittal **(a)** and transverse **(b)** ultrasound scans through the pylorus show increased thickness (5 mm) and increased length (1.9 cm) of the hypoechogenic muscle layer of the pylorus. The echogenic mucosa of the pyloric channel is normal in thickness.

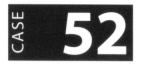

CASE 52 Pneumatosis cystoides intestinalis

Heike E. Daldrup-Link

Imaging description

A nine-year-old girl with cystic fibrosis presented with chronic constipation. The patient did not have any other clinical symptoms. A radiograph of the abdomen demonstrated multiple focal, rounded lucencies along the course of the colon consistent with extensive colonic pneumatosis (Fig. 52.1). A different, asymptomatic patient was found to have pneumatosis intestinalis on a routine radiograph of the abdomen after chemotherapy and bone marrow transplant. In this case, the pneumatosis was linear in configuration, outlining the colonic wall (Fig. 52.2).

Importance

Benign pneumatosis cystoides intestinalis is a rare form of pneumatosis, characterized by multiple thin-walled microvesicular gas collections in the subserosa or submucosa of the colon. Some authors postulate that the cystic-bubbly type of pneumatosis refers to subserosal air while a linear configuration of intramural air refers to submucosal air. Radiographs demonstrate multiple small, round or linear gas collections along the course of the bowel. An ultrasound can often confirm the presence and location of the intramural air (Fig. 52.3) and may be useful for follow-up studies. A CT is rarely needed to confirm the diagnosis in asymptomatic patients. The etiology of benign pneumatosis is thought to be twofold: (1) in patients with cystic fibrosis or other obstructive pulmonary disorders, gas may dissect from ruptured alveoli along vessels and bronchi into the mediastinum, then along major vessels into the retroperitoneum and via the mesentery to the subserosa of bowel loops; (2) intramural gas may originate from intraluminal gas in the bowel, which enters the bowel wall either through a mucosal defect (trauma, ulcer, tear) or as a result of increased intraluminal pressure. In benign idiopathic pneumatosis, the specific underlying cause is typically not identified and the pneumatosis is an isolated radiologic diagnosis without associated clinical symptoms, therefore allowing conservative treatment. A well-documented complication is spontaneous rupture of a gas cyst and formation of an asymptomatic pneumoperitoneum. Treatment is usually still unnecessary. Because the cysts contain high levels (70–75%) of nitrogen, hyperbaric oxygen therapy can be beneficial if the pneumatosis does not resolve spontaneously.

Typical clinical scenario

Benign pneumatosis cystoides intestinalis typically does not cause any symptoms and presents as an incidental finding on imaging studies. However, a variety of mild coexisting clinical findings have been described, including diarrhea, constipation, passage of mucus per rectum, vague abdominal discomfort, abdominal pain, urgency, malabsorption, weight loss, and excessive flatus. It is more likely that these symptoms may lead to an imaging study, which then reveals the coexisting benign pneumatosis rather than confirming a causal association.

Differential diagnosis

Benign, idiopathic pneumatosis has to be differentiated from secondary pneumatosis intestinalis, which may be due to a variety of defined pathologies. Some of these may also be benign and generally asymptomatic including: (1) obstructive pulmonary diseases or chest trauma, with air entering the mesentery as described above; (2) disruption of the mucosa of the small or large bowel, e.g. due to blunt trauma, surgery, or endoscopy; (3) increased intraluminal pressure, such as in intestinal obstructions, including pyloric stenosis and Hirschsprung's disease; and (4) increased mucosal permeability, such as in patients after chemotherapy, steroid therapy, bone marrow transplantation, and graft-versus-host disease.

More concerning and more likely to be symptomatic and require treatment is pneumatosis associated with inflammatory conditions, such as Crohn's disease, ulcerative colitis, parasites, radiation enteritis, and enterocolitis in immunosuppressed patients (Fig. 52.3), as well as bowel ischemia and necrosis due to vascular stenoses, necrotizing enterocolitis, and/or connective tissue diseases (scleroderma, dermatomyositis, systemic lupus erythematosus).

Some authors argue that all cases of pneumatosis are secondary and that the cause could just not be detected in the so-called primary cases, due to lack of timing or sensitivity of the applied diagnostic techniques. Gas in the portal venous system, located in the periphery of the liver (as opposed to biliary air, which is centrally located), is only seen in patients with secondary pneumatosis, has a high association with ischemic bowel, and warrants further clinical and/or imaging workup and intervention. In most neonates and young infants, plain films and ultrasound are usually sufficient to generate a comprehensive diagnosis. CT scan may be helpful in older children to identify additional details that may guide therapeutic interventions, such as vascular stenosis, obstruction or thrombosis, abnormal or absent wall enhancement, mesenteric stranding, edema or hemorrhage, vascular engorgement, ascites, perforation, abscess, and portomesenteric gas.

A diagnostic pitfall on conventional radiographs may be intraluminal gas around fecal or contrast material. This gas can simulate pneumatosis. The intraluminal location of the gas can be confirmed by ultrasound evaluation, although the distinction of intraluminal from intramural gas can be difficult. Imaging while changing patient position is helpful; intraluminal air changes its position, always rising to the highest point in the lumen, while intramural air would not change its location. Radiographs with decubitus positioning (same concept) or, rarely, CT scan may also be useful.

Teaching point

Benign pneumatosis cystoides intestinalis may present as an incidental finding on imaging studies in an asymptomatic patient. The radiologist plays an important role in diagnosing pneumatosis and differentiating between benign pneumatosis intestinalis and secondary causes, which may require surgical or medical intervention.

REFERENCES

1. Micklefield GH, Kuntz HD, May B. Pneumatosis cystoides intestinalis: case reports and review of the literature. *Mater Med Pol* 1990;**22**(2):70–2.
2. Zülke C, Ulbrich S, Graeb C, *et al.* Acute pneumatosis cystoides intestinalis following allogeneic transplantation: the surgeon's dilemma. *Bone Marrow Transplant* 2002;**29**(9):795–8.

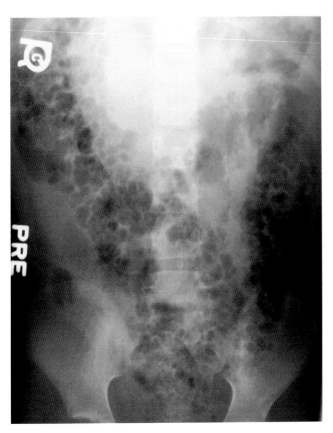

Figure 52.1. A nine-year-old girl with cystic fibrosis and chronic constipation. A radiograph of the abdomen/pelvis shows numerous rounded focal lucencies throughout the course of the colon consistent with the diagnosis of pneumatosis cystoides intestinalis.

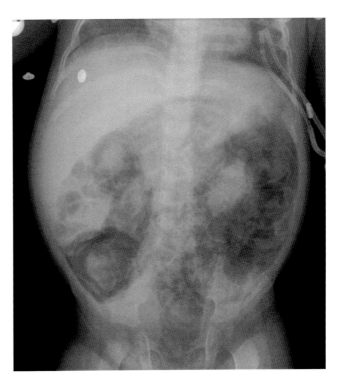

Figure 52.2. A 27-month-old infant with juvenile myelomonocytic leukemia (JMML), status post bone marrow transplant. Benign pneumatosis after chemotherapy, presenting as linear lucencies, which outline the colonic wall.

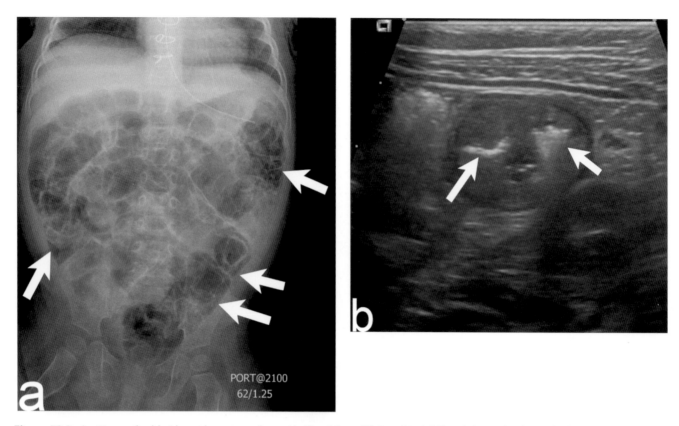

Figure 52.3. An 11-month-old girl post heart transplant with *Clostridium difficile* colitis. **(a)** The abdominal radiograph demonstrates extensive linear and bubbly colonic pneumatosis (arrows). **(b)** Ultrasound image of the left flank demonstrates thickened colonic wall with intramural echogenic foci of air (arrows).

53 Desmoplastic small round cell tumor

Heike E. Daldrup-Link

Imaging description

A teenage boy presented with increasing abdominal girth and diffuse abdominal pain. Clinical exam revealed a palpable mass in the lower abdomen and pelvis. A CT scan demonstrated a large, predominantly solid mass in the pelvis with evidence of mesenteric and nodal metastases (Fig. 53.1). A biopsy confirmed the suspected diagnosis of a desmoplastic small round cell tumor.

Importance

A desmoplastic small round cell tumor is a very aggressive type of soft tissue sarcoma, which typically presents in adolescent white boys. Ninety percent of the affected patients are males and 85% are white. The tumor shows clinical and imaging characteristics similar to malignant ovarian cancers in women. It grows very fast and often remains unnoticed or misdiagnosed for a long time. When finally diagnosed, most tumors are very large and have already spread, leading to an overall dismal five-year survival rate of less than 15%. Treatment consists of aggressive surgical resection, chemotherapy, and sometimes irradiation. A complete surgical resection is the single most effective intervention to improve outcomes. Thus, an earlier diagnosis is critical to improve the prognosis of these patients.

Typical clinical scenario

Desmoplastic small round cell tumors represent aggressive soft tissue sarcomas with histopathologic characteristics of the Ewing's sarcoma family type of tumors. The diagnosis can be proven based on a unique chromosomal translocation (t11;22) (p13;q12).

The tumor initially causes no discernable symptoms, leading to late presentations with marked abdominal distention, abdominal or back pain, anemia, chronic constipation or diarrhea, lack of appetite, weight loss, and/or cachexia.

Ultrasound, CT, and MRI studies demonstrate a heterogeneous, bulky, solid mass, usually located in the pelvis, less frequently located in the abdomen. The majority of the mass enhances after contrast media injection, with possible delineation of some areas of necrosis. In about half of the patients, peritoneal or omental implants are noted at the time of diagnosis. The tumor spreads directly via the mesentery or via lymphatic and hematogenous routes. Thus, sites of metastases include visceral organs in the pelvis and abdominal cavity, particularly the liver, lymph node metastases, as well as metastases in lungs, bones, and the brain. PET/CT has been found to be useful in the early detection of tumor relapse after multimodality therapy.

Differential diagnosis

Differential diagnoses in boys include lymphoma, germ cell tumors (in particular testicular cancer), other soft tissue sarcomas, and–less likely in teenagers–rhabdomyosarcoma or neuroblastoma. On the rare occasion of a presentation in a female patient, ovarian cancer is the main differential diagnosis, in addition to the above mentioned tumor types. A peritoneal mesothelioma is another differential consideration, although very rare in teenagers.

> ### Teaching point
>
> In adolescent boys who present with an aggressive pelvic mass, a desmoplastic small round cell tumor should be considered in the differential diagnosis. Avoiding delay in establishing the correct diagnosis is crucial to improving the dismal prognosis of patients with this disease.

REFERENCES

1. Gerald WL, Haber DA. The EWS-WT1 gene fusion in desmoplastic small round cell tumor. *Semin Cancer Biol* 2005;**15**(3):197–205.
2. Kushner BH, Laquaglia MP, Gerald WL, *et al.* Solitary relapse of desmoplastic small round cell tumor detected by positron emission tomography/computed tomography. *J Clin Oncol* 2008;**26**(30):4995–6.
3. Lal DR, Su WT, Wolden SL, *et al.* Results of multimodal treatment for desmoplastic small round cell tumors. *J Pediatr Surg* 2005;**40**(1):251–5.
4. Saab R, Khoury JD, Krasin M, *et al.* Desmoplastic small round cell tumor in childhood: the St. Jude Children's Research Hospital experience. *Pediatr Blood Cancer* 2007;**49**(3):274–9.

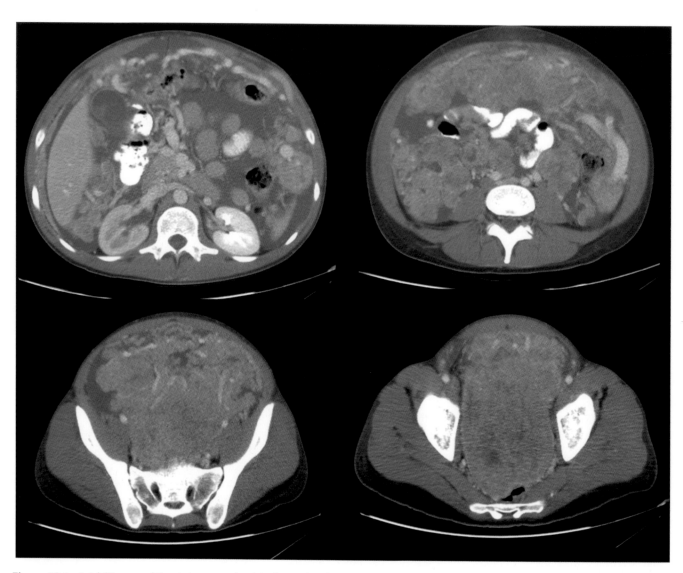

Figure 53.1. Axial CT scans of the abdomen and pelvis after oral and intravenous contrast media administration demonstrate a large, ill-defined, heterogeneous, contrast-enhancing mass in the pelvis, which encases the iliac vessels. Images of the abdomen demonstrate extensive "omental caking," consistent with mesenteric tumor spread. Many enlarged mesenteric lymph nodes are also noted, consistent with nodal metastases. Ascites is seen throughout the abdomen and pelvis. The right kidney shows asymmetric, delayed enhancement compared to the left kidney, possibly due to compression of the right ureter by the mass.

Post-transplantation lymphoproliferative disorder

Khun Visith Keu and Andrei Iagaru

Imaging description

A 14-year-old female with a prior history of double lung transplantation for end-stage cystic fibrosis presented with abdominal pain, constipation, and fever. A non-contrast CT scan (not shown) demonstrated nodular gastric wall thickening, intra-abdominal lymphadenopathy, and bilateral lung nodules. These findings were concerning for post-transplantation lymphoproliferative disorder (PTLD). A subsequent staging ^{18}F-FDG PET/CT showed intense ^{18}F-FDG uptake within the lesions noted on the non-contrast CT and also identified additional ^{18}F-FDG-avid sites of disease within the bowel and the left kidney that were not apparent on the corresponding or previous non-contrast CT images (Fig. 54.1). The diagnosis of Epstein–Barr virus (EBV)-positive PTLD was confirmed by biopsy. Serial ^{18}F-FDG PET/CT studies were then performed to monitor the disease, which initially demonstrated complete response to treatment, only to be followed by subsequent recurrence within the liver (Fig. 54.2).

Importance

PTLD is a rare but serious complication of chronic immunosuppression occurring in the setting of either solid organ or bone marrow transplantation. PTLD represents a spectrum of lymphoproliferative disorders, ranging from abnormal lymphoid hyperplasia to frank malignant lymphoma. PTLD is the most common post-transplant neoplasm in children.

The overall incidence of PTLD has risen over the past few decades and continues to vary depending on multiple factors such as age, type of organ transplanted, and degree of immunosuppression. For example, the incidence of PTLD is highest in lung, small bowel, and heart–lung transplant patients (5–20%), while significantly lower for kidney transplants (1–5%), likely relating to the degree of immunosuppression. However, the most important and best-characterized risk factor for PTLD in the pediatric population is development of a primary EBV infection in an EBV-seronegative transplant recipient, increasing the risk of disease 3–24-fold. The fact that most pediatric transplant patients are initially EBV-seronegative while most adults have been exposed to the virus by the time of transplantation may account for the higher incidence of PTLD in the pediatric population. Primary EBV infection can result from donor organs, blood transfusions, or community acquisition. Generally, most early PTLD lesions are EBV-positive (50–70%), while later presenting disease is often EBV-negative.

When polymorphic benign PTLD is diagnosed early in children, most cases are treated only with decreased immunosuppression and respond very well. Of course, this entails balancing immunosuppression needed to prevent transplant rejection. By comparison, monomorphic lymphoma tends to behave more aggressively and leads to poorer outcomes.

Typical clinical scenario

The diagnosis of PTLD can be challenging as the clinical features are often vague and vary widely depending on disease extent and location. Patients often present with non-specific signs and symptoms, such as fatigue, malaise, weight loss, fevers, and sweats, mimicking a non-specific viral syndrome or even allograft rejection. On the other hand, more specific clinical findings may help target a particular site of involvement, such as nausea and vomiting with gastrointestinal involvement or seizures with intracranial lesions.

While the evaluation of EBV viral load or serology in the post-transplantation patient may be useful for monitoring risk of developing PTLD, it is not diagnostic. In the setting of rising or elevated EBV titers without obvious disease on physical exam, a search for occult disease is necessary. Therefore, a high degree of clinical suspicion must be maintained at all times in order to detect early rather than late disseminated disease.

Likewise, the imaging appearance and distribution of PTLD also varies widely, with nodal and/or extranodal lesions found in virtually any location. Typical imaging findings range from lymphadenopathy to discrete or infiltrating, ill-defined masses. Isolated nodal disease is rare, with extranodal involvement in up to 75–85% of cases of PTLD. In approximately 50% of cases there is multiorgan involvement at presentation, most commonly within the gastrointestinal tract. The imaging findings of PTLD are related to the type of allograft transplanted and degree of immunosuppression, as lesions frequently occur near or within the transplanted organ. Other common disease locations include the liver, lung, and gastrointestinal tract; splenic involvement and central nervous system lesions are less common.

Various imaging modalities are useful in the evaluation of known or suspected PTLD. These patients will typically undergo initial evaluation with contrast-enhanced CT and/or possibly MRI or US, depending on disease location or symptoms. ^{18}F-FDG PET/CT has shown high sensitivity for staging of PTLD and malignant lymphomas, albeit with relatively high radiation exposure. ^{18}F FDG-PET/CT can be used to detect occult lesions, suggest malignancy in equivocal lesions, or monitor therapeutic response to disease. ^{18}F-FDG PET/CT is especially useful for detecting extranodal sites of disease, as those lesions are traditionally more difficult to detect on conventional imaging studies.

Differential diagnosis

The differential diagnosis for PTLD is complex, and varies according to the imaging appearance and distribution of the lesions. The main differential diagnosis is malignant lymphoma and other lymphoproliferative disorders. Graft-versus-host disease (GVHD) can present with isolated bowel involvement in the setting of allogeneic bone marrow transplantation.

However, GVHD usually does not cause mass-like lesions. Other entities to consider include infection, particularly fungal or other opportunistic infections, and allograft rejection.

Teaching point

The imaging findings and clinical presentation of PTLD are often non-specific and vary widely, depending on many factors. General imaging features include lymphadenopathy or solid or infiltrating masses in any location, especially in or close to the transplanted organ. A high degree of clinical suspicion should be maintained at all times in any post-transplant patient, particularly in the face of rising EBV titers. While conventional contrast-enhanced CT or MR studies are often the initial diagnostic imaging tools utilized in the workup of known or potential PTLD, ^{18}F-FDG PET/CT can add additional information, especially in staging and identifying occult or equivocal lesions and appears very important for early monitoring of treatment response.

REFERENCES

1. Bakker NA, van Imhoff GW, Verschuuren EA, et al. Presentation and early detection of post-transplant lymphoproliferative disorder after solid organ transplantation. Transpl Int 2007;20(3):207–18.

2. Blaes AH, Cioc AM, Froelich JW. Positron emission tomography scanning in the setting of post-transplant lymphoproliferative disorders. Clin Transplant 2009;23(6):794–9.

3. Borhani AA, Hosseinzadeh K, Almusa O, et al. Imaging of post-transplantation lymphoproliferative disorder after solid organ transplantation. Radiographics 2009;29(4):981–1000; discussion 1000–2.

4. Dharnidharka VR, Araya CE. Post-transplant lymphoproliferative disease. Pediatr Nephrol 2009;24(4):731–6.

5. Evans IV, Belle SH, Wei Y, et al. Post-transplantation growth among pediatric recipients of liver transplantation. Pediatr Transplant 2005;9(4):480–5.

6. Gallego S, Llort A, Gros L, et al. Post-transplant lymphoproliferative disorders in children: the role of chemotherapy in the era of rituximab. Pediatr Transplant 2010;14(1):61–6.

7. Green M, Webber S. Posttransplantation lymphoproliferative disorders. Pediatr Clin North Am 2003;50(6):1471–91.

8. Maecker B, Jack T, Zimmermann M, et al. CNS or bone marrow involvement as risk factors for poor survival in post-transplantation lymphoproliferative disorders in children after solid organ transplantation. J Clin Oncol 2007;25(31):4902–8.

9. O'Conner AR, Franc BL. FDG PET imaging in the evaluation of post-transplant lymphoproliferative disorder following renal transplantation. Nucl Med Commun 2005;26(12):1107–11.

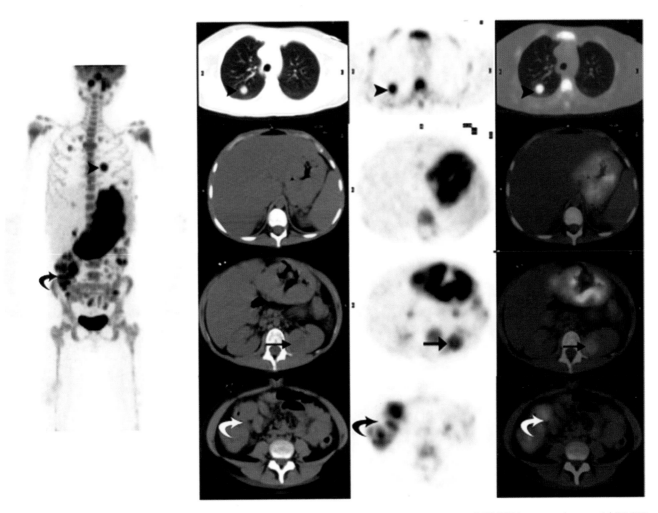

Figure 54.1. A 14-year-old female after double lung transplant with PTLD. Maximum intensity projection (MIP) PET image and transaxial CT, PET, and fused PET/CT images from the initial staging scan demonstrate intense ^{18}F-FDG uptake within several lung nodules (arrowheads) and a nodular thickened stomach. PET/CT was also able to detect additional intense ^{18}F-FDG uptake within the left kidney (arrows) and right-sided bowel (curved arrows).

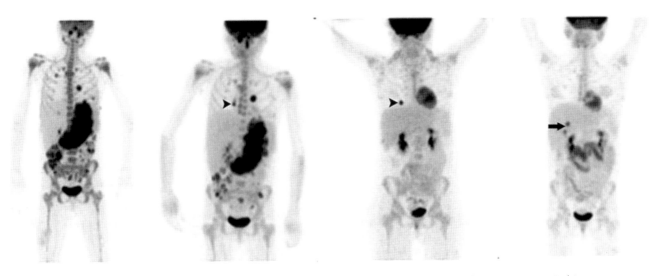

Figure 54.2. Serial MIP PET images show complete metabolic response to treatment, followed by disease recurrence in biopsy-proven ^{18}F-FDG-avid liver lesions (arrow). Arrowheads mark tracer present at the injection port.

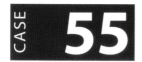

Traumatic pancreatic injury

Matthew Schmitz and Beverley Newman

Imaging description

A 10-year-old boy with a history of a motor vehicle accident presented with abdominal pain and distension. On physical examination he had multiple bruises on his anterior abdominal wall and left flank. CT of the abdomen and pelvis with intravenous contrast (Fig. 55.1) demonstrated a linear area of hypoattenuation extending across the body of the pancreas as well as a small collection of fluid situated between the pancreas and splenic vein. Given the patient's history of trauma, these findings were consistent with pancreatic fracture.

Importance

The rapid diagnosis of traumatic pancreatic injury either in isolation or in multisystem trauma is essential for limiting the risk of significant morbidity or mortality in pediatric patients. Traumatic injury to the pancreas, especially when associated with injuries to other abdominal organs or rapid intra-abdominal hemorrhage, has a high early mortality rate in children.

Early detection of injury to the pancreatic duct is important as early surgical or medical intervention in the setting of major ductal injury can lessen the risk of pseudocyst, speed overall recovery, and lessen the risk of secondary infection.

Both blunt and penetrating trauma can result in pancreatic fracture or other injury, with blunt trauma being far more common. In children, the most common causes of pancreatic trauma are related to handlebar injuries, motor vehicle accidents, sports injuries, non-accidental trauma, and falls. The mechanism of injury from blunt trauma can be due to a direct blow to the upper abdomen impacting the pancreas, compression of the pancreas against the spine, shearing of pancreatic vasculature, or injury from other deformed structures such as broken ribs.

Typical clinical scenario

Most cases of pancreatic traumatic injury will present with a history of a direct blow to the upper abdomen and upper abdominal pain. However, children who are too young or disabled to communicate effectively, victims of non-accidental trauma, or patients who have sustained a high-velocity injury such as from a fall or motor vehicle accident may not present with this classic history or classic symptomatology. Young children may present with generalized abdominal pain and any patient with pancreatic injury may have referred back pain.

On physical examination, right upper quadrant or epigastric tenderness, abdominal wall hematoma or skin abrasions, abdominal distension, and/or signs of hypovolemic shock (tachycardia, hypotension, decreased urine output, altered mental status) may be present. Occasionally, patients may have a delayed presentation and could then also exhibit findings related to pancreatic pseudocyst such as a palpable abdominal mass.

Laboratory studies are notoriously unreliable for assessment of traumatic pancreatic injury in the acute setting, with "normal" laboratory results (including lipase and amylase) not uncommon despite significant injury.

CT with intravenous contrast is generally accepted as the best imaging modality for evaluation of pancreatic injury and could be the first imaging test chosen if there is high suspicion of pancreatic injury. However, ultrasound (US) and plain radiograph of the abdomen are often obtained first in patients with non-classic presentations in order to spare radiation dose.

Plain radiographs of the abdomen will most often be normal in patients with only pancreatic injury. Dilated bowel loops from ileus caused by pancreatic juice spillage could be seen, though this finding is very non-specific for pancreatic injury.

US imaging capabilities have improved dramatically in recent years and the pancreas can often be well assessed, especially in thin patients. The findings of traumatic pancreatic injury can be similar to those seen in acute pancreatitis, with an enlarged, hypoechoic pancreas, adjacent free fluid, or a fluid collection/pseudocyst.

Initial CT can often be negative in patients with traumatic pancreatic injury. The spectrum of CT findings can range from peripancreatic fluid and inflammation (especially fluid between the pancreas and splenic vein), to focal or diffuse abnormal pancreatic enhancement and contour, to active hemorrhage, to a fracture line separating the pancreas along its short or long axis. Unfortunately, there may be little change in parenchymal density and minimal separation of pancreatic fragments during the acute phase – making detection sometimes difficult.

Thickening of the anterior pararenal fascia of the left kidney, fluid around the superior mesenteric artery, or fluid in the lesser sac may also point to a pancreatic injury on CT. Pseudocysts (Fig. 55.2) can be seen in the patient with delayed presentation. In addition, CT is effective at demonstrating injuries to other abdominal organs, which are not uncommon in the setting of pancreatic injury.

Specific types of injuries to the pancreas can be differentiated on CT, including contusion (focal hypoattenuation and decreased enhancement), hematoma (mixed or increased attenuation focus within or adjacent to the pancreas), laceration (linear hypoattenuating band, usually anteroposterior, does not extend across entire width of pancreas), fracture or transection (hypoattenuating linear focus with separation of the pancreas into two portions, fluid anterior to the splenic vein).

MRI can demonstrate peripancreatic fluid, heterogeneous enhancement of the pancreas, or non-enhancing fluid collections. Magnetic resonance cholangiopancreatography (MRCP) or endoscopic cholangiopancreatography (ERCP) can determine the integrity of the pancreatic duct.

Differential diagnosis

Acute inflammatory pancreatitis can have imaging findings that closely mimic traumatic pancreatic injury, with peripancreatic fluid, non-enhancing fluid collections, and heterogeneous parenchymal enhancement all being seen in both entities (Fig. 55.3). Clinical history is important for differentiation. Acute pancreatitis in children is frequently associated with anomalies of the pancreatic duct, including an abnormal junction with the common bile duct and pancreas divisum. These anomalies can be elucidated on MRCP and ERCP.

Duodenal injuries can result in peripancreatic fluid and pancreatic contour irregularities due to duodenal edema. Pancreas injuries are often seen concurrently.

Generalized abdominal hypoperfusion can result in abnormally heterogeneous or intense contrast enhancement of the pancreas (shock pancreas). The adrenals, kidneys, and bowel wall may also show abnormally intense enhancement, the bowel may be dilated and fluid filled, the aorta may be decreased in caliber, and the inferior vena cava may be collapsed.

Teaching point

CT is the most effective imaging modality for accurate radiologic detection of traumatic pancreatic injury in pediatric patients. Identification of the specific type of pancreatic injury (contusion, hematoma, laceration, or fracture) is important for appropriate and prompt management and is often possible with CT. Other imaging modalities can have specific functions, especially MRCP or ERCP to assess the integrity of the pancreatic duct.

REFERENCES

1. Linsenmaier U, Wirth S, Reiser M, *et al.* Diagnosis and classification of pancreatic and duodenal injuries in emergency radiology. *Radiographics* 2008;**28**(6):1591–602.
2. Pariset JM, Feldman KW, Paris C. The pace of signs and symptoms of blunt abdominal trauma to children. *Clin Pediatr (Phila)* 2010; **49**(1):24–8.
3. Recinos G, DuBose JJ, Teixeira PG, *et al.* Local complications following pancreatic trauma. *Injury* 2009;**40**(5):516–20.

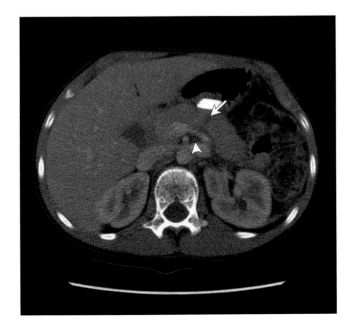

Figure 55.1. Axial contrast-enhanced CT demonstrates a low attenuation line traversing the entire width of the body of the pancreas (arrow), consistent with pancreatic transection in this 10-year-old boy with a history of a motor vehicle accident. Also seen is a small collection of fluid between the pancreas and splenic vein and adjacent to the superior mesenteric artery (arrowhead), often seen in patients with traumatic pancreatic injury.

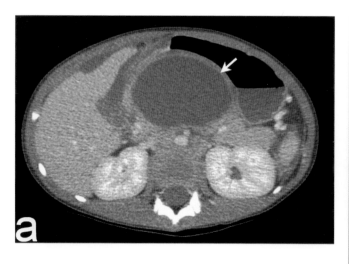

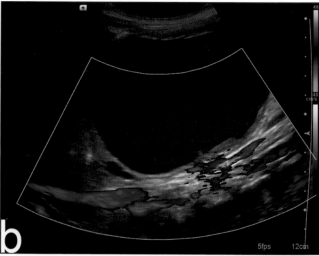

Figure 55.2. **(a)** Contrast-enhanced axial CT image in a five-year-old boy with handlebar injury and pancreatic transection several weeks prior, now with newly diagnosed large, encapsulated peripancreatic fluid collection consistent with a pseudocyst (arrow) as well as some free fluid around the liver. **(b)** US image of the upper midline abdomen in the sagittal plane demonstrates a large pseudocyst measuring at least 12 cm in greatest dimension. The fluid contains low-level echoes and is encapsulated by a thin wall. This is consistent with a pancreatic pseudocyst.

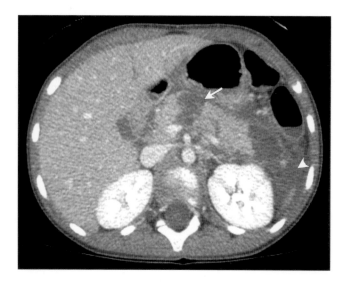

Figure 55.3. Contrast-enhanced CT in a five-year-old boy. Large area of low attenuation in the area of the pancreatic neck (arrow) with a large amount of free peripancreatic fluid (arrowhead) in this patient with acute necrotizing pancreatitis and no history of traumatic injury.

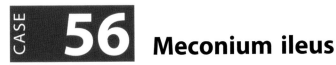

Meconium ileus

Amy Neville and Beverley Newman

Imaging description

A 36-week gestational age male presented clinically with failure to pass meconium at birth. Radiographs of the abdomen demonstrated abdominal distension and findings of mid to distal bowel obstruction (Fig. 56.1a). The clinical presentation was not unexpected since a prenatal ultrasound (US) performed at 19 weeks gestational age identified echogenic bowel, prompting further evaluation with a prenatal MRI at 27 weeks. The MRI findings of dilated bowel and a small rectum suggested the presence of distal bowel obstruction (Fig. 56.1b, c). A water-soluble contrast enema at two days of age (performed with Cysto-Conray II) demonstrated a microcolon containing multiple small filling defects/plugs (Fig. 56.1d). Contrast reached the cecum and appendix, located in the right upper quadrant. Contrast could not be refluxed into the terminal ileum. A decubitus view demonstrated many dilated small bowel loops without air–fluid levels, suggesting meconium ileus as the most likely diagnosis (Fig. 56.1e). However, ileal atresia, malrotation with small bowel volvulus, and total colonic Hirschsprung's disease were also considerations. Surgical exploration at two days of age demonstrated severe meconium ileus extending into the mid small bowel causing marked jejunal dilatation secondary to the impacted meconium. Multiple plugs of inspissated meconium were removed surgically. However, postoperatively he continued to have bowel obstruction and inspissated bowel contents indicative of ongoing meconium ileus. He underwent a total of five water-soluble contrast enemas with a final successful enema, utilizing Gastrografin and Mucomyst, which relieved his obstruction (Fig. 56.1f).

Importance

Meconium ileus is a cause of low intestinal obstruction due to abnormally thick and tenacious meconium causing mechanical obstruction usually at the level of the distal ileum. It constitutes approximately 20% of cases of neonatal intestinal obstruction. Almost all infants with meconium ileus have cystic fibrosis, and up to 20% of cystic fibrosis cases present with meconium ileus.

Cystic fibrosis is inherited as an autosomal recessive mutation of the CFTR (cystic fibrosis transmembrane conductance regulator) gene, due to one of nearly 1900 mutations. The resultant deficient chloride transport affects all secretory glands in the body, with the predominant clinically significant effects on the respiratory and gastrointestinal systems. The altered electrolyte content in tubular structures lined by the affected epithelium leads to dessication and decreased clearance of secretions. In the intestine, this causes water to move out of the intestinal lumen with inspissation of bowel contents,

and subsequent bowel obstruction. A microcolon results from failure of small bowel contents (succus entericus) to pass into the colon during fetal life.

Meconium ileus is considered complicated in approximately 50% of cases in association with intestinal perforation, segmental volvulus, obstructing mesenteric bands, and/or acquired small bowel atresia. Prenatal perforation may result in ascites and diffuse peritonitis, cystic meconium peritonitis, and focal or diffuse peritoneal calcifications.

Bowel obstruction, whether caused by meconium ileus, bowel atresia, volvulus, meconium peritonitis, or other obstructing lesion, such as an intestinal duplication cyst, is frequently first suspected on in utero US screening examinations. The diagnosis of fetal bowel obstruction is often difficult before 24 weeks of gestation, but in the third trimester, with increased fetal bowel peristalsis, loops become progressively more dilated and easier to evaluate. Dilated fetal bowel loops, generally characterized as more than 7 mm in diameter and more than 15 mm in length, often with mural thickness more than 3 mm, suggest the presence of a bowel obstruction. The abdominal circumference may also be disproportionately increased due to the resultant abdominal distention. Increased bowel echogenicity is most suggestive of meconium ileus as the cause of obstruction. The number of dilated loops may help to localize the site of obstruction as jejunal (when only a few dilated loops are present) or more distal (when multiple dilated loops are identified). Other findings may suggest perforation, including ascites, extraluminal meconium, or scattered peritoneal calcifications.

Fetal MRI may also be used in the assessment of bowel obstruction, possibly offering more accurate findings than US in the assessment of bowel obstruction or atresia. As with US, dilated small bowel loops may be identified measuring 13–30 mm in caliber. The signal characteristics will vary based on the gestational age, and the number and location of dilated bowel loops may suggest the level of obstruction, similar to US. Meconium is readily identified on MR as it has very bright signal on T1-weighted images. Meconium is expected to be present in the colon and rectum by 20 weeks of gestation. The presence of a microcolon is also important in assessing the severity and type of bowel obstruction. Meconium peritonitis may be diagnosed based on the finding of scattered extraluminal fluid collections within the abdomen. MRI offers the advantage of being able to better distinguish meconium cysts from adjacent bowel due to their characteristic signal intensities. However, US remains more sensitive and specific in detecting peritoneal calcifications.

Plain radiographs are usually the first postnatal imaging study performed in cases of suspected intestinal obstruction, although on neonatal radiographs, it is often difficult to clearly differentiate small and large bowel. Characteristic findings of meconium ileus on plain radiographs include varying-sized loops of distended bowel, a relative absence of air–fluid levels, and a "soap-bubble" or mottled appearance of portions of the bowel (Neuhauser's sign, reflecting viscid meconium mixed with air), most often in the right lower quadrant. This soap-bubble appearance can be difficult to distinguish from the intramural bubbles of pneumatosis intestinalis, and the clinical setting of a full-term infant may help to favor meconium ileus, particularly if the finding is identified within the first day after delivery as pneumatosis is more often seen in sick premature infants after the first few days of life. The radiographic findings of meconium ileus also overlap with other causes of low intestinal obstruction.

Meconium peritonitis as a complication of meconium ileus or other causes of bowel obstruction or ischemia should be considered upon identification of abdominal calcifications, particularly along peritoneal surfaces, including the inferior liver, flanks, and inguinal canal/scrotum (Fig. 56.2). A peripherally calcified mass may represent cystic meconium peritonitis; free intraperitoneal air suggests more recent bowel perforation.

Contrast enema remains the diagnostic study of choice in further evaluating low intestinal obstructions postnatally. Most commonly, a lower osmolar water-soluble contrast agent, such as Omnipaque 300 (672 mOsm/kg, can be diluted one-third with water) or Cysto-Conray II (403 mOsm/kg), is used initially (normal plasma osmolarity is 285 mOsm/kg). In the case of meconium ileus as well as other longstanding low intestinal obstructions a contrast enema will usually demonstrate a microcolon, and may allow for specific identification of the level of obstruction. The presence of plugs of meconium in the colon is common in meconium ileus but is non-specific and often present in other causes of microcolon. Reflux of contrast into the terminal and distal ileum may demonstrate filling defects reflecting the inspissated meconium. This reflux of contrast into the ileum containing large plugs of meconium helps to differentiate meconium ileus from other causes of a microcolon, including small bowel atresia (Fig. 56.3a, b) or volvulus, which tend to show an abrupt termination of contrast, and total colonic Hirschsprung's disease (Fig. 56.4), characterized by a small rectum, redundant loops of microcolon, and easy reflux into a dilated terminal ileum, usually without significant meconium filling defects. However, if contrast cannot be refluxed into the distal ileum due to a competent ileocecal valve or markedly inspissated meconium, then a confident radiologic diagnosis may not be possible. In the case of meconium ileus, the purpose of the enema is both diagnostic and therapeutic, with relief of the obstruction frequently successful, thus obviating the need for surgical disimpaction. Multiple enema attempts may be needed to disimpact meconium ileus.

Gastrografin, a first generation hyperosmolar water-soluble contrast media (1940 mOsm/kg) has been used for a long time (with or without Mucomyst [acetylcysteine], a mucolytic agent) to disimpact meconium ileus. Solutions of 25–50%

Gastrografin are typically used. This agent draws fluid into the intestinal lumen, hydrating the meconium and producing a transient osmotic diarrhea to resolve the meconium obstruction. Due to potentially increased risks of hypovolemic shock associated with these large fluid shifts, great care must be taken when employing this agent and many radiologists prefer at least initial use of a more iso-osmolar contrast agent to avoid potentially deleterious fluid shifts, given the neonate's limited reserve.

Postnatal US imaging is generally non-specific in uncomplicated meconium ileus; findings may include hyperechoic meconium within dilated distal small bowel, findings of bowel obstruction, and poor visualization of the gallbladder. US findings are more specific in the situation of meconium peritonitis or pseudocyst. Sonographic features include clumped or diffuse echogenic shadowing foci due to calcified meconium and free or loculated echogenic fluid or a pseudocyst containing fluid and/or bowel loops, often with peripheral calcification.

Typical clinical scenario

Intestinal obstruction in infants with meconium ileus is generally evident within the first 48 hours following delivery. In some cases the diagnosis may be delayed for a prolonged time period when the infant is not fed orally (Fig. 56.3). Many of these infants are small-for-dates, but meconium ileus is rare in premature infants. Similar to other causes of low intestinal obstruction, meconium ileus may be suspected by failure to pass meconium, abdominal distention, and vomiting. Occasionally a dilated and meconium filled intestinal loop may be palpated on exam. In the setting of complicated meconium ileus the infant may present with severe abdominal distention and respiratory distress. On occasion, abnormal prenatal imaging studies may trigger investigation in an otherwise asymptomatic infant.

In the setting of uncomplicated meconium ileus, non-operative intervention is strongly preferred. Success rates of treatment with contrast enema reach up to 70–80%, with bowel perforation complicating 1–3%. It is generally thought that keeping the infants well-hydrated helps decrease complications by counteracting the fluid and electrolyte shifts that can occur, particularly with more hyperosmolar agents.

In the setting of complicated meconium ileus, or simple meconium ileus that is not successfully treated after multiple contrast enemas, surgical intervention is warranted.

When the diagnosis of bowel obstruction is made on fetal imaging, a careful search for associated anomalies should be performed. Early prenatal diagnosis allows for parental counseling and preparation. Meconium ileus or bowel atresia alone are not indications to alter the route of delivery, but delivery should be planned at a center with appropriate neonatal care.

Gastrointestinal obstruction in cystic fibrosis, similar to meconium ileus, now termed distal intestinal obstruction syndrome (DIOS), may persist into adulthood in 10–47% of cystic fibrosis patients, depending on the criteria used to make the diagnosis. DIOS is most common in adolescents or adults but can occur in younger children. DIOS is often recurrent, caused by inspissated intestinal contents that completely or partially block the small bowel, most commonly at the ileocecal junction. In contrast to constipation, DIOS causes a more acute obstruction and though most patients also have constipation, they may have diarrhea or no appreciable change in their stool pattern. It is more common in patients with a history of meconium ileus, and there is no relationship between the development of DIOS and the pulmonary manifestations of cystic fibrosis.

Other later gastrointestinal complications of cystic fibrosis include intussusception, colonic stricture, rectal prolapse, pancreatitis, pancreatic insufficiency, and malabsorption as well as liver and biliary disease, including obstruction, stones, cholangitis, cirrhosis, and portal hypertension.

The pulmonary manifestations of cystic fibrosis, including recurrent pulmonary infection, mucous plugging, and bronchiectasis, begin later in infancy or childhood and are not manifest early in life. Currently, many asymptomatic cases of cystic fibrosis are diagnosed postnatally on early genetic screening studies.

Differential diagnosis

Causes of a failure to pass meconium after birth include imperforate anus, ileal atresia (Fig. 56.3), colonic atresia, meconium ileus (Fig. 56.1), Hirschsprung's disease (Fig. 56.4), and functional immaturity of the colon such as meconium plug syndrome and small left colon syndrome (associated with gestational diabetes). Most of these are associated with a small caliber of either a segment or the entire colon. A microcolon is most commonly associated with ileal atresia, meconium ileus, or long segment Hirschsprung's disease. Anorectal malformations are also an important cause of distal bowel obstruction but are generally diagnosed on physical examination. Other causes of mid to distal bowel obstruction in neonates include gastroschisis/omphalocele (both pre- and postoperatively), congenital and acquired bands/adhesions, inguinal hernia, intussusception (usually with a pathologic lead point such as a Meckel's diverticulum), intestinal duplication cyst, internal hernia, necrotizing enterocolitis, and obstruction by an abdominal mass.

While meconium ileus is a prominent cause of bowel obstruction and in utero perforation with meconium peritonitis, other causes of in utero bowel obstruction and/or perforation include bowel atresia, volvulus, and incarcerated hernia.

Teaching point

Meconium ileus is a common first presentation of cystic fibrosis prenatally or in the early postnatal period. Approximately 50% of patients with meconium ileus may develop complicated meconium ileus with in utero bowel perforation and meconium peritonitis. Consequences may include meconium pseudocyst, acquired small intestinal atresia or stenosis, small bowel volvulus, and mesenteric bands or adhesions.

REFERENCES

1. Berrocal T, Lamas M, Gutieérrez J, et al. Congential anomalies of the small intestine, colon, and rectum. *Radiographics* 1999;**19**(5):1219–36.

2. Bloom DA, Slovis TL. Congenital anomalies of the gastrointestinal tract. In: Slovis TL, ed. *Caffey's Pediatric Diagnostic Imaging*, 11th edition. Philadelphia: Mosby Elsevier, 2008; 188–236.

3. Burke MS, Ragi JM, Karamanoukian HL, et al. New strategies in nonoperative management of meconium ileus. *J Pediatr Surg* 2002;**37**(5):760–4.

4. Farhataziz N, Engels JE, Ramus RM, et al. Fetal MRI of urine and meconium by gestational age for the diagnosis of genitourinary and gastrointestinal abnormalities. *AJR Am J Roentgenol* 2005;**184**(6): 1891–7.

5. Kao SC, Franken EA Jr. Nonoperative treatment of simple meconium ileus: a survey of the Society for Pediatric Radiology. *Pediatr Radiol* 1995;**25**(2):97–100.

6. Kraus SJ. Controversies in the treatment of uncomplicated meconium ileus. Sunrise Session Materials, Society for Pediatric Radiology 43rd Annual Meeting, Naples, FL, Apr-May 2000.

7. Neal MR, Seibert JJ, Vanderzalm T, et al. Neonatal ultrasonography to distinguish between meconium ileus and ileal atresia. *J Ultrasound Med* 1997;**16**(4):263–6.

8. Veyrac C, Couture A, Saguintaah M, et al. MRI of fetal GI tract abnormalities. *Abdom Imaging* 2004;**29**(4):411–20.

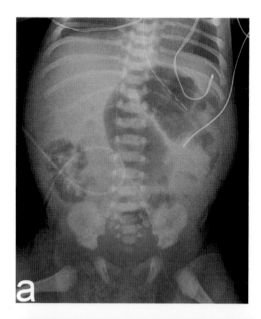

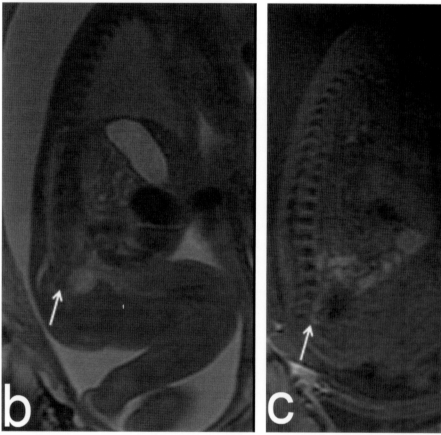

Figure 56.1. Meconium ileus. **(a)** Frontal radiograph of the abdomen taken on the first day of life of this 36-week gestational age infant demonstrated marked dilatation of several loops of small bowel, suggestive of a mid to distal bowel obstruction. **(b, c)** Sagittal T2- (b) and T1-weighted (c) fetal MR images obtained at 27 weeks' gestation demonstrated a very small rectum (arrows) without the normal bright T1 meconium signal. There are several dilated loops of bowel seen anteriorly (T2-hypointense and T1-hyperintense, i.e. containing meconium), with more proximal loops of non-dilated small bowel seen behind the stomach. It was not clear whether the dilated loops reflected distal small bowel or proximal colon. This constellation of findings was suggestive of distal bowel obstruction, and was thought to most likely be Hirschsprung's disease or meconium ileus.

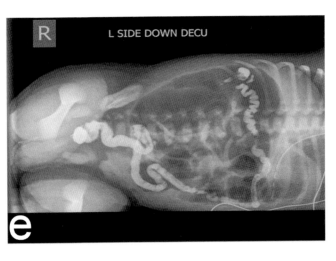

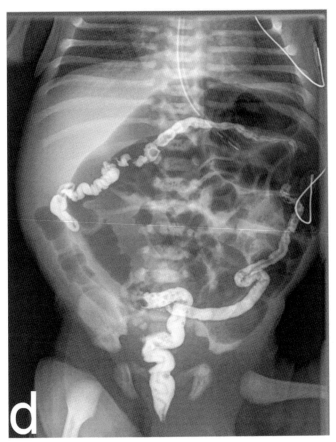

Figure 56.1. (cont.) **(d)** Initial water-soluble contrast enema performed at two days of age. A frontal radiograph of the abdomen obtained at the completion of the contrast enema demonstrated small filling defects throughout the colon with contrast extending to the level of the cecum, which was located in the right upper quadrant. The colon was diffusely small in caliber. Contrast did not reflux into the terminal ileum. Loops of small bowel were more dilated than they had been on the previous day (a). **(e)** Left side down decubitus radiograph of the abdomen obtained after the completion of the first contrast enema again demonstrated contrast extending to the cecum and appendix, which are located within the right upper quadrant. The colon is diffusely small in caliber. There are multiple loops of gaseous dilated small bowel with no air–fluid levels, a feature suggestive of meconium ileus.

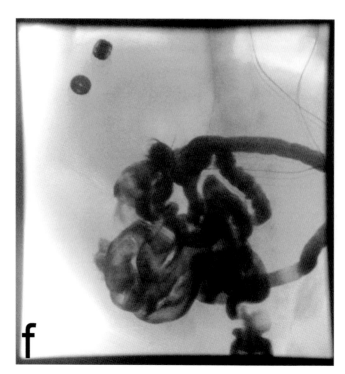

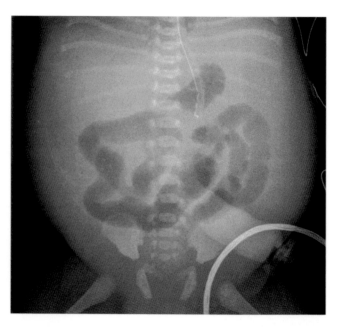

Figure 56.1. (cont.) **(f)** Image from the final successful contrast enema, performed with Gastrografin and Mucomyst at 28 days of life, demonstrated reflux of contrast into multiple loops of small bowel. Several distal loops of bowel are decompressed, with more dilated proximal loops containing inspissated meconium. The large bowel again has the appearance of a microcolon.

Figure 56.2. Meconium peritonitis. Frontal radiograph of the abdomen obtained on the first day of life for this 32-week gestational age male demonstrated a central location of the bowel loops and widened flanks, suggestive of ascites. Thin peritoneal calcifications along the right lateral abdomen are suggestive of meconium peritonitis.

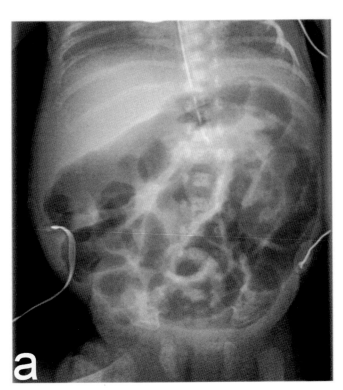
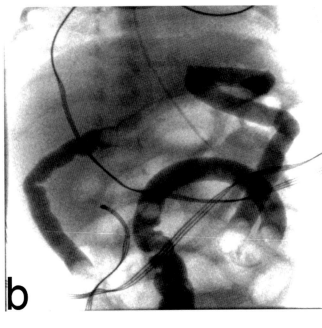

Figure 56.3. Ileal atresia. **(a)** A four-week-old, 27-week gestational age premature female with clinically suspected bowel obstruction based on abdominal distention and poor stooling. There were multiple loops of gaseous distended bowel suggestive of a possible bowel obstruction. There was no free intraperitoneal air or peritoneal calcifications. Clinically occult necrotizing enterocolitis with stricture was considered the most likely diagnosis in this premature infant given the patient age of four weeks. **(b)** Single frontal spot image of the abdomen obtained during a water-soluble contrast enema demonstrated an unexpected diffusely small caliber colon with a few scattered filling defects and abrupt termination of contrast in the region of the cecum. No contrast refluxed into the distal small bowel. At subsequent surgical exploration, ileal atresia was found. It was postulated that this infant's extreme prematurity led to very little oral feeding in the first few weeks of life such that signs and symptoms of bowel obstruction were only manifest later.

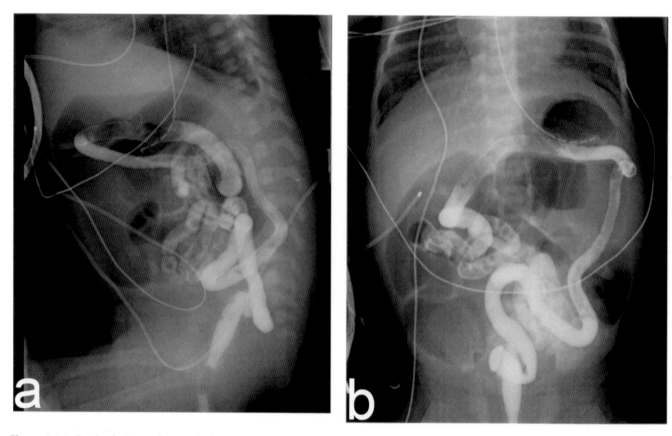

Figure 56.4. Total colonic Hirschsprung's disease. Spot lateral **(a)** and frontal **(b)** images obtained during a water-soluble contrast enema show a redundant microcolon including a small caliber rectum. A few filling defects/plugs are present within the colon and terminal ileum. The distal terminal ileum is not distended. There is marked dilatation of multiple more proximal loops of distal small bowel, compatible with a low obstruction. Biopsy confirmed the diagnosis of total colonic and distal ileal Hirschsprung's disease.

Renal cysts in tuberous sclerosis

Heike E. Daldrup-Link

Imaging description

A 14-year-old girl presented with seizures. The clinical examination revealed wart-like, small 4–5 mm, brownish nodules of the face with a bimalar distribution as well as palpable flank masses bilaterally. An ultrasound of the kidneys demonstrated multiple renal cysts bilaterally (Fig. 57.1a). Color Doppler evaluation did not reveal any vascular abnormality (Fig. 57.1a). A CT confirmed the cystic nature of the renal lesions (Fig. 57.1b); there was no evidence for solid renal masses. Tuberous sclerosis was suggested as the most likely diagnosis.

Criteria for uncomplicated renal cysts on ultrasound scans include the presence of an anechoic, round or oval structure with sharply circumscribed smooth walls and enhanced through-transmission. On CT scans, criteria for a cyst include a round or oval well-defined lesion with water attenuation, sharply circumscribed smooth walls, and lack of enhancement or fat attenuation. On MR images, a cyst is defined as a lesion that demonstrates fluid signal intensity on T1- (dark) and T2- (bright) weighted images, with round, well-defined borders and sharply circumscribed smooth walls, and no contrast enhancement.

Importance

Tuberous sclerosis complex (TSC) is an autosomal dominant disorder that affects many organ systems such as skin, brain, kidneys, lungs, heart, and bones. Approximately 50% of cases are inherited and at least 50% are sporadic. Two genes for TSC have been identified: *TSC1*, located on chromosome 9q34, encodes for hamartin and *TSC2*, on chromosome 16p13, encodes the protein tuberin.

Renal manifestations in TSC are common. Over 80% of older patients have angiomyolipomas, with cysts being most common in infants and children. Other renal lesions include malignant angiomyolipomas and renal cell carcinoma (RCC). Malignant renal lesions are rare in children with TSC, occurring in 1–2% of patients. Thus, screening for malignant lesions is not performed on a routine basis.

Typical clinical scenario

The classical clinical triad of TSC includes hypopigmented skin lesions (facial angiofibromas, previously called "adenoma sebaceum"), mental retardation, and seizures. Renal cysts in TSC patients usually present as an incidental finding. They may increase in size over time or resolve through childhood. It is important to differentiate renal cysts from vascularized, fat-containing angiomyolipomas, which can progressively enlarge, leading to hemorrhage and impaired renal function.

Differential diagnosis

Simple renal cysts occur in more than 50% of adults but are uncommon in childhood. Differential considerations that should be carefully considered in imaging studies include hydronephrosis (a dysplastic obstructed upper pole in a duplex kidney can easily be mistaken for a cyst) and caliceal diverticulum (may see communication with collecting system and contrast filling on delayed CT/MR images). Differential considerations for multiple renal cysts include normal hypoechoic medullary pyramids (sometimes mistaken for cysts in neonates), hydronephrosis, multicystic dysplastic kidney (multiple non-communicating cysts of varying sizes, little or no renal parenchyma), cystic renal dysplasia (small peripheral cysts), polycystic kidney disease (Figs. 57.2 and 57.3), syndromes associated with renal cystic disease (see below), medullary cystic disease (small echogenic kidneys with medullary or corticomedullary cysts), cystic neoplasms, e.g. multilocular cystic nephroma (see image in Case 64, Figure 64.6), acquired renal cysts (AIDS, hemodialysis), and renal abscess.

Renal cysts in pediatric patients with TSC can be indistinguishable from autosomal dominant polycystic kidney disease (ADPCKD) (Fig. 57.3). The similarity has been related to a combined deletion of the *PKD1* and *TSC2* genes, which lie close together on chromosome 16 and is called the TSC2 and PKD1 contiguous gene syndrome. Family history as well as atypical additional clinical findings, such as an adenoma sebaceum and seizures in TSC patients versus progressive renal insufficiency, cysts in other organs (especially liver and pancreas), and cerebral aneurysms in patients with ADPCKD, can help to differentiate these conditions (Fig. 57.3). In infants with ADPCKD the kidneys may be normal or enlarged and echogenic with tiny cysts (indistinguishable from the autosomal recessive disease [ARPCKD]) (Fig. 57.2). The typical appearance of nephromegaly with multiple macroscopic cysts in ADPCKD usually only starts to become apparent in adolescence. ARPCKD has a spectrum of abnormality with an inverse relationship between renal involvement (polycystic disease–tubular ectasia) and hepatic involvement (hepatic fibrosis). Renal involvement predominates in the infantile form and hepatic disease in the older (juvenile) age group.

Patients with von Hippel–Lindau disease can also present with multiple renal cysts. These cysts have a neoplastic endothelial lining, which can give rise to renal cell carcinomas. About one-third of patients with von Hippel–Lindau disease die from clear cell carcinomas of the kidneys.

Thus, patients with von Hippel–Lindau disease undergo regular screening ultrasound exams of the kidneys, with careful evaluation of the cysts for any new nodular lesions. Other syndromes associated with renal cysts in childhood include Turner's syndrome, Jeune's syndrome, oro-facial-digital syndrome, and Meckel's syndrome. The specific diagnosis usually hinges on correlation with clinical findings.

Angiomyolipomas in patients with TSC typically show marked contrast enhancement as well as hyperechogenic areas and/or areas of low attenuation value on CT studies, which are indicative of fat components. In TSC patients, angiomyolipomas are rarely solitary lesions, but tend to be numerous when present. If they contain little or no fat, they are indistinguishable from other renal tumors. Angiomyolipomas can grow substantially in adults and lead to hemorrhage and impaired renal function. It has been suggested that lesions larger than 4 cm are at risk of spontaneous hemorrhage and should undergo prophylactic embolization. Ultrasound imaging surveillance in TSC patients usually starts in the second or third decade and concentrates on growth evaluation of the angiomyolipomas.

Teaching point

Simple incidental renal cysts are uncommon in children; other differential possibilities should be sought as detailed above.

Renal cysts are the most common renal finding in infants and children with tuberous sclerosis while angiomyolipomas are most common in adolescents and adults. Patients with TSC have a slightly increased incidence of RCC, which arise from the renal parenchyma and not from the cysts and which typically present in adulthood. Angiomyolipomas >4 cm in adult TSC patients may bleed and cause renal failure.

REFERENCES

1. Breysem L, Nijs E, Proesmans W, *et al.* Tuberous sclerosis with cystic renal disease and multifocal renal cell carcinoma in a baby girl. *Pediatr Radiol* 2002;**32**(9):677–80.
2. Casper KA, Donnelly LF, Chen B, *et al.* Tuberous sclerosis complex: renal imaging findings. *Radiology* 2002;**225**(2):451–6.
3. Dähnert W. Brain disorders. In: *Radiology Review Manual.* Philadelphia: Lippincott Williams & Wilkins, 2011; 272–3.
4. Siegel MJ, ed. *Pediatric Sonography.* Philadelphia: Lippincott Williams & Wilkins, 2011.

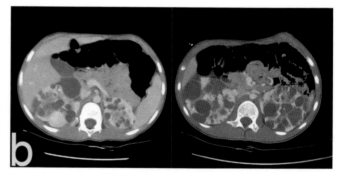

Figure 57.1. Tuberous sclerosis in a 14-year-old girl. **(a)** Longitudinal ultrasound images of the kidneys demonstrate multiple well-defined, hypoechoic round lesions of the kidneys bilaterally, with posterior acoustic enhancement, compatible with multiple bilateral renal cysts. **(b)** Axial contrast-enhanced CT scans through the kidneys confirm renal enlargement with multiple bilateral renal cysts. The cysts are well delineated, of variable size, and do not show any contrast enhancement. The visualized kidney parenchyma and the renal vessels show normal enhancement.

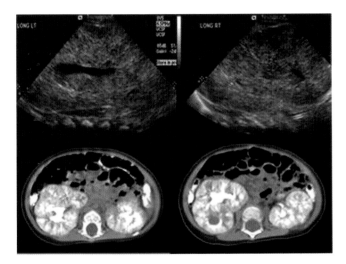

Figure 57.2. Autosomal recessive polycystic kidney disease (ARPCKD) in an infant. Ultrasound scans (upper row) demonstrate enlarged, diffusely hyperechogenic kidneys bilaterally, with diminished corticomedullary differentiation. A corresponding CT scan after intravenous administration of iodinated contrast media confirms enlarged kidneys bilaterally with striated nephrograms, a typical finding in ARPCKD and important differential diagnosis to a pyelonephritis, especially in the absence of fever.

ARPCKD ADPCKD

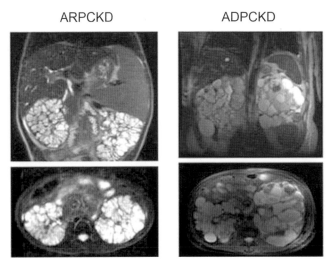

Figure 57.3. Coronal (upper rows) and axial (lower rows) T2-weighted fast spin echo sequences of two adult patients with autosomal recessive polycystic kidney disease (ARPCKD) and autosomal dominant polycystic kidney disease (ADPCKD). In ARPCKD, the cysts are relatively smaller and the shape of the kidney is preserved. In ADPCKD, the cysts are relatively larger, and additional cysts are noted in liver and pancreas.

Prune belly syndrome

Heike E. Daldrup-Link

Imaging description

A newborn baby boy presented with a broad flabby-appearing abdomen and apparent absence of the musculature of the abdomen. A radiograph of the chest and abdomen confirmed marked bulging of the bilateral flanks, flaring of the lower ribs, and flared iliac wings (Fig. 58.1). An ultrasound examination showed marked hydronephrosis and very dilated, tortuous ureters. The findings are characteristic for prune belly syndrome.

On ultrasound, the renal parenchyma is often dysplastic and hyperechoic, with small subcapsular cortical cysts. The calices are dilated and dysplastic. The ureters are markedly distended and tortuous. The bladder appears markedly dilated and trabeculated, with possible urachal remnants. The posterior urethra may appear dilated, with a prominent prostatic utricle (associated with hypoplastic or absent prostate). In addition, there is nearly always accompanying cryptorchidism (undescended testes).

Radiographs of the chest and abdomen typically demonstrate markedly bulging flanks, flaring of the lower ribs, and hypoplastic lungs (Fig. 58.2). Possible findings on voiding cystourethrogram (VCUG) include urethral stenosis or atresia, megalourethra, dilated prostatic utricle, dilated urinary bladder with trabeculated borders, bladder diverticula, patent urachus, vesicoureteral reflux, markedly tortuous hydroureters, and hydronephrosis. In addition, calcifications in the bladder or urachus may be present due to stasis of urine. A ^{99m}Tc DMSA (dimercaptosuccinic acid) scan can help to evaluate renal function.

Importance

Prune belly syndrome is a rare anomaly, typically occurring in baby boys, who present with deficient abdominal musculature and urinary tract abnormalities. The etiology is not fully understood. However, there is evidence to suggest at least two separate mechanisms: (1) a primary obstructing lesion of the urethra, which leads to chronic intrauterine abdominal distention and pressure atrophy of the abdominal muscle; and (2) a primary deficiency of the abdominal muscular wall due to a mesenchymal insult to the fetus at about six weeks of gestation, with resultant secondary functional abnormalities of the urinary system (without urethral obstruction). Many children with prune belly syndrome are stillborn or die shortly after birth. Those that survive usually do not have urinary tract obstruction postnatally but varying degrees of hydroureteronephrosis with poor muscular function of the ureters and bladder. They frequently have chronic renal insufficiency or failure and recurrent urinary tract infections. Similar to other conditions with a dilated urinary system (e.g. ureteropelvic junction obstruction), there is an increased risk of urinary tract injury/rupture with even relatively minor abdominal trauma (Fig. 58.3).

Typical clinical scenario

The classic triad of prune belly syndrome comprises: (1) a deficient abdominal wall, (2) urinary tract abnormalities, and (3) cryptorchidism. The diagnosis is usually suspected based on a prenatal ultrasound. Severe cases of prenatal abdominal distension and renal insufficiency may lead to oligohydramnios and lung hypoplasia, with severe respiratory problems postpartum. Other possible complications of oligohydramnios include bone deformities, such as clubfeet, hip dislocation, and limb hypoplasia or aplasia. The diagnosis is confirmed postnatally based on clinical and imaging findings on conventional radiographs, ultrasound, and VCUG. Other anomalies associated with prune belly syndrome include gastrointestinal disorders (malrotation, atresia, imperforate anus, Hirschsprung's disease) and congenital heart disease. Prune belly syndrome is associated with other syndromes including chromosomal anomalies (Turner's, Down's, trisomy 13 and 18).

Differential diagnosis

Differential diagnoses include posterior urethral valves with severe hydroureteronephrosis and dilated trabeculated bladder which may have a pseudo-prune belly appearance of the abdominal wall (Fig. 58.4). Additionally, megacystis-microcolon intestinal hypoperistalsis syndrome can resemble prune belly syndrome. Megacystis-microcolon syndrome occurs typically in girls, the abdominal wall is less hypoplastic, the bladder is much larger and not trabeculated, and the bowel is hypoplastic.

Teaching point

Prune belly syndrome presents with typical clinical and imaging features, as described above. The classic triad comprises: (1) a deficient abdominal wall, (2) urinary tract abnormalities, and (3) cryptorchidism. Many cases do not survive infancy and those that do have numerous medical problems. While the major clinical and imaging focus may be on the urinary tract, other primary or secondary organ system involvement including respiratory, gastrointestinal, musculoskeletal, and cardiac abnormalities may be important.

REFERENCES

1. Barnewolt CE, Paltiel HJ, Lebowitz RL, *et al*. Genitourinary tract. In: Kirks DR, Griscom NT, eds. *Practical Pediatric Imaging: Diagnostic Radiology of Infants and Children*. Philadelphia: Lippincott-Raven Publisher, 1998; 1120–2.
2. Caldamone AA, Woodard JR. Prune belly syndrome. In: Wein AJ, ed. *Campbell-Walsh Urology*, 9th edition. Philadelphia: Saunders Elsevier, 2007; Chapter 118.
3. Swischuk LE. Genitourinary tract and adrenal glands. In: Swischuk LE, ed. *Imaging of the Newborn, Infant, and Young Child*. Baltimore, Maryland: Lippincott Williams & Wilkins, 1997; 635–7.

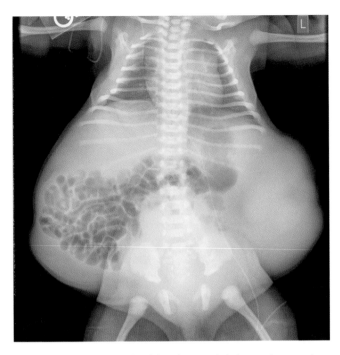

Figure 58.1. A radiograph of the chest and abdomen in a newborn baby demonstrates small thorax and lung volumes, elevated diaphragm, and marked bulging of the lateral contours of the abdomen with wavy deformity of the lower ribs, compatible with prune belly syndrome.

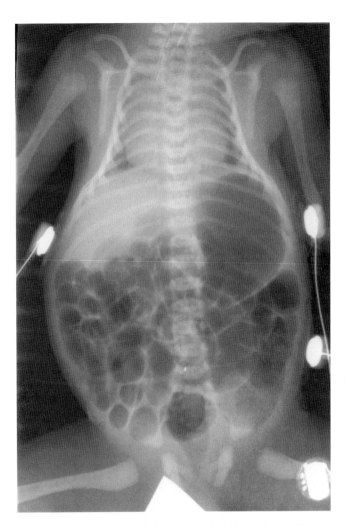

Figure 58.2. Radiograph of the chest and abdomen in a different newborn with prune belly syndrome demonstrates bulging flanks, gaseous distension of bowel loops, flaring of the lower ribs, and hypoplastic lungs.

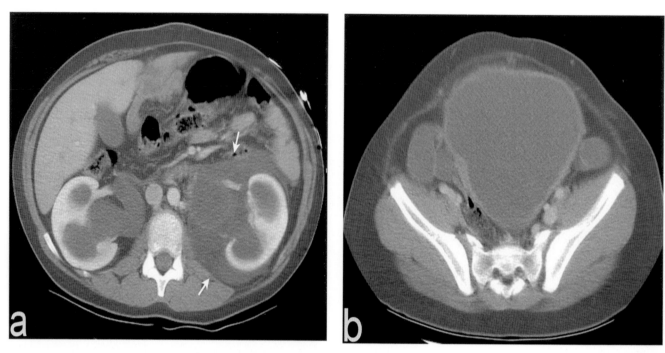

Figure 58.3. An 11-year-old boy with known prune belly syndrome with left flank pain after minor trauma (punched in the belly). **(a, b)** Axial contrast-enhanced CT images of the kidneys and bladder demonstrate bilateral ureteropelvocaliectasis and a dilated bladder. Note the very thin anterior abdominal wall with virtually absent musculature. There is symmetric opacification of the thinned cortices and no intrarenal laceration or contusion was seen. There is a left paranephric and parapelvic fluid collection consistent with hematoma/urinoma (arrows). This was thought to likely be a traumatic rupture of the left renal pelvis which subsequently healed spontaneously.

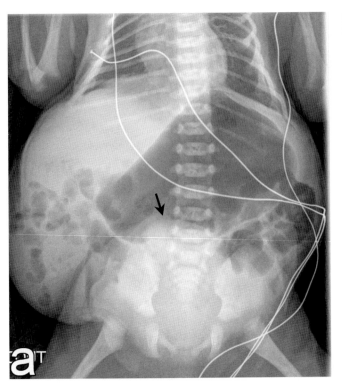

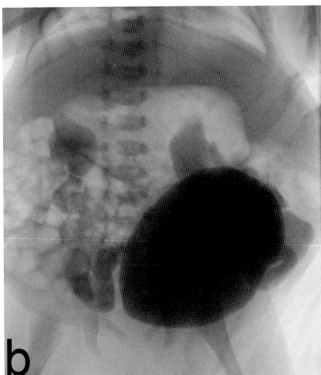

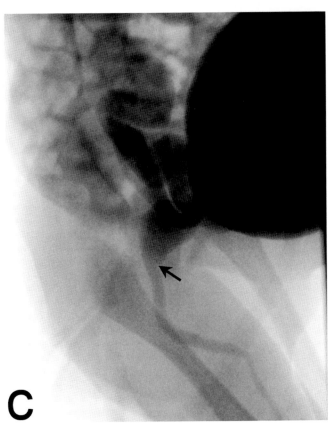

Figure 58.4. A five-day-old male infant diagnosed as probable prune belly syndrome in utero. (a) VCUG scout abdominal radiograph. Note the typical bulging flanks, small thorax and distended bladder (arrow), and bilateral dislocated hips. (b, c) VCUG demonstrating a dilated bladder, reflux bilaterally into tortuous dilated ureters and dilated collecting systems (b), and dilated posterior urethra with partially obstructing posterior urethral valves (c, arrow).

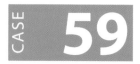

Renal vein thrombosis

Kriengkrai Iemsawatdikul and Heike E. Daldrup-Link

Imaging description

An infant presented with hematuria and thrombocytopenia. An ultrasound and subsequent CT scan demonstrated a thrombus in the right renal vein with an enlarged edematous right kidney (Fig. 59.1). The CT demonstrated diminished contrast enhancement of the medial/posterior aspect of the kidney (Fig. 59.1b) and a thrombus in the inferior vena cara (IVC), which extended into the right renal vein.

Importance

Renal vein thrombosis is the most common vascular pathology of the newborn kidney. Predisposing factors in a neonate include dehydration, sepsis, birth asphyxia, maternal diabetes, polycythemia, adrenal hemorrhage, and the presence of an indwelling catheter. In older children, renal vein thrombosis is associated with nephrotic syndrome and membranous glomerulonephritis, renal tumor (most commonly Wilms' tumor; see Case 64), phlebitis, renal amyloidosis, hereditary thrombophilia, and other hypercoaguable states as well as trauma and burns. The prognosis for the affected kidney is very poor. Anticoagulant and fibrinolytic therapies rarely lead to successful reperfusion. In a few patients, the kidney may recover completely. However, much more frequently, late sequelae are observed, such as focal or complete atrophy of the kidney, impaired renal function, and arterial hypertension.

Typical clinical scenario

The most common clinical presentations include gross hematuria, enlarged, palpable kidneys, and thrombocytopenia.

As opposed to renal vein thrombosis in older children, neonatal renal vein thrombosis (except those associated with umbilical venous catheters) commences in the arcuate or interlobular veins. On ultrasound, the first signs are highly echogenic streaks in the kidney parenchyma due to interlobular and interlobar thrombus and perivascular hemorrhage. These streaks commence in a peripheral, focal segment of the involved kidney and spread to involve the intermedullary vessels (interlobar veins). It is important to recognize these echogenic streaks as they represent the initial phase of renal vein thrombosis and only persist for a few days. After the first week, the echogenic streaks are usually no longer detectable, but there is progressive edema of the kidney, leading to enlargement and heterogeneous loss of corticomedullary differentiation. Occasionally, thrombus may be visualized directly in the renal vein or IVC.

Duplex and color Doppler ultrasound may be used in addition to gray-scale examination. In the early stage of renal vein thrombosis, intrarenal and renal venous flow and pulsatility may be absent and renal arterial diastolic flow may be decreased or reversed, with an increased resistive index.

Subsequently, some retraction of the venous thrombus may occur and venous collaterals form at the renal hilum and around the capsule. These processes lead to some venous flow in the kidney, which can cause diagnostic confusion. If color flow is detected in the renal vein, the degree of pulsatility should be determined. Any obstruction will cause a decrease in right atrial pulsation and the flow will either be steady or of reduced pulsatility. The development of collateral flow also renders the measurement of resistive index from renal and intrarenal arterial vessels insensitive and non-specific.

A contrast-enhanced CT or MR can be obtained to evaluate renal perfusion and function (Fig. 59.2) and confirm a thrombus in a thick-walled renal vein with or without extension into the IVC (Fig. 59.3a). In the chronic phase, the affected renal vein becomes attenuated due to retraction of the clot and development of extensive collateral vessels (Fig. 59.3b). Multiplanar reconstruction images may be useful in demonstrating the extent of the thrombus. Delayed scans may improve visualization of the IVC.

Differential diagnosis

Different possible causes for renal vein thrombosis are listed above. Other causes of a swollen, edematous, enlarged, and/or hypoperfused kidney/s include infection/inflammation such as pyelonephritis, abscess, and glomerulonephritis, trauma, tumors (including Wilms' tumor, lymphoma, nephroblastomatosis), as well as hereditary and metabolic disorders such as autosomal recessive polycystic kidney disease and renal amyloidosis.

Teaching point

Ultrasound is the modality of choice for evaluation of suspected renal vein thrombosis in a newborn. Typical signs include echogenic streaks in the kidney parenchyma in the early phase and an enlarged kidney with loss of corticomedullary differentiation in the subacute phase. Color and Doppler ultrasound may show absent flow or decreased pulsatility in the renal vein. In equivocal cases, CT and/or MR may be helpful in detecting a renal thrombus directly.

REFERENCES

1. Barnewolt CE, Paltiel HJ, Lebowitz RL, Kirks DR. Genitourinary tract. In: Kirks DR, Griscom NT, eds. *Practical Pediatric Imaging: Diagnostic Radiology of Infants and Children*. Philadelphia: Lippincott-Raven Publisher, 1998; 1150–1.

2. Hibbert J, Howlett DC, Greenwood KL, Macdonald LM, Saunders AJS. Pictorial review: the ultrasound appearances of neonatal renal vein thrombosis. *Br J Radiol* 1997;**70**:1191–4.

3. Kawashima A, Sandler CM, Ernst RD, *et al*. CT evaluation of renovascular disease. *Radiographics* 2000;**20**:1321–40.

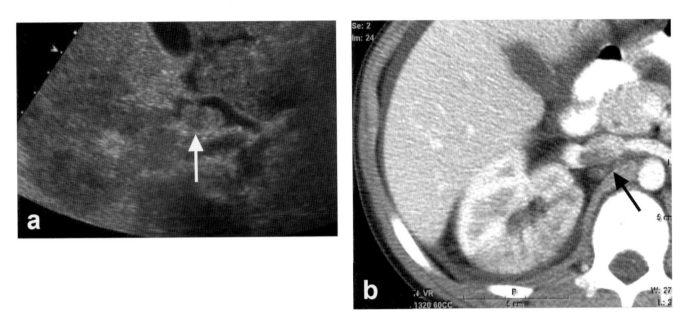

Figure 59.1. (a) Transverse ultrasound image of the right upper abdomen demonstrates enlargement of the right kidney with loss of corticomedullary differentiation. **(b)** Contrast-enhanced CT scan demonstrates cortical enhancement of the anterior and lateral portions of the right kidney, with diminished enhancement of medial and posterior portions. A thrombus is noted in the right renal vein and IVC in both the ultrasound and CT (arrows).

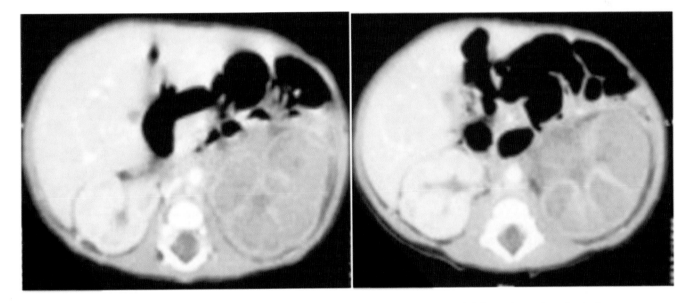

Figure 59.2. Axial contrast-enhanced CT images through the kidneys in a different patient with left renal vein thrombosis demonstrate marked enlargement of the left kidney with very decreased, peripheral contrast enhancement. The right kidney shows normal parenchymal enhancement.

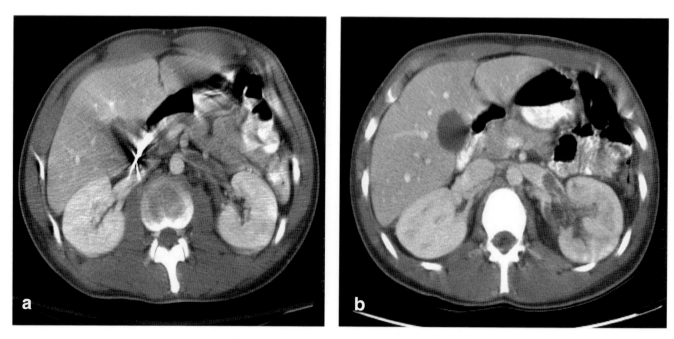

Figure 59.3. Axial, contrast-enhanced CT scan of an acute thrombus in a thick-walled left renal vein **(a)**. In the chronic phase **(b)**, the affected renal vein becomes attenuated due to retraction of the clot along with development of collateral vessels. Note asymmetric contrast enhancement of the kidneys, with delayed parenchymal opacification on the left.

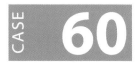

60 Acute bacterial pyelonephritis

Heike E. Daldrup-Link

Imaging description

A 16-year-old female patient presented with a two-week history of increasing fever, back pain, and dysuria. The clinical evaluation revealed tenderness in the left flank, an elevated C-reactive protein, and leukocytosis. An ultrasound (US) of the kidneys demonstrated a focal lesion of uncertain etiology in the left kidney. A CT scan was obtained for further evaluation and showed two focal wedge-shaped hypodense lesions in the left kidney (Fig. 60.1) suggestive of acute focal pyelonephritis. The patient was placed on antibiotic treatment, which led to resolution of the lesions.

In the clinical setting of fever and laboratory signs of an infection, focal lesions in the kidneys as described above should be considered to be acute bacterial pyelonephritis, previously called "lobar nephronia."

Renal US examination in a child with acute pyelonephritis is often completely normal and is less sensitive than other imaging modalities such as CT, MR, or nuclear scintigraphy. There may be focal hypo- or hyperechoic areas, depending on the degree of associated edema and/or hemorrhage. In some cases, the focal area of inflammation may produce mass effect on adjacent structures. Color Doppler US, especially power Doppler, tends to show decreased flow in these areas. Diffuse renal involvement may produce diffuse enlargement with hypo- or hyperechogenicity, loss of corticomedullary differentiation, and uro-epithelial thickening. There may be additional features of an underlying renal obstructive anomaly predisposing to infection, including an obstructed duplicated upper pole collecting system, ureteropelvic or ureterovesical obstruction.

On CT scans, pyelonephritis produces focal or diffuse swelling with poorly marginated hypodense wedge-shaped areas with no or minimal enhancement. Perirenal fat stranding or thickening of the adjacent Gerota's fascia is occasionally seen.

On DMSA scintigraphy, acute pyelonephritis produces a focal region(s) of photopenia.

Importance

Acute bacterial pyelonephritis may produce diffuse or focal inflammation with edema, small vein thrombosis, and potential areas of hemorrhage. Especially if the lesion(s) affects a renal pole or one moiety of a duplex kidney, it may initially be misdiagnosed as tumor(s). It is important to recognize this process as an infection so that the patient receives prompt antibiotic therapy. Cases that are treated inadequately or too late or which are resistant to antibiotic therapy may progress to renal abscess and/or renal scarring. Renal abscess is a rare complication of acute pyelonephritis, seen mostly in children with diabetes, sickle cell disease, or immune compromise. On US an abscess appears as an anechoic rounded region with through-transmission and on CT a well-defined non-enhancing area is seen, with variable wall thickness (Fig. 60.2).

Typical clinical scenario

Pyelonephritis in children often presents clinically with unexplained fever, with or without systemic symptoms and abdominal or back pain. Urinalysis and blood and urine cultures may not be abnormal. Common organisms that cause acute bacterial pyelonephritis include *Eschericia coli*, *Klebsiella pneumoniae*, *Pseudomonas aeruginosa*, and *Staphylococcus aureus*. When clinical and/or imaging findings are equivocal and/or resistance to antibiotic therapy occurs, the diagnosis may be further confirmed by fine-needle aspiration under US or CT guidance.

Differential diagnosis

Differential diagnoses of focal hypo- or hyperechogenic or low attenuating lesions with decreased vascularity compared to the adjacent kidney parenchyma include renal lymphoma, nephroblastomatosis, angiomyolipomas, renal infarction, and renal abscesses. Occasionally, a complex renal cyst, focally dilated collecting system, or caliceal diverticulum might also enter into the differential diagnosis. Fungal renal infections, predominantly due to *Candida albicans*, are seen mostly in premature infants and immunocompromised children. US may be useful in confirming renal candida infection when urine cultures are positive. US findings may be normal or non-specific; the kidneys may be enlarged, with diffuse or focal echogenic or hypoechoic areas. The presence of a fungal ball(s) in the collecting system is the most useful US finding.

> ### Teaching point
>
> The finding of a focal renal lesion on imaging does not always indicate a neoplastic condition. It is important to consider focal pyelonephritis in the appropriate clinical setting.

REFERENCES

1. Chapman S, Nakielny R. Urinary tract. In: *Aids to Radiological Differential Diagnosis*, 3rd edition. London: W.B. Saunders Company Limited, 1995; 307.

2. Currarino G, Wood B, Majd M. The genitourinary tract and retroperitoneum. In: Silverman FN, Kuhn JP, eds. *Caffey's Pediatric X-Ray Diagnosis: An Integrated Imaging Approach*, 9th edition. St Louis: Mosby, 1993; 1331.

3. Klar A, Hurvitz H, Berkun, *et al.* Focal bacterial nephritis (lobar nephronia) in children. *J Pediatr* 1996;**128**(6):850–3.

4. Rohrschneider WK, Weirich A, Rieden K, *et al.* US, CT and MR imaging characteristics of nephroblastomatosis. *Pediatr Radiol* 1998;**28**(6):435–43.

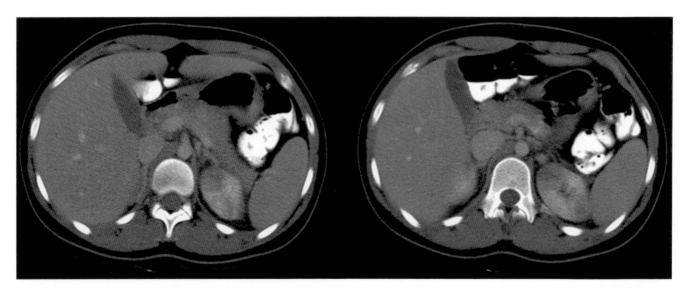

Figure 60.1. A 16-year-old female with fever and multifocal pyelonephritis. Axial CT scans after oral and intravenous contrast media administration demonstrate two focal wedge-shaped hypodense lesions in the left kidney with no or minimal enhancement compared to the normally enhancing kidney parenchyma. The anterior lesion shows mild mass effect on the collecting system.

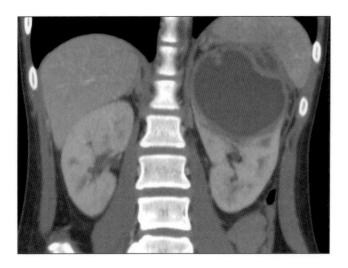

Figure 60.2. Renal abscess in a 14-year-old previously healthy girl with a 10-day history of fever, chills, and left flank pain. Both US (not shown) and CT demonstrated a large multiloculated cystic mass in the left upper pole. The CT also showed moderate perinephric inflammatory changes. The large renal abscess was drained, with no evidence seen of an underlying lesion.

Ectopic ureterocele

Heike E. Daldrup-Link

Imaging description

A three-year-old boy presented with recurrent urinary tract infection. An ultrasound of the urinary bladder and kidneys demonstrated a left-sided ureterocele, hydroureter, and upper pole hydronephrosis (Fig. 61.1a–d). The left kidney demonstrated evidence of a duplicated collecting system with a dilated, obstructed upper pole collecting system and a non-dilated lower pole collecting system (not shown). Echogenic debris in the dilated left upper pole collecting system and ureter suggested the possibility of superimposed pyohydronephrosis. A subsequent voiding cystourethrogram (VCUG) confirmed the ureterocele and showed grade 2 reflux into a non-dilated left lower pole ureter and renal collecting system (Fig. 61.1e, f). The findings are consistent with a duplicated collecting system with a dilated, obstructed upper pole moiety, which ends in an ectopic ureterocele and a non-dilated lower pole moiety, which shows vesicoureteral reflux.

Imaging findings of a duplicated kidney with duplicated ureters comprise the following:

1. Duplicated collecting systems and parenchymal bridge identified on ultrasound. Both upper and lower poles may be normal if there is a partial duplication (bifid pelvis or ureters join) or the two ureters both terminate at or close to the normal orifice.
2. Hydronephrosis on ultrasound, often much more prominent in the upper pole collecting system than the lower pole collecting system.
3. Upper pole moiety: hydronephrosis, tortuous hydroureter, ectopic ureterocele.
4. Lower pole moiety: orthotopic ureter; may show reflux.
5. Drooping lily sign on a VCUG: downward displacement of lower pole calices by a hydronephrotic upper pole moiety.
6. Nubbin sign: scarring, atrophy, and decreased function of the lower pole moiety may simulate a renal mass.
7. Ureterocele disproportion sign: very subtle dysplastic upper pole with a mildly dilated ectopic ureter and ureterocele.

Importance

An ectopic ureterocele is a cystic protrusion of the distal dilated ureter with an obstructed orifice at a non-physiologic ureteral insertion site, including the lower urinary bladder, the urethra, vagina, the seminal vesicle, vas deferens, or rectum. Ectopic ureteroceles are almost always associated with a duplicated collecting system of the ipsilateral kidney. The ectopic ureterocele typically originates from the upper pole ureter of the duplicated kidney. The Weigert–Meyer rule states that in duplicated kidneys, the lower pole moiety inserts at or near normal position, while the upper pole ureter inserts ectopically medially and inferiorly to the normal position. The more ectopic the insertion of the ureter, the more dysplastic the associated upper pole parenchyma is likely to be. The upper pole ureter is commonly obstructed (often associated with a ureterocele), while an abnormal lower pole ureter is most often associated with vesicoureteral reflux.

Typical clinical scenario

Ureteroceles occur in approximately 1 in 4000 children and are most common in females and whites. Approximately 10% of ureteroceles are bilateral. Ureteroceles may be asymptomatic or present with a wide range of clinical symptoms, including recurrent fever and urinary tract infections, urosepsis, bladder outlet obstruction or perineal mass (ureterocele prolapsing into the urethra), recurrent abdominal, flank or pelvic pain, failure to thrive, or renal insufficiency.

The most common current treatment is an endoscopic incision of the ureterocele. It is important to understand possible implications of this intervention for the duplicated system. The upper pole hydronephrosis may be decompressed, remain unchanged, or may increase due to new ipsilateral upper pole reflux. Likewise, the lower pole reflux may remain unchanged or improve due to resolution of ureterocele-induced alterations of the bladder wall.

Differential diagnosis

An orthotopic ureterocele defines a cystic ureteral protrusion at the normal insertion site of the ureter into the bladder. It usually arises from a single renal unit with one collecting system, is usually asymptomatic and, thus, more commonly diagnosed in adults.

Ectopic ureters may insert in anatomic structures distal to the bladder. The most common sites in girls are the urethra and vagina. The most common site in boys is the prostatic urethra, rarely the rectum. A retrograde urogram, a vaginogram, or an MR urogram can confirm the diagnosis. A ureterocele may have a varied appearance on imaging, often related to filling of the bladder or voiding. On a cystogram, the ureterocele is usually best seen with early filling as with increased bladder pressure it may be compressed or obscured by the dense contrast-filled bladder. The ureterocele may also evert, producing an appearance simulating a bladder diverticulum, or prolapse into the urethra, producing bladder outlet obstruction simulating posterior urethral valves. A ureterocele is a smooth, rounded, variably sized, thin-walled defect in the bladder and is usually not confused with other rare bladder masses in children, which tend to be more irregular.

Other causes for dilated ureter/s without a ureterocele include bladder outlet obstruction such as posterior urethral valves, vesicoureteral reflux, congenital ureterovesical junction obstruction (primary megaureter), prune belly syndrome, and acquired ureteral obstruction.

Teaching point

An ectopic ureterocele is almost always associated with a duplicated collecting system. According to the Weigert–Meyer rule, the ectopic ureterocele usually connects to an obstructed upper pole collecting system, while the lower pole collecting system inserts via an orthotopic ureter which is prone to vesicoureteral reflux.

REFERENCES

1. Barnewolt CE, Paltiel HJ, Lebowitz RL, *et al.* Genitourinary tract. In: Kirks DR, Griscom NT, eds. *Practical Pediatric Imaging: Diagnostic Radiology of Infants and Children*. Philadelphia: Lippincott-Raven Publisher, 1998; 70–8.
2. Dahnert W. Renal, adrenal, ureteral, vesical, and scrotal disorders. In: Dahnert W, ed. *Radiology Review Manual*. Philadelphia: Lippincott Williams & Wilkins, 1996; 815.
3. Kriss VM. Congenital renal abnormalities. In: Kriss VM, ed. *Handbook of Pediatric Radiology*. St Louis: Mosby, 1998; 199–200.

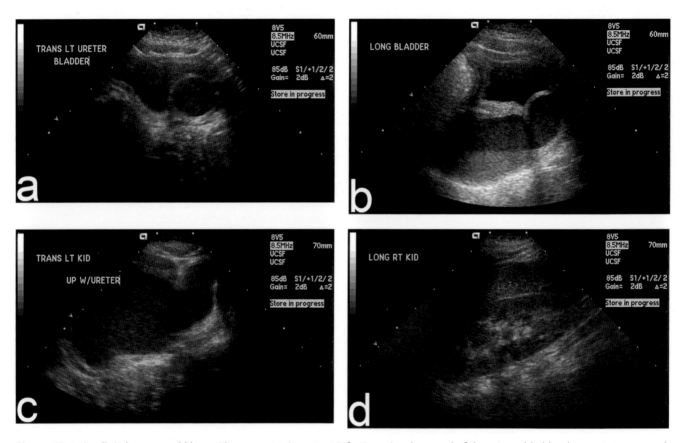

Figure 61.1. (a–d) A three-year-old boy with recurrent urinary tract infections. An ultrasound of the urinary bladder demonstrates a round, fluid-filled structure, protruding into the left side into the bladder (a). A longitudinal view of this fluid-filled structure shows continuity with a dilatated left ureter (b), which can be followed into a markedly dilated left upper pole collecting system (c). There is echogenic debris in the hydronephrotic left upper pole and ureter suggestive of possible pyohydronephrosis. The right kidney is normal (d).

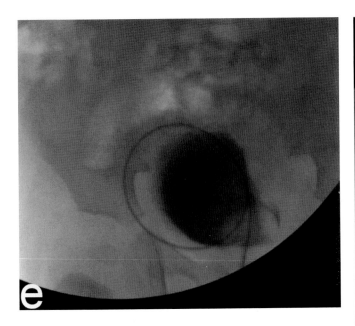
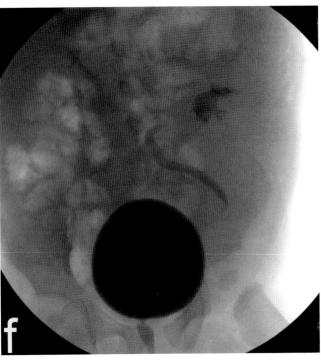

Figure 61.1. (cont.) **(e, f)** A VCUG in the same patient demonstrates a filling defect in the left lower bladder during the early retrograde filling phase with iodinated contrast media (e). The filling defect disappears with further contrast filling of the bladder due to increased pressure in the bladder. During the voiding phase, grade 2 reflux is noted into a non-dilatated ureter and a non-dilatated lower pole collecting system of the left kidney (f). The ureter is slightly redundant and the lower pole collecting system has a slight downward orientation, consistent with a "drooping lily" sign indicative of mass effect from the non-visualized obstructed hydronephrotic upper pole.

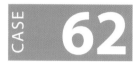

Nephroblastomatosis

Gregory Cheeney, Rakhee Gawande, Beverley Newman, and Heike E. Daldrup-Link

Imaging description

A four-year-old boy presented with large palpable flank masses bilaterally. An ultrasound (not shown) revealed bilaterally enlarged kidneys with homogeneous low echogenicity, resembling renal cortex. A contrast-enhanced CT was performed which showed a thick rim of non-enhancing, homogeneous soft tissue, surrounding centrally enhancing renal parenchyma (Fig. 62.1). Bilateral homogeneous non-enhancing soft tissue surrounding the renal parenchyma is a typical finding in diffuse bilateral nephroblastomatosis. Another patient with a similar presentation is shown in Figure 62.2. In this case, axial contrast-enhanced CT images demonstrate multiple lenticular, uniform, non-enhancing lesions in the renal cortex (Fig. 62.2), consistent with the more common multifocal type of nephroblastomatosis. On CT, focal nephroblastomatosis appears as low attenuation, subcapsular, or intraparenchymal lesions with poor enhancement relative to that of adjacent normal renal parenchyma. On MRI, focal nephroblastomatosis demonstrates low to intermediate signal intensity foci on both T1- and T2-weighted sequences. Both types of nephroblastomatosis typically resemble the normal renal cortex with regard to their echogenicity on ultrasound, and density and signal intensity on unenhanced CT and MRI. After contrast media injection, however, the lesions typically show no or only minimal enhancement. Contrast administration is helpful in differentiating nephroblastomatosis from Wilms' tumor. The latter is typically inhomogeneous and enhances after contrast media administration.

Importance

Nephroblastomatosis refers to the continuation of nephrogenic rests beyond 36 weeks of gestation. Nephrogenic rests arise from the metanephros, the embryonic origin of the renal cortex (Fig. 62.3). As shown in these cases, nephroblastomatosis may be characterized as diffuse or multifocal, with further classification of the focal subtype into perilobar or intralobar. Nephroblastomatosis can regress spontaneously; benign lesions can grow substantially and/or develop into a Wilms' tumor. Thirty to forty percent of unilateral and 99% of bilateral Wilms' tumors are thought to arise from these nephrogenic rests. Intralobar nephroblastomatosis has a higher association with Wilms' tumor compared to the perilobar type. The presence of nephroblastomatosis is associated with several congenital syndromes. Intralobar nephroblastomatosis is associated with Drash syndrome and sporadic aniridia. In contrast, perilobar nephroblastomatosis is associated with trisomy 18, Beckwith–Wiedemann syndrome, and hemihypertrophy. Imaging is essential for following the evolution of the often bilateral and multifocal lesions, as well as the preoperative assessment of both the affected and contralateral kidneys if surgery is performed to remove a suspected Wilms' tumor.

Typical clinical scenario

Nephroblastomatosis is most common in neonates, with the peak age ranging from six to 18 months. Patients may present incidentally or with a palpable flank or abdominal mass. Special consideration must be given to rule out congenital syndromes.

Differential diagnosis

Given the concurrence of Wilms' tumor with nephroblastomatosis, it is essential to distinguish the two (Fig. 62.4). The key differences are the size of the lesion, the homogeneity of the tissue, and the contrast enhancement. Wilms' tumors tend to be large and inhomogeneous due to areas of necrosis/hemorrhage within the variably vascularized tumor, while untreated nephroblastomatosis is homogeneous and relatively avascular. However, renal cysts can be associated with nephroblastomatosis, leading to an apparent "inhomogeneous" picture (Fig. 62.4). In addition, empiric therapy in doubtful cases of growing lesions leads to inhomogeneities of benign nephroblastomatosis, which may then be difficult to differentiate from a Wilms' tumor. Development of inhomogeneity in previously homogeneous, untreated nephroblastomatosis is highly suggestive of malignant transformation. Additionally, diffusion-weighted MR scan can help in the differential diagnosis. Wilms' tumors are characterized by restricted diffusion of the solid tumor component (low apparent diffusion coefficient [ADC] values), while benign nephroblastomatosis shows only minimally restricted diffusion.

Other differential diagnoses include mesoblastic nephroma (typically affecting children less than one year of age) as well as renal metastases and lymphoma (typically affecting children >4–5 years of age), and other less common pediatric renal masses.

Teaching point

Diffuse nephroblastomatosis is usually seen as reniform enlargement with a thick peripheral rind of soft tissue that may show no or minimal enhancement. Focal nephroblastomatosis appears as ovoid or lenticular non-enhancing masses, typically multifocal and peripherally located in the renal cortex; the lesions may contain small cysts. Nephroblastomatosis is a precursor to Wilms' tumor and is associated with several congenital syndromes. Rapid growth, inhomogeneity, and increasing enhancement are concerning features for malignant transformation.

REFERENCES

1. Cormier PJ, Donaldson JS, Gonzalez-Crussi F. Nephroblastomatosis: missed diagnosis. *Radiology* 1988;**169**(3):737–8.

2. Lowe LH, Isuani BH, Heller RM. Pediatric renal masses: Wilms tumor and beyond. *Radiographics* 2000;**20**(6):1585–603.

3. Lowe LH, Taboada EM. Pediatric kidney cancer. In: Baert AL, Sartor LK, eds. *Imaging of Kidney Cancer*. Berlin: Springer, 2006; 351–70.

4. Rohrschneider WK, Weirich A, Rieden K, *et al.* US, CT and MR imaging characteristics of nephroblastomatosis. *Pediatr Radiol* 1998;**28**(6):435–43.

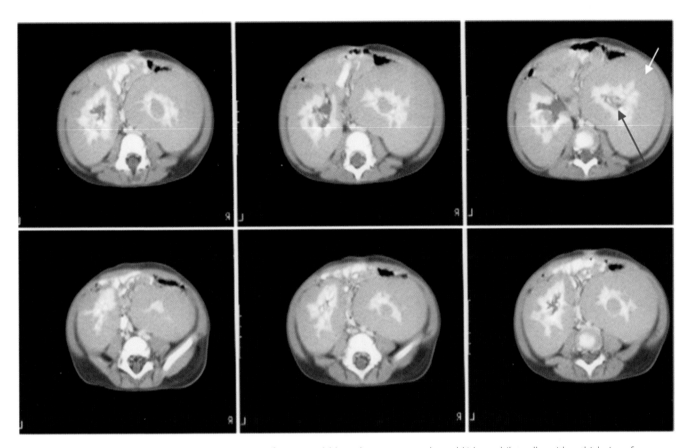

Figure 62.1. Axial contrast-enhanced CT images in a four-year-old boy demonstrate enlarged kidneys bilaterally, with a thick rim of non-enhancing soft tissue (white arrow) surrounding central enhancing renal tissue (blue arrow). In a young child, the finding is characteristic of nephroblastomatosis.

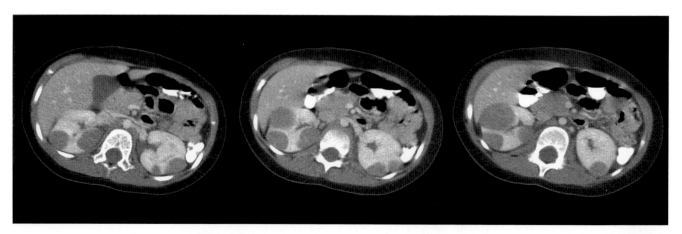

Figure 62.2. Axial contrast-enhanced CT images show several focal, well-defined, hypodense, non-enhancing masses in the right kidney (white arrows), which represent intralobar multifocal nephroblastomatosis.

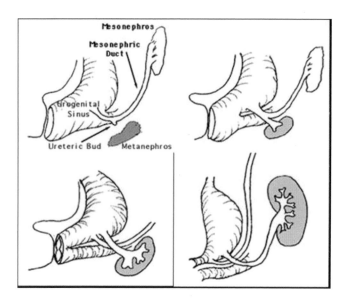

Figure 62.3. Demonstrates the embryonic development of the kidney and its collecting system. The metanephros is mesodermal tissue that originates inferior to the mesonephros. At around five weeks of development the ureteric bud will form and advance towards the metanephros. This interaction will induce differentiation of the metanephros into the specialized cells of the kidney. Nephrogenic rests are remnants of metanephros that persist. (Illustration from: www.meddean.luc.edu/lumen/MedEd/urology/unldevb.htm, ©David A. Hatch, M.D., 1996. Teaching website of Loyola University. With permission.)

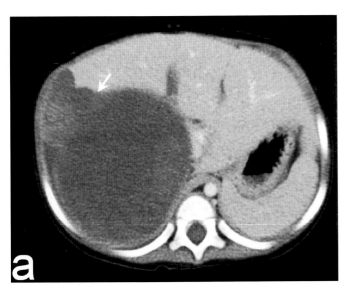
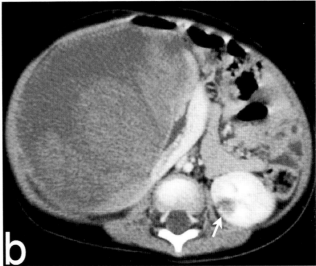
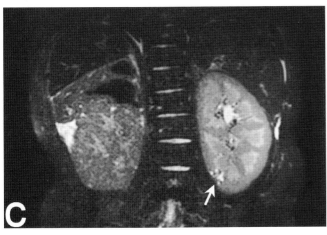

Figure 62.4. A 12-month-old girl with ruptured Wilms' tumor of the right kidney and nephrogenic rest (nephroblastoma) in the left kidney. **(a, b)** Axial contrast-enhanced CT images show a large hypodense heterogeneous combined solid and cystic/necrotic mass arising from the right kidney. The anterolateral margin of the tumor shows an area of focal bulging with adjacent free fluid (arrow), suspicious for tumor capsule disruption. A ruptured Wilms' tumor was found at surgery. (b) A lower image demonstrates a small remnant of normal parenchyma of right kidney medially with a claw sign around the tumor and denser contrast enhancement similar to the contralateral normal kidney. In the left kidney a small hypodense lesion is visible in the lower pole (arrow), thought to likely represent a nephrogenic rest. **(c)** Postoperative coronal T2-weighted MR image shows a small lesion in the medial lower pole of the left kidney with a T2- isointense center and multiple adjacent tiny T2-hyperintense cysts (arrow), likely representing the same nephrogenic rest. The right kidney has been surgically removed and large bowel is located in the right renal fossa.

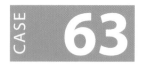
Urachal mass

Rakhee Gawande and Beverley Newman

Imaging description

A 35-year-old lady in her first trimester of pregnancy presented with abdominal pain and a palpable anterior abdominopelvic mass. Ultrasound (US) of the pelvis (Fig. 63.1a, b) demonstrated a gravid uterus with multiple uterine fibroids (not shown). In addition, a hypoechoic solid mass with moderately prominent vascularity was noted superior to the uterus, extending up to the umbilicus, raising the suspicion of a pedunculated fibroid. An MRI of the pelvis (Fig. 63.1c, d) also revealed a large heterogeneously enhancing mass beneath the anterior pelvic wall, extending up to the umbilicus. The mass was resected and histopathological analysis revealed a squamous cell carcinoma of a urachal remnant. The pregnancy continued successfully to term.

Importance

The urachus is a three-layered remnant of the embryonic allantois (innermost layer of transitional epithelium, an intermediate layer of fibroconnective tissue, and outer smooth muscle layer). The urachus extends from the dome of the bladder to the umbilicus and gets progressively obliterated by four to five months of gestation, leaving behind a fibrous cord called the median umbilical ligament. The complete obliteration of the urachus was originally thought to be a prenatal process; however, recent literature has indicated that the involution may continue in the first few months of life. Failure of this obliteration may result in different types of urachal remnant anomalies, including a completely patent urachus (vesicoumbilical fistula, 48%), vesicourachal diverticulum (3%), umbilical-urachal sinus (18%), and urachal cyst (31%). A normal urachal remnant is quite commonly seen as an incidental finding on pelvic US in children as a small hypoechoic structure, superior to the urinary bladder (Fig. 63.2). A patent urachus can be seen as a tubular connection between the bladder and the umbilicus on sagittal us (Fig. 63.3). An umbilical-urachal sinus can be seen as a blind-ending midline tubular structure below the umbilicus, and may occasionally become infected, resulting in umbilical drainage. A vesicourachal diverticulum is generally asymptomatic and can be incidentally detected on imaging as a midline cystic structure at the superior aspect of the bladder. Occasionally, a large diverticulum may result in stasis, aberrant micturition, infection, or stone formation. Urachal diverticulum as well as other urachal anomalies are particularly associated with prune belly syndrome (see Case 58). A urachal cyst is formed when the urachus closes at both the umbilical and bladder ends and remains patent in between. It is seen on US or CT as a midline extraperitoneal cystic structure beneath the anterior abdominal wall; multiple cysts may be present, thought to be related to segmental partial urachal obliteration.

Urachal neoplasms are rare; benign tumors include adenoma, fibroma, myoma, and hamartoma. The urachus is lined by transitional epithelium; however, the majority of malignant neoplasms are adenocarcinomas thought to be due to metaplasia of the transitional epithelium. Approximately 30% of bladder carcinomas in adults are urachal in origin. Urachal tumors are more common in males and most often occur between 40 and 70 years of age; they are extremely rare in childhood. The majority of the urachal cancers arise in the juxta-vesical region with very few occurring near the umbilical end. They are seen as heterogeneous superficial masses on CT with low attenuation due to high mucin content. Calcifications are extremely common in urachal cancers.

Typical clinical scenario

The most common symptom of a patient with a patent urachus is umbilical drainage. The other congenital urachal anomalies are usually asymptomatic unless they become infected, which occurs quite commonly with urachal cysts and sinuses (Fig. 63.4). An infected urachal remnant may present with abdominal pain, mass, umbilical drainage, urinary tract infections, fever, and rarely, peritonitis. A superficial midline infra-abdominal mass in a child should raise suspicion for an infected urachal remnant, much less likely a urachal neoplasm, although the lesions can be very heterogeneous in appearance (Fig. 63.4).

Asymptomatic urachal remnants may undergo spontaneous regression during the first six months of life and can be monitored by serial follow-up US examinations. Due to the extreme rarity of malignant transformation, excision is usually not considered to be necessary, although symptomatic urachal remnants are generally excised. Urachal anomalies are associated with other genitourinary and gastrointestinal anomalies, including prune belly syndrome, hypospadias, meatal stenosis, umbilical and inguinal hernia, omphalocele, anal atresia, ureteroplevic junction obstruction, and most frequently, vesicouretral reflux.

Urachal neoplasms may present as midline abdominal masses. Due to their extraperitoneal location, tumors may be clinically asymptomatic initially, leading to a more advanced stage at presentation. Patients may present with hematuria due to urinary bladder involvement. Metastases may occur to the pelvic lymph nodes, lung, brain, liver, and bone.

Differential diagnosis

An infected urachal remnant may mimic other midline abdominal or pelvic inflammatory pathologies. A urachal carcinoma may be confused with a primary vesical cancer, which is usually seen as a mass arising from the bladder mucosa, with a smaller extravesical component than a urachal tumor.

Other tumors that arise from or can involve the bladder in childhood include rhabdomyosarcoma (most common usually arising from the bladder base or prostate, or uterus/vagina and involving the bladder), leiomyosarcoma, pheochromocytoma, and leukemia/lymphoma. Benign bladder neoplasms are very rare and include hemangioma, neurofibroma, fibroepithelial polyps, and inflammatory pseudotumor (Fig. 63.5).

The other umbilical embryonic remnants that may be present are the spectrum of omphalomesenteric duct anomalies. These arise from the vitelline duct and have a similar spectrum to that of the urachal remnants, including a patent omphalomesenteric duct connection from the umbilicus to the distal ileum (Fig. 63.6), umbilcal sinus, ileal (Meckel's) diverticulum (most common), and vitelline duct cyst. These remnants may cause umbilical drainage, become infected, bleed (gastric mucosa), perforate, and cause intestinal obstruction, intussusception, or volvulus.

Teaching point

A urachal remnant can undergo spontaneous involution in the first few months of life. Asymptomatic cases can be followed by serial US examinations. Urachal abnormality should be considered when a midline superficial infra-umbilical abdominopelvic lesion is present. Complications of urachal remnants in childhood include umbilical drainage, diverticulum, cystic mass, infection, and very rarely, carcinoma. While congenital lesions and their complications are generally more often encountered or actually considered in infants and children, there is a continuum into adulthood and long-term complications of congenital lesions need to be appropriately added to differential diagnoses.

REFERENCES

1. Cacciarelli AA, Kass EJ, Yang SS. Urachal remnants: sonographic demonstration in children. *Radiology* 1990;**174**(2):473–5.
2. Choi YJ, Kim JM, Ahn SY, *et al.* Urachal anomalies in children: a single center experience. *Yonsei Med J* 2006;**47**(6):782–6.
3. Cuda SP, Vanasupa BP, Sutherland RS. Nonoperative management of a patent urachus. *Urology* 2005;**66**(6):1320.
4. Galati V, Donovan B, Ramji F, *et al.* Management of urachal remnants in early childhood. *J Urol* 2008;**180**(4):1824–6; discussion 1827.
5. Lipskar AM, Glick RD, Rosen NG, *et al.* Nonoperative management of symptomatic urachal anomalies. *J Pediatr Surg* 2010;**45**(5):1016–9.
6. Yapo BR, Gerges B, Holland AJ. Investigation and management of suspected urachal anomalies in children. *Pediatr Surg Int* 2008;**24**(5): 589–92.
7. Yu JS, Kim KW, Lee HJ, *et al.* Urachal remnant diseases: spectrum of CT and US findings. *Radiographics* 2001;**21**(2):451–61.
8. Zieger B, Sokol B, Rohrscheider WK, *et al.* Sonomorphology and involution of the normal urachus in asymptomatic newborns *Pediatr Radiol* 1998;**28**:156–161.

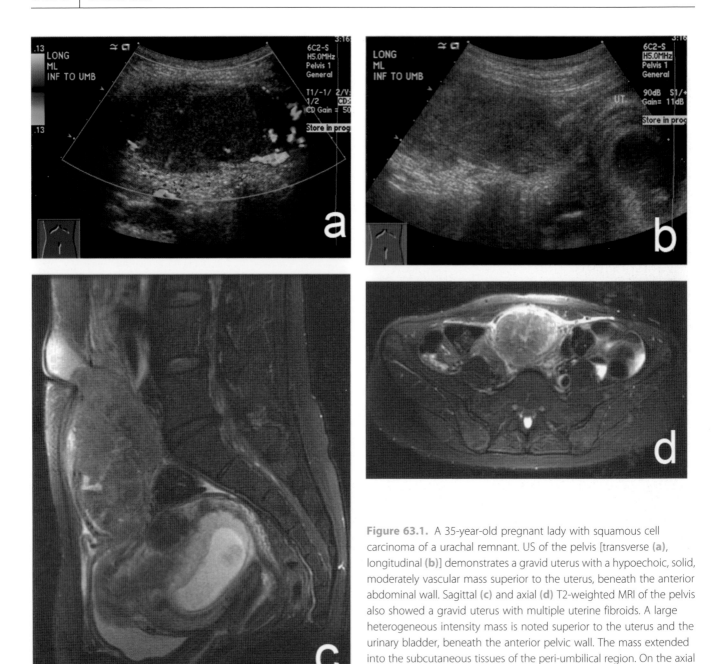

Figure 63.1. A 35-year-old pregnant lady with squamous cell carcinoma of a urachal remnant. US of the pelvis [transverse (a), longitudinal (b)] demonstrates a gravid uterus with a hypoechoic, solid, moderately vascular mass superior to the uterus, beneath the anterior abdominal wall. Sagittal (c) and axial (d) T2-weighted MRI of the pelvis also showed a gravid uterus with multiple uterine fibroids. A large heterogeneous intensity mass is noted superior to the uterus and the urinary bladder, beneath the anterior pelvic wall. The mass extended into the subcutaneous tissues of the peri-umbilical region. On the axial image, at least part of the mass appears to be superficial, questionably extraperitoneal.

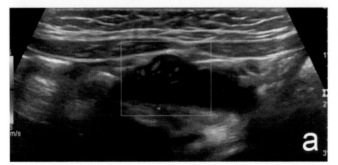

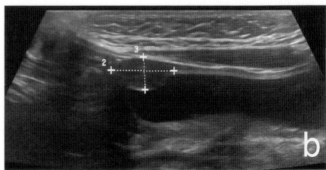

Figure 63.2. one-month-old infant with umbilical discharge. Transverse (a) and longitudinal (b) US images of the pelvis reveal a small oval hypoechoic structure superior to the urinary bladder, just beneath the anterior abdominal wall. The lesion demonstrated mild internal vascularity and was thought to be a normal urachal remnant.

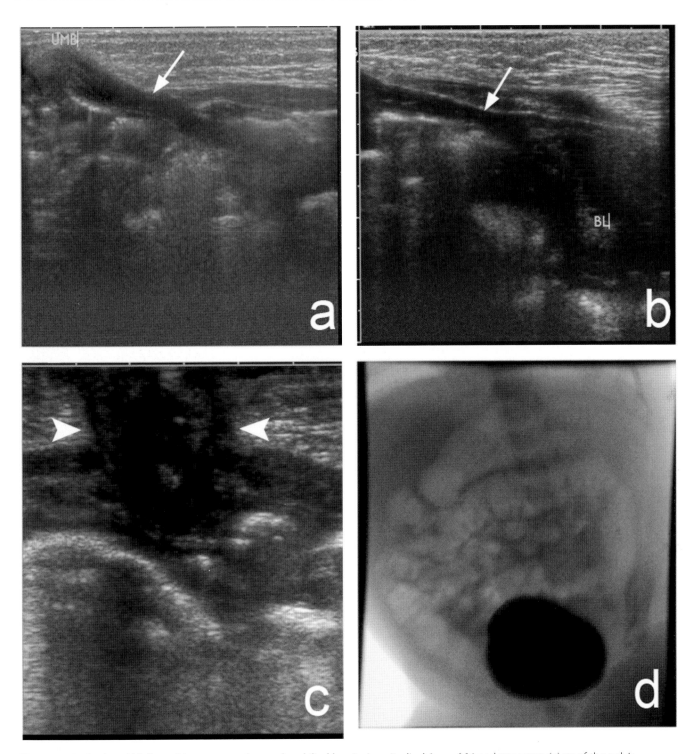

Figure 63.3. 31-day-old infant with patent urachus and umbilical hernia. Longitudinal (a and b) and transverse (c) us of the pelvis demonstrates a linear hypoechoic tract extending from the dome of the bladder to the umbilicus [arrows (a),(b)]. An abdominal wall defect is noted in the umbilical region with herniation of bowel loops [arrows, (c)]. Voiding cystourethrogram two months later demonstrated a normal urinary bladder.

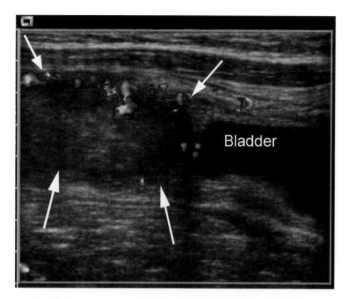

Figure 63.4. Three-year-old girl presenting with fever and abdominal pain. Urachal abscess. Sagittal US demonstrates a prominent superior diverticular extension of the bladder consistent with a urachal diverticulum. Superior to this, there is an echogenic superficial walled-off oval mass (arrows). The central echogenic portion is avascular with a hyperemic wall and good posterior wall through transmission consistent with a fluid/debris containing collection. The provisional diagnosis of an infected urachal cyst/urachal abscess was confirmed surgically.

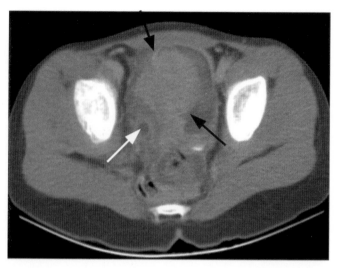

Figure 63.5. Four-year-old boy with hematuria and bladder mass on US. Inflammatory pseudotumor. Axial CT slice post contrast demonstrates a large homogeneously enhancing intravesical mass (black arrows) arising from the region of the right trigone and encasing the distal right ureter, which is dilated (white arrow). The most likely diagnosis in this age group would be bladder rhabdomyosarcoma; however, this proved to be a very unusual benign lesion; inflammatory pseudotumor.

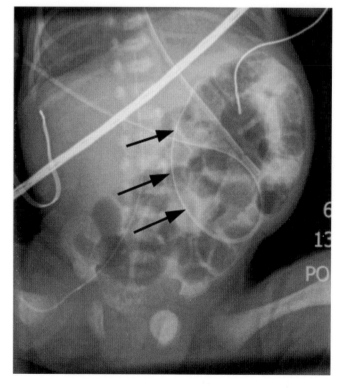

Figure 63.6. 10-day-old male infant with persistent umbilical drainage. US and a voiding cystourethrogram obtained to evaluate for a patent urachus were normal. A small catheter was threaded into the umbilicus and carefully advanced. A small amount of water soluble contrast was injected, demonstrating a patent connection between the umbilicus and bowel (arrows). At surgery, a patent omphalomesenteric duct was found, extending from the umbilicus to the mid ileum.

Wilms' tumor

Rakhee Gawande, Kriengkrai Iemsawatdikul, Heike E. Daldrup-Link, and Beverley Newman

Imaging description

A 22-month-old female presented with a history of vomiting and a palpable right abdominal mass. An abdominal ultrasound (not shown) and an MRI of the abdomen (Fig. 64.1) demonstrated a large mass involving the right kidney, with distortion of the pelvicalyceal system. In addition a large tumor thrombus was noted in the right renal vein, extending into the inferior vena cava (IVC) to the level of the mid liver with marked dilatation of these vessels. The tumor thrombus also extended into the left renal vein, up to the renal hilum (Fig. 64.1). A renal biopsy confirmed the diagnosis of a Wilms' tumor (WT).

Importance

WT is the most common renal neoplasm in children, with 95% of cases occurring between 2 and 5 years of age. Five to seven percent of children have bilateral disease with 7% of cases being multicentric (Fig. 64.2). Nephrogenic rests, which are thought to be precursors of WT, are seen in 1% of neonates and it is believed that only 1% of these transform into WT. Histologically, WTs are of triphasic cell lineage comprising blastemal, stromal, and epithelial cells and about 7% are anaplastic. Favorable histology WT have absence of anaplasia, have a better prognosis, and are more responsive to chemotherapy. Unfavorable histology WTs exhibit anaplasia, are chemotherapy resistant, and are associated with an increased risk of recurrence.

On imaging studies, WT are typically large intrarenal masses with a pseudocapsule and with distortion of the pelvicalyceal system. Tumors are heterogeneous due to the presence of hemorrhage, necrosis, calcification (10%), and fat. Occasionally WT can be predominantly cystic. The tumor spreads by direct extension and typically displaces adjacent anatomic structures but does not encase or elevate the aorta. Vascular extension of the tumor occurs in approximately 6% of cases into the renal veins, IVC, liver veins, and even into the right atrium. The most common site of metastases is the lungs, followed by liver and regional lymph nodes. The presence of peritumoral fluid or discontinuity of the pseudocapsule should raise suspicion for tumor rupture.

Ultrasound is usually the initial imaging study obtained with a suspected abdominal mass and is useful in confirming that a mass is truly present as opposed to a normal structure or benign entity such as an adrenal hemorrhage or hydronephrotic kidney. Doppler ultrasound is also often helpful in evaluating the vessels associated with a mass and especially the location and patency of hepatic, portal, and renal veins and IVC. MR or CT imaging with contrast is usually required for more detailed anatomic assessment of neoplastic masses.

Typical clinical scenario

WT is usually discovered incidentally as a palpable abdominal mass or after coincidental abdominal trauma. Rarely, pain and hematuria may occur. Hypertension may be present in 25% of cases due to production of renin.

WT and its precursor, nephroblastomatosis (see Case 62), are associated with a number of syndromes including sporadic aniridia, WAGR syndrome (Wilms' tumor, Aniridia, Genitourinary abnormalities and mental Retardation), Denys–Drash syndrome (Fig. 64.2), trisomy 18, and Beckwith–Wiedemann syndrome. Regular ultrasound screening until about 8 years of age is recommended in children at risk for developing WT.

Unilateral WT is treated by surgical resection followed by chemotherapy; however, several courses of chemotherapy may precede surgery if the tumor is very large and/or there is extensive tumor thrombus. Residual tumor thrombus may also be removed surgically. The presence of tumor spillage, tumor rupture, or peritoneal implants is an indication for complete abdominal radiation therapy. Preoperative chemotherapy is important in patients with bilateral WT as resolution of disease in one kidney may allow surgery on the other with eventual cure. Tumor resection with sparing of normal parenchyma is generally carried out for bilateral disease.

Children undergo follow-up imaging at regular intervals. In our hospital, we obtain MR of the abdomen rather than CT for follow-up of most abdominal neoplasms, including WT, in order to limit ionizing radiation exposure. When chest imaging is needed for metastatic surveillance, CT is used since MR imaging is currently less sensitive for pulmonary nodules and parenchymal lung disease.

Differential diagnosis

Nephroblastomatosis consists of multifocal or diffuse involvement of both kidneys by persistent embryonic nephrogenic rests. These are low-density peripheral lesions on CT and most often resolve spontaneously but have potential for malignant transformation into WT (Fig. 64.2). Differentiating WT from nephroblastomatosis can be difficult both on imaging and histology. Large size, inhomogeneity, restricted diffusion, rapid growth, and increasing enhancement are suspicious signs of malignant transformation.

Mesoblastic nephroma (Fig. 64.3) is the most common renal mass in a neonate. It was originally believed to be a congenital WT, but is now recognized as a renal hamartoma. Ninety percent of cases are seen in the first year, with most occurring in the first three months after birth. On imaging it is a solid renal mass indistinguishable from WT, which involves the renal sinus and may contain hemorrhagic, cystic, and necrotic areas and may have perinephric infiltration. Treatment is nephrectomy with need for wide local excision due to the presence of infiltration. It is usually benign but hypercellularity histologically may denote a more aggressive lesion that may recur locally or very rarely metastasize to the lungs, brain, or bone. Diffusion-weighted imaging may help to differentiate highly cellular malignant lesions from benign lesions. Malignant tumors have restricted diffusion (bright signal) and very low ADC values in comparison to benign and cystic lesions (Fig. 64.3).

Metanephric stromal tumor has been described relatively recently as a renal neoplasm that occurs in young infants. This is thought to also be a benign lesion but somewhat more aggressive than mesoblastic nephroma, perhaps a form of well-differentiated WT. This tumor is characterized by aggressive local spread, including growth down the ureter.

Renal cell carcinoma is rare in children, accounting for less than 7% of renal tumors, most in older children. The tumor mass is usually smaller than WT and may be indistinguishable preoperatively. There is an increased incidence of this tumor in von Hippel–Lindau disease and tuberous sclerosis (multiple renal cysts occur in both also).

Clear cell sarcoma accounts for 4–5% of pediatric renal tumors and is an aggressive unilateral renal tumor seen at 1–4 years of age, with male predominance. This tumor has a higher rate of recurrence, metastasis, and mortality than WT. Generally indistinguishable from WT on imaging, clear cell sarcoma is usually unilateral, rarely has vascular extension, and commonly has skeletal metastases.

Rhabdoid tumor of the kidney (Fig. 64.4) is a highly aggressive renal malignancy accounting for 2% of childhood renal tumors. It usually occurs in children less than two years of age and confers a very poor prognosis. These are usually large renal masses involving the renal hilum with tumor lobules separated by necrosis or hemorrhage, linear calcifications outlining tumor lobules, and subcapsular fluid collections. The central intrarenal location and lobulated appearance helps differentiate a rhabdoid tumor from WT. Vascular invasion and early metastases to lymph nodes and/or visceral organs are common. The association of a rhabdoid tumor of the kidney with synchronous or metachronous cerebral tumors is described in about 20% of patients (Fig. 64.4). These tumors include teratoid/rhabdoid tumors as well as medulloblastoma, astrocytoma, glioma, primitive neuroepithelial tumor, ependymoma, and pinealocytoma. Malignant rhabdoid tumors are not associated with the syndromes seen in concert with WT.

Renal medullary carcinoma is a very rare aggressive renal tumor seen in teenage or young adult males with sickle cell disease (Fig. 64.5). This unilateral tumor tends to encase the renal pelvis, causing caliectasis and commonly has metastases at diagnosis (lymph nodes, lung, bone, and central nervous system).

Multilocular cystic nephroma is another rare renal tumor seen as a well-marginated multicystic mass with thin septae (Fig. 64.6). The lesion may appear solid if cystic spaces are small. In young children (usually boys) the lesion may have blastemal elements in the cyst walls and is considered a partially differentiated nephroblastoma. This can be associated with a hereditary tumor predisposition (*DICER1* gene mutation) occurring along with other tumors, especially pleuropulmonary blastoma. Older patients (usually women) typically have well-differentiated cystic nephromas.

Children with tuberous sclerosis frequently have renal cysts (see Case 57) that tend to resolve with age. They may also have solid renal masses most of which are angiomyolipomas (small well-defined solid lesions containing fat) but they may also develop WT or renal cell carcinoma.

Other large intra-abdominal masses may be difficult to differentiate from an intrarenal tumor. This is especially true for a neuroblastoma that has infiltrated the kidney. Neuroblastomas typically encase vessels and grow behind the aorta. This helps to distinguish neuroblastoma from WT. Other useful distinctions are the more common presence of calcification in neuroblastoma (50–60%), intraspinal extension of neuroblastoma, and absence of vascular tumor thrombus. Metastatic renal tumor involvement is very uncommon, lymphoma (non-Hodgkin's) being the most likely.

Occasionally a renal infection including focal pyelonephritis or a renal abscess may mimic a renal tumor or vice versa (see Case 60, Fig. 60.2). Clinical history and evolution of the lesion as well as the imaging appearance will usually serve to differentiate. As in other locations, a cystic or necrotic tumor may also become secondarily infected, sometimes creating greater diagnostic difficulty in separating tumor from infection.

Teaching point

WT is the most common renal neoplasm in children usually arising in precursor embryonic nephrogenic rests. There are a number of syndromes that are associated with a predisposition to WT as well as other intra-abdominal neoplasms; these children require close monitoring. Other renal neoplasms in children have imaging features similar to WT and a thorough knowledge of specific clinical and imaging differentiating features is important in suggesting the most likely diagnosis. Aside from metastatic spread, specific childhood renal tumors are associated with primary tumors elsewhere; examples include the association of renal rhabdoid tumor with central nervous system neoplasms and multilocular cystic nephroma with pleuropulmonary blastoma.

REFERENCES

Bhole S, Rigsby C, Sake M. *ACR Case in Point Case. Metanephric Stromal Tumor.* http://www.ACR.org (accessed April 25, 2012).

Geller E, Kochan PS. Renal neoplasms of childhood. *Radiol Clin North Am* 2011;**49**(4):689–709, vi.

Han TL, Kim MJ, Yoon HK, *et al.* Rhabdoid tumor of the kidney: imaging findings. *Pediatr Radiol* 2001;**31**(4):233–7.

Kaste SC, Dome JS, Babyn PS, *et al.* Wilms tumour: prognostic factors, staging, therapy and late effects. *Pediatr Radiol* 2008;**38**(1):2–17.

Lowe LH, Isuani BH, Heller RM, *et al.* Pediatric renal masses: Wilms tumor and beyond. *Radiographics* 2000;**20**(6):1585–603.

Owens CM, Brisse HJ, Olsen ØE, *et al.* Bilateral disease and new trends in Wilms tumour. *Pediatr Radiol* 2008;**38**(1):30–9.

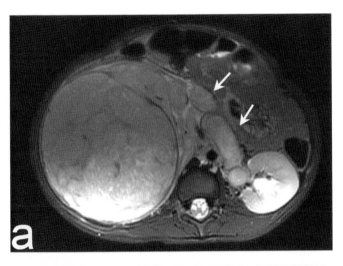

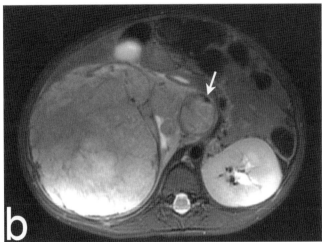

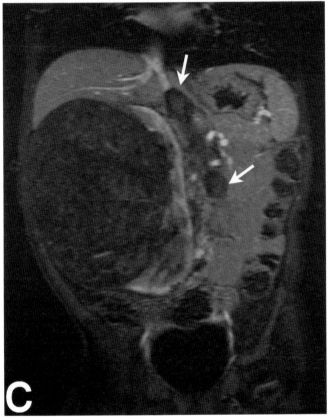

Figure 64.1. A 22-month-old girl with right renal Wilms' tumor. Axial T2-weighted MRI of the abdomen **(a, b)** reveals a large solid mass in the right kidney, distorting the pelvicalyceal system. On a post contrast coronal image **(c)** the lesion demonstrates poor heterogeneous enhancement. The mass displaces the abdominal aorta, inferior vena cava (IVC), and mesenteric vessels, without encasement. A large tumor thrombus extends into and expands the right and left renal veins and the IVC to the level of the mid liver (arrows).

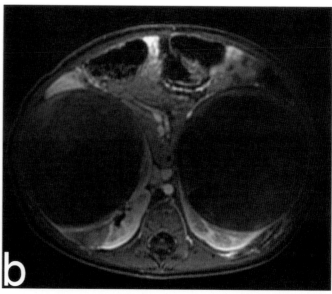

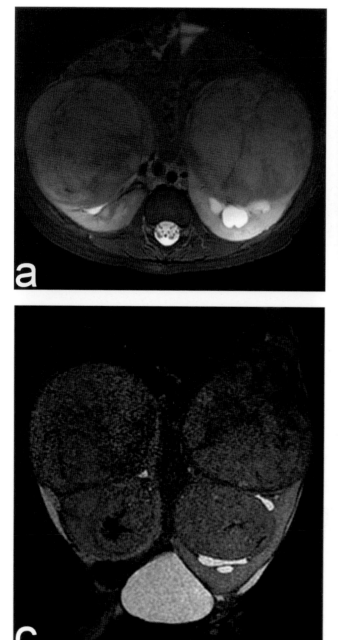

Figure 64.2. A nine-month-old female with ambiguous genitalia, bilateral Wilms' tumors, and Denys–Drash syndrome. Axial T2-weighted (a) and postcontrast (b) MRI images of the abdomen demonstrate large inhomogeneous masses in both kidneys with a T2 signal similar to renal parenchyma and heterogeneous enhancement. The masses appear to be multicentric on the coronal T2-weighted image (c).

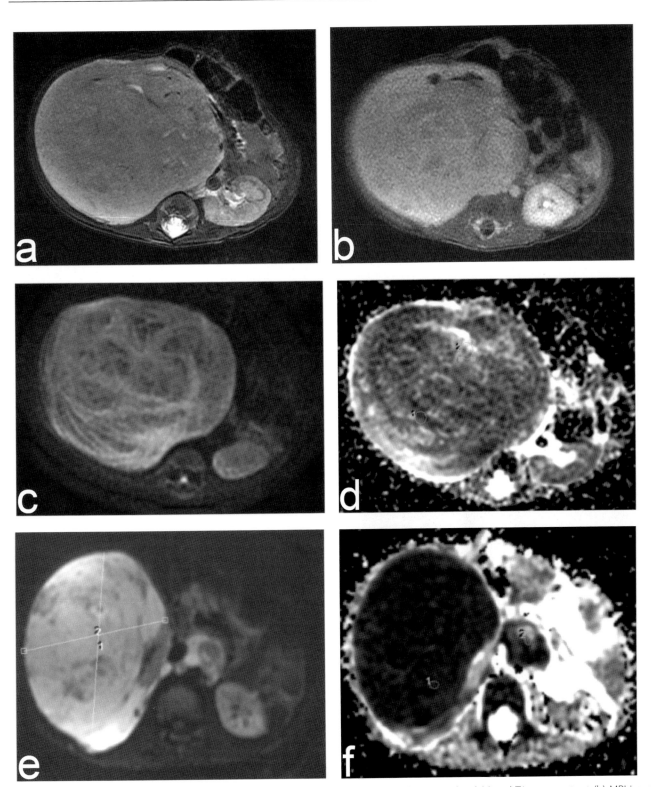

Figure 64.3. A seven-day-old neonate with congenital mesoblastic nephroma **(a–d)**. T2-weighted (a) and T1 post contrast (b) MRI images of the abdomen demonstrate a large right renal mass extending across the midline. The mass appears predominantly isointense to renal parenchyma on the T2-weighted image with a few small T2-hyperintense cystic regions and demonstrates homogeneous enhancement on the contrast-enhanced T1-weighted image. The mass appears heterogeneous on the diffusion-weighted image (c) and ADC map (d), with a high ADC value of 1.6×10^{-3} mm²/sec. In contrast, a Wilms' tumor, being highly cellular, demonstrates a restricted diffusion signal (bright signal) **(e)** with a very low ADC value of 0.6×10^{-3} mm²/sec **(f)**. (Figures 64.3c–f: Reprinted from *Pediatric Radiology*, Vol. **43**(7), 2013:836–45, Role of diffusion-weighted imaging in differentiating benign and malignant pediatric abdominal tumors, Gawande RS, Gonzalez G, Messing S, *et al.*, Figures 4a, b, 3a, b, with kind permission from Springer Science and Business Media.)

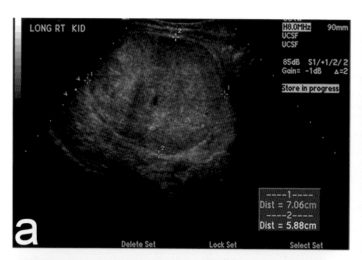

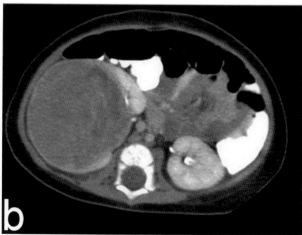

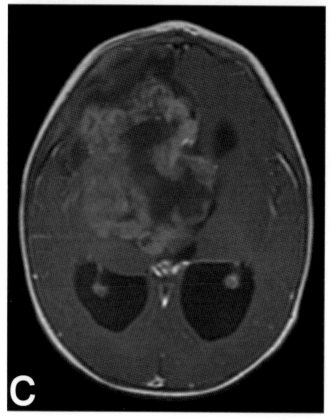

Figure 64.4. A six-month-old child with a right flank mass. An ultrasound of the right kidney (a) shows a very large, ill-defined, solid inhomogeneous mass in the right flank, appearing to arise from the right kidney. Axial contrast-enhanced CT scan of the abdomen confirmed a large, solid, inhomogeneous, enhancing mass in the right kidney with claw sign of the surrounding enhancing normal kidney parenchyma (b). There was no evidence for a tumor thrombus or lymph node metastases. Contrast-enhanced axial T1-weighted MR image of the brain (c) revealed a large, heterogeneously enhancing mass in the right frontal lobe, obstructing the foramen Monroe and causing hydrocephalus. Biopsy confirmed rhabdoid tumors of the kidney and the brain.

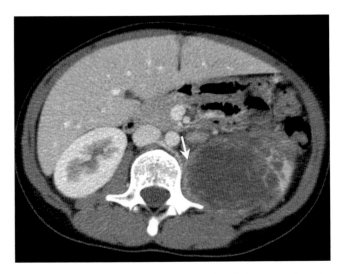

Figure 64.5. A 14-year-old male with sickle cell disease and renal medullary carcinoma. The contrast-enhanced axial CT image demonstrates a heterogeneously enhancing renal mass in the lower pole of the left kidney which invades the adjacent psoas muscle (arrow). There was marked caliectasis in the remainder of the kidney (not shown). Several prominent retroperitoneal lymph nodes were reactive nodes on histology. However, pulmonary and hepatic metastases were present at diagnosis.

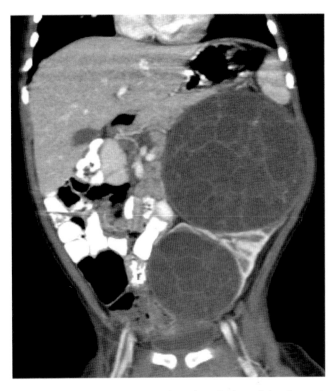

Figure 64.6. A 10-month-old male with multiple multilocular cystic nephromas. *DICER1* gene positive. Coronal CT reconstruction shows two large multicystic rounded masses with thin septae in the left kidney. The *DICER1* gene is associated with a hereditary tumor predisposition; the most common lesions are pleuropulmonary blastoma and multilocular cystic nephroma. Tumors can occur concurrently or at different times.

Ureteropelvic junction obstruction

Rakhee Gawande, Heike E. Daldrup-Link, and Beverley Newman

Imaging description

A nine-year-old boy presented with intermittent episodic left flank pain consistent with Dietl's crisis (=sudden attack of acute lumbar and abdominal pain accompanied by nausea and vomiting, caused by distension of the renal pelvis due to kinking of the ureter or other obstruction of urine flow from the kidney to the ureter). An initial ultrasound showed moderate left renal pelvocaliectasis (Fig. 65.1a). A follow-up study one month later showed mild dilatation of the left renal pelvis (Fig. 65.1b) and a follow-up ultrasound six months later when the child was again acutely symptomatic showed moderate hydronephrosis with marked dilatation of the renal pelvis (Fig. 65.1c). A review of serial ultrasounds of the kidneys revealed fluctuating mild to moderate hydronephrosis of the left kidney over several years. The imaging appearance was strongly suggestive of intermittent ureteropelvic junction (UPJ) obstruction.

Importance

UPJ obstruction is the most common cause of hydronephrosis in children and accounts for approximately 64% of cases. It is defined as a partial or total obstruction at the point where the renal pelvis narrows to form the ureter. It is found more commonly in boys and frequently involves the left kidney. It can be bilateral in 10–40% of cases. Ipsilateral vesicoureteral reflux is seen in about 10% of patients with UPJ obstruction. Various congenital renal anomalies may be associated with UPJ obstruction, including contralateral multicystic dysplastic kidney (MCDK), renal agenesis, duplicated renal collecting system, horseshoe kidney (Fig. 65.2), and ectopic kidney. Other associated congenital anomalies include imperforate anus, congenital heart disease, esophageal atresia, and VATER syndrome.

UPJ obstruction can be congenital or acquired. Congenital UPJ obstruction may occur due to intrinsic or extrinsic causes. Various theories have been proposed to explain intrinsic causes, including failure of recanalization of the UPJ, presence of an aperistaltic segment at the level of the UPJ, improper innervation, or muscular discontinuity. Uncommon intrinsic causes also include valvular folds or fibroepithelial polyps. Extrinsic causes include presence of aberrant crossing vessels, kinks, or fibrous bands. Rarely, a secondary UPJ obstruction may occur due to iatrogenic causes, inflammation, and tumors.

Congenital UPJ obstruction is often found during the antenatal period by measuring the anteroposterior dimension of the renal pelvis. A clinically significant obstruction is more likely to be present if there is grade 3–4 hydronephrosis and if the renal pelvis diameter is more than 10mm. A postnatal ultrasound (US) is usually performed 48–72 hours following delivery. If performed earlier, results may not be accurate due to physiologic neonatal dehydration and oliguria. If the US is negative, a repeat study is performed within 4–6 weeks. The most common cause of an abdominal mass in a neonate is a large hydronephrotic kidney, which may be secondary to a UPJ obstruction.

A longstanding UPJ obstruction can lead to progressive functional impairment of the affected kidney, poor growth in infants, and hypertension. Urinary stasis may lead to frequent urinary tract infections (UTI), pyelonephritis, and stone formation (Fig. 65.3). The dilated renal pelvis is susceptible to rupture following blunt abdominal trauma (Fig. 65.4).

Intermittent hydronephrosis and acute dilatation of the renal pelvis due to UPJ obstruction can lead to acute symptoms of nausea, pain, vomiting, and hematuria, referred to as Dietl's crisis. The actual pathophysiology of intermittent obstruction is not clear and 40% of cases may be related to increased fluid intake (beer drinker's kidney) or use of diuretics. The cause of the pain is stretching of the renal capsule. Extrinsic mechanical disturbances, such as kinking around a crossing vessel, that occur alone or in combination with intrinsic causes can predispose the kidney to intermittent obstruction.

Tc-99m-MAG3 diuretic renography is the most commonly used test to assess the degree of obstruction and differential renal function. The time required for normal clearance of radionuclide is <10 minutes. A clearance time of radiotracer from the renal pelvis of more than 20 minutes is suggestive of obstruction. The diuretic is employed to increase urine flow and may also precipitate quiescent intermittent obstruction. US and other imaging studies can also be coupled with the use of diuretics. It is helpful to obtain the US study emergently when the individual has acute pain as the kidney may appear normal or near normal when the patient is asymptomatic (Fig. 65.1), making the diagnosis quite elusive.

An MRI may be used to evaluate the renal anatomy, renal blood flow, and contrast agent excretion in more detail (Fig. 65.5). MRI or CT angiography and Doppler sonography may be performed to evaluate extrinsic causes of UPJ, such as an extrinsic crossing vessel. A CT scan may be performed in cases of acute trauma and hematuria, with suspected rupture of a dilated renal pelvis secondary to UPJ obstruction (Fig. 65.4).

Typical clinical scenario

Congenital UPJ obstruction is usually diagnosed during antenatal US. It may present in infants as a large palpable abdominal mass, failure to thrive, sepsis, and frequent UTI. In older children, it may present as episodic flank pain, nausea, vomiting, UTI, and hematuria. Similar to other causes of prolonged severe prenatal renal obstruction, UPJ obstruction may be associated with renal dysplasia (often manifested by small peripheral cysts), poor renal function, or even pelvocalyceal rupture and perirenal urinoma.

Indications for surgical management (usually dismembered pyeloplasty) include presence of symptoms such as pain, infection, stones; deterioration of renal function; grade 3 or 4 dilatation; asymptomatic obstruction when differential function <35–40% and pelvis dimension >20 mm.

Differential diagnosis

UPJ obstruction should be differentiated from other causes of antenatal hydronephrosis, including vesicouretric reflux (VUR), posterior urethral valves, congenital megaureter, and obstructed duplicated kidney. VUR may coexist with UPJ obstruction in 10% of cases and is important to identify, as these children are at higher risk for severe infections. Differential considerations also include congenital megacalyces and extrarenal pelvis (a normal finding). The typically non-communicating cysts seen in an MCDK (Fig. 65.6) may sometimes be difficult to distinguish from the dilated communicating calyces associated with UPJ obstruction, especially when severe hydronephrosis is present.

Teaching point

UPJ obstruction is the most common cause of antenatal hydronephrosis in children. It can be associated with various renal anomalies, including MCDK, renal ectopia, contralateral UPJ obstruction, and horseshoe kidney. It may be associated with VUR, which leads to increased risk of frequent and severe infection. Long-term stasis can also lead to stone formation. Intermittent or acute UPJ obstruction can present with acute symptoms and can be very difficult to diagnose. It is important to image the patient when symptoms are present as the kidney can appear normal or have only subtle abnormality during asymptomatic periods.

REFERENCES

1. Calder AD, Hiorns MP, Abhyankar A, *et al*. Contrast-enhanced magnetic resonance angiography for the detection of crossing renal vessels in children with symptomatic ureteropelvic junction obstruction: comparison with operative findings. *Pediatr Radiol* 2007;**37**(4):356–61.
2. McDaniel BB, Jones RA, Scherz H, *et al*. Dynamic contrast-enhanced MR urography in the evaluation of pediatric hydronephrosis: Part 2, anatomic and functional assessment of uteropelvic junction obstruction. *AJR Am J Roentgenol* 2005;**185**(6):1608–14.
3. Sheu JC, Koh CC, Chang PY, *et al*. Ureteropelvic junction obstruction in children: 10 years' experience in one institution. *Pediatr Surg Int* 2006;**22**(6):519–23.
4. Tsai JD, Huang FY, Lin CC, *et al*. Intermittent hydronephrosis secondary to ureteropelvic junction obstruction: clinical and imaging features. *Pediatrics* 2006;**117**(1):139–46.

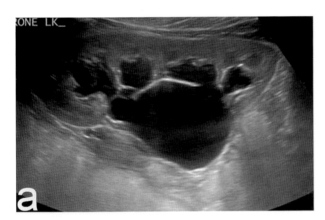

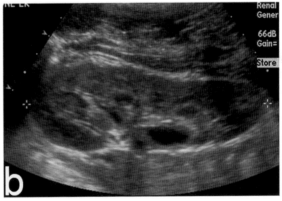

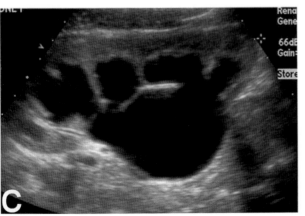

Figure 65.1. A nine-year-old boy with intermittent UPJ obstruction. Sagittal prone US image of the left kidney (**a**) shows moderate left pelvocaliectasis with marked dilatation of the left renal pelvis, consistent with UPJ obstruction. Repeat US one month later (**b**) showed resolution of the hydronephrosis with mild residual fullness of the renal pelvis. Six months later the patient again presented with left flank pain and repeat US showed (**c**) moderate left hydronephrosis.

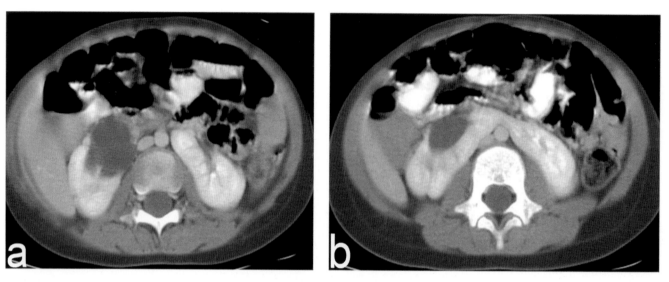

Figure 65.2. A four-year-old male with horseshoe kidney and mild to moderate UPJ obstruction of the right moiety. CT contiguous axial slices **(a, b)** show decreased enhancement and slow excretion of contrast in the right kidney. This was an incidental finding on a CT done for abdominal pain after a motor vehicle accident. Horseshoe kidney often has a dilated extrarenal pelvis with malrotated kidney. Obstruction is less common, but can occur.

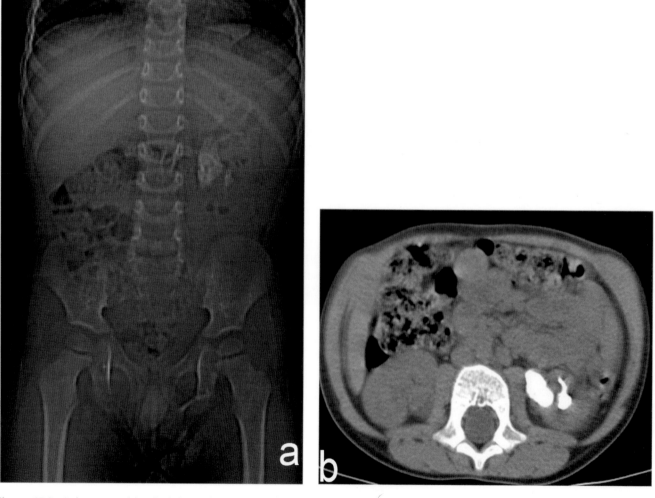

Figure 65.3. A three-year-old with abdominal pain. CT scout image **(a)** and axial non-contrast CT image **(b)** shows congenital left UPJ obstruction and large staghorn calculus.

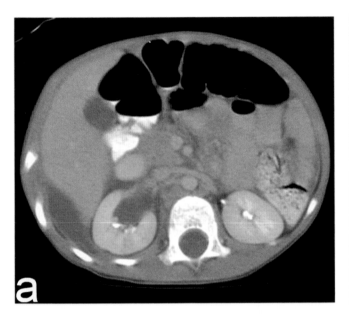

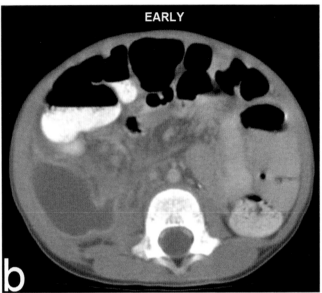

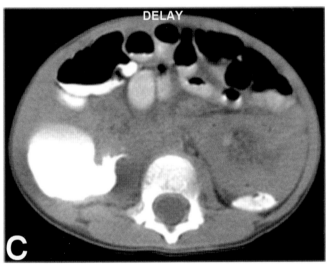

Figure 65.4. A three-year-old child presented with acute abdominal pain. CT ordered to rule out appendicitis showed a dilated right renal pelvis with slightly decreased nephrogram and delayed excretion on the right (a). Right inferior perirenal fluid, free fluid adjacent to the liver, and a loculated fluid collection in the right lower quadrant was noted (b). The appendix was not seen. Initially it was thought the findings might represent ruptured appendicitis but because of the abnormal right kidney, delayed images were obtained showing filling of the right lower quadrant collection with excreted renal contrast (c). The diagnosis of abdominal trauma with a rupture at the UPJ with probable underlying UPJ obstruction was suggested and proven surgically. The father confirmed that they had been "rough-housing" and he had punched the boy in the stomach.

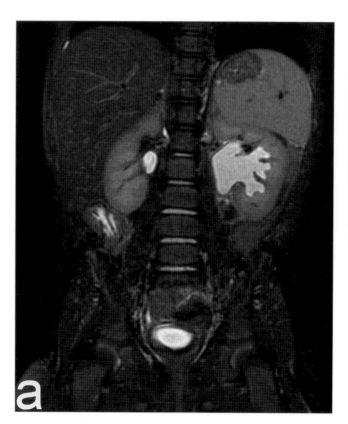
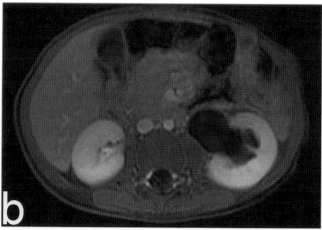

Figure 65.5. A two-year-old with UPJ obstruction. Sagittal T2-weighted CUBE **(a)** and contrast-enhanced axial LAVA **(b)** images show moderate left hydronephrosis with delayed contrast excretion in left kidney secondary to UPJ obstruction. MRI can accurately define renal anatomy, calculate differential renal function, and assess urinary tract obstruction.

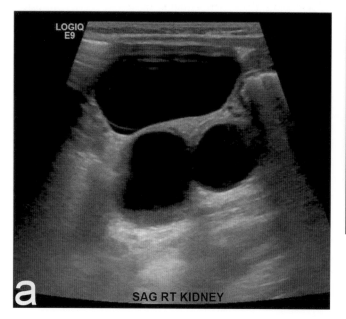
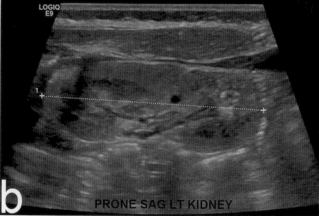

Figure 65.6. A one-month-old with right MCDK first visualized on prenatal US. The right kidney **(a)** is larger than the normal appearing left kidney **(b)**. The right kidney consists of several large non-connecting renal cysts with no visible parenchyma, consistent with MCDK. MCDK is typically associated with high grade in utero obstruction, often ureteral atresia. The natural history postnatally is gradual involution.

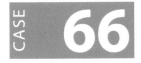

CASE 66

Oxalosis in an 11-year-old boy

Heike E. Daldrup-Link

Imaging description

An 11-year-old boy presented with end-stage renal disease (ESRD). A radiograph of the abdomen demonstrated multiple focal calcifications, projecting over the bilateral kidneys (Fig. 66.1a). An ultrasound confirmed echogenic calcifications in the deep parenchyma of the kidneys bilaterally, consistent with medullary nephrocalcinosis (Fig. 66.1b). An X-ray of the left hand showed dense metaphyseal bands on the metaphyseal side of the growth plates of the radius and ulna as well as focal cystic rarefactions and sclerotic margins of the metaphyses of the radius and ulna (Fig. 66.1c).

Importance

Oxalosis is a condition in which calcium oxalate crystals are deposited in renal and extrarenal tissues. The underlying pathology is hyperoxaluria, excessive oxalate excretion in the urine (>40 mg/mL), which leads to chronic renal failure. Once oxalate cannot be excreted due to impaired renal function, insoluble calcium oxalate crystals are deposited in bone, bone marrow, blood vessels, central nervous system, peripheral nerves, retina, skin, and thyroid.

Hyperoxaluria can be due to three major conditions:

1. Primary hyperoxaluria, a rare autosomal recessive disorder with defective glyoxylate metabolism in the liver, resulting in increased production and urinary excretion of oxalate and glyoxylate (type 1) or oxalate and L-glycerate (type 2).
2. Secondary hyperoxaluria due to reduced excretion, excessive dietary intake, and/or increased gut absorption of oxalate.
3. Idiopathic hyperoxaluria.

Typical clinical scenario

Clinical manifestations of hyperoxaluria are nephrocalcinosis and nephrolithiasis, caused by saturation of calcium oxalate in the urine. When left untreated, hyperoxaluria will ultimately lead to end-stage renal failure. Complications of bone involvement include bone deformities and fractures.

Imaging findings in patients with oxalosis are caused by a combination of crystalline calcium oxalate deposition, and renal osteodystrophy due to secondary hyperparathyroidism (Fig. 66.2). The most common findings in the long bones are condensations (dense bands) on the metaphyseal side of the growth plates. End-stage renal failure may lead to additional translucent metaphyseal bands between the epiphysis and the dense bands. Additional changes in long bones may include cystic rarefaction and erosions on the concave side of metaphyses and a bone-in-bone appearance. The vertebrae may show dense end plates and lucent centers (rugger-jersey-spine).

The extent of radiographic bone changes correlates with the presence and duration of terminal kidney failure. Other, less specific findings include subperiosteal resorption osteolysis of the distal phalanges, periosteal apposition, spondylolysis, and generalized osteopenia. With progressive disease, oxalosis can lead to obliteration of the bone marrow space and pancytopenia.

Nephrocalcinosis is caused by intratubular deposition of oxalate crystals and leads to increasing density of the kidneys on radiographic imaging tests and increased echogenicity of the renal parenchyma on ultrasound examinations. The amplitude of echoes is greater than that encountered in renal parenchymal disease, such as renal vein thrombosis or infantile polycystic kidneys. Pathognomonic ultrasound findings are normal sized kidneys with increased cortical echogenicity. However, ultrasound examinations may also show medullary nephrocalcinosis, either isolated or as a progression of cortical nephrocalcinosis. It has been reported that creatinine levels and risk of renal failure tend to be higher in patients with cortical nephrocalcinosis than in those with isolated medullary nephrocalcinosis. In advanced diseases, calcium oxalate stones may also be noted, with acoustic shadowing.

Differential diagnosis

Differential diagnosis includes other causes of rickets and renal osteodystrophy. The combination of hyperoxaluria and radiographic findings resembling rickets together with osteosclerotic changes are indicative of the diagnosis of oxalosis.

Diffuse cortical nephrocalcinosis is also seen in paraneoplastic hypercalciuria, Alport's syndrome, and acquired immunodeficiency syndrome-associated infections such as cytomegalovirus and *Mycobacterium avium-intracellulare* infections. Medullary nephrocalcinosis is associated with medullary sponge kidney, hyperparathyroidism, and renal tubular acidosis.

Soft tissue calcification can also occur in progressive systemic sclerosis, parasitic infestations, calcifying cavernous hemangioma, heterotopic calcifications after burn injuries, tumoral calcinosis, and Thibierge–Weissenbach syndrome (a form of scleroderma that is a combination of calcinosis, Raynaud's phenomenon, esophageal motility disorders, sclerodactyly, and telangiectasia).

Teaching point

Oxalosis should be considered in cases of impaired renal function, cortical or medullary nephrocalcinosis, and radiographic bone findings resembling rickets/osteodystrophy with superimposed osteosclerotic changes.

REFERENCES

1. Akhan O, Ozmen MN, Coskun M, *et al.* Systemic oxalosis: pathognomonic renal and specific extrarenal findings on US and CT. *Pediatr Radiol* 1995;**25**:15–16.

2. Diallo O, Janssens F, Hall M, Avni EF. Type 1 primary hyperoxaluria in pediatric patients: renal sonographic patterns. *AJR Am J Roentgenol* 2004;**183**:1767–70.

3. Elmståhl B, Rausing A. A case of hyperoxaluria; radiological aspects. *Acta Radiol* 1997;**38**(6):1031–4.

4. Kuo LW, Horton K, Fishman EK. CT evaluation of multisystem involvement by oxalosis. *AJR Am J Roentgenol* 2001;**177**:661–3.

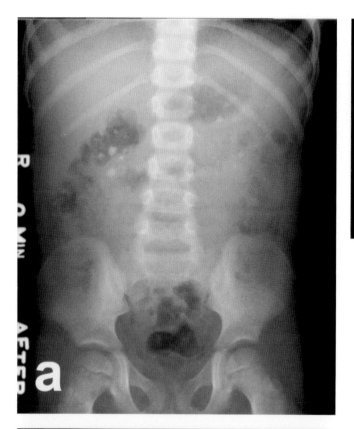

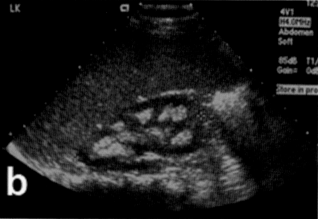

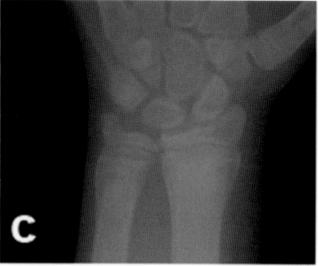

Figure 66.1. **(a)** Radiograph of the abdomen of an 11-year-old boy shows multiple focal calcifications, projecting over the bilateral kidneys. **(b)** An ultrasound of the left kidney shows markedly increased echogenicity of the deep parenchyma of the kidneys bilaterally, consistent with medullary nephrocalcinosis. **(c)** An X-ray of the left hand shows dense metaphyseal bands on the metaphyseal side of the growth plates of the radius and ulna, and focal cystic rarefactions of the metaphyses of the radius and ulna.

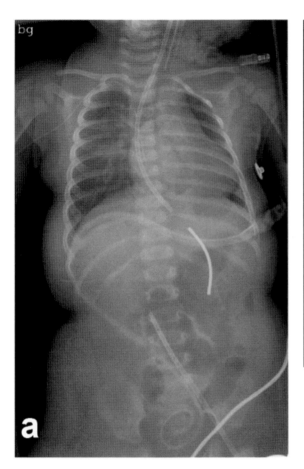

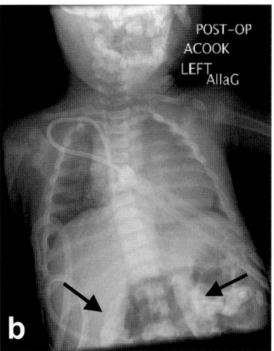

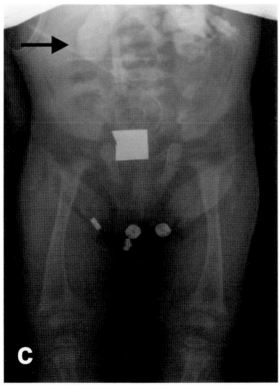

Figure 66.2. Patient with primary hyperoxaluria and primary renal insufficiency. (a) Day 1: a radiograph of the abdomen shortly after birth demonstrates no evidence for renal calcifications or osteodystrophy (day 1). (b, c) 10 months: (b) A follow-up radiograph shows bilateral nephrocalcinosis (arrows). The bones show signs of renal osteodystrophy with dense bands and widening of the metaphyses of the proximal humeri, distal femura, and proximal tibiae bilaterally.

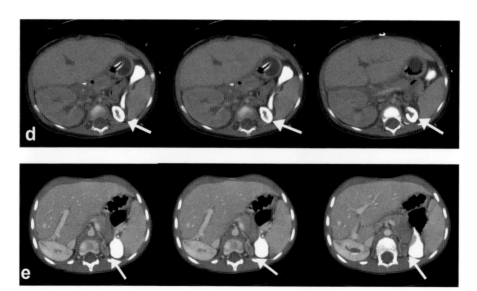

Figure 66.2. (cont.) **(d)** An initial non-enhanced CT of the abdomen directly after an orthotopic right kidney transplant shows increased density and decreased size of the native left kidney, compatible with nephrocalcinosis. **(e)** Follow-up contrast-enhanced CT scan several months after kidney and liver transplant shows resolution of kidney calcinosis due to resolution of the underlying metabolic defect.

Pediatric Graves' disease

Sami M. Akram and Andrei Iagaru

Image description

A 15-year-old girl presenting with tachycardia, heat intolerance, and goiter is found to have elevated free thyroxin (FT4) and low thyroid-stimulating hormone (TSH) (FT4 = 6 ng/mL [normal: 2–4 ng/mL], serum TSH = 0.01 μIU/mL [normal: 1–5 μIU/mL]). The iodine-123 (^{123}I) uptake and scan showed homogeneously increased radiotracer uptake. The isthmus and the pyramidal lobe were prominent. The 24 hours ^{123}I neck uptake was 70% (normal: 10–30%) (Fig. 67.1). These features are typical of Graves' disease.

Importance

Graves' disease is an autoimmune disorder of multifactorial etiology and is the commonest cause of hyperthyroidism in children. The classic clinical triad of Graves' disease includes hyperthyroidism, orbitopathy, and dermatopathy and is four to five times more frequent in girls. Peak incidence of Graves' disease occurs in early adolescence. There is a familial predisposition; however, the hereditary component has not been clearly defined. Untreated Graves' disease can lead to arrhythmia, heart failure, and cardiovascular collapse.

Typical clinical scenario

Graves' disease is an autoimmune disorder in which thyroid-stimulated immunoglobulin binds to receptors for TSH. It presents in children between the ages of 5 and 18 years with symptoms of hyperthyroidism such as rapid heart rate, nervousness, intense perspiration, and weight loss. Girls may have menstrual irregularities. An enlarged thyroid gland is noted on physical examination. Children may present with behavioral changes, poor performance in school, and other neuropsychiatric symptoms.

Graves' disease is associated with a number of specific features. The Graves' orbitopathy is mild in children compared to adults although it occurs with the same frequency. In adults it is associated with smoking; the mechanism is unknown. The incidence of pretibial myxedema in pediatric Graves' disease is not known but appears to be less common than the orbitopathy. Thyroid acropathy occurs infrequently and refers to clubbing, tightness of the skin of fingers and toes along with pain in distal small joints associated with periosteal reaction seen on x-rays. Vitiligo when present is often seen in a younger age group (mean age of 4 ± 0.7 years) and the diagnosis of vitiligo often precedes that of the thyroid disease by about 2 years. Frequently, the patients may have other autoimmune disorders. Thyroid hormones shorten the lifespan of platelets and thrombocytopenia is noted in untreated Graves' disease patients.

Differential diagnosis

Due to the presence of neuropsychiatric symptoms the diagnosis of Graves' disease may be delayed in children. The patients are evaluated for anxiety disorders, attention deficit hyperactivity disorder, and drug abuse. Other causes of hyperthyroidism such as pituitary tumors secreting TSH, recent infection leading to subacute thyroiditis, struma ovarii (teratoma containing functioning thyroid tissue), and factitious hyperthyroidism (excessive exogenous intake of thyroid hormone) are also included in the differential diagnoses.

Diffuse thyroid enlargement in a euthyroid or hypothyroid patient is most often due to a multinodular goiter (gross nodularity) or Hashimoto's thyroiditis (familial autoimmune disorder associated with collagen vascular disease, thyroid enlargement on ultrasound, and radionuclide studies with occasional nodules; 10% are hyperthyroid).

Ultrasound imaging is often the initial study in a child with focal or diffuse thyroid enlargement. It is useful in characterizing thyroid versus non-thyroid origin of the lesion, cystic versus solid, number of lesions, size, and vascularity of a lesion or gland (diffusely hyperemic in Graves' disease) and presence of neck adenopathy.

> ## Teaching points
>
> The ^{123}I uptake and scan separates the hyperthyroid patients who have high iodine uptake from those with low iodine uptake in the thyroid gland, thereby determining further management of hyperthyroid patients. It is important to have a high index of suspicion for Graves' disease in children due to their atypical presentation. Additionally, pediatric Graves' disease is often resistant to anti-thyroid drugs, requiring early definitive therapy with surgery or iodine-131 radioablation.

REFERENCES

1. Cho SB, Kim JH, Cho S, et al. Vitiligo in children and adolescents: association with thyroid dysfunction. J Eur Acad Dermatol Venereol 2011;25(1):64–7.

2. Gogakos AI, Boboridis K, Krassas GE. Pediatric aspects in Graves' orbitopathy. Pediatr Endocrinol Rev 2010;7(Suppl 2):234–44.

3. Hemminki K, Li X, Sundquist J, et al. The epidemiology of Graves' disease: evidence of a genetic and an environmental contribution. J Autoimmun 2010;34(3):J307–13.

4. Horwitz DL, Refetoff S. Graves' disease associated with familial deficiency of thyroxine-binding globulin. J Clin Endocrinol Metab 1977;44(2):242–7.

5. Iagaru A, McDougall IR. Treatment of thyrotoxicosis. *J Nucl Med* 2007;**48**(3):379–89.

6. Ishizawa T, Sugiki H, Anzai S, *et al*. Pretibial myxedema with Graves' disease: a case report and review of Japanese literature. *J Dermatol* 1998;**25**(4):264–8.

7. Prindaville B, Rivkees SA. Incidence of vitiligo in children with Graves' disease and Hashimoto's thyroiditis. *Int J Pediatr Endocrinol* 2011;**2011**(1):18.

8. Zimmerman D, Lteif AN. Thyrotoxicosis in children. *Endocrinol Metab Clin North Am* 1998;**27**(1):109–26.

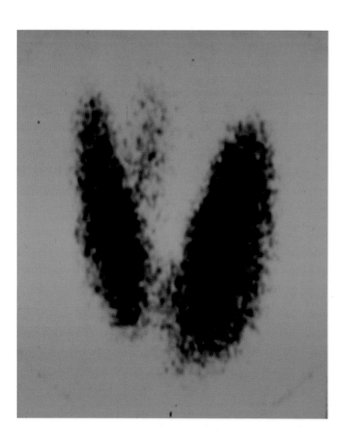

Figure 67.1. A 15-year-old girl with Graves' disease. [123]I scintiscan image obtained at 24 hours shows homogeneously increased uptake in both lobes of the thyroid gland. Visualization of the pyramidal lobe and very low background uptake are commonly seen in Graves' disease.

Thyroglossal duct cyst

Richard A. Barth

Imaging description

A four-year-old girl presented with a tender midline neck mass. Sonogram of the neck demonstrated a normal thyroid gland anterior to the trachea (Fig. 68.1a). Sonographic images obtained cranial to the thyroid gland at the level of the hyoid bone demonstrated a predominately hypoechoic mass associated with septations and small anechoic components (Fig. 68.1b, c). The mass demonstrated posterior acoustic enhancement most consistent with a cystic lesion as opposed to a solid nodule. The most likely diagnosis for a cystic midline neck mass in a child is a thyroglossal duct cyst (TGDC). The septations within the mass suggest associated inflammation and/or infection. Findings in this case are most consistent with a TGDC complicated by an inflammatory process.

Importance

TGDCs are the most common cause of a congenital neck cyst in a child and are typically located in the midline either at the level of the hyoid bone or in an infra-hyoid location. The thyroglossal duct defines the normal migration path of the developing thyroid gland in the fetus from the base of the tongue caudally to the thyroid's normal position anterior to the trachea in the lower neck. The thyroglossal duct normally involutes, leaving a remnant in the tongue known as the foramen cecum. If some or all of the thyroid tissue fails to descend in normal fashion, ectopic thyroid tissue will be located in the arrested position. TGDCs result from failure of normal ablation of the thyroglossal duct during thyroid development and occur along the course of the duct from the foramen cecum to the thyroid bed. The majority of TGDCs are located at or near the midline of the neck. On sonography TGDC are usually cystic but they may contain solid components or appear complex with septations. In children TGDCs can range in echogenicity from hypoechoic to heterogeneous. The presence of a thick wall and internal septations correlates with the presence of inflammation. Inflammation may result in increased echogenicity, mimicking a solid lesion. The presence of septations and posterior acoustic enhancement on ultrasound characterizes the lesion as a cystic mass as opposed to a solid nodule and confirms the most likely diagnosis as a TGDC. Treatment consists of complete resection of the cyst and duct up to the level of the foramen cecum and is usually curative.

Typical clinical scenario

Most TGDCs present as a painless midline anterior neck swelling with approximately 90% presenting before age 10 years. Infected cysts will present as a painful or tender mass. The latter often present in later childhood or adulthood when they become infected.

Differential diagnosis

A TGDC is the most likely diagnosis for a midline cystic neck mass presenting in a child. Differential diagnosis of a TGDC includes a dermoid cyst, branchial cleft cyst, hemangioma, and enlarged lymph nodes. The primary differential diagnosis is a dermoid cyst, which is often mistaken for a TGDC. Dermoid cysts occur as a developmental cystic lesion in the midline or in a paramedian location in the neck. Only 7% of dermoid cysts occur in the head and neck. Approximately 12% of dermoid cysts located in the head and neck are positioned in the floor of the mouth. The latter appear as thin-walled cystic masses located in the submandibular and sublingual space. The presence of fat within a cyst is pathognomic for a dermoid cyst and allows for differentiation from a TGDC. Midline lymph nodes can also appear hypoechoic on sonography and mimic a cystic mass; however, the echogenic hilum within an enlarged lymph node on sonography, absence of posterior acoustic enhancement, and internal Doppler flow will correctly characterize the lymph node as a solid mass as opposed to a cystic lesion. The close proximity of a TGDC to the hyoid bone is also a key feature for distinguishing lesions. Branchial cleft cysts may also mimic a TGDC; however, they are often non-midline and positioned in a lateral location in the neck. It is important to note that TGDCs may also sometimes be in a non-midline lateral location. Congenital teratomas may also present as an anterior midline neck mass, most often as a complex solid and cystic lesion usually diagnosed prenatally or at birth.

Teaching point

The presence of an anechoic or hypoechoic cystic lesion in the midline of the neck at the level of the hyoid bone or slightly below should be considered a TGDC until proven otherwise. It is important to note that some TGDCs will have low to intermediate level internal echos, mimicking a solid lesion. Demonstration of posterior acoustic enhancement should allow confirmation of the cystic nature of the lesion and suggest the correct diagnosis.

REFERENCES

1. Ahuja AT, King AD, Metreweli C. Sonographic evaluation of thyroglossal duct cysts in children. *Clin Radiol* 2000;**55**(10):770–4.

2. Harnsberger HR. Cystic masses of the head and neck: rare lesions with characteristic radiologic features. In: *Handbook of Head and Neck Imaging*, 2nd edition. St Louis, MO: Mosby-Year Book, 1999.

3. Kutuya N, Kurosaki Y. Sonographic assessment of thyroglossal duct cysts in children. *J Ultrasound Med* 2008;**27**(8):1211–19.

4. Som PM, Curtin HD. Congenital lesions. In: *Handbook of Head and Neck Imaging*, 4th edition. St Louis, MO: Mosby-Year Book, 2003.

5. Wadsworth DT, Siegel MJ. Thyroglossal duct cysts: variability of sonographic findings. *AJR Am J Roentgenol* 1994;**163**(6):1475–7.

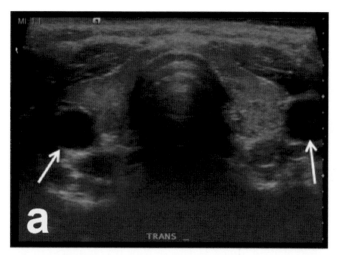

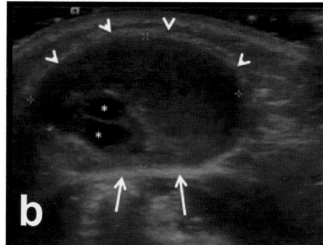

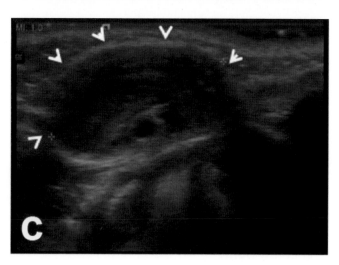

Figure 68. 1. (a) A four-year-old girl with a thyroglossal duct cyst. Axial plane sonogram through the thyroid bed demonstrates a normal thyroid gland. Carotid arteries (arrows). **(b, c)** Axial and longitudinal sonograms craniad to the thyroid gland at the level of the hyoid bone demonstrate a predominately hypoechoic mass (arrowheads) associated with septations and small anechoic components (*). The mass demonstrated posterior acoustic enhancement (arrows) most consistent with a cystic lesion with internal echoes.

Thyroid colloid cyst

Richard A. Barth

Imaging description

An 11-year-old child was found to have a palpable thyroid nodule as an incidental finding on routine clinical examination. The child was asymptomatic and thyroid function tests including thyroid hormone levels and thyroid stimulating hormone (TSH) were normal. An outside ultrasound study raised concern for a malignant thyroid nodule and the patient was referred for ultrasound-guided fine-needle aspiration for cytology. A pre-biopsy repeat ultrasound exam demonstrated a thyroid gland with multiple hypoechoic nodules and a dominant $4 \times 3 \times 1.5$ mm hypoechoic cystic nodule containing multiple punctate hyperechogenic foci associated with comet tail artifact in the right lobe of the gland (Fig. 69.1). These findings are most consistent with a benign colloid cyst and not indicative of a thyroid carcinoma. The biopsy was cancelled and a follow-up ultrasound in 3 months was scheduled to assess lesion stability.

Importance

Approximately 2% of children develop solitary thyroid nodules. The majority of thyroid nodules in children are benign (85%) and approximately 15% are malignant. Follicular adenomas are the most common cause of a benign thyroid nodule. Thyroid nodules are usually evaluated by ultrasound, which characterizes the nodule as cystic, solid, or complex (contains both cystic and solid components). It is not unusual for additional thyroid nodules to be detected on ultrasound in addition to the index lesion that results in the patient referral. In one study of multinodular thyroid glands in 16 children, multiple nodules were seen on ultrasound in all subjects whereas several of the patients had only one palpable nodule. The majority of cystic thyroid nodules represent benign degenerating thyroid adenomas and purely cystic lesions rarely contain cancer. Complex thyroid nodules with both cystic and solid components increase the risk for cancer and are malignant in approximately 5% of patients. The likelihood for cancer decreases as the proportion of the nodule that is cystic increases. A solid or hypoechoic nodule with internal microcalcifications should raise a high concern for malignancy and needs to be distinguished from the echogenic foci and comet tail artifact associated with a colloid cyst (Fig. 69.1, 2). The presence of a comet tail artifact in a cystic thyroid nodule occurs secondary to microcrystals and is highly specific for a benign colloid cyst. In contrast to microcalcifications, the echogenic foci in a colloid cyst are not associated with acoustic shadowing. The strict criteria for a comet tail in a benign colloid cyst is the identification of a linear echo with unequivocal ring-down artifact. Comet tail artifact is a form of reverberation. In this artifact, the two reflective interfaces and sequential echos are closely spaced. On the display screen the sequential echos may be so close together that individual echos are not perceivable. In addition, the later echos in a ring-down artifact may have decreased amplitude secondary to attenuation, which display as decreased width. If the comet tail artifact is not identified in association with hyperechogenic foci in a nodule, there should be consideration for fine-needle aspiration to rule out malignancy. Fine-needle aspiration is the single most useful test in separating benign lesions from cancer and is of high diagnostic accuracy in children. Fine-needle aspirations are often performed under ultrasound guidance for smaller nodules that are not readily palpable.

Typical clinical scenario

Cystic thyroid nodules most often come to attention when discovered by the patient, detected as an incidental finding during a routine physical examination, or diagnosed on an imaging exam of the neck, as a so-called "thyroid incidentaloma." Most patients are euthyroid; however, a positive family history of thyroid disease is elicited in up to 30% of cases. Thyroid nodules can be solitary or multiple, giving rise to a multinodular thyroid gland.

Differential diagnosis

Given the predominately cystic nature of the thyroid nodule in this case and the presence of comet tail artifacts, the diagnosis is highly specific for a colloid cyst with no other significant considerations. The presence of a hypoechoic cystic lesion in the thyroid gland is most consistent with a degenerating thyroid adenoma. When a cystic lesion contains a solid component, the risk for malignancy is increased and close clinical follow-up is warranted. It is important to evaluate the entire thyroid gland to ensure that no other lesions of higher suspicion are identified.

> ## Teaching point
>
> The presence of a cystic nodule in the thyroid gland with hyperechogenic foci associated with a comet tail artifact is highly specific for a benign colloid cyst and should not be confused with the microcalcifications associated with papillary thyroid carcinoma.

REFERENCES
1. Ahuja A, Chick W, King W, *et al.* Clinical significance of the comet-tail artifact in thyroid ultrasound. *J Clin Ultrasound* 1996;**24**(3):129–33.
2. Babcock DS. Thyroid disease in the pediatric patient: emphasizing imaging with sonography. *Pediatr Radiol* 2006;**36**(4):299–308, quiz 372–3.
3. Davies SM. Subsequent malignant neoplasms in survivors of childhood cancer: Childhood Cancer Survivor Study (CCSS) studies. *Pediatr Blood Cancer* 2007;**48**(7):727–30.

4. Feldman MK, Katyal S, Blackwood MS. US artifacts. *Radiographics* 2009;**29**(4):1179–89.

5. Hogan AR, Zhuge Y, Perez EA, *et al.* Pediatric thyroid carcinoma: incidence and outcomes in 1753 patients. *J Surg Res* 2009;**156**(1):167–72.

6. Hung W. Solitary thyroid nodules in 93 children and adolescents. a 35-years experience. *Horm Res* 1999;**52**(1):15–18.

7. Taylor AJ, Croft AP, Palace AM, *et al.* Risk of thyroid cancer in survivors of childhood cancer: results from the British Childhood Cancer Survivor Study. *Int J Cancer* 2009;**125**(10):2400–5.

8. Wiersinga WM. Management of thyroid nodules in children and adolescents. *Hormones (Athens)* 2007;**6**(3):194–9.

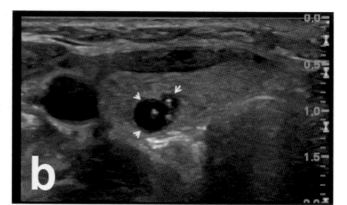

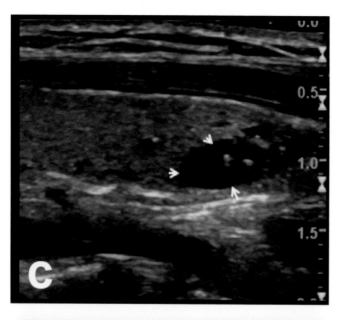

Figure 69.1. Colloid cyst in an 11-year-old girl. **(a)** Axial sonogram demonstrates a heterogeneous gland with numerous small hypoechoic nodules. **(b, c)** Axial and sagittal sonograms show a dominant hypoechoic cystic nodule in the right lobe of the gland (arrows) with internal hyperechogenic foci associated with comet tail artifact diagnostic for a colloid cyst.

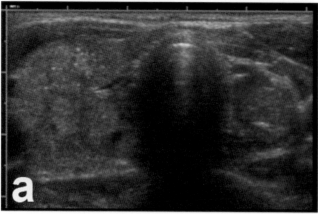

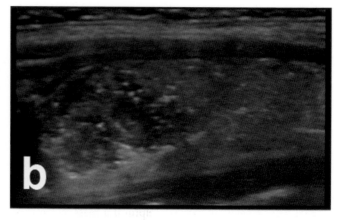

Figure 69.2. Papillary thyroid carcinoma. **(a, b)** Axial and longitudinal sonograms demonstrate a heterogeneous nodule in the right lobe of the thyroid gland with multiple punctate hyperechogenic foci with acoustic shadowing, microcalcifications, which are highly suggestive of a malignant thyroid nodule. Of note, there is no evidence for comet tail artifact associated with the hyperechogenic foci.

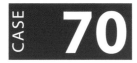

Adrenal hemorrhage

Rakhee Gawande, Rosalinda Castaneda, and Heike E. Daldrup-Link

Imaging description

A seven-day-old neonate presented with a history of birth asphyxia and abdominal distension. A routine abdominal-renal ultrasound demonstrated incidental heterogeneous lesions in the bilateral suprarenal regions (Fig. 70.1). The lesions were relatively well defined, with mild compression of the upper poles of both kidneys. A review of prenatal ultrasound images (not shown) did not reveal any evidence for adrenal masses. The finding is most consistent with bilateral adrenal hemorrhages. A neuroblastoma is much less likely due to the bilateral nature of the lesions and the history of an acute occurrence.

Importance

The adrenal gland in neonates is large and susceptible to hemorrhage due to rapid regression of the fetal cortex during the neonatal period and markedly engorged vascular channels in the primitive cortex. Adrenal hemorrhage is postulated to occur either due to ischemic hemorrhagic infarction because of reflex vascular redistribution in response to asphyxia or rupture of engorged veins related to increased abdominal pressure and inferior vena cava (IVC) compression. A significant hemorrhage can result in hypovolemic shock and may present as a life-threatening emergency. In neonates, the development of adrenal insufficiency is rare.

Ultrasound is the diagnostic modality of choice; the sonographic appearance varies depending on the age of the hemorrhage. The most common appearance is an anechoic avascular suprarenal mass with variable compression and displacement of the kidneys. Less commonly, the hematoma will be an echogenic or complex mass, making it difficult to differentiate from neonatal neuroblastoma. Sequential sonographies can demonstrate the evolution and resolution of a hematoma: an early lesion appears relatively homogeneous and iso- or hyperechoic, followed by subsequent liquefaction and mixed echogenicity with a central hypoechoic region. Within 2 weeks following the hemorrhage, clots and rim-like calcifications may be seen. Subsequently, the mass will attenuate and eventually resolve completely. Rarely, a persistent adrenal pseudocyst may be present with or without calcifications. Absence of internal flow on Doppler examinations can confirm that the lesion is fluid rather than solid.

CT or MR scans are usually not needed to diagnose an adrenal hemorrhage but may be helpful if a mass lesion is of concern. On MR scans, a typical evolution of the hematoma can be recognized as follows: In the acute phase (few days), the hematoma typically appears T1-isointense and T2-hypointense due to intracellular deoxyhemoglobin. In the subacute phase (several weeks), the hematoma appears T1- and T2-hyperintense due to free methemoglobin. The high T1 signal appears first in the periphery of the hematoma and gradually expands towards the center over several weeks. In the chronic stage (several months), a T1- and T2-hypointense rim is noted due to hemosiderin deposition. MR imaging is also helpful in excluding any enhancing soft tissue component of the mass.

Typical clinical scenario

Clinical manifestations vary; small adrenal hemorrhage at birth is common and often will go unnoticed or only be found incidentally; more extensive hemorrhage including large unilateral or bilateral extensive bleeding may result in a palpable flank mass, anemia, jaundice due to hemolysis from an enclosed hemorrhage, and retroperitoneal, intraperitoneal, or scrotal hematoma (extracapsular rupture of adrenal hematoma). Very large and/or bilateral hemorrhages may result in hypovolemic shock or complete exsanguination.

Although the etiology is not clear, adrenal hemorrhage occurs most commonly after a traumatic delivery, a neonatal course complicated by hypoxia, dehydration, hypotension, or coagulopathy, or in large infants with Beckwith–Wiedemann syndrome or maternal diabetes.

The majority of cases are unilateral on the right side while 10% of cases occur bilaterally. The higher frequency of right-sided adrenal hemorrhage is attributed to a greater likelihood of right adrenal compression between the liver and spine and because the right adrenal vein often drains directly into the IVC and is more susceptible to variations in venous pressure.

Surgical intervention is not usually required for adrenal hemorrhage except when a secondary infection occurs, which may lead to an adrenal abscess. Abscess formation in the adrenal gland is rare, but neonates with a pre-existing adrenal hemorrhage are at risk for hematogenous bacterial seeding which results in abscess formation elsewhere. Infecting organisms include *Neisseria meningitides*, *Escherichia coli*, and group B hemolytic streptococci.

Differential diagnosis

The most common differential diagnosis is adrenal neuroblastoma (Fig. 70.2), especially the cystic form, which is typical in neonates. In most cases an adrenal hemorrhage can be distinguished from a neonatal neuroblastoma by the clinical presentation and imaging/Doppler appearance, but sometimes the distinction may be very difficult, especially since a neuroblastoma may also bleed. Since the prognosis of neonatal neuroblastoma is very good, serial ultrasonography and/or MRI are appropriate to help with making this distinction. Evaluation of urinary excretion of vanillylmandelic acid (VMA) can help in the differentiation as increased levels of VMA are seen in over 90% of neuroblastoma cases.

Other less common differential considerations for a neonatal suprarenal mass include subdiaphragmatic extralobar pulmonary sequestration (Fig. 70.3) (almost always left-sided, frequently identified in utero, echogenic often with cysts, and may have a prominent aortic arterial supply) and renal duplication anomalies.

Renal vein thrombosis in a neonate may be associated with adrenal hemorrhage. The presence of hematuria and azotemia suggests a coexistent renal vein thrombosis, which can be confirmed sonographically.

Teaching point

In most instances, adrenal hemorrhage presents as an incidental suprarenal mass without significant clinical abnormality. These cases can be treated conservatively. Occasionally an adrenal hemorrhage may present as an emergency in the neonatal ICU unit, including rapid abdominal distension, decreasing hematocrit, acidosis, or shock. The extent, evolution, and resolution of adrenal hemorrhage can be diagnosed and followed with ultrasound studies. The imager should be aware of and on the lookout for possible concomitant renal vein thrombosis.

When there is uncertainty regarding the etiology of a suprarenal mass, serial ultrasound imaging will often be helpful showing progressive evolution and resolution of hemorrhage versus a solid or cystic mass.

REFERENCES

1. Abdu AT, Kriss VM, Bada HS, et al. Adrenal hemorrhage in a newborn. Am J Perinatol 2009;26(8):553–7.
2. Hosoda Y, Miyano T, Kimura K, et al. Characteristics and management of patients with fetal neuroblastoma. J Pediatr Surg 1992;27(5):623–5.
3. Kawashima A, Sandler CM, Ernst RD, et al. Imaging of nontraumatic hemorrhage of the adrenal gland. Radiographics 1999;19(4):949–63.
4. Simon DR, Palese MA. Clinical update on the management of adrenal hemorrhage. Curr Urol Rep 2009;10(1):78–83.
5. Westra SJ, Zaninovic AC, Hall TR, et al. Imaging of the adrenal gland in children. Radiographics 1994;14(6):1323–40.

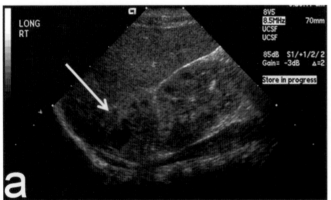

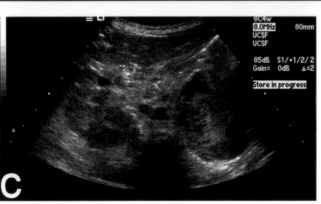

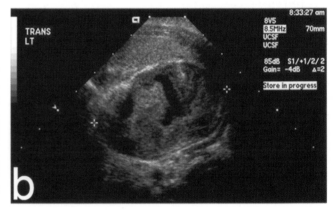

Figure 70.1. A seven-day-old neonate with bilateral adrenal hemorrhages. A longitudinal sonographic image demonstrates a heterogeneous, triangular to rounded hyperechoic mass located in the suprarenal region of the right kidney (arrow) **(a)** as well as a similar lesion in the suprarenal region above the left kidney **(b)**. The masses compressed the upper poles of both kidneys without evidence of invasion of the renal parenchyma. A transverse view of both sides **(c)** emphasizes the bilateral suprarenal masses, which are most consistent with bilateral adrenal hemorrhages.

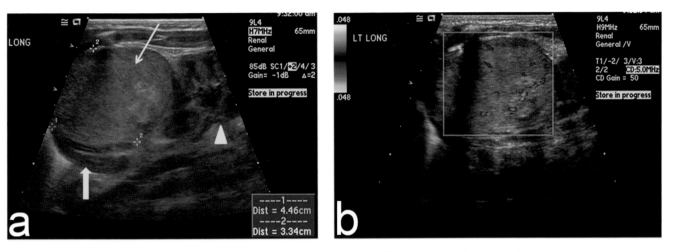

Figure 70.2. A two-day-old neonate with left suprarenal neuroblastoma. Longitudinal gray-scale **(a)** and color Doppler **(b)** sonographic images demonstrate a hyperechoic solid vascular mass (thin arrow) contiguous with the left adrenal gland (thick arrow) and superior to the left kidney (arrowhead), likely representing a neuroblastoma. Histopathologic evaluation confirmed the diagnosis of left adrenal neuroblastoma.

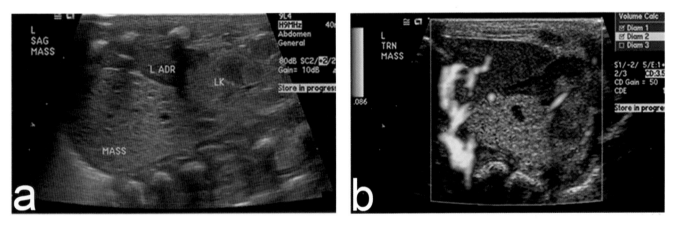

Figure 70.3. A five-day-old female with left subdiaphragmatic sequestration. Longitudinal gray-scale **(a)** and transverse color Doppler **(b)** sonographic images demonstrate an echogenic mass with small cystic areas, supero-medial to the left adrenal gland and superior to the left kidney, with mobility during respiration, likely representing an extralobar sequestration and less likely a neuroblastoma. Histopathologic evaluation confirmed the diagnosis of an extralobar sequestration.

Khun Visith Keu and Andrei Iagaru

Imaging description

A three-year-old child presented with back pain and inability to stand or walk. CT and MRI demonstrated epidural masses in the midthoracic and lumbar spine causing cord compression, as well as a large right adrenal mass (Fig. 71.1a–c). Iodine-123 (^{123}I) metaiodobenzylguanidine (MIBG) planar scintigraphy and SPECT/CT showed a large area of focal radiotracer uptake in the right adrenal gland and disseminated bone marrow involvement involving the axial and appendicular skeleton (Fig. 71.1d). Technetium-99m (^{99m}Tc) methyl diphosphonate (MDP) bone scintigraphy demonstrated destructive cortical lesions in the axial and appendicular skeleton (Fig. 71.1e). Biopsies of the adrenal mass and bone marrow confirmed metastatic neuroblastoma (NB).

Importance

NB is an embryonic tumor of the sympathetic nervous system and is the most common extracranial solid tumor in childhood. At the time of diagnosis, nearly half of the patients have distant metastases, commonly to the bone cortex and bone marrow, which confers a poor prognosis. However, involvement of the bone marrow does not always correlate with cortical bone involvement, or vice versa. The combination of ^{123}I-MIBG scintigraphy and ^{99m}Tc-MDP bone scans gives the highest sensitivity for the evaluation of skeletal lesions. ^{123}I-MIBG is taken into cells via the norepinephrine transporter, which allows for a sensitive and specific method for assessing disease extent in both the soft tissues and bone marrow. However, the ^{123}I-MIBG scan alone may underestimate the extent of bone involvement. ^{99m}Tc-MDP bone scans, which better evaluate the cortical lesions, provide complementary information to ^{123}I-MIBG scintiscans. They are based on the increased rate of calcium turnover at the site of injury, which can begin as early as 24 hours after the triggering event. During follow-up, ^{99m}Tc-MDP bone scans can remain positive for more than 6 months during the healing process whereas ^{123}I-MIBG scans are only positive in viable, functioning lesions. Thus, MIBG is more suitable for monitoring response to therapy.

Typical clinical scenario

NB is more commonly seen in young children, with 50% presenting before age two and more than 90% by age five years. Presentation of NB is very variable, dependent on the location and extent of the primary tumor, as well as the presence of metastatic disease. The most common primary site is in the retroperitoneum, often involving the adrenal glands (35%) or paraspinal ganglia (35%). Other common sites involve the posterior mediastinum (20%), pelvis (<5%), and neck (<5%). Systemic symptoms are common because of the high incidence of metastases at presentation. Common metastatic sites include lymph nodes, liver, subcutaneous tissues, bone marrow, and cortical bone. Metastatic bone lesions are typically multifocal and may involve a symmetrical pattern in the metaphyseal regions of the long bones. Involvement of the skull, vertebrae, ribs, and pelvis are also common. Both lytic and sclerotic bone lesions may be present. Clinically, children frequently present with a palpable abdominal mass although newborns may just have abdominal distension. Bruising around the eyes or proptosis is also not uncommon and is due to metastatic involvement of the bones and soft tissues around the orbits. Some children present with symptoms similar to leukemia: pallor, anemia, fever, and bone pain. Older children may exhibit a limp or joint pain suggestive of arthritis. Paraspinal tumors can result in cord compression and large abdominal or pelvic masses may cause urinary obstruction. If there is excessive catecholamine secretion, hypertension and diarrhea can also be seen. Opsoclonus–myoclonus is an unusual but distinct paraneoplastic presentation of NB (see Case 16). NB has a widely variable clinical course ranging from spontaneous regression, to differentiation into benign ganglioneuromas, to rapid and progressive fatal disease. The natural history of NB is closely linked to the child's age at presentation. Patients younger than 12 months of age, even with metastatic disease, have a better prognosis. The majority of children older than 12 months of age with advanced disease will die from progressive disease. Stage IV-S disease is a distinct subtype of neuroblastoma with a benign course, typically resulting in spontaneous resolution. This is usually seen in young children and is characterized by a small primary lesion and focal or diffuse involvement at specific sites that include liver, skin, and bone marrow, but not cortical bone.

Differential diagnosis

Based on clinical symptoms alone, the differential diagnosis can be broad and may include Wilms' tumor, rhabdomyosarcoma, leukemia, and juvenile rheumatoid arthritis, but none of these entities are expected to have increased ^{123}I-MIBG uptake. However, a positive ^{123}I-MIBG is not only specific to NB. Pheochromocytomas, ganglioneuroblastomas, ganglioneuromas, paragangliomas, carcinoid tumors, medullary thyroid carcinomas, and Merkel cell tumors also take up ^{123}I-MIBG. Lastly, ^{99m}Tc-MDP bone scans are positive in an even wider array of pathologies including metabolic disorders, trauma, infection, and various malignancies. In children, evaluating skeletal metastatic disease by ^{99m}Tc-MDP bone scintigraphy is most commonly performed in sarcomas and NB.

Teaching point

NB is the most common extracranial solid tumor in childhood and roughly half of patients demonstrate distant metastasis at the time of diagnosis. Metastatic involvement of the bone cortex and bone marrow confers a worse prognosis. ^{123}I-MIBG scintigraphy and ^{99m}Tc-MDP bone scans are complementary studies that together offer the greatest sensitivity for the evaluation of skeletal disease.

REFERENCES

1. Barai S, Bandopadhayaya GP, Malhotra A, *et al*. Does I-131-MIBG underestimate skeletal disease burden in neuroblastoma? *J Postgrad Med* 2004;**50**(4):257–60; discussion 260–1.

2. Howman-Giles R, Shaw PJ, Uren RF, *et al*. Neuroblastoma and other neuroendocrine tumors. *Semin Nucl Med* 2007;**37**(4):286–302.

3. Matthay KK, Shulkin B, Ladenstein R, *et al*. Criteria for evaluation of disease extent by (123)I-metaiodobenzylguanidine scans in neuroblastoma: a report for the International Neuroblastoma Risk Group (INRG) Task Force. *Br J Cancer* 2010;**102**(9):1319–26.

4. Ziessman HA, O'Malley JP, Thrall JH. *Nuclear Medicine: The Requisites*, 3rd edition. Philadelphia: Mosby Elsevier Health Sciences, 2005.

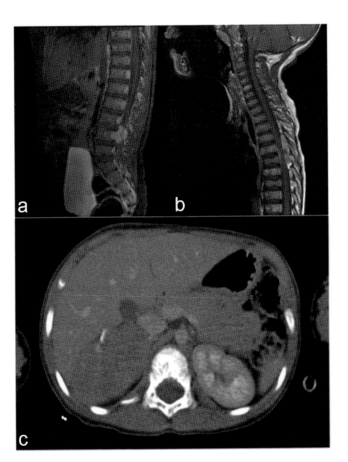

Figure 71.1. A three-year-old child with diffuse metastatic neuroblastoma. Sagittal MRI T1 post-gadolinium images **(a, b)** shows multiple heterogeneously enhancing irregular and flattened vertebral bodies denoting bone metastases. There were several associated enhancing epidural masses in the midthoracic and lumbar spine causing cord compression. CT **(c)** revealed a large hypodense right adrenal mass, which was the primary site of malignancy.

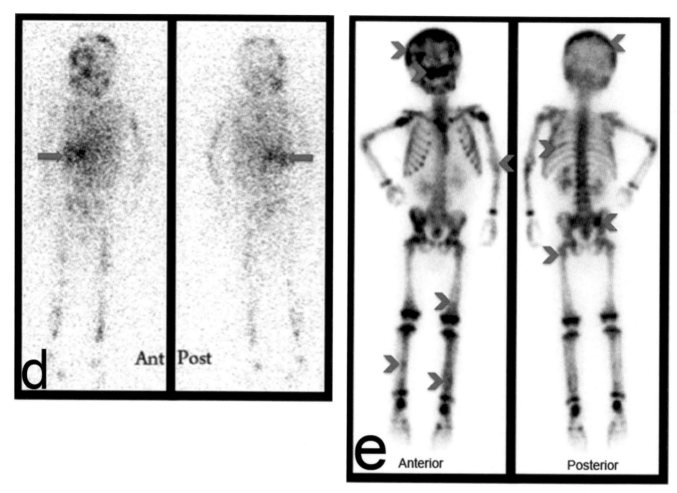

Figure 71.1. (cont.) ¹²³I-MIBG scintigraphy **(d)** showed a large area of tracer uptake in the right adrenal gland (arrow) and disseminated bone marrow involvement of the skull, long bones, and vertebrae. ⁹⁹ᵐTc-MDP bone scintigraphy **(e)** identified destructive cortical lesions in the axial and appendicular skeleton (arrowheads).

Ovarian torsion in childhood

Atalie Thompson and Beverley Newman

Imaging description

A two-month-old girl presented with fussiness and a tender mass located in the left labia majora. A longitudinal ultrasound (US) of the labial mass revealed an enlarged hypoechoic left ovary with multiple peripheral enlarged follicles (Fig. 72.1). The labial location suggested herniation of the ovary into a patent pouch of peritoneum known as the canal of Nuck. Irreducibility along with the abnormal appearance of the ovary and absent venous waveforms with bidirectional arterial flow still present on Doppler US suggested incarceration of the herniated ovary and partial rather than complete ovarian torsion (Fig. 72.1b). Transverse views demonstrated a normal right ovary of smaller size (Fig. 72.1c). Surgical intervention confirmed the diagnosis of partial torsion, with successful detorsion and hernia repair.

Importance

Ovarian torsion is a rare though serious cause of abdominal pain in female children. Delayed diagnosis and treatment is common because of non-specific symptoms and can lead to necrosis and loss of the ovary, resulting in decreased fertility. Due to the higher incidence of functional ovarian cysts as well as pregnancy, girls entering their reproductive years are at greatest risk. However, even infants can present with torsion, especially if a large ovarian tumor or cystic mass initiates twisting of the vascular pedicle.

A patent canal of Nuck in girls is the anatomic equivalent of a patent processus vaginalis in boys predisposing to indirect inguinal hernia. This peritoneal pouch extends from the peritoneal cavity adjacent to the round ligament to its distal attachment on the labia majora. A variety of peritoneal contents can herniate into the canal of Nuck, particularly the ovary, with the resultant risk of incarceration and/or torsion.

Both US and CT or MRI can help to differentiate torsion from the wide array of other causes of abdominal and pelvic pain in female children. Decreased vascular flow on Doppler and presence of an enlarged ovary or ovarian mass provide clues to the diagnosis and need for prompt surgical management.

Typical clinical scenario

Ovarian torsion occurs when the ovary compromises its own blood supply by twisting on its supporting ligaments. The presenting signs and symptoms can be non-specific, though several studies have concluded that the only constant and ubiquitous symptom is pain from the ischemic event. Classically, this pain has a sharp severe quality, and localizes to either lower quadrant. It may be accompanied by a palpable mass and/or peritoneal signs such as rebound tenderness.

Non-verbal infants and children may simply be irritable or inconsolable. Urinary symptoms, fever, and waves of nausea with emesis may also be associated. If the ovary is only intermittently torsed, there may be alternating periods of pain and relief, which can further cloud the clinical picture. Ovarian torsion and infarction can even occur in utero. In this situation, as well as in the case of a missed postnatal torsion, an infarcted amputated ovary may be seen as a small mobile calcified abdominal mass.

Torsion is the primary complication of ovarian tumors, ranging from 3–16% in incidence. Thus, the finding of an ovarian cystic or solid mass on pelvic imaging greatly increases the likelihood of torsion (Fig. 72.2). Pediatric populations more commonly present with germ cell (GCT) rather than epithelial tumors, with benign cystic teratomas being the most prevalent. Calcifications on imaging indicative of teeth or bone accompanying other mesodermal or ectodermal tissue, particularly fat, within a complex cystic mass can clinch the diagnosis (Figs. 72.3, 72.4) but does not definitively separate benign from malignant germ cell tumors. It is thought that benign tumors may be more likely to torse because they lack the degree of adhesions or local invasion that malignant tumors frequently possess. However, even malignant neoplasms can be associated with ovarian torsion. Findings of a solid mass, and any features of invasion or metastases such as omental caking on CT or MRI, should prompt the ordering of additional tumor markers, alpha-fetoprotein (AFP) and beta human chorionic gonadotropin (beta-HCG).

More common than tumors, rapidly growing ovarian cysts also predispose to torsion, especially those exceeding 5 cm in diameter (Fig. 72.2a,c). Imbalance of gonadotropic hormones during adolescence or pregnancy can trigger the development of functional follicular, luteal, or theca lutein cysts. The neonatal period can also generate follicular cysts, especially in the context of maternal diabetes, pre-eclampsia, or rhesus immunization. A history of precocious puberty, polyostotic fibrous dysplasia, and café-au-lait spots on exam can imply hormonally active autonomous cysts such as those found in the McCune–Albright syndrome. When there is a large ovarian cyst or mass, the ovary can migrate into the pouch of Douglas (the space between the uterus and rectum) or out of the pelvis into the abdomen above the bladder (Figs. 72.2 and 72.4); frequently the uterus is deviated to the side of the displaced ovary.

Torsion of normal adnexa is uncommon. Purported causes range from elongated fallopian tubes, mesosalpingeal vessels, and supportive ligaments, to spasm of the fallopian tube, to sudden changes in intra-abdominal pressure from coughing or vomiting.

Gray-scale real-time US is the primary tool to evaluate a female child with abdominal pain. It is not only cost-effective and non-invasive, but also able to elicit local reaction to tenderness. In young children, the technique is limited to the suprapubic approach, which is usually accurate, although transvaginal imaging can provide additional more detailed views in older sexually active adolescents. The most common sonographic finding in ovarian torsion is an enlarged unilateral ovary (>4cm). Approximately three-fourths of cases reveal a complex mass that is solid, cystic, or both. Heterogeneous stroma may indicate edema and hemorrhage. Thickened cyst walls can signify chronic inflammation (Fig. 72.2c). A "string of pearls" sign with multiple small follicles lining the periphery of an engorged ovary is a useful imaging feature of ovarian torsion although this finding may be present in normal ovaries and other entities without torsion notably polycystic ovarian syndrome (Fig. 72.2a). Other pertinent findings include pelvic free fluid and a twisted vascular pedicle, which appears as an echogenic mass with concentric hypoechoic stripes (whirlpool sign). Comparison to the contralateral ovary provides an important frame of reference and should always be performed (Figs. 72.1c and 72.2). Addition of color Doppler flow can further aid in the diagnosis of torsion, although the results are less consistent (Fig. 72.1b). The pathognomonic finding is absent arterial flow (73%), yet decreased venous flow has been documented significantly more frequently (93%) and often times the waveforms are normal depending on the degree of vascular obstruction.

Occasionally, additional imaging modalities are needed to verify the diagnosis, especially in subacute cases or when the US images are non-diagnostic. Criteria for torsion on CT and MRI, however, are not as well defined. Both can detect smooth wall thickening of a cystic mass, as well as fallopian tube thickening, a deviated uterus, and ascites. MRI avoids the radiation exposure of CT, and can show engorged blood vessels on the side of the torsion (Fig. 72.2a,c), hematoma, and absence of postcontrast enhancement indicative of hemorrhagic infarction.

Differential diagnosis

The differential diagnosis for ovarian torsion presenting as acute lower abdominal pain ranges from appendicitis and renal colic to ectopic pregnancy, pelvic inflammatory disease, and ruptured ovarian cyst. Several important distinctions can narrow the diagnosis. Visualization of an enlarged, fluid-filled, and non-compressible hyperemic appendix confirms appendicitis. Tenderness at the costovertebral angle and visualization of renal or ureteral shadowing echogenic foci with accompanying hydronephrosis suggests nephrolithiasis. An even greater mimic of ovarian torsion is any ovarian mass that could itself lead to torsion, such as a hemorrhagic cyst. In such

cases absent arterial or venous flow on Doppler can provide additional insight, although a normal Doppler does not effectively rule out torsion. Following rupture of an ovarian cyst, however, the child may experience some reprieve from symptoms that would be uncharacteristic of torsion. Rupture of an ectopic pregnancy can escalate pain, and an elevated beta-HCG would further confirm this etiology. The onset of pain in pelvic inflammatory disease is more gradual than in torsion, though it may be suspected if the patient is sexually active. A palpable groin or labial mass can provide evidence that an inguinal hernia may be present with or without the presence of an ovary and incarceration/torsion, although hydrocele of the canal of Nuck, lymphadenopathy, Bartholin's cyst, or tumor can present in similar fashion.

Teaching points

Ovarian torsion is a rare though important diagnosis in the female child with abdominopelvic pain. The non-specific nature of the clinical signs and symptoms make the timely use of US all the more critical. Presence of an enlarged ovary, peripheral ovarian cysts, adjacent free fluid, accompanying large cyst/s or mass, and diminished vascular flow on Doppler can confirm the diagnosis, though Doppler is not highly sensitive or specific. Rarely, herniation of the ovary into the canal of Nuck can lead to incarceration or torsion, and can be suspected on physical exam and confirmed on US. In the setting of subacute torsion, or ambiguous US findings, the assistance of CT and particularly MR can elucidate the pathologic process. Postcontrast enhancement can provide further insight regarding the viability of the torsed ovary. Prompt diagnosis and surgical intervention can prevent necrosis of the ovary, systemic infection, and decreased fertility.

REFERENCES

1. Chang HC, Bhatt S, Dogra VS. Pearls and pitfalls in diagnosis of ovarian torsion. *Radiographics* 2008;**28**(5):1355–68.
2. Jedrzejewski G, Stankiewicz A, Wieczorek AP. Uterus and ovary hernia of the canal of Nuck. *Pediatr Radiol* 2008;**38**(11):1257–8.
3. Kokoska ER, Keller MS, Weber TR. Acute ovarian torsion in children. *Am J Surg* 2000;**180**(6):462–5.
4. Pienkowski C, Cartault A, Carfagna L, *et al.* Ovarian cysts in prepubertal girls. *Endocr Dev* 2012;**22**:101–11.
5. Rha SE, Byun JY, Jung SE, *et al.* CT and MR imaging features of adnexal torsion. *Radiographics* 2002;**22**(2):283–94.
6. Saito JM. Beyond appendicitis: evaluation and surgical treatment of pediatric acute abdominal pain. *Curr Opin Pediatr* 2012;**24**(3):357–64.

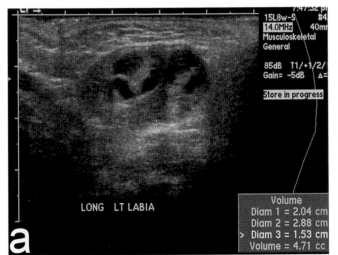

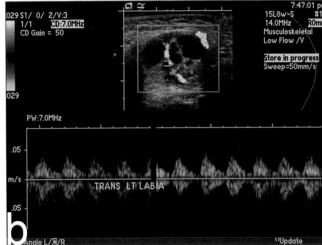

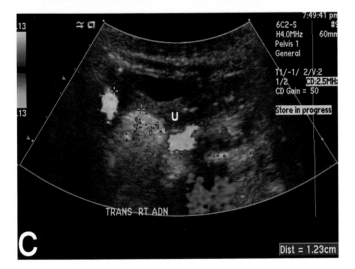

Figure 72.1. A two-month-old girl with fussiness and a tender mass in the left labia. Herniation of left ovary (calipers) into the canal of Nuck with partial ovarian torsion. **(a)** Longitudinal US image of the left labial mass demonstrates an enlarged hypoechoic left ovary with multiple peripheral enlarged follicles. **(b)** Doppler US of the herniated left ovary demonstrates bidirectional arterial flow. Absence of venous waveforms (not shown) in the ovary suggested partial torsion. This diagnosis was confirmed surgically and the ovary was found to be still viable. **(c)** Transverse US image of the pelvis demonstrating the uterus (U) and normal, much smaller right ovary (calipers).

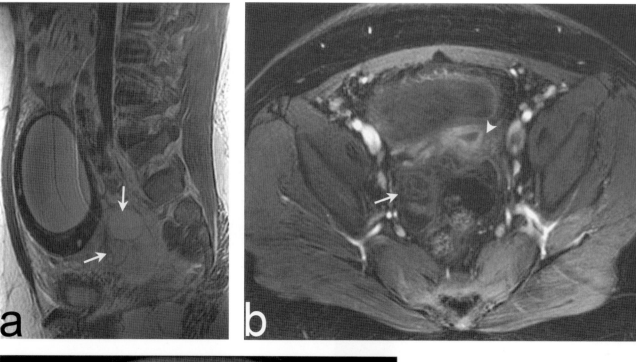

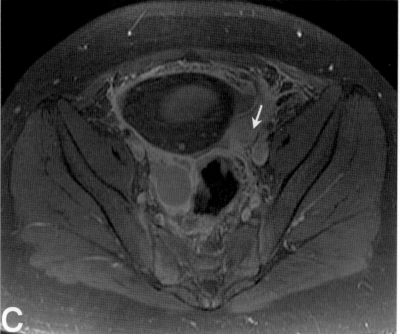

Figure 72.2. A 12-year-old girl with severe recurrent abdominal pain and subsequently diagnosed polycystic ovarian syndrome. Outside US (not shown) incorrectly suggested hematometra (obstructed blood-filled uterus) as the diagnosis. **(a)** Sagittal T2-weighted MR image demonstrates the right ovary positioned posteriorly (arrows) containing multiple peripheral follicles, with a larger cyst located superiorly and surrounded by free pelvic fluid. There is a giant thick-walled cyst anteriorly that was thought to arise from the left ovary. The uterus was normal (not shown). **(b)** Axial T1-weighted MR postcontrast demonstrating the enhancing right ovary (arrow) and uterus containing small fluid (arrowhead) behind the bladder. **(c)** Axial T1-weighted MR postcontrast demonstrates the right ovarian cyst positioned posteriorly and what was thought to be some normal enhancing left ovarian tissue (arrow) adjacent to the thick-walled anterior cyst. In retrospect this may represent a whirlpool sign indicative of a twisted vascular pedicle. Note that there is marked pericyst and pelvic sidewall enhancement, suggestive of inflammation. The wall of the left ovarian cyst does not enhance although there are intramural engorged veins (see also in (a)). The contents of the cyst are suggestive of hemorrhage (bright signal on both T1 and T2). Left ovarian torsion (possibly partial or repetitive torsion/detorsion) was of concern because of the thick-walled unenhancing cyst and marked pelvic inflammatory changes. Intraoperatively the left ovary including the cyst was found to be torsed, with marked surrounding inflammation. The ovary was viable and was detorsed; the cyst containing hemorrhagic contents was resected.

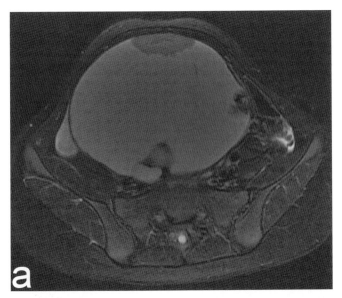

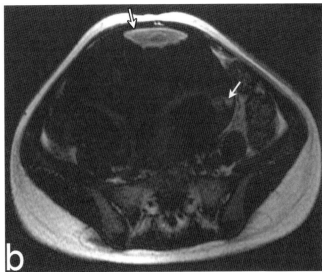

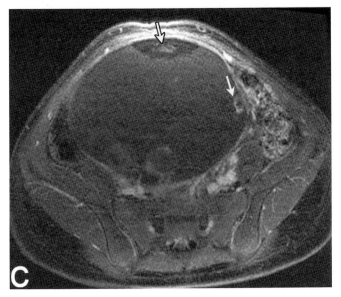

Figure 72.3. A12-year-old girl with a pelvic mass diagnosed as a mature left ovarian teratoma on pathology. **(a)** Axial T2-weighted MR image demonstrates a large predominantly cystic abdominopelvic mass that appears to arise from the left ovary, with a normal right ovary seen (not shown). There are several heterogeneous peripheral solid and partially cystic nodules. **(b)** Axial image at the same level reconstructed as a "fat"-specific image. Note the areas that were relatively gray on the fat-saturated T2 image follow the same signal as subcutaneous fat and are now very bright (arrows). **(c)** Axial postcontrast image with fat saturation at the same level demonstrates enhancement of solid non-fatty components of the nodules (arrows) and confirms dark saturated fat signal elsewhere in the nodules.

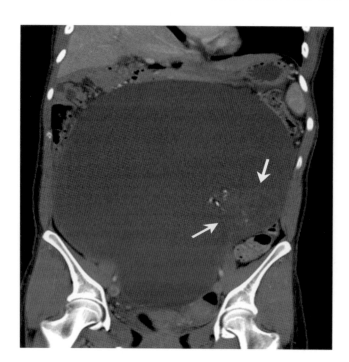

Figure 72.4. A 16-year-old girl with progressive abdominal distention. Immature teratoma in the right ovary confirmed pathologically. Coronal CT image of the abdomen demonstrates a huge predominantly cystic mass that has risen out of the pelvis and now occupies most of the abdomen. There is a large enhancing peripheral solid nodule (arrows) with small hypodense fatty and hyperattenuating calcific components. A normal appearing uterus and left ovary are seen in the pelvis. No separate right ovary was identified.

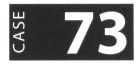

CASE 73 Torsion of the appendix testis

Rakhee Gawande, Heike E. Daldrup-Link, and Beverley Newman

Imaging description

A longitudinal ultrasound of the right scrotum (Fig. 73.1) in a 13-year-old boy with gradual onset of testicular pain demonstrates a well-defined oval hypoechoic avascular structure located in the groove between the testis and epididymis. There was mild hyperemia of the testis and epididymis, which were otherwise normal in appearance. A moderate hydrocele and scrotal wall edema was also noted. These findings were suggestive of torsion of the appendix testis.

Importance

Testicular appendages are remnants of embryonic mesonephric and paramesonephric ducts and consist of vascularized connective tissue. Five types of appendages have been identified. The appendix testis is a tiny structure, 1–7 mm in size, located at the upper pole of the testis, in the groove between the testis and epididymis. It has similar echogenicity to the testis and may be oval or sessile and less commonly pedunculated. It is present in 92% of patients and is the commonest appendage to undergo torsion. The appendix epididymis is located at the head of the epididymis, is commonly pedunculated, and is less frequently seen on ultrasound. The other appendages are difficult to identify on ultrasound imaging.

Torsion of a testicular appendage is the most common cause of acute scrotal pain in prepubertal boys and is usually managed conservatively. The clinical presentation of pain and swelling may mimic testicular torsion or acute epididymo-orchitis. Color Doppler ultrasound will help to differentiate between these conditions.

Typical clinical scenario

Gradual or sudden onset of pain usually localized to the upper pole of the testis. A firm nodule superior to the testis may be palpated with bluish discoloration of the skin (blue dot sign).

On ultrasound, a twisted appendage is seen as a small round extratesticular mass of mixed or increased echogenicity with lack of color Doppler signal. Adjacent inflammation may be noted with enlargement and hypervascularity of the epididymis, reactive hydrocele, and thickening of scrotal skin. The torsed appendage may infarct, calcify, and become detached, leaving a scrotal calcification known as a scrotolith or scrotal pearl.

Differential diagnosis

The main differential diagnoses for acute scrotal pain include epididymo-orchitis, torsion of a testicular appendage, and testicular torsion (Fig. 73.2). A strangulated inguinal hernia (Fig. 73.3) and trauma are other causes of acute inguinoscrotal pain. Patient history is clearly essential to guide the clinical workup and differential considerations.

Ultrasound including Doppler imaging is the primary imaging method used to differentiate scrotal pathology. While absence of testicular flow is strongly suggestive of testicular torsion, incomplete torsion may be accompanied by reduced rather than absent flow and torsion/detorsion may produce testicular hyperemia simulating epididymo-orchitis. It is helpful to image the inguinal canal as a twisted spermatic cord may be directly visible. In the case of appendage torsion, associated inflammatory changes of the testis, epididymis, and scrotal wall may be very prominent but should not divert attention away from a careful examination to identify the characteristic small avascular superior mass (Fig. 73.1).

Other inguinal and paratesticular masses occur; most are larger, cystic, or vascular. Also, with the exception of an incarcerated hernia, most paratesticular masses/neoplasms do not present clinically with scrotal pain.

Teaching point

Torsion of the testicular appendage is the most common cause of acute scrotal pain in prepubertal children and is usually managed conservatively. Ultrasound with spectral and color Doppler will help to differentiate this condition from testicular torsion, which requires prompt surgical intervention. Scrotal wall edema/hyperemia is a useful sonographic feature of vascular, inflammatory, or traumatic scrotal lesions.

REFERENCES

1. Aso C, Enríquez G, Fité M, et al. Gray-scale and color Doppler sonography of scrotal disorders in children: an update. Radiographics 2005;25(5):1197–214.
2. Rakha E, Puls F, Saidul I, Furness P. Torsion of the testicular appendix: importance of associated acute inflammation. J Clin Pathol 2006;59(8):831–4.
3. Sellars NE, Sidhu PS. Ultrasound appearances of the testicular appendages: pictorial review. Eur Radiol 2003;13:127–35.

(a)

(b)

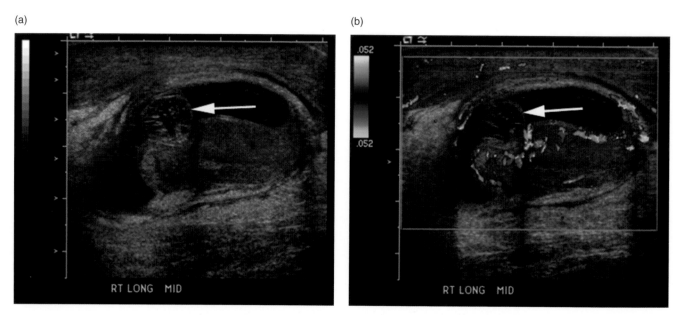

Figure 73.1. A 13-year-old boy with right scrotal pain and torsion of the appendix testis. Longitudinal ultrasound of the right scrotum without (a) and with (b) color Doppler demonstrates a well-defined oval hypoechoic avascular lesion in the groove between the testis and the epididymis (arrows). A moderate hydrocele and scrotal wall edema/hyperemia is also noted. Mildly prominent color Doppler flow is seen in both the testis and epididymis (b).

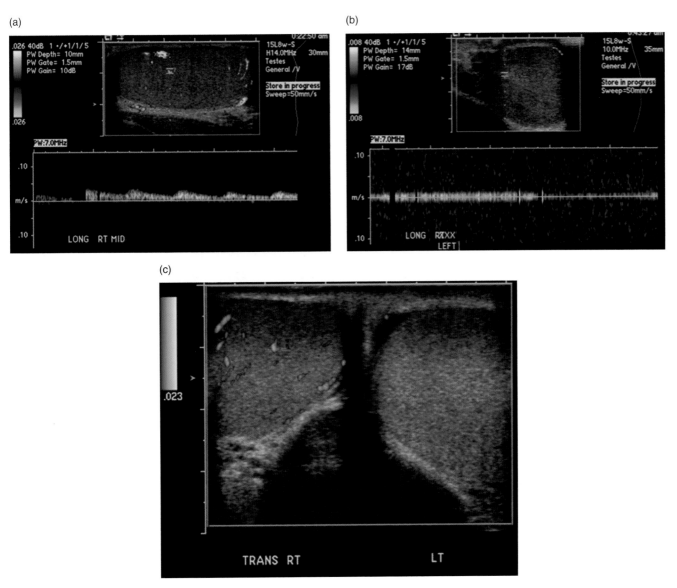

Figure 73.2. A 15-year-old boy with acute left scrotal pain and testicular torsion. Longitudinal and transverse spectral and color Doppler images of both testes (a: right and b: left, c: transverse – both) demonstrate normal right **(a)** but absent vascular flow (just noise on spectral Doppler) in the left testis **(b, c)** consistent with acute left testicular torsion. The left testis also appears to be enlarged with left scrotal wall edema (c).

(a)

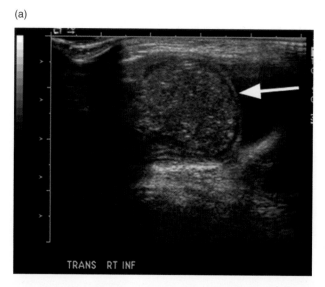

(b) (c)

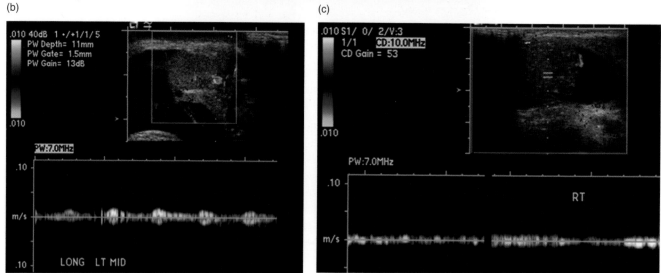

Figure 73.3. A three-year-old with right incarcerated inguinal hernia. A dilated bowel loop is noted in the right inguinal region (arrow) **(a)**, suggestive of an inguinal hernia. Scrotal wall edema is noted. Bilateral hydroceles are present **(b, c)**. The left testis (b) appears normal in size with normal vascularity. The right testis (c) appears enlarged and heterogeneous with decreased vascularity, suggestive of testicular ischemia/torsion. A strangulated right inguinal hernia was found at surgery with an edematous right testes; there was no evidence of testicular torsion.

Intratesticular neoplasms

Hedieh K. Eslamy and Beverley Newman

Imaging description

A 23-month-old male presented with a six-month history of a right scrotal mass that had been increasing in size. Alpha-fetoprotein was markedly elevated and the beta human chorionic gonadotropin level was within normal limits. Scrotal ultrasound (US) demonstrated a right intratesticular mass, replacing the right testicle and measuring 5.5 × 6.4 × 8.4 cm (volume of 152 mL). The mass was heterogeneously echogenic and hypervascular (Fig. 74.1). The normal left testicle measured 1.3 × 0.7 × 1.5 cm (volume of 0.7 mL). The patient underwent CT of the chest, abdomen, and pelvis which did not demonstrate metastatic disease. Radical orchiectomy was performed and pathology was consistent with a yolk sac tumor.

Importance

US is the initial imaging modality for the evaluation of suspected intrascrotal pathology and is used to confirm the presence and evaluate the nature of abnormalities. A systematic approach to the interpretation of scrotal US includes:

1. Determine structure of origin:
   a. intratesticular
   b. extratesticular: epididymis, testicular appendage, epididymal appendage, tunica albuginea and tunica vaginalis, spermatic cord, scrotal wall, and intraperitoneal (herniated bowel or omentum)
2. Determine characteristics of lesion(s): structural characteristics (solid, cystic/fluid, or complex; presence of calcification), vascularity, size, and presence of peristalsis (seen in herniated loops of bowel).
3. Evaluate testicles for:
   a. flow: testicular ischemia may be a complication of diverse pathologies.
   b. longitudinal axis of testis: abnormal longitudinal axis of testis and position of mediastinum testis, and superior traction of epididymis and mediastinum may be seen in testicular torsion.
4. Correlate US findings with patient age, clinical presentation, and serum testicular tumor markers:
   a. alpha-fetoprotein: may be elevated in yolk sac tumors (in >90%), teratomas, and embryonal carcinoma.
   b. beta subunit of human chorionic gonadotropin: may be elevated in pure or mixed embryonal carcinoma and choriocarcinoma.

Typical clinical scenario

The most common clinical presentation of intratesticular neoplasms is a painless scrotal mass (>90%), with <10% having a history of trauma, bruising, hydrocele, or hernia. An associated hydrocele is seen in up to 50% of cases. Cases with associated intratumoral hemorrhage or torsion will present with a painful scrotal mass. Sex cord-stromal tumors may produce estrogen (Sertoli cell tumors, Leydig cell tumors) or testosterone, progesterone, and/or corticosteroids (Leydig cell tumors) and present with gynecomastia, precocious puberty, or Cushing's syndrome.

In contrast, the child or adolescent male with an acute scrotum presents with acute painful swelling of the scrotum or its contents, with or without swelling and erythema. The differential diagnoses of an acute scrotum include: spermatic cord torsion, torsion of testicular appendages, epididymo-orchitis, and trauma. A correct diagnosis is mandatory as treatment options depend on the disease process, with spermatic cord torsion requiring immediate surgical intervention to avoid testicular loss.

Intratesticular neoplasms have a bimodal age distribution, with a large peak in young adults and a small peak in the first 3 years of life. Prepubertal testicular neoplasms are rare and are distinct from postpubertal and adult testicular neoplasms. Prepubertal testicular neoplasms include germ cell tumors (mature teratomas, epidermoid cyst, and yolk sac tumors) and stromal tumors (juvenile granulosa cell, Leydig cell, and Sertoli cell tumors); yolk sac tumors and mature teratomas make up the majority of neoplasms in this age group (Figs. 74.1 and 74.2). Epidermoid cysts (Fig. 74.3) are benign germ cell tumors that arise from the ectoderm. Prepubertal testicular neoplasms have low mortality rates, with a five-year survival rate of 99%.

Testicular neoplasms seen in the postpubertal male (embryonal carcinomas, mixed germ cell tumors, teratocarcinomas, and choriocarcinomas) tend to be more aggressive, with lymphatic and hematogenous spread.

Differential diagnosis

The differential diagnosis of a scrotal mass in the pediatric patient includes: congenital lesions, intratesticular and extratesticular neoplasms, and non-neoplastic intratesticular and extratesticular masses (see List 1, Figs. 74.4–74.7). In the approach to the differential diagnosis of an intratesticular mass in the pediatric patient population, the radiologist should consider congenital etiologies (polyorchidism, testicular ectopia, testicular size asymmetry, cystic dysplasia of the testis, splenogonadal fusion) (Figs. 74.4 and 74.5) and non-neoplastic intratesticular masses (Leydig cell hyperplasia, testicular adrenal rests). These lesions may not be definitively distinguished from a neoplasm on imaging.

In general, extratesticular lesions are more likely to be benign and intratesticular lesions more likely to be malignant. US is 90–100% accurate in differentiating intratesticular from extratesticular pathologies. While US imaging has excellent sensitivity for defining the presence of a testicular neoplasm, the specific tumor type may not be distinguishable.

US is the initial modality of choice to image scrotal masses. MRI (preferred due to lack of ionizing radiation) and CT may be used for staging. Testicular masses tend to have a non-specific appearance of a solid or complex mass on all cross-sectional imaging modalities. Color Doppler sonography can determine the vascularity of a mass and may help to distinguish it from testicular torsion. Hypervascularity is present in 85% of neoplasms, although smaller tumors (<1.5 cm) are often avascular or hypovascular. Avascularity of the testis, an unusual finding in neoplasms, suggests a diagnosis of chronic testicular torsion. However, intact blood flow in cases of perinatal torsion is not uncommon (Fig. 74.6), and the torsion–detorsion sequence may appear as testicular hyperemia on color Doppler US due to reperfusion following detorsion. Scrotal wall thickening is uncommon in association with testicular tumors and is more likely to be secondary to spermatic cord torsion (Fig. 74.6), trauma, or epididymo-orchitis.

MRI may be a valuable problem-solving tool in cases with equivocal or inconclusive findings on US and allows differentiation of intra- and extratesticular origin and further characterizes the lesion as likely benign vs. malignant and thus help to guide therapy (testis-preserving surgery versus orchiectomy).

Testis-preserving surgery (mass enucleation) for testicular tumors is indicated in:

- Benign intratesticular neoplasms: epidermoid cysts, Leydig cell tumors (these are most often small, avascular, or hypovascular lesions)
- Synchronous or metachronous bilateral intratesticular germ cell tumors
- Unilateral testicular germ cell tumor in a solitary testicle.

In patients with small solid intratesticular tumors, negative serum testicular tumor markers, and benign histology on intraoperative frozen-section analysis of the enucleated tumor, the tumor-bearing testicle may be preserved.

List 1 – Differential diagnosis of a scrotal mass in the pediatric patient (pre- and postpubertal)

1. Congenital: polyorchidism, testicular ectopia, testicular size asymmetry, cystic dysplasia of the testis, splenogonadal fusion
2. Intratesticular neoplasms
   a. Primary (refer to List 2)
   b. Secondary: lymphoma, leukemia, metastases (rare)
3. Extratesticular neoplasms: benign and malignant
   a. Extratesticular lipoma
   b. Melanotic neuroectodermal tumor of infancy
   c. Hemangioma
   d. Adenomatoid tumor
   e. Papillary cystadenoma
   f. Extratesticular rhabdomyosarcoma

4. Non-neoplastic intratesticular masses: Leydig cell hyperplasia, testicular adrenal rests, fibrous pseudotumor
5. Non-neoplastic extratesticular masses
   a. Solid masses: meconium periorchitis, fibrous pseudotumor
   b. Cystic masses: hydrocele, hematocele, pyocele; inguinal hernia; epididymal cyst and spermatocele, testicular cyst; lymphatic malformation

List 2 – Primary intratesticular tumors: classified by tissue of origin

- **Germ cell tumors** (up to 90%)
  - Non-seminomatous: yolk sac tumors, teratoma, teratocarcinoma, embryonal carcinoma, choriocarcinoma, and mixed germ cell tumors
  - Seminomatous: rare in pediatric population
  - Epidermoid cyst
- **Sex cord-stromal tumors**
  - Sertoli cell tumor
  - Leydig cell tumor
  - Juvenile granulosa cell tumor (most common testicular tumor in neonates)
- **Mixed germ cell/sex cord tumors**: gonadoblastoma
- **Originating from testicular supporting tissues**: rare and mostly benign
  - Leiomyoma, fibroma, hemangioma
  - Leiomyosarcoma, fibrosarcoma

Teaching point

Ultrasound is the appropriate initial imaging modality for the evaluation of suspected intrascrotal pathology and is used to confirm its presence and evaluate the structure of origin and characteristics of the lesion. Ultrasound and MRI often cannot diagnose the specific tumor type in intratesticular primary neoplasms but will help to exclude extratesticular cystic and solid masses, congenital abnormalities, spermatic cord torsion, and epididymo-orchitis. A comprehensive approach to the interpretation of scrotal US requires correlation of patient age, clinical presentation, and serum testicular tumor markers with imaging features to avoid radical surgery and allow consideration of observation or enucleation (testis-sparing surgery) in specific lesions.

REFERENCES
1. Ahmed HU, Arya M, Muneer A, et al. Testicular and paratesticular tumours in the prepubertal population. Lancet Oncol 2010;**11**(5):476–83.
2. Cole BD, Jayanthi VR. Imaging scrotal lumps in children. In: Bertolotto M, Trombetta C, eds. Scrotal Pathology. Heidelberg: Springer, 2012; 191–206.

3. Heidenreich A, Angerer-Shpilenya M. Organ-preserving surgery for testicular tumours. *BJU Int* 2012;**109**(3):474–90.

4. Mirone V, Verze P, Arcaniolo D. Acute scrotal pain: clinical features. In: Bertolotto M, Trombetta C, eds. *Scrotal Pathology*. Heidelberg: Springer, 2012; 85–90.

5. Shah RU, Lawrence C, Fickenscher KA, *et al*. Imaging of pediatric pelvic neoplasms. *Radiol Clin North Am* 2011;**49**(4):729–48, vi.

6. Tsili AC, Argyropoulou MI, Giannakis D, *et al*. MRI in the characterization and local staging of testicular neoplasms. *AJR Am J Roentgenol* 2010;**194**(3):682–9.

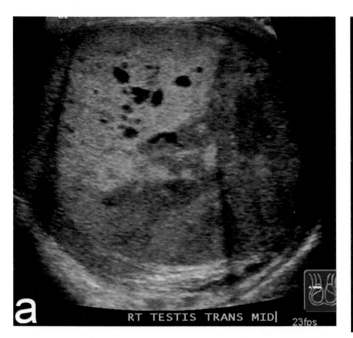

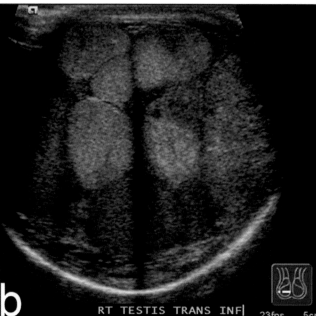

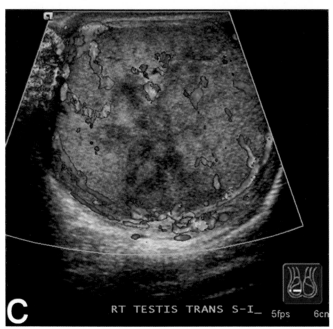

Figure 74.1. Yolk sac tumor of right testis. **(a, b)** Gray-scale US images of the right scrotum demonstrate a heterogeneously echogenic, large right intratesticular mass replacing almost the entire testis. **(c)** Color Doppler demonstrates that the mass is hypervascular.

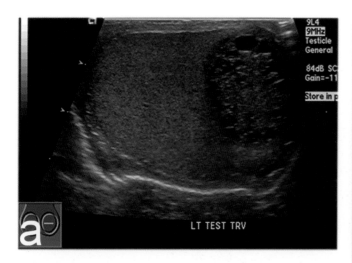
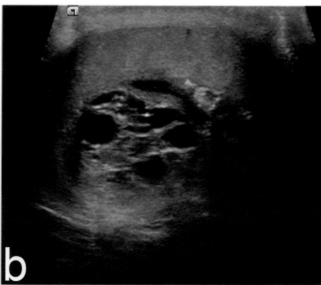

Figure 74.2. Mixed germ cell tumors. **(a, b)** Transverse gray-scale US images of testicles demonstrate complex intratesticular masses in two different patients (solid components were hypervascular on Doppler US – not shown).

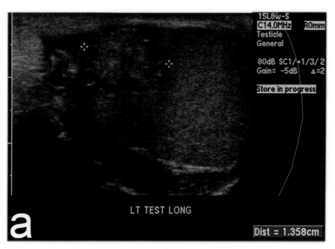
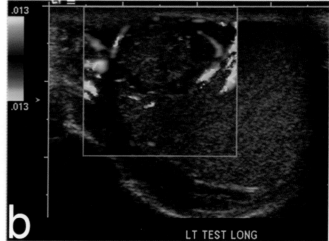

Figure 74.3. Epidermoid cyst. Longitudinal gray-scale **(a)** and color Doppler US **(b)** images of the left testis demonstrate a heterogeneously echogenic, avascular intratesticular mass.

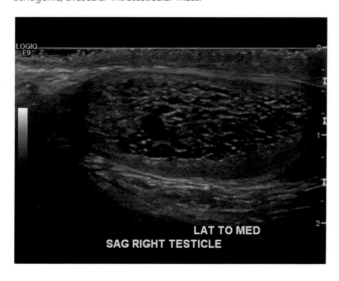

Figure 74.4. Cystic dyplasia of right testicle in a 1-month-old boy with right multicystic dysplastic kidney. Gray-scale longitudinal ultrasound demonstrates multiple cysts replacing most of the enlarged right testicle; this mass was avascular on Doppler (not shown).

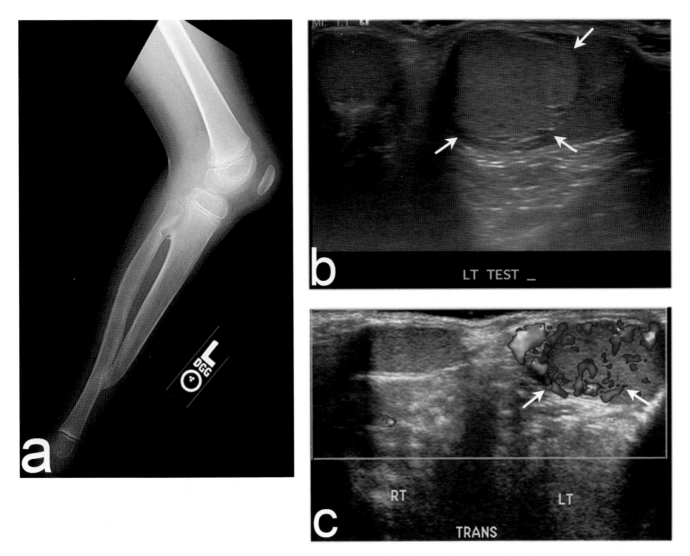

Figure 74.5. Splenogonadal fusion, discontinuous type. A 9-year-old male with a left testicular mass palpated on a routine physical exam. **(a)** Patient also had a past medical history of congenital terminal transverse arrest of left lower extremity (dysplasia of left tibia, synostosis of proximal tibia and fibula, and absence of ankle and foot). **(b, c)** Transverse US images of the testicles demonstrate a homogeneously hyperechoic and hypervascular, left intratesticular mass. Pathology specimen after orchiectectomy was consistent with splenogonadal fusion. Splenogonadal fusion may be of the continuous or discontinuous type (classified based on continuity of the gonadal tissue with either the anatomic spleen or accessory/ectopic spleen respectively). Splenogonadal fusion has been associated with other congenital anomalies, most commonly defects of the limbs.

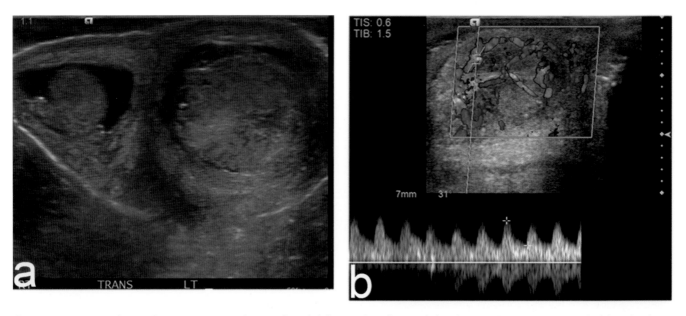

Figure 74.6. Neonatal testicular torsion in a newborn male with left scrotal swelling and discoloration. Transverse gray-scale **(a)** and color Doppler US **(b)** images demonstrate asymmetrically enlarged left testis with heterogeneous echogenicity, intraparenchymal flow, and scrotal wall thickening. Testicular torsion was confirmed on pathology.

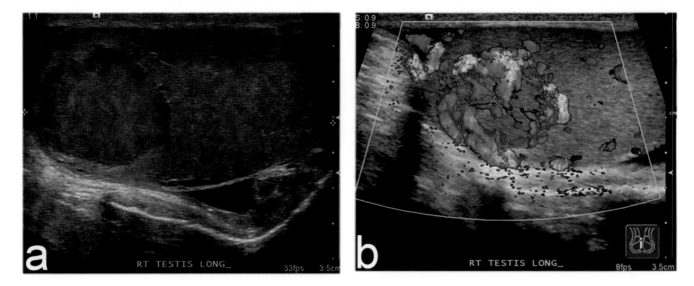

Figure 74.7. Fibrous pseudotumor. A six-year-old boy presents with a right scrotal mass. Longitudinal gray-scale **(a)** and color Doppler **(b)** images of the right testis demonstrate a slightly heterogeneous, mildly hypoechoic, hypervascular intratesticular mass. Pathology of the orchiectomy specimen was consistent with a fibrous pseudotumor.

Fetal lymphatic malformation

Erika Rubesova

Imaging description

A 32-year-old patient at 22 weeks of gestation was referred carrying a female fetus that had previously been diagnosed with a left thigh mass on ultrasound (US). Repeat US demonstrated a hypoechoic cystic soft tissue mass of the left thigh, most consistent with a lymphatic malformation (Fig. 75.1a). The mass was well circumscribed in the subcutaneous soft tissues and anterior muscle, but follow-up US demonstrated extension of the mass into the retroperitoneum. Displacement of the fetal bladder to the right and mild hydronephrosis in the left kidney was noted. Follow-up US studies were performed on a weekly basis to follow the size of the mass and check for development of hydrops fetalis. These showed progression of the lymphatic malformation with further extension into the retroperitoneum. A fetal MRI at 32 weeks showed a high T2- and low T1-signal cystic mass of the left thigh with an extensive retroperitoneal component (Fig. 75.1b, c), infiltrating the pelvic structures. Postnatally, the mass appeared as a multi-septated hypoechoic mass infiltrating most of the soft tissues of the left thigh, labia, and perineum, and extending into the retroperitoneum, surrounding the ureters (Fig. 75.1d). Slow Doppler flow was detected in the septations; the diagnosis of lymphatic malformation was confirmed, and sclerotherapy was begun.

Importance

Lymphangiomas are malformations of the lymphatic vessels or lack of communication between the lymphatic pathways and the venous system. Most lymphatic malformations are located in the neck and axilla and diagnosed during the first trimester screening US as an enlarged nuchal translucency. They are usually associated with chromosomal abnormalities. Lymphangiomas are infiltrative and may cause obstruction of the vascular structures of the neck or the upper airways.

Lymphangiomas of the abdomen and retroperitoneum are much less common and are typically not associated with chromosomal abnormalities. They are more frequently diagnosed on the anatomy scan around 20 weeks of gestational age. They may present as ascites but more frequently appear as an infiltrative hypoechoic mass with thin septations in the retroperitoneum that may extend into the limbs. US is the main modality used to diagnose and follow lymphangiomas; however, fetal MRI has been shown to be helpful for better delineation of the extent of the mass and involvement of the abdominal and retroperitoneal structures.

On color Doppler, the lesions show minimal or slow flow in the septa of the lesions. Lymphangiomas are part of a spectrum of vascular malformations, with variable degrees of lymphatic and venous components.

Large lymphangiomas involving the thigh have been described in the context of several syndromes such as Klippel–Weber syndrome.

Klippel–Weber syndrome is characterized by lymphatic or venous malformations associated with limb hypertrophy and port-wine stains.

Typical presentation

Lymphatic malformations are usually seen prenatally in the neck area and they are often associated with congenital or chromosomal abnormalities such as Down, Turner's and Noonan's syndromes. Abdominal or retroperitoneal lymphangiomas often extend into the leg. Lymphangiomatous lesions tends to grow progressively in utero but in spite of their infiltrative nature and growth, they are considered benign lesions. However, prognosis will depend on the degree of infiltration or compression of vital organs.

The lesions may be micro- or macrocystic depending on the nature and density of the tissue in which they occur. On imaging there may be prominent fluid–fluid levels and the fluid within the lesion may be echogenic on US, hyperdense on CT, or bright on T1-weighted MRI, related to the proteinaceous nature of the fluid and/or intralesional hemorrhage. Large lesions may require specific delivery planning that may include C-section or ex utero intrapartum treatment (EXIT) if the airway is compromised.

Differential diagnosis

- Neuroblastoma: The most common retroperitoneal tumor in fetuses. Usually arises from the adrenal gland or paraspinal region. It is most often a solid mass but may also be cystic to a variable degree. The cystic neuroblastoma usually has more well-defined borders than a lymphangioma.
- Adrenal hemorrhage: Adrenal hemorrhage appears as a hypoechoic mass or heterogeneous mass with septations in the adrenal area. If a fetal MRI is performed, it may demonstrate high T1 signal depending on the age of the hemorrhage.
- Teratoma: Teratoma is usually a heterogeneous mass that may be mostly cystic in the fetus. It is usually well circumscribed, displacing the adjacent structures, and may contain fat and calcifications. They can occur in the retroperitoneum and mimic a lymphangioma.
- Other vascular soft tissue lesions can include venocapillary lesions and arteriovenous malformations. These lesions contain enlarged branching vascular elements rather than the fluid-filled septated cysts typical of a lymphatic malformation. There is however overlap with lymphatic and venous lesions, quite often coexisting. Infantile hemangiomas are solid vascular lesions in the soft tissues or viscera that are usually small at birth but may rapidly enlarge in the first few months of life and tend to spontaneously involute subsequently.

- Fetal hydrops: Fetuses with hydrops will have subcutaneous edema, well seen around the calvarium, pleural effusions, and ascites. Fetuses with retroperitoneal lymphangioma may also develop fetal hydrops.

Teaching point

Lymphatic malformations are the most common cystic soft tissue mass in babies. They may grow rapidly both in utero and after birth and compress and displace vital organs, creating a relatively poor prognosis for a benign lesion. Accurate diagnosis and assessment of the extent of the lesion is essential for appropriate parental counseling, as well as pre- and postnatal management.

REFERENCES

1. Cozzi DA, Olivieri C, Manganaro F, et al. Fetal abdominal lymphangioma enhanced by ultrafast MRI. *Fetal Diagn Ther* 2010;**27**(1): 46–50.
2. Gonçalves LF, Rojas MV, Vitorello D, et al. Klippel-Trenaunay-Weber syndrome presenting as massive lymphangiohemangioma of the thigh: prenatal diagnosis. *Ultrasound Obstet Gynecol* 2000;**15**(6): 537–41.
3. Rohrer SE, Nugent CE, Mukherji SK. Fetal MR imaging of lymphatic malformation in a twin gestation. *AJR Am J Roentgenol* 2003;**181**(1): 286–7.

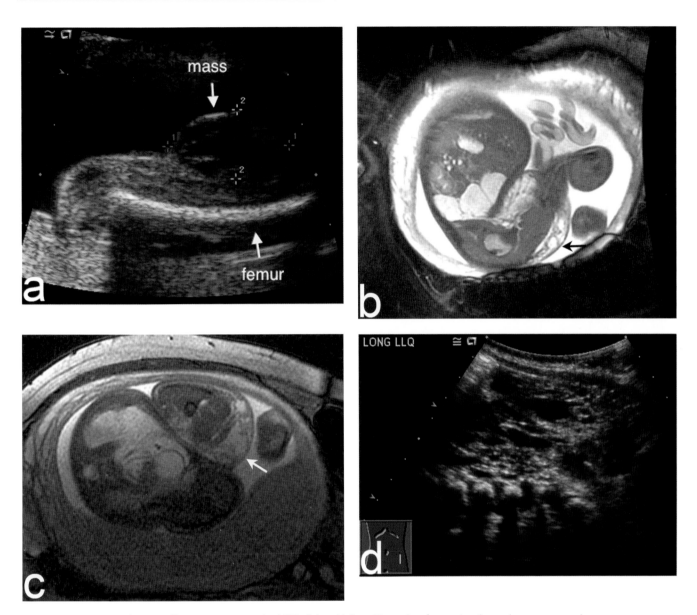

Figure 75.1. (a) Lymphatic malformation. Longitudinal US of the thigh at 22 weeks of gestational age demonstrates a heterogeneous multicystic mass arising from the soft tissues of the right thigh. The mass was well-defined, affecting anterior subcutaneous tissues and muscle. Subsequent US demonstrated extension of the mass into the fetal retroperitoneum. **(b, c)** Fetal MR at 32 weeks. Sagittal and axial views on the fetal MRI (Fiesta, GE) of the fetal abdomen and leg demonstrate the enlarging bright T2 signal lymphatic malformation extending from the thigh (arrows) into the retroperitoneum. **(d)** Postnatal longitudinal US of the left flank demonstrates the extension of the lymphangioma into the retroperitoneum. Doppler studies demonstrated some venous and arterial flow in the septa of the lesion (not shown).

Anal atresia with urorectal fistula

Erika Rubesova

Imaging description

A 21-year-old patient with twin pregnancy at 19 weeks of gestational age (GA) was referred for echogenic bowel on ultrasound (US) in one of the two male fetuses. On repeat US some mildly distended loops of bowel were noted and the presence of echogenic bowel was confirmed. A fetal MRI was performed at 22 weeks of GA. T1-weighted images failed to demonstrate normal high signal meconium in the rectum (Fig. 76.1a). The fluid-sensitive sequences demonstrated distended fluid-filled colon, including the rectum, and within the fluid multiple low signal intensity pellets were noted. The diagnosis of imperforate anus with urorectal fistula was made based on these findings. The follow-up US and MRI at 32 weeks of gestational age confirmed the findings (Fig. 76.1b, c). A newborn abdominal radiograph demonstrated discrete oval to rounded calcifications along the course of the colon, consistent with intraluminal calcified meconium. The infant was treated surgically for imperforate anus with urorectal fistula.

Importance

In the fetus, meconium is formed primarily by the accumulation of dehydrated amniotic fluid swallowed by the fetus, bile salts, and desquamation of enteric cells. On US, meconium has intermediate echogenicity while on MRI images meconium has high T1 and low T2 signal. Since fetuses apparently do not pass large amounts of meconium during pregnancy, meconium accumulates in the rectum, which is the largest meconium-filled area of the fetal bowel. Anal atresia is therefore difficult to diagnose prenatally by US or MRI if there is not an associated urorectal fistula. Anal atresia is typically differentiated into two types: low atresia (below the levator ani muscle) and high atresia (above the levator ani muscle). An urorectal fistula is typically associated with high anal atresia, mainly in boys (ratio boys:girls = 6:1). In girls, imperforate anus is most frequently associated with urogenital sinus or a cloaca. Cloaca usually presents with a fluid-filled bladder and vagina and with a rudimentary sigmoid colon.

In anal atresia with urorectal fistula, the mixing of urine with meconium may result in the precipitation and calcification of intraluminal meconium. It is not clearly understood why the meconium calcifies but some authors suggest that the calcification of meconium is the result of changes in pH due to the presence of alkaline urine in the bowel. Precipitated and calcified meconium appears on imaging as small pellets called enteroliths that are floating in the urine-filled bowel. They are echogenic on US and have low T1 and T2 signal intensity on MRI. This finding is strongly suggestive of anal atresia with urorectal fistula, but can also occur in other types of urorectal malformation where urine is in contact with meconium.

Enteroliths are only rarely seen in the fetal colon in a female with a cloacal anomaly.

It is important to pay special attention to the rectum in the fetus to assess normal echogenicity of meconium and rule out any urorectal malformation.

Typical clinical scenario

The diagnosis of a bowel abnormality may be suggested prenatally on a screening anatomic US, usually between 18 and 22 weeks GA. US may demonstrate dilated loops of bowel with hypoechoic content and echogenic pellets within the bowel lumen, suggesting the likely diagnosis of high imperforate anus with urorectal fistula. If a fetal MRI is performed, T1-weighted images demonstrate a lack of high T1 meconium signal at the level of the fetal rectum. Absence of meconium in the rectum should always raise a concern for bowel abnormality in a fetus beyond 20 weeks, GA. Fluid-sensitive images demonstrate the presence of fluid in the rectum, which is also always abnormal in a fetus at any GA. The calcified pellets can also be seen on the prenatal MRI as low T2 signal structures within the bowel lumen.

Differential diagnosis

1. Echogenic bowel: Is a soft marker in prenatal US and is seen in fetuses with cystic fibrosis and meconium ileus, with chromosomal abnormalities, or viral infections; the bowel will appear diffusely echogenic, similar to adjacent bone.

2. Meconium ileus: Is often observed in fetuses with cystic fibrosis. Meconium ileus usually manifests with dilated loops of distal small bowel filled with very echogenic meconium. On fetal MRI, microcolon will be noted, with a relatively small rectum, with absence of both meconium and fluid in the colon and rectum.

3. Meconium peritonitis: When an in utero bowel perforation has occurred (most commonly associated with meconium ileus), calcifications will be seen in the peritoneal cavity or a fluid, and meconium-filled cyst. The calcifications associated with meconium peritonitis tend to be clustered along peritoneal surfaces and the edge of intraperitoneal organs such as the liver. Particularly on postnatal radiographs, meconium peritonitis should not be confused with intraluminal calcified meconium, which is discrete calcific pellets that follow the course of the colon (Fig. 76.1d).

4. Distal ileal atresia: Dilated loops of distal small bowel and microcolon may be seen. The rectum is usually small and difficult to identify without normal meconium signal or fluid.

5. Congenital chloride diarrhea: Is a rare anomaly of transmembrane chloride transport in the fetal bowel and presents with diffuse distention of the bowel by fluid, including the colon and the rectum. Meconium is not identified on

T1-weighted images nor are enteroliths seen in the fluid-filled bowel.

6. Hirschsprung's disease is included in the causes of fetal and neonatal distal bowel obstruction with a small caliber rectum without normal meconium. With long segment Hirschsprung's disease there is a variable length of microcolon with dilatation of bowel proximal to the transition point between ganglionic and aganglionic bowel. Hirschsprung's disease has been difficult to definitively identify prenatally.

Teaching point

A small or fluid-filled rectum in a fetus is always abnormal. High T1 signal meconium should be identified in the rectum by the third trimester. Presence of fluid-filled sigmoid and rectum-containing enteroliths is strongly suggestive of high anal atresia with urorectal fistula or other urorectal malformation with fecal/urine mixing.

REFERENCES

1. Lubusky M, Prochazka M, Dhaifalah I, *et al.* Fetal enterolithiasis: prenatal sonographic and MRI diagnosis in two cases of urorectal septum malformation (URSM) sequence. *Prenat Diagn* 2006;**26**(4): 345–9.

2. Rubesova E, Vance CJ, Ringertz HG, *et al.* Three-dimensional MRI volumetric measurements of the normal fetal colon. *AJR Am J Roentgenol* 2009;**192**(3):761–5.

3. Veyrac C, Couture A, Saguintaah M, *et al.* MRI of fetal GI tract abnormalities. *Abdom Imaging* 2004;**29**(4):411–20.

4. Walker AJ. Caecal faecolith; a report on two cases. *Br J Surg* 1948 **36**(141):55–8.

5. Zizka J, Elias P, Hodik K, *et al.* Liver, meconium, haemorrhage: the value of T1-weighted images in fetal MRI. *Pediatr Radiol* 2006;**36**(8): 792–801.

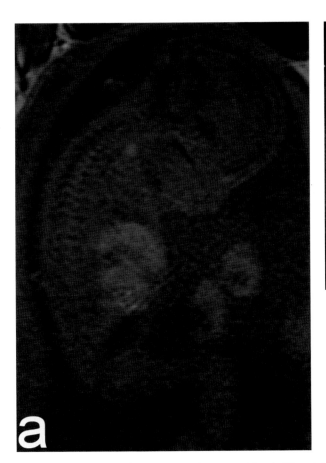
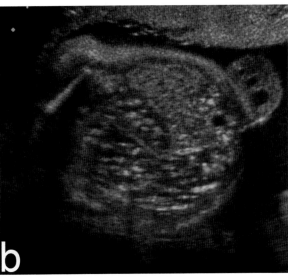

Figure 76.1. (a) Imperforate anus with urorectal fistula. T1-weighted image of the fetus at 22 weeks of GA demonstrates absence of high T1 signal meconium in the rectum. Note high signal content in more proximal dilated loops of bowel, a reversal of the normal appearance on a T1-weighted image. **(b)** Axial US image through the abdomen of the fetus at 32 weeks of GA demonstrates dilated bowel filled with fluid and echogenic pellets consistent with enteroliths. This is pathognomonic for intraluminal meconium that calcifies in contact with urine.

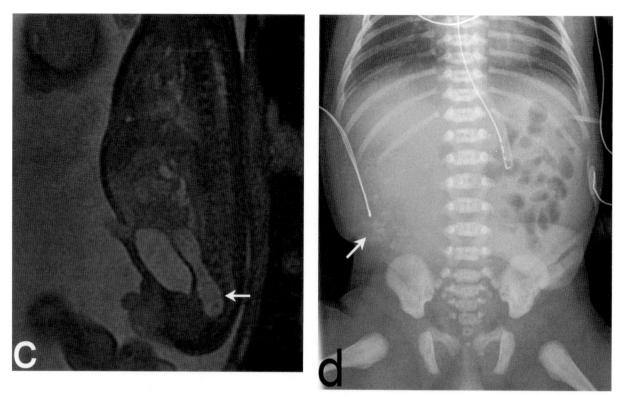

Figure 76.1. (cont.) **(c)** T2-weighted sagittal image of the fetus at 32 weeks of GA demonstrates a distended fluid-filled rectum (arrow) containing low signal intensity pellets. **(d)** Postnatal abdominal film demonstrates presence of calcified intraluminal meconium best visualized in the dilated cecum and ascending colon (arrow).

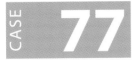
Cystic dysplasia of the kidneys

Erika Rubesova

Imaging description

A 16-year-old patient was diagnosed at 22 weeks of gestational age (GA) with a fetus with multicystic dysplastic kidney (MCDK). The contralateral kidney appeared slightly echogenic but otherwise normal on ultrasound (Fig. 77.1a,b). Fetal MRI confirmed large disorganized cortical cysts of different size in the right kidney but also demonstrated the presence of small subcortical cysts in the left kidney (Fig. 77.1c). However, the amount of amniotic fluid remained normal throughout the pregnancy and the patient carried the baby to term. At birth, ultrasound of the kidneys confirmed a right MCDK that got progressively smaller over time (Fig. 77.1d, f), but failed to demonstrate the small subcortical cysts in the left kidney (Fig. 77.1e). A dysplastic appearance of the left kidney with subcortical cysts was only noticed on follow-up ultrasound at the age of 1 year (Fig. 77.1g). The renal function was mildly decreased postnatally.

Importance

Renal cystic dysplasia is usually unilateral and may affect an entire kidney, a segment of a kidney, or a pole of a duplex kidney. Recent studies demonstrate that MCDK and obstructive dysplasia may have a similar pathogenesis, with glomerular cysts being the initial dysplastic event in the kidneys. Early prenatal studies show that MCDK appear as normal kidneys on ultrasound up to 14 weeks of gestational age despite complete obstruction. They are often diagnosed at the routine anatomic scan around 20 weeks of gestational age. Small subcortical cysts in the setting of obstructive dysplasia may appear later in pregnancy or after birth and are often more difficult to diagnose prenatally than MCDK.

During pregnancy, a single functioning kidney is usually sufficient to produce a normal amount of amniotic fluid. If the MCDK is unilateral, most newborns will have normal or only slightly impaired renal function at birth.

When both kidneys are affected there may be poor renal function in utero manifesting as oligo- or anhydramnios. It is important to evaluate the contralateral kidney in fetuses with unilateral MCDK since about 20% of contralateral kidneys to MCDK may have some dysplasia, obstruction, or vesicoureteral reflux. When bilateral renal dysplasia is present, parental counseling and fetal management will be significantly different than in a fetus with a contralateral normal kidney. The definitive role of fetal MRI in the evaluation of MCDK prenatally has not yet been clearly established; however, at our institution, we have noticed that small subcortical cysts are better seen on fetal MRI than ultrasound and therefore we encourage clinicians to order fetal MRI in cases of unilateral MCDK for detailed evaluation of the contralateral kidney.

Postnatally the newborn will undergo additional examinations such as voiding cystourethrogram (VCUG) and renal ultrasound to assess the growth and normality of the non-affected kidney. It is imperative to examine the kidneys carefully using a high-resolution linear transducer in order to appreciate subtle abnormalities such as tiny subcortical cysts.

Typical clinical presentation

The diagnosis of cystic dysplasia is usually suggested on the prenatal anatomic screening ultrasound around 20 weeks of gestational age. Cysts of variable size will be noticed in the affected fetal kidney. It is important to pay special attention to increased renal echogenicity, loss of corticomedullary differentiation, and presence of small subcortical cysts. Hydronephrosis (pelvis measuring in transverse diameter more than 4 mm before 32 weeks and more than 7 mm after 32 weeks) may or may not be present. When the diagnosis is challenging, especially in patients with a large body habitus or oligohydramnios, MRI may be helpful to visualize the small subcortical cysts and make the diagnosis of subtle cystic renal dysplasia.

Differential diagnosis

1. Hydronephrosis: Renal pelvis and the renal calyces interconnect as opposed to discrete separate cysts. The collecting system may be markedly dilated but there is usually some visible surrounding cortex. The cortex may be echogenic and small peripheral dysplastic cysts may be present. Common causes of obstruction in utero include ureteropelvic junction obstruction, ureterovesical junction obstruction, posterior urethral valves, and obstructed ectopic upper pole of a duplicated collecting system.
2. Cystic neuroblastoma: A congenital tumor arising from the adrenal gland and appears as a cystic lesion that displaces the kidney inferiorly.
3. Mesoblastic nephroma: A heterogeneous lesion of the kidney; is usually predominantly solid but may have some cystic or hemorrhagic components.
4. Autosomal recessive polycystic kidney disease: Hereditary disease where the kidneys are affected bilaterally; they appear large for GA and echogenic due to the reflection of the ultrasound beam at the many cyst–parenchyma interfaces.
5. Autosomal dominant polycystic kidney disease: Hereditary disease affecting both kidneys. Although the cysts usually appear in adulthood, it may be detected in some instances prenatally. Few macrocysts may be present later; both kidneys are affected with cysts in the cortex and medulla.
6. Syndromal cysts: Cystic renal disease can be seen in several syndromes such as Meckel's syndrome, tuberous sclerosis,

von Hippel–Lindau disease, and Lawrence–Moon–Biedl–Bardet syndrome.

Teaching point

It is essential to perform careful examination of the renal cortex in order to assess the echogenicity of the renal parenchyma and presence of small subcortical cysts. Bilateral renal dysplasia raises concern for impaired renal function both pre- and postnatally.

REFERENCES

1. Aslam M, Watson AR; Trent & Anglia MCDK Study Group. Unilateral multicystic dysplastic kidney: long-term outcomes. *Arch Dis Child* 2006;**91**(10):820–3.
2. Cambio AJ, Evans CP, Kurzrock EA. Non-surgical management of multicystic dysplastic kidney. *BJU Int* 2008;**101**(7):804–8.
3. Kuwertz-Broeking E, Brinkmann OA, Von Lengerke HJ, *et al.* Unilateral multicystic dysplastic kidney: experience in children. *BJU Int* 2004;**93**(3):388–92.
4. Nagata M, Shibata S, Shu Y. Pathogenesis of dysplastic kidney associated with urinary tract obstruction in utero. *Nephrol Dial Transplant* 2002;**17**(Suppl 9):37–8.

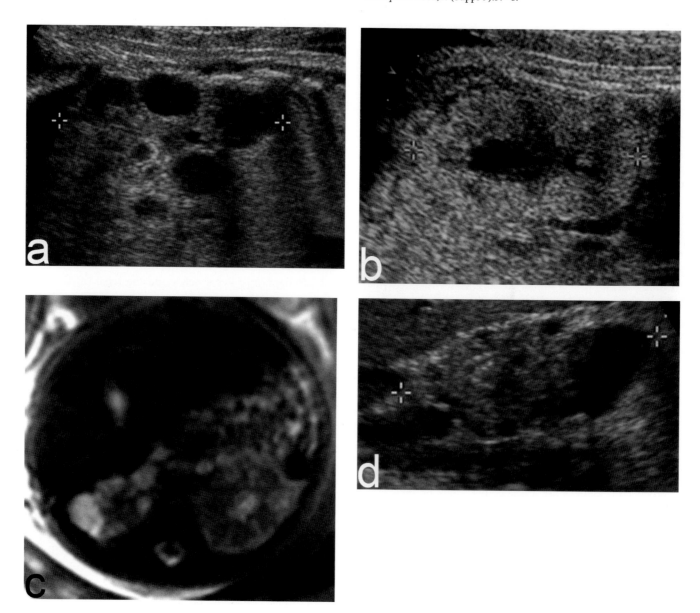

Figure 77.1. Cystic renal dysplasia. Prenatal ultrasound at 22 weeks of gestational age demonstrated a right MCDK (a) and a slightly echogenic but otherwise normal appearing left kidney (b). A subsequent fetal MRI, axial T2-weighted image (c) demonstrated multiple subcortical cysts in the left kidney and confirmed disorganized cysts of various sizes on the right consistent with MCDK. Longitudinal postnatal ultrasound images at birth (d, e) and at the age of 1 year (f, g) confirmed a progressively atrophying MCDK on the right. The subcortical cysts in the left kidney were not visualized at birth (e) but only at 1 year of age (calipers in g) when a high-resolution linear transducer was utilized.

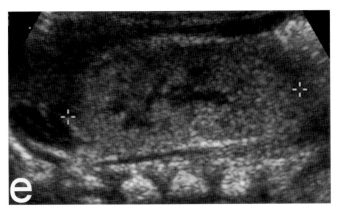

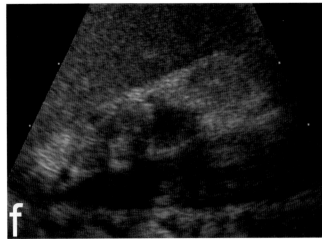

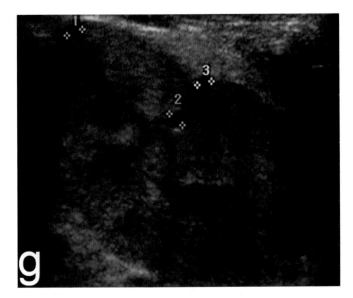

Figure 77.1. (cont.)

Gastroschisis

Binh Huynh and Erika Rubesova

Imaging description

Gastroschisis is a para-umbilical, anterior abdominal wall defect, resulting in the herniation of bowel, and occasionally other organs, such as stomach and liver, into the amniotic cavity. The defect is usually to the right of midline and the umbilicus insertion (Figs. 78.1a–f and see 78.3a, b). There is no membrane covering the herniated structures and, as a result the extracorporeal loops of bowel are directly exposed to amniotic fluid. This causes an inflammatory, fibrous coating on the bowel, called peel; additionally, there is thickening of the muscularis propria and atrophy of the mucosa (Fig. 78.1b).

During fetal gastrointestinal development, the midgut elongates rapidly, such that at the sixth week of gestation, developing loops of bowel project into the extra-embryonic coelom, causing physiologic herniation of bowel into the umbilicus (Fig. 78.2a and b). The intestines return into the fetal abdominal cavity after 11 weeks of gestation. As a result, the diagnosis of an anterior abdominal wall defect should not be made until after this event is expected to have occurred.

Importance

The prenatal diagnosis of gastroschisis warrants close interval fetal monitoring to assess for the development of complications, such as bowel atresia, infarction, and perforation. The inflammatory changes that result from exposure of bowel to amniotic fluid may cause decreased bowel motility, and possibly bowel atresia. Constriction of bowel at the site of the abdominal wall defect will lead to bowel dilatation, and possibly bowel necrosis (Fig. 78.3c). The inherent malrotation of the bowel increases the risk of volvulus. Significant postnatal morbidity may occur as a result of short gut syndrome. The prognosis for gastroschisis depends on the severity of prenatal and neonatal bowel injury. Intra-abdominal dilatation has been associated with poorer prognosis but there have been no definitive prenatal sonographic findings, including bowel wall thickness, degree of dilatation, or Doppler flow, to predict bowel atresia or postnatal gastrointestinal dysfunction.

Associated anomalies are rarely seen in fetuses with gastroschisis, unlike other anterior abdominal wall defects, such as omphaloceles. When evaluated independent of these anomalies, patients with gastroschisis actually have a poorer prognosis secondary to the severity of the bowel complications.

Typical clinical scenario

The diagnosis of gastroschisis is typically made prenatally with routine fetal ultrasound and screening maternal serum alpha-fetoprotein levels, which are elevated. The incidence is 0.5–1.0 cases per 10 000 births. The most common epidemiologic factor has been young maternal age, generally less than 20 years old, with associated factors including environmental teratogens, such as cigarette smoking and drug abuse.

Differential diagnosis

The differential considerations for gastroschisis include omphalocele and especially ruptured omphalocele. Imaging characteristics of an omphalocele include a midline, anterior abdominal mass surrounded by a membrane, made of amnion, Wharton jelly, and parietal peritoneum. The cord insertion is seen at the apex of the mass. Over 50% of omphalocele cases are associated with other physical, genetic, and chromosomal anomalies, which determine the prognosis of these patients.

Other less common anterior abdominal wall defects include bladder exstrophy which manifests by absence of bladder on prenatal ultrasound. Bladder exstrophy is part of a spectrum of anomalies ranging from epispadias to cloacal exstrophy.

Ectopia cordis is a rare but severe abnormality of the thoracoabdominal wall where the heart is partially or completely herniated ouside the fetal chest. The most extreme form of abdominal wall defect is the limb–body wall complex that manifests with severe scoliosis, limb anomalies, abdominal and thoracic wall defects, as well as craniofacial anomalies.

Teaching point

The diagnosis of gastroschisis should be made when a para-umbilical, anterior abdominal wall defect is seen with herniation of non-membrane covered bowel, after 11 weeks of gestation. The prognosis of gastroschisis depends on the severity of bowel injury and is infrequently associated with other anomalies.

REFERENCES

1. Callen PW, ed. *Ultrasonography in Obstetrics and Gynecology*, 4th edition. Philadelphia: W.B. Saunders, 2000.

2. Christison-Lagay ER, Kelleher CM, Langer JC. Neonatal abdominal wall defects. *Semin Fetal Neonatal Med* 2011;**16**(3):164–72.

3. Slovis TL, ed. *Caffey's Pediatric Diagnostic Imaging*, 11th edition. Philadelphia: Mosby Elsevier, 2008.

4. Wilson RD, Johnson MP. Congenital abdominal wall defects: an update. *Fetal Diagn Ther* 2004;**19**(5):385–98.

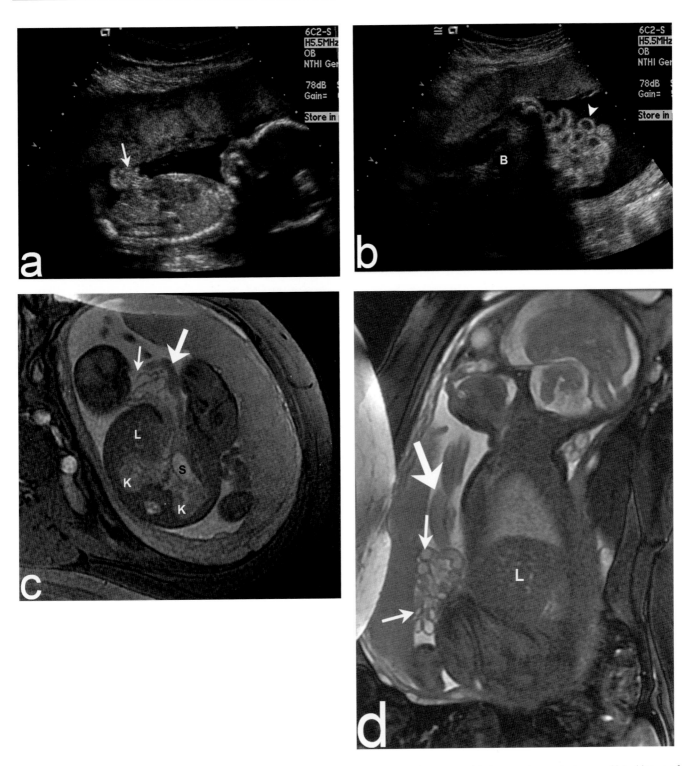

Figure 78.1. Gastroschisis. (a, b) Longitudinal (a) and zoomed transverse (b) gray-scale sonographic images demonstrate non-dilated loops of bowel (arrow) herniating through an anterior abdominal wall defect in this fetus with gastroschisis at 29 weeks' gestation to a mother of young maternal age, 17 years old. The bowel is not covered by a membrane and is directly exposed to amniotic fluid. This causes an inflammatory, fibrotic coating on the bowel, called peel, resulting in thickened, echogenic bowel wall (arrowhead). (c, d, e) Transverse (c) and sagittal FIESTA (d) and transverse SSFSE MR (e) images in the same fetus at the same gestational age demonstrate herniation of small bowel (thin arrows) and colon (curved arrow) through an anterior abdominal wall defect to the right of the umbilical cord (bold arrow). The loops of small bowel are not dilated and contain T2-hyperintense fluid. (f) Sagittal T1-weighted image demonstrates the hyperintense meconium contents of the colon. The rectosigmoid colon is in the abdominal cavity while the more proximal colon is seen herniating through the defect (B = urinary bladder, L = liver, K = kidneys, S = stomach).

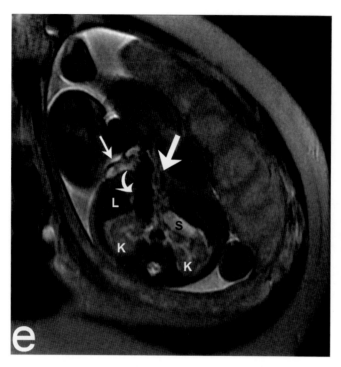

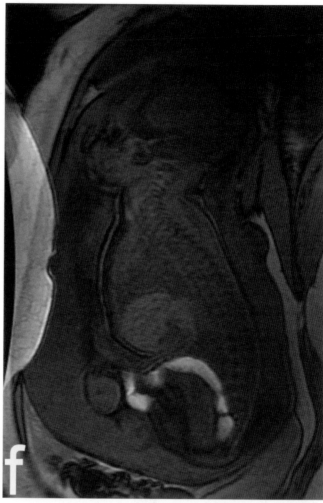

Figure 78.1. (cont.)

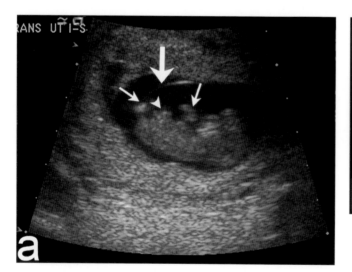

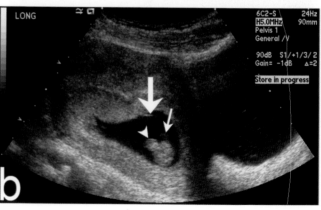

Figure 78.2. Physiologic bowel herniation into the umbilical cord in early gestation. Longitudinal **(a)** and transverse **(b)** gray-scale sonographic images demonstrate an echogenic mass external to the anterior abdominal wall (arrowhead). Real-time cine images revealed the echogenic mass was contained by the extra-embryonic coelom and was in continuity with the cord and placenta. In this fetus of 9 weeks' gestation, the amniotic membrane is still visible (bold arrow). This mass was no longer present on follow-up prenatal ultrasound and represented physiologic herniation of bowel into the umbilical cord. The diagnosis of an anterior abdominal wall defect, such as gastroschisis or omphalocele, should not be made until after 11 weeks of gestation, following the expected return of bowel into the abdominal cavity (arrows = fetal limbs).

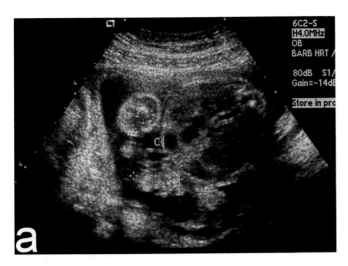

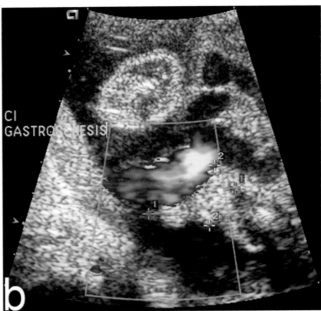

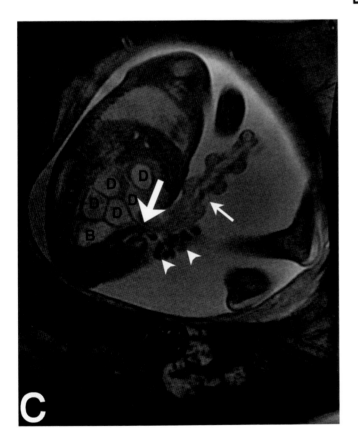

Figure 78.3. **(a, b)** Transverse gray-scale (a) and Power Doppler (b) sonographic images demonstrate non-dilated echogenic loops of bowel (calipers) herniating through an anterior abdominal wall defect, in this fetus with gastroschisis. The defect is located to the right of the umbilical cord insertion (CI) which is demonstrated by the Power Doppler flow. This fetus is 26 weeks' gestation to an 18-year-old mother. **(c)** Sagittal SSFSE fetal MR image of the same fetus at 31 weeks' gestation demonstrates interval development of dilated intra-abdominal bowel loops (D), with the site of obstruction at the anterior abdominal wall defect (bold arrow). The herniated loops of bowel are decompressed (arrowheads), and are not covered by a membrane, with direct exposure to amniotic fluid (arrow = umbilical cord, B = urinary bladder).

Fetal osteogenesis imperfecta

Jordan Caplan and Erika Rubesova

Imaging description

A 37-year-old G2P1 white female presented for a fetal anatomic survey at 19 weeks 3 days gestational age. She had been previously seen by the Genetic Counseling Service to discuss prenatal diagnosis options due to maternal age. She chose to proceed with sequential screening by nuchal translucency and first and second trimester biochemical analysis. Results of the sequential screening were negative.

Fetal ultrasound images showed an abnormal triangular-shaped calvarium (Fig. 79.1a) which demonstrated deformity on compression by the ultrasound probe (Fig. 79.1b). The fetal chest was abnormally shaped, with irregular contour of the ribs (Fig. 79.1c). The fetal humeri and femora were extremely short, with the length corresponding to a 13- to 14-week fetus (Fig. 79.1d, e). The head circumference, by comparison, reflected the true gestational age of 19 weeks 3 days (images not shown). The findings were strongly suggestive of osteogenesis imperfecta (OI).

After genetic counseling the couple decided to undergo termination of the pregnancy. Tissue was sent for mutation analysis of the *COL1A1* and *COL1A2* genes.

The fetus was heterozygous for the mutation Gly529Asp, a nucleotide G to A substitution that converted a codon for glycine to a codon for aspartic acid. Although this exact mutation had not been previously reported, similar mutations in this region have been identified in patients diagnosed with OI types II and III. DNA analysis of the parents showed this mutation to be a *de novo* fetal mutation.

Importance

Osteogenesis imperfecta is a genetic disorder of the bones and connective tissues that is characterized by bone fragility. The basic mechanism is abnormal synthesis of the type I collagen molecule caused by mutations in the *COL1A1* and *COL1A2* genes. Seven subtypes of OI have been described, although types I–IV account for approximately 95% of cases (Table 79.1).

Skeletal dysplasias comprise a group of genetic conditions characterized by variable bony involvement. Abnormalities of the skeleton may include the shape of bones, the number of bones, bone length, and bone density.

Typical clinical scenario

OI is one of the most common genetic diseases affecting the skeleton, occurring worldwide without gender preference. The disease occurs in approximately one in every 10 000 live births and affects between 25 000 and 50 000 patients in the US.

Diagnosis of OI and other skeletal dysplasias is usually made during fetal sonography. OI type II and other lethal skeletal dysplasias can be diagnosed at 14–16 weeks gestational age by ultrasound and earlier by DNA- or protein-based methods. Molecular diagnosis is available which will detect approximately 90% of OI mutations.

It may not be possible to reach a specific diagnosis in cases of skeletal dysplasia; however, a lethal disorder may be diagnosed with high confidence. Lethality in OI is caused by pulmonary hypoplasia secondary to an abnormally formed, restrictive thorax.

Criteria used to diagnose lethal skeletal dysplasia

- Early, severe micromelia
- Femur length:abdominal circumference <0.16
- Thoracic circumference <5th percentile
- Thoracic circumference:abdominal circumference <0.79
- Cardiac circumference:thoracic circumference >0.60

Differential diagnosis

Of the over 200 skeletal dysplasias, the four most commonly diagnosed prenatally are: thanatophoric dysplasia, achondrogenesis, achondroplasia, and OI type II. Of these, only achondroplasia is non-lethal.

Achondroplasia is the most common non-lethal skeletal dysplasia and manifests with the combination of mainly rhizomelia and to a lesser degree of mesomelia, and acromelia.

Fetal findings in achondrogenesis range from short limbs to extreme micromelia, with variable degrees of under mineralization of the bones and particularly the axial skeleton.

Thanatophoric dysplasia is an autosomal dominant lethal condition that presents with short limbs and characteristic "telephone receiver femurs."

Hypophosphatasia causes profound undermineralization of the skeleton with limb deformities.

Trisomies 13 and 18 present with short long bones secondary to intrauterine growth restriction but without osseous undermineralization. Trisomy 21 may present with mild shortening of the humeri and femora.

Teaching points

- When a skeletal dysplasia is discovered in utero, a multidisciplinary approach to diagnosis and treatment is recommended, including consultation with medical genetics, maternal–fetal medicine, neonatology, and pathology.
- OI is a genetic disorder caused by abnormal synthesis of type I collagen that affects the bones and soft tissues and is characterized by bone fragility.
- OI type II is lethal in the perinatal period, and OI type III is severe, causing short stature with progressive deformity and scoliosis.

REFERENCES

1. Byers PH, Krakow D, Nunes ME, *et al.* Genetic evaluation of suspected osteogenesis imperfecta (OI). *Genet Med* 2006;**8**(6):383–8.

2. Cassart M. Suspected fetal skeletal malformations or bone diseases: how to explore. *Pediatr Radiol* 2010;**40**(6):1046–51.

3. Lachman RS. Skeletal dysplasias. In: Slovis TL, ed. *Caffey's Pediatric Diagnostic Imaging*, 11th edition. Philadelphia: Mosby Elsevier, 2008; 2613–70.

4. Martin E, Shapiro JR. Osteogenesis imperfecta: epidemiology and pathophysiology. *Curr Osteoporos Rep* 2007;**5**(3):91–7.

5. McCarthy EF. Genetic diseases of bones and joints. *Semin Diagn Pathol* 2011;**28**(1):26–36.

6. Shapiro JR, Sponsellor PD. Osteogenesis imperfecta: questions and answers. *Curr Opin Pediatr* 2009;**21**(6):709–16.

7. Teele RL. A guide to the recognition of skeletal disorders in the fetus. *Pediatr Radiol* 2006;**36**(6):473–84.

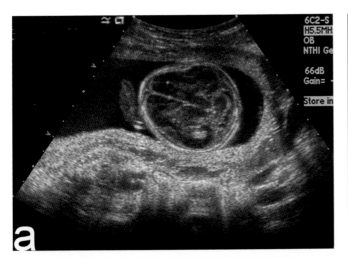

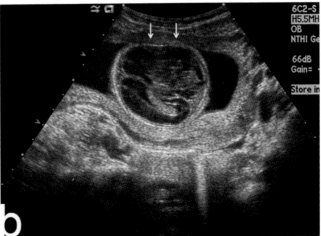

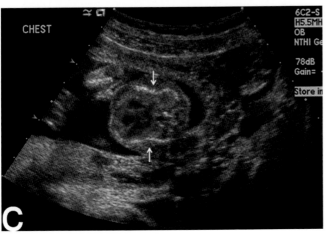

Figure 79.1. Osteogenesis imperfecta. (a) Axial ultrasound image of the fetal calvarium at 19 weeks 3 days demonstrates an abnormal triangular configuration. (b) Axial ultrasound image with gentle compression by the sonographer demonstrates deformation of the calvarium (arrows), indicating abnormal osseous fragility. (c) Axial ultrasound image through the fetal thorax shows the ribs to be irregularly shaped (arrows). (d) Measurement of the fetal humerus at 19 weeks 3 days gestational age shows abnormal shortening, corresponding to a gestational age of 13 weeks 5 days. (e) Measurement of the fetal femur also shows relative shortening, with additional abnormal angulation.

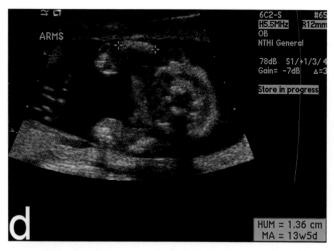
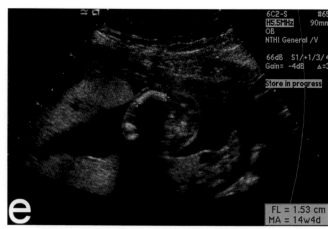

Figure 79.1. (cont.)

Table 79.1

Type	Genetics	Clinical findings	Ultrasound findings in utero
OI I	Autosomal dominant	Fractures with little or no limb deformity, blue sclerae, normal stature, hearing loss, dentinogenesis imperfecta (DI)	Rarely, long bone bowing or fracture
OI II	Autosomal dominant	Lethal perinatal type: undermineralized skull, micromelic bones, "beaded" ribs on x-ray, bone deformity, platyspondyly	Undermineralization; broad, crumpled, and shortened limbs; thin beaded ribs; fractures; angulation or bowing of long bones; normal appearing hands; deformable calvarium
OI III	Autosomal dominant	Progressively deforming type: moderate deformity of limbs at birth, scleral hue varies, very short stature, DI	Thin ribs, short curved limbs, fractures, undermineralized calvarium
OI IV	Autosomal dominant	Normal sclerae, mild/moderate limb deformity with fracture, variable short stature, DI, some hearing loss	Rarely, long bone bowing and/or fracture
OI V	Autosomal dominant	Similar to OI IV plus calcification of interosseous membrane of forearm, radial head dislocation, hyperplastic callus formation	Unknown
OI VI	Unknown	More fractures than OI type IV, vertebral compression fractures, no DI	Unknown
OI VII	Autosomal recessive	Congenital fractures, blue sclerae, early deformity of legs, coxa vara, osteopenia	Unknown

Adapted from Byers PH, Krakow D, Nunes ME, *et al.* Genetic evaluation of suspected osteogenesis imperfecta (OI). *Genet Med* 2006;**8**(6):383–8.

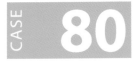

Congenital diaphragmatic hernia

Vy Thao Tran and Erika Rubesova

Imaging description

Antenatal screening ultrasound (US) demonstrated multiple echogenic rounded foci within the left chest causing mass effect on the heart. The stomach was not noted to be in its expected location within the left upper abdomen. Longitudinal US images demonstrated the stomach above the diaphragm and the heart shifted towards the right side of the chest (Fig. 80.1a, b). T2-weighted MR sequences demonstrated multiple rounded hyperintense (fluid-filled) bowel loops in the left chest and the heart shifted towards the right aspect of the chest (Fig. 80.1c–e). The diagnosis of left congenital diaphragmatic hernia (CDH) was suggested. Immediate postnatal chest radiograph in a different patient with CDH demonstrated both opacification of the left hemithorax and multiple rounded lucencies in the left thorax, representing a combination of herniated tissues and gaseous distended bowel loops (Fig. 80.2).

Importance

CDH affects 1/3000 live births. The diaphragm is completely formed at eight weeks of gestation by the septum transversum and the pleuroperitoneal membranes. A defect in formation of the diaphragm leads to CDH. Approximately 85–90% of diaphragmatic hernias occur on the posterolateral left side, referred to as a Bochladek hernia, 5% occur in the anteromedial region, referred to as a Morgagni hernia. Morgagni hernias are frequently small and asymptomatic and discovered incidentally postnatally. The following discussion refers to the Bochdalek hernia as CDH. Despite advances in antenatal and perinatal care, when CDH is associated with morphologic or genetic anomalies, there is a high overall mortality rate of up to 50%. Severe pulmonary hypoplasia and pulmonary hypertension are the main etiologies for one-third of neonatal deaths from CDH. The administration of antenatal steroids, use of extracorporeal membrane oxygenation (ECMO), new modes of ventilation, timing of the hernia repair, as well as ex utero intrapartum treatment (EXIT) to ECMO along with intermittent in utero fetal tracheal occlusion have provided neonatologists and surgeons with various modes of management. Surgical repair consists of a subcostal incision, reduction of the hernia, and primary surgical repair with a prosthetic patch if the defect is large. Because the synthetic material lacks the ability for growth, hernia recurrences can occur. In addition to the pulmonary hypoplasia that occurs bilaterally from mass effect from the herniated abdominal contents and mediastinal shift, infants with CDH often have increased pulmonary vascular resistance. This may be due to a hypoplastic vascular bed and abnormal arterial muscular structure as well as functional abnormalities of the pulmonary vasculature. Persistence of pulmonary hypertension is associated with an increased risk for early death.

Several US and MRI findings are associated with poor outcomes. Liver position is one of the most important prognostic factors. Liver herniation into the chest is associated with a mortality rate of 57%. The severity of pulmonary hypoplasia is also an important determinant of survival. The lung to head ratio (LHR) is an US measurement performed by obtaining orthogonal dimensions of the unaffected lung at the level of the four-chamber heart view and dividing by the head circumference to attempt to correct for gestational age. LHR is most reliable at predicting outcome when performed between 24 and 34 weeks (Fig. 80.3). Because the lung grows faster than the head circumference, other means of measuring LHR include the observed to expected LHR, which takes the measured LHR and divides it by the mean LHR of the same lung in a normal fetus of a given gestational age. Utilizing this method, fetuses with observed/expected (O/E) LHR of less than 15% do not survive, O/E LHR of less than 25% is associated with a survival rate of <20%, and fetuses with O/E LHR greater than 45% have a survival rate of >75%. Because MRI provides excellent soft tissue delineation, it is useful to help identify any additional pathologies and extremely helpful in confirming liver up or down morphology. Quantifying liver herniation and comparing it as a percentage to total thoracic volume is also predictive of postnatal survival. Additionally, MRI is the method of choice in volumetric analysis of the lungs (Fig. 80.4). To acquire lung volumes, axial images are obtained at slice thicknesses of 3–5 mm without an intersection gap. The lung tissue is outlined by free hand to obtain a computer-generated region of interest or area. The mediastinum and hila are excluded. The areas from contiguous sections are summed and then multiplied by the section thickness to obtain the total fetal lung volume in cubic centimeters. Charted ranges of fetal lung volumes in normal fetuses can be obtained; however, there is significant overlap in the measurements for normal fetuses and fetuses with CDH, with higher variability at later gestational ages. Other methods for standardizing normal lung volume involve obtaining a thoracic volume and subtracting the mediastinal volume to obtain an estimate of the expected lung volume. The actual lung volume is then divided by the expected lung volume to yield a percent predicted lung volume (PPLV). Research has shown that a PPLV of 20% has been shown to have 100% survival whereas a PPLV of less than 15% has a 40% survival. It is important to note that although various prognostic measurements are provided in the literature, different limits for survival have been quoted and overlap between fetuses with CDH and normal fetuses have been reported, making accurate predictions about outcome unclear.

Typical clinical scenario

Routine antenatal screening US will typically be the first modality to detect an underlying CDH either by visualization of an intrathoracic mass containing bowel, stomach, liver, or kidney, or by indirect evidence such as a scaphoid abdomen. Rarely, the mother may present with a uterus with enlarged fundal measurements due to polyhydramnios that is caused by a large CDH causing compression on the esophagus. Because both lung and liver are echogenic, utilizing Doppler of the hepatic vasculature or umbilical vein may be helpful. A dedicated fetal survey with US should ensue after the diagnosis of a CDH is made, including fetal echo evaluation, as there are associated cardiac, renal, central nervous system, and gastrointestinal anomalies. Aneuploidy is noted in approximately one-third of all CDH cases and hence amniocentesis and genetic consultation for chromosomal anomalies is advised for any patient with a CDH. MRI is used to complement US and for improved anatomic delineation of the contents of the hernia. Radiologists play an important role in helping clinicians determine if there are associated congenital anatomic anomalies and in the assessment of lung hypoplasia.

Differential diagnosis

The differential diagnosis for an echogenic chest mass seen on prenatal US would include a CDH, a cystic pulmonary adenomatoid malformation (CPAM), sequestration, congenital lobar overinflation (CLO), bronchogenic cyst, or bronchial atresia. Additionally, hybrid lesions that include both a CPAM/sequestration or CLO and bronchial atresia can exist. Rarely, primary pulmonary neoplasms such as a pleuropulmonary blastoma, congenital peribronchial myofibroblastic tumor, or fibrosarcoma can present in utero.

Teaching point

CDH is an uncommon but important entity as it is associated with high morbidity and mortality. Imaging plays an important role in terms of prenatal counseling and management and should focus on finding any additional anomalies, determining the contents of the hernia, particularly the liver, as this is associated with decreased survival. US is the mainstay for evaluation as it provides a means for neonatal wellbeing screening, provides the initial underlying suspicion for CDH, is used for fetal biometry, and is the mainstay for fetal cardiac assessment. MRI can better assess the type and contents of the hernia and is more accurate for the assessment of pulmonary volumes. Infants with CDH should be delivered in a tertiary care hospital where there is a multidisciplinary team approach to help optimize the care of the patient.

REFERENCES

1. Barnewolt CE, Kunisaki SM, Fauza DO, et al. Percent predicted lung volumes as measured on fetal magnetic resonance imaging: a useful biometric parameter for risk stratification in congenital diaphragmatic hernia. J Pediatr Surg 2007;42(1):193–7.

2. Cannie M, Jani J, Chaffiotte C, et al. Quantification of intrathoracic liver herniation by magnetic resonance imaging and prediction of postnatal survival in fetuses with congenital diaphragmatic hernia. Ultrasound Obstet Gynecol 2008;32(5):627–32.

3. CDC. Hospital stays, hospital charges, and in-hospital deaths among infants with selected birth defects – United States, 2003. MMWR 2007;56(2):25–29.

4. Harrison MR, Adzick NS, Estes JM, et al. A prospective study of the outcome for fetuses with diaphragmatic hernia. JAMA 1994;271(5):382–4.

5. Kline-Fath BM. Congenital diaphragmatic hernia. Pediatr Radiol 2012;42(Suppl 1):S74–90.

6. Kotecha S, Barbato A, Bush A, et al. Congenital diaphragmatic hernia. Eur Respir J 2012;39(4):820–9.

7. Langham MR Jr, Kays DW, Ledbetter DJ, et al. Congenital diaphragmatic hernia: epidemiology and outcome. Clin Perinatol 1996;23(6):671–88.

8. Mehollin-Ray AR, Cassady CI, Cass DL, et al. Fetal MR imaging of congenital diaphragmatic hernia. Radiographics 2012;32(4):1067–84.

9. Morini F, Goldman A, Pierro A. Extracorporeal membrane oxygenation in infants with congenital diaphragmatic hernia: a systematic review of the evidence. Eur J Pediatr Surg 2006;16(6):385–91.

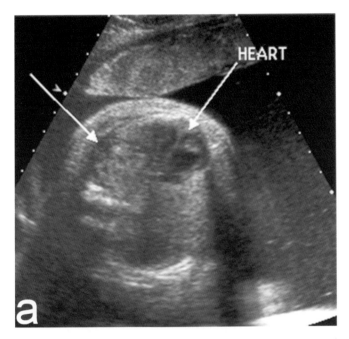

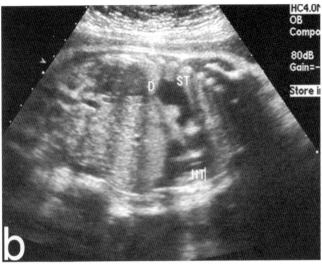

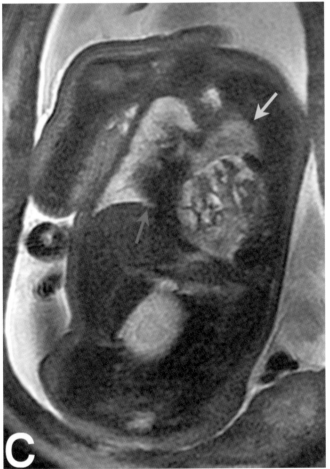

Figure 80.1 (a, b) Left CDH. Transverse and longitudinal sonographic images of a 34-week gravid patient through the fetal chest demonstrating the fetal heart shifted towards the right side of the chest and multiple echogenic serpiginous appearing foci in the left chest which represent loops of bowel. The longitudinal sonographic image demonstrates the stomach (ST) at the same level as the heart (HT), above the level of the diaphragm (D). **(c, d)** T2-weighted fetal MRI images from a 34-week gravid patient confirming the presence of a left-sided CDH with mediastinal shift from left to right. Note the heart is within the right aspect of the chest (red arrow). The left lung is hypoplastic and of lower signal intensity (yellow arrow). **(e)** Sagital T2-weighted image in the same 34-week gravid patient demonstrates that a portion of the left kidney is included in the contents of the hernia (blue arrow).

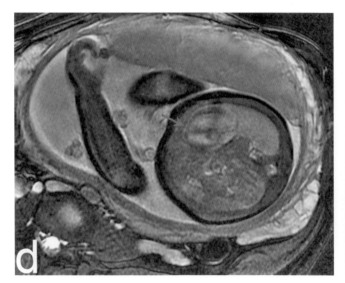

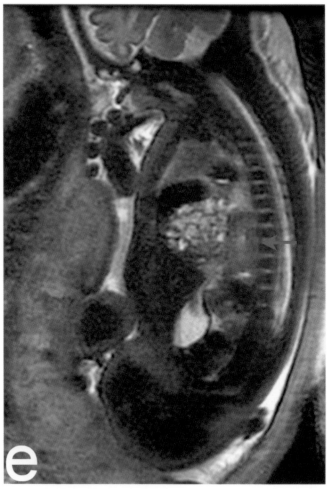

Figure 80.1. (cont.)

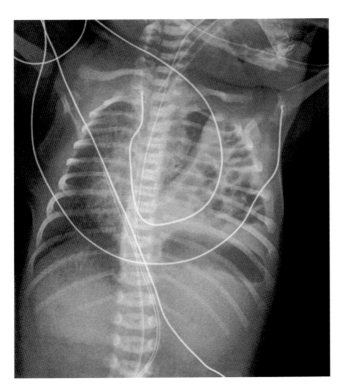

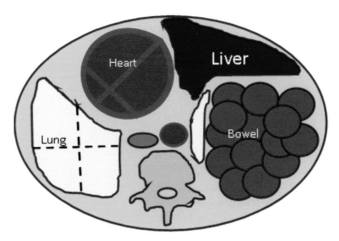

Figure 80.3. To calculate the lung to head ratio (LHR) utilizing the San Francisco method, the area of the contralateral lung, or the lung that is not involved with the CDH, is measured in two orthogonal planes at the level of the four-chamber heart (dashed black lines). This measurement (mm) is divided by the head circumference (mm). An LHR of < 1 portends a poor prognosis and an LHR of > 1.4 portends a favorable prognosis. (Art by Vy Thao Tran.)

Figure 80.2. Immediate postnatal chest X-ray in a different patient with CDH demonstrating multiple air-filled cystic spaces in the left chest compatible with bowel loops. The exact components of the herniated tissue is better delineated on the prenatal MRI. The left lung field is hypoplastic with minimal aeration at the left lung apex and there is mediastinal shift from left to right causing a component of right lung hypoplasia as well.

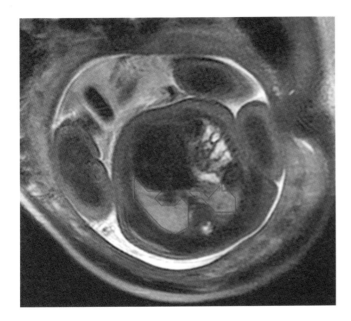

Figure 80.4. Axial T2 MRI demonstrating the hyperintense lung field outlined utilizing free hand region of interest (ROI). The areas from contiguous sections are summed and then multiplied by the section thickness to obtain the total fetal lung volume in cubic centimeters. Charted ranges of fetal lung volumes in normal fetuses can be obtained; however, there is significant overlap in the normal fetuses and fetuses with CDH and there is higher variability at later gestational age sometimes making accurate prediction for poor outcome difficult.

Hydrops fetalis

Kriengkrai Iemsawatdikul and Heike E. Daldrup-Link

Imaging description

A term infant presented with generalized anasarca, pleural effusion, and acites. A radiograph of the chest and abdomen/pelvis confirmed marked, generalized soft tissue swelling and bilateral pleural effusions (Fig. 81.1). There were several focal, round calcifications projecting below the right 12th rib, at the expected location of the gallbladder. An ultrasound confirmed numerous gallstones in the gallbladder (Fig. 81.2). There was no evidence of gallbladder wall thickening, pericholecystic fluid, cholestasis, or other abnormalities of the bile ducts.

Importance

A hydrops fetalis is defined by the presence of fluid accumulation in at least two anatomic compartments in the fetus or newborn. Based on its etiology, two types of hydrops fetalis are distinguished: immune hydrops and non-immune hydrops. Gallstones are frequently noted in patients with immune-mediated hydrops, but not in patients with non-immune causes of hydrops. Hydrops fetalis is a serious condition, which can result in death of the infant shortly before or after delivery.

Typical clinical scenario

Prenatally, hydrops fetalis may present with increased amniotic fluid and an abnormally large placenta as well as fluid accumulation in the fetus, including pleural and pericardial effusions, anasarca, ascites, and increased size and edema of liver, spleen, heart, and lungs.

Postnatally, clinical and imaging findings include anasarca, pleural effusions, pericardial effusions, ascites, hepatosplenomegaly, respiratory distress, heart failure, bruising of the skin, and jaundice.

Cholelithiasis in neonates and infants may not be recognized clinically until perforation of the biliary tree occurs. Imaging studies are important to recognize and follow for development of gallstones in patients with various risk factors. In adults, 80% of gallstones are composed primarily of cholesterol. By contrast, in children, pigment stones are more common. Pigment stones have 25% or less cholesterol and form when unconjugated bile pigments precipitate and form calcium-copper polymers. Beta-glucuronidase deconjugates bilirubin back into its insoluble form, allowing it to form metal salts with calcium and copper. Normal bile contains glucaric acid, an inhibitor of the enzyme. Pigment stones are formed when the balance of these two moieties change in light of an increasing bilirubin load or infection.

Differential diagnosis

Classical causes of immune-mediated hydrops fetalis include Rh incompatibility and incompatibilities against the minor blood types (e.g. Kell, Duffy, MNSs). The incidence of immune-mediated hydrops has significantly decreased with the wide use of passive immunization using Rh immunoglobulin for Rh-negative mothers. Examples of conditions that can lead to non-immune hydrops fetalis include primary cardiomyopathy, high output cardiac failure, impaired liver perfusion and/or function (leading to decreased production of albumin and decreased colloid oncotic pressure), tissue hypoxia or sepsis (leading to increased capillary permeability), as well as venous or lymphatic obstructions.

Acquired gallstones in the neonate or infant are associated with the following risk factors: (1) conditions associated with cholestasis, such as prematurity, fasting states and total parenteral nutrition, diuretics (furosemide leads to decreased bile flow), abnormalities of the biliary tree, and cystic fibrosis; (2) conditions associated with excessive direct bilirubin–(a) hemolytic disorders, such as immune-mediated hemolysis, congenital spherocytosis, sickle cell disease, thalassemia syndrome, phototherapy products, and large hematomas and (b) short bowel syndrome and after terminal ileum resection; and (3) hydrolysis of conjugated bilirubin or phospholipid by bacteria in the setting of infection.

Congenital cholelithiasis without hydrops or other pathologies differs from acquired neonatal cholelithiasis in etiology, presentation, and significance. Routine prenatal ultrasonography in obstetrics has brought about the incidental recognition of gallstones in some fetuses. The etiology is not well understood. One theory is that in utero cholelithiasis develops secondary to a silent in utero infection. Congenital gallstones are apparently asymptomatic, causing no detectable fetal distress. The stones are usually transient, as they commonly either disappear or pass spontaneously without evidence of hemolysis or cholestasis at birth.

> ## Teaching point
>
> Hydrops fetalis is a serious, multifactorial condition that can lead to the death of the infant. The combination of a hydrops fetalis with pigment stones in the gallbladder may indicate an immune incompatibility or other pathologies that lead to hemolysis. It is important to differentiate acquired neonatal cholelithiasis from incidental congenital cholelithiasis. Acquired neonatal cholelithiasis requires treatment of the underlying pathology, such as hemolysis, infection, or biliary stasis. Congenital cholelithiasis without hydrops or other pathologies can be an incidental finding and may resolve spontaneously.

REFERENCES

1. Adzick NS, Holzgreve W. The fetus with nonimmune hydrops fetalis. In: Harrison MR, Evans MI, Adzick NA, Holzgreve W, eds. *The Unborn Patient. The Art and Science of Fetal Therapy*, 3rd edition. Philadelphia: W.B. Saunders, 2001; 513–80.

2. Colon AR, Dipalma JS, Leftridge CA, *et al.* Biliary tract and gall bladder. In: Colon AR, ed. *Textbook of Pediatric Hepatology*, 2nd edition. Chicago: Year Book Medical Publishers, 1990; 182–207.

3. Klingensmith WC 3rd, Cioffi-Ragan DT. Fetal gallstones. *Radiology* 1988;**167**(1):143–4.

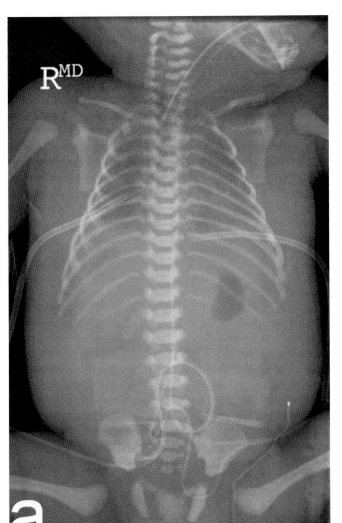

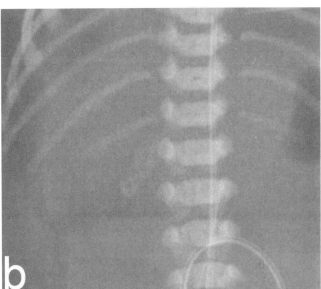

Figure 81.1. Newborn infant with hydrops fetalis. A radiograph of the chest and abdomen/pelvis shows marked, generalized soft tissue swelling and bilateral pleural effusions (a). Pleural drains project over the lower hemithorax bilaterally. There is a non-specific paucity of bowel gas. There are several focal, round calcifications projecting below the right 12th rib, at the expected location of the gallbladder (b).

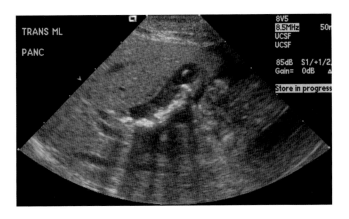

Figure 81.2. An ultrasound of the gallbladder demonstrates numerous calcified gallstones.

Bo Yoon Ha

Imaging description

A 16-month-old girl with bilateral foot deformities since birth had radiographs that demonstrated marked hindfoot and forefoot varus abnormalities bilaterally consistent with bilateral clubfeet (Fig. 82.1a). The talocalcaneal angles measured 0 degrees bilaterally on AP radiographs. The angle between the talus and the first metatarsal measured more than 20 degrees. Lateral views of both feet demonstrated decreased talocalcaneal angles bilaterally. In addition, the right foot demonstrated a fixed hindfoot equinus deformity (plantar flexed calcaneus) whereas the left calcaneus was able to be forcibly dorsiflexed (Fig. 82.1b).

Importance

Clubfoot (talipes equinovarus) is a congenital deformity consisting of hindfoot equinus, hindfoot varus (inversion), and forefoot varus (adduction) deformities. Clubfoot deformities affect three joints of the foot to varying degrees, including inversion of the subtalar joint, adduction of the talonavicular joint, and plantarflexion of the calcaneus relative to the tibia, resulting in "toe walking." Clubfoot deformities can involve one foot or both. Bilateral involvement is found in 30–50% of cases. Clubfoot deformities can be classified as either postural or structural. Postural or positional clubfoot is not defined as true clubfoot. Structural clubfoot can be subdivided into either a flexible type, which is correctable without surgery, or a resistant type, which requires surgical release.

Clubfoot is a common birth defect, occurring in about one in every 1000 live births. The incidence differs among ethnicities, with as many as six to seven cases per 1000 live births in the Polynesian islands. The male-to-female ratio is 2–2.5:1. There is a 10% chance of a subsequent sibling being affected. The true etiology of congenital clubfoot is unknown. Most cases are considered to be idiopathic. However, there are teratogenic causes such as myelodysplasia, arthrogryposis, and amyoplasia as well as associated syndromes such as diastrophic dysplasia and Larsen syndrome. Additionally, acquired forms of clubfoot can develop in patients with cerebral palsy.

The standard imaging modality for evaluation of clubfeet is the plain radiograph, which should be taken in the most anatomic or corrected position. Forced dorsiflexion of the foot should be obtained to evaluate if the equinus deformity is flexible. Important measurements on weight-bearing radiographs include talocalcaneal and talo-first metatarsal angles. The talocalcaneal angle normally measures 20–40 degrees on the AP view and 35–50 degrees on the lateral view, and is decreased to 0–10 degrees on the AP view and −10 to 20

degrees on the lateral view in the case of clubfoot deformity. The talo-first metatarsal angles normally measure 0–15 degrees on the AP view, and are typically increased to 20–40 degrees in the case of clubfoot deformity due to forefoot varus. The talus is laterally rotated within the ankle joint and the calcaneus is medially rotated. The talonavicular joint may show medial subluxation of the navicular bone and the calcaneo-cuboid joint may demonstrate medial subluxation of the cuboid bone.

Plain radiographs have the disadvantage of exposing the patient to ionizing radiation and being dependent on proper positioning. Additionally, as clubfoot is a congenital condition, the lack of ossification in some of the involved bones is another limitation for the interpretation. In neonates, only the talus and calcaneus are ossified. The navicular bone does not ossify until two to three years of age. CT or MR imaging is sometimes obtained to provide additional information prior to surgery. It has been noted that the anterior tibial artery is hypoplastic or absent in 85% of severe clubfoot cases.

Typical clinical scenario

Most patients present with the characteristic clubfoot deformity at birth. Acquired forms may present later. Advantages and disadvantages of non-surgical versus surgical treatments are controversial. For the idiopathic clubfoot, non-surgical approaches using the Ponseti and French methods may be the first line of treatment up to about three to 12 months of age. The Ponseti method consists of manipulation and casting. The French method consists of physiotherapy, taping, and continuous passive motion. Surgical options include posteromedial and lateral soft tissue release, osteotomies, and tendon transfer. However, surgical management can result in residual deformity, stiffness, and pain in some children. Careful evaluation of techniques and results of these two approaches may minimize the use of surgical management and associated morbidity resulting from extensive releases.

Differential diagnosis

Other associated conditions should be carefully evaluated. Similar deformities could be seen with underlying amniotic band syndrome, myelodysplasia, and arthrogryposis. Metatarsus adductus is an isolated forefoot varus deformity without other findings of clubfoot.

Congenital vertical talus is a severe rigid foot deformity that can exist as an isolated condition but usually accompanies severe neurologic abnormalities and some syndromes, including trisomy 13–15, trisomy 16–18, and arthrogryposis. It is characterized by a convex everted plantar arch (rockerbottom foot), forefoot dorsiflexion, hindfoot valgus, calcaneal equinus, vertical orientation of the talus, and frequently talonavicular dislocation (Fig. 82.2a, b). A rockerbottom foot type deformity (convex plantar arch like a "Persian slipper") can also be seen after clubfoot repair.

Cavovarus foot deformity is most commonly associated with underlying neurologic abnormality and also seen occasionally after treated clubfoot. It is characterized by calcaneal dorsiflexion and simultaneous forefoot plantarflexion creating an exaggerated plantar arch.

Planovalgus foot deformity is characterized by flattened plantar arch plus/minus hindfoot and forefoot abduction. The talus may have a more vertical orientation but without talonavicular dislocation. There are flexible (idiopathic or hereditary) and more rigid (associated with cerebral palsy and tarsal coalition) forms of this entity (see Fig. 82.3). Calcaneonavicular coalition is demonstrated as one type of tarsal coalition (Fig. 82.3a, b).

Teaching point

Clubfoot (talipes equinovarus) is usually a congenital deformity consisting of hindfoot equinus, hindfoot varus, and forefoot varus deformities and is distinct from other congenital and acquired foot deformities. Plain radiographs are the diagnostic and follow-up imaging modality of choice. Careful monitoring of non-surgical or surgical treatment is recommended, with frequency depending on the patient's age and severity of the deformity.

REFERENCES

1. Cummings RJ, Davidson RS, Armstrong PF, *et al*. Congenital clubfoot. *Instr Course Lect* 2002;**51**:385–400.

2. Harty MP. Imaging of pediatric foot disorders. *Radiol Clin North Am* 2001;**39**(4):733–48.

3. Noonan KJ, Richards BS. Nonsurgical management of idiopathic clubfoot. *J Am Acad Orthop Surg* 2003;**11**(6):392–402.

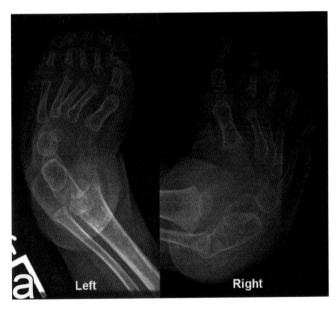 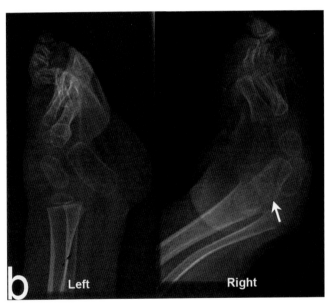

Figure 82.1. A 16-month-old girl with bilateral clubfoot deformities. **(a)** AP views of both feet demonstrate hindfoot varus (inversion), and forefoot varus (adduction). The talocalcaneal angle measures about 0 degrees bilaterally (parallel talus and calcaneus). The talo-first metatarsal angles measure more than 20 degrees. **(b)** Lateral views of both feet demonstrate decreased talocalcaneal angles bilaterally. Hindfoot equinus deformity (plantarflexed calcaneus) of the right foot is noted (arrow) whereas that of the left foot is overcome with forced dorsiflexion.

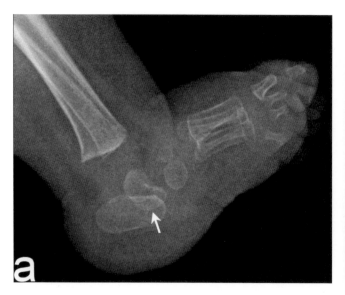
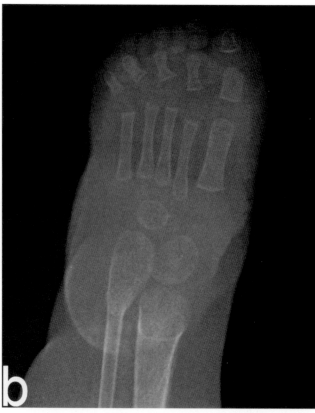

Figure 82.2. A three-month-old girl, infant of a diabetic mother, subsequently found to have an absent sacrum and caudal regression. She had congenital vertical talus bilaterally. **(a)** Lateral view of the left foot demonstrates calcaneal and forefoot plantarflexion, flattened to everted plantar arch (rockerbottom foot) and vertical orientation of the talus (arrow) with talonavicular dislocation. **(b)** AP view of the left foot demonstrates mild hindfoot and forefoot valgus.

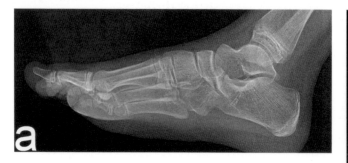
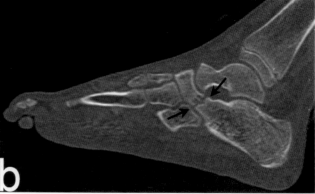

Figure 82.3. **(a)** Lateral view of the left foot demonstrates a flattened plantar arch (pes planus) and anterior beaking of the distal talus, suspicious for underlying tarsal coalition. There is possible sclerosis of the anteroinferior calcaneus adjacent to the navicular bone without definite tarsal coalition identified on this or oblique view (not shown). **(b)** Reconstructed sagittal CT image demonstrates irregularity, cystic change, and mild sclerosis in the anterior calcaneus and posterior navicular bones (arrows) indicative of calcaneonavicular tarsal coalition. This would be a fibrous coalition as no bony fusion is seen. There is no normal joint between these two bones. Talocalcaneal and calcaneonavicular coalitions are the most common types of tarsal coalition.

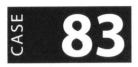

Developmental dysplasia of the hip

Vanessa Starr and Bo Yoon Ha

Imaging description

Case 1

A one-month-old girl had a physical examination suggesting developmental dysplasia of the hip (DDH). A coronal sonographic image through the right hip in neutral position, performed at one month of age, demonstrated an abnormal alpha angle of 47 degrees and less than 50% coverage of the femoral head under the acetabular roof (Fig. 83.1a). Pelvic AP radiograph at three months of age demonstrated a steep right acetabular roof with asymmetrically delayed ossification of the right femoral head (Fig. 83.1b).

Case 2

A three-year-old girl with a chromosomal deletion syndrome presented with bilateral hip pain and difficulty with abduction. Pelvic AP radiograph demonstrated dysplastic acetabulae with bilateral femoral head dislocation, pseudoacetabula formation, and valgus deformity (Fig. 83.2a). Frog leg view demonstrated that the hips did not relocate with abduction (Fig. 83.2b). This appearance is typical of secondary neurogenic hip dislocation related to muscle imbalance and overactive hip adductors.

Importance

DDH is a spectrum of disease affecting the femoral head and its acetabulum, ranging from slight hip laxity to irreducible hip dislocation. The reported incidence varies from 1.5–20 per 1000 births. Joint laxity, femoral head position, and acetabular development are all interdependent entities. For example, a normal acetabulum enables the femoral head to develop normally and conversely, a normal femoral head position stimulates normal acetabular development. Joint laxity during the perinatal period can result in migration of the femoral head, resulting in abnormal dysplastic acetabular development. If this process is uncorrected, muscle contractures form and fibrofatty tissue (pulvinar) in the medial acetabulum thickens, further preventing proper location of the femoral head. Various risk factors for DDH that have been described include breech delivery, family history, female, first born, and oligohydramnios. It has been proposed that maternal estrogens during the perinatal period may predispose to joint laxity. The left hip is affected more frequently than the right hip.

Ultrasound is the preferred imaging modality for infants up to four to five months old. Current ACR (American College of Radiology) guidelines combine a static acetabular morphology method proposed by Graf and a dynamic stress technique proposed by Harcke. Standard sonographic evaluation of the hip evaluates the position of the femoral head relative to the acetabulum at rest and stress and the morphology of the acetabulum. Three anatomic landmarks in the coronal plane include the iliac line, the triradiate cartilage in the deep medial acetabulum, and the echogenic lateral tip of the cartilaginous acetabular roof (the labrum). These anatomic landmarks are used to measure the alpha and beta angles. The Graf alpha angle is defined by the angle formed between the vertical cortex of the ilium and acetabular roof in the coronal plane (Fig. 83.1a). A Graf alpha angle greater than 60 degrees is considered normal. The beta angle is defined by the angle formed between the vertical cortex of the ilium and the cartilaginous acetabular labrum, measuring the elevation of the acetabular labrum in the coronal plane. A Graf beta angle less than 55 degrees is considered normal. With lateral and superior femoral head displacement, the labrum is elevated, increasing the beta angle. While standard examination with static two views meets ACR standards, the Harcke method consists of four views, incorporating more dynamic testing. Coronal and axial images are obtained from the lateral aspect of the hip in neutral position with approximately 20 degrees of hip flexion (physiologic in infants) and at 90 degrees of hip flexion. The goal of the Harcke method is to evaluate the acetabular development and to determine the position and stability of the femoral head during dynamic stress manipulation. Acetabular development can also be assessed by the amount of acetabular coverage of the femoral head. Percentage of coverage reflects acetabular depth, and is normally greater than 50%. With DDH, shallow acetabulae result in a decreased percentage of the coverage of the femoral head. The modified Graf grading classification takes into account the alpha angle and acetabular roof coverage, with the following morphologic types:

Type 1: Normal, mature hip with greater than 50% acetabular roof coverage. Alpha angle is greater than 60 degrees.

Type 2: Subtypes include types a–c, as described below. Most of the less severe type 2 will become normal by 3 months of age; however, 1–2% will ultimately require treatment.

Type 2a: Physiologic immaturity at <3 months; alpha angle is 50–59 degrees.

Type 2b: Immature at age >3 months; alpha angle is 50–59 degrees.

Type 2c: Extremely deficient bony acetabulum; femoral head is still concentric, but unstable. Alpha angle is 43–49 degrees. Beta angle remains <77 degrees.

Type D: Femoral head grossly subluxed, alpha angle is difficult to measure but roughly 43–49 degrees. Beta angle is >77 degrees, indicating an everted labrum.

Type 3: Dislocation with a shallow acetabulum, as indicated by a Graf alpha angle of less than 43 degrees. Treatment is typically necessary.

Type 4: Dislocation, a severely shallow and dysplastic acetabulum with inverted labrum. Treatment is typically necessary.

Once the femoral head ossification begins to obscure sonographic landmarks by about four to six months of age, radiographs become easier and more reliable for detection of DDH. An AP radiograph of the hips in neutral position is preferred to evaluate for DDH. A frog leg lateral position can serve as an adjunct to determine whether a subluxed hip reduces. The acetabular morphology, femoral head ossification, and position are assessed. Femoral head ossification can be seen on radiographs and should be assessed for symmetry and degree of ossification for patient's given age. Femoral head ossification is typically delayed with DDH. The acetabular contour should also be assessed. With DDH, the acetabulum is more shallow and with a steeper roof. The combination of joint laxity and shallow acetabulum can result in subluxation and dislocation of the femoral head. There are specified lines such as Hilgenreiner's, Perkin's, and Shenton's, which are used to determine the degree of hip dysplasia (Fig. 83.3a). The Hilgenreiner's line is a horizontal line across both triradiate cartilages. The acetabular angle measures the steepness of the acetabular roof and is formed by the intersection of the Hilgenreiner's line and a line drawn tangential to the acetabular roof. A normal acetabular angle is less than 30 degrees in newborns and 22 degrees at one year of age. The Perkin's line is a vertical line drawn perpendicular to the Hilgenreiner's line, intersecting the lateral rim of the acetabular roof. The normally located femoral head should be in the inferior medial quadrant of the intersecting Hilgenreiner's and Perkin's line. Deviations from this indicate the degree of subluxation and percentage of acetabular coverage of the femoral head. When the femoral head ossification center is not yet present, the Perkin's line intersecting the medial third of the femoral metaphysis indicates that the hip is not dislocated (Fig. 83.3a). The Shenton's line is drawn along the inferior border of the superior pubic ramus and should normally form a smooth arc along the medial aspect of the femoral neck. The Shenton's line is discontinuous with subluxation. Once the femoral head ossifies, femoral head subluxation or dislocation can be quantified by the percentage of the femoral head with osseous acetabular roof coverage or by the center-edge (CE) angle. The CE angle is formed by a vertical line through the center of the femoral head and another line from the center to the lateral edge of the acetabular roof. An angle greater than 25 degrees is considered normal and an angle less than 20 degrees indicates dysplasia (Fig. 83.3b).

Typical clinical scenario

Current practice guidelines recommend that all newborns are screened by physical exam. The goal is to detect all patients with DDH early, when therapy is most effective and non-invasive, although not all hip dislocations are present at birth. Physical examination in a patient with DDH may reveal asymmetric gluteal folds, apparent leg length discrepancy,

and restricted motion. The Ortolani and Barlow tests are abduction/adduction stress maneuvers that are used to assess hip stability in the newborn. Older infants and children can present clinically with leg length discrepancies, gait disturbances such as limping, and possibly associated knee and hip pain. If it is untreated, DDH can result in hip deformity, avascular necrosis, or early degenerative joint disease. Initial treatment consists of bracing with a Pavlik harness in patients younger than six months. If this is not effective or a diagnosis is made at a later age, surgical hip reduction and casting are typically recommended. The final treatment option may consist of either femoral and/or iliac osteotomies in severe DDH, to achieve acetabular coverage of the femoral head both anteriorly and superiorly.

Differential diagnosis

Differential diagnostic considerations of DDH include cerebral palsy, congenital coxa valga, and neuromuscular disease. In these disorders, subluxation or dislocation (Fig. 83.2) is caused by abnormal muscular tension rather than by ligamentous laxity and bony abnormalities. Septic arthritis of infancy may cause temporary joint dislocation and can be distinguished clinically as well as by ultrasound and joint aspiration. Proximal focal femoral deficiency is a rare congenital malformation, which is due to failure of development of the upper femur and in the differential consideration for a severely shallow and dysplastic acetabulum.

Teaching points

Early detection of DDH is important to ensure more efficient treatment options and prevent complications. All newborns should be screened by physical exam. Ultrasound is the imaging modality of choice in infants younger than 4 months, in which both static and dynamic methods are used for the assessment. Radiographs are a reliable imaging technique for infants older than four months. Various measurements may assist with assessment. The combination of coxa valga and bilateral hip subluxation or dislocation is strongly suggestive of neurogenic hip abnormality, which tends to be progressive.

REFERENCES

1. American Academy of Pediatrics. Clinical practice guideline: early detection of developmental dysplasia of the hip. Committee on Quality Improvement, Subcommittee on Developmental Dysplasia of the Hip. *Pediatrics* 2000;**105**(4 Pt 1):896–905.

2. Dezateaux C, Rosendahl K. Developmental dysplasia of the hip. *Lancet* 2007;**369**(9572):1541–52.

3. Roposch A, Graf R, Wright JG. Determining the reliability of the Graf classification for hip dysplasia. *Clin Orthop Relat Res* 2006;**447**:119–24.

4. Slovis T, ed. *Caffey's Pediatric Diagnostic Imaging*. 11th edn. Philadelphia: Mosby, 2007.

5. Wheeless CR. *Textbook of Orthopaedics,* online edition. Original text by Wheeless CR. Last updated by Data Trace Staff on Dec 27, 2011. http://www.wheelessonline.com (accessed February 5, 2013).

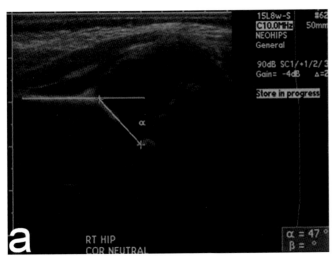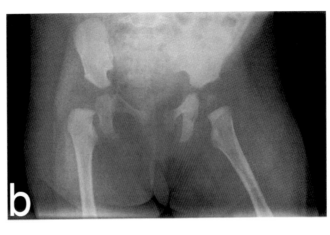

Figure 83.1. Right hip DDH. **(a)** Coronal sonographic image through the right hip in neutral position, performed at one month of age, demonstrates an abnormal alpha angle of 47 degrees and less than 50% coverage of the femoral head under the acetabular roof. **(b)** Right hip DDH. Pelvic AP radiograph at three months of age demonstrates a shallow acetabulum with a steep right acetabular roof with asymmetrically delayed ossification of the right femoral head.

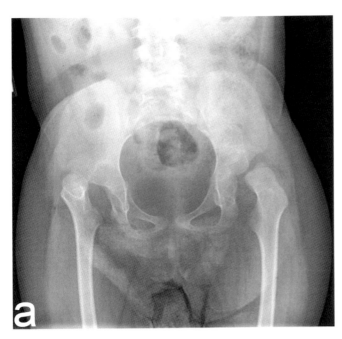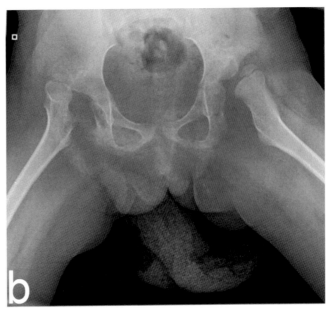

Figure 83.2. **(a)** A three-year-old with a chromosomal deletion syndrome. Pelvic AP radiograph demonstrates dysplastic acetabulae with complete dislocation of the bilateral femoral heads, pseudoacetabula formation, and valgus deformity. This represents an acquired form of neurologic hip subluxation/dislocation related to muscle imbalance (adductor overactivity). **(b)** Frog leg view demonstrates that the hips do not relocate with abduction.

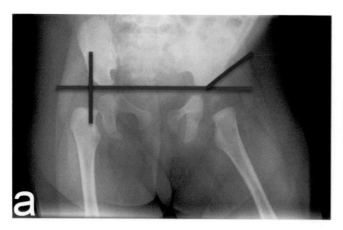
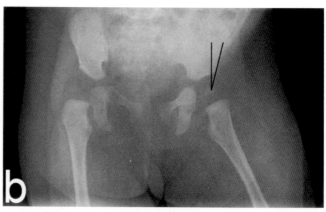

Figure 83.3. (a) Standard lines. Ideally both hips should be in straight AP position with no pelvic rotation. This left hip is slightly abducted and the pelvis is rotated (asymmetric obturator foramina). Blue line indicates Hilgenreiner's line (a horizontal line across both triradiate cartilages). Red line indicates Perkin's line (a vertical line drawn perpendicular to the Hilgenreiner's line, intersecting the lateral rim of the acetabular roof). Acetabular angle is formed by intersection of Hilgenreiner's line and purple line through acetabular roof. A normal acetabular angle is less than 30 degrees in newborns and 22 degrees at 1 year of age. There is an angle of 24 degrees in this normal left hip. Although the right acetabulum is dysplastic, the right hip is not dislocated as evidenced by the vertical Perkin's line intersecting the medial right femoral metaphysis. **(b)** CE angle. The CE angle is formed by a vertical line through the center of the femoral head and another line from the center to the lateral edge of the acetabular roof. An angle greater than 25 degrees is considered normal and an angle less than 20 degrees indicates dysplasia. Thin black lines illustrate CE angle of 26 degrees, indicating normal coverage of this femoral head.

Legg–Calve–Perthes disease

Vy Thao Tran and Bo Yoon Ha

Imaging description

A seven-year-old boy presented with right leg pain. Plain film of the hips demonstrated sclerosis, flattening, and fragmentation of the bilateral femoral capital epiphyses as well as shortening and widening of the femoral necks with metaphyseal irregularity including cystic changes. There was involvement of the lateral pillars bilaterally, worse on the right compared to the left (Fig. 84.1). Additionally, slight lateral subluxation of the right hip was demonstrated, consistent with non-containment of the right femoral head within the acetabulum (Fig. 84.1). Findings were considered diagnostic of Legg–Calve–Perthes disease (LCPD).

Importance

LCPD is a condition characterized by idiopathic osteonecrosis of the capital femoral epiphysis. It affects approximately 4 to 15.6 per 100 000 children. Almost all are between three and 12 years old, with the peak incidence occurring around 7 years of age. Boys are affected four to five times more often than girls. Those diagnosed at a younger age typically experience a more benign course than those diagnosed at an older age, who often require increased rates of intervention. Both hips are involved in 10–20% of cases, usually successively rather than simultaneously. It is hypothesized that rapid growth of the bone in relation to the developing blood supply of the secondary ossification centers results in an interruption of adequate blood flow, making these areas prone to avascular necrosis.

Radiography is the primary imaging modality for the evaluation of LCPD. Early plain films show widening of the joint space caused by thickening of the cartilage, the presence of a joint effusion, and/or joint laxity. Another early finding is failure of epiphyseal growth. Later findings include a radiolucent "crescent sign," representing a subchondral fracture, which may be followed by coxa plana and coxa magna related to fragmentation and collapse of the femoral head during the necrotic phase and enlargement or deformation of the femoral head with incomplete containment in the acetabulum during the healing phase. Early recognition of LCPD is important because it enables the orthopedic surgeon to initiate potential joint-preserving therapies. MRI can detect LCPD earlier than plain film, allowing for better accuracy in staging the disease, and may reveal other unsuspected causes of hip pain. It also can be used to assess the success of orthopedic invasive or non-invasive hip containment procedures. Bone scintigraphy and MRI findings correlate well; however, MRI depicts the anatomic detail of the femoral head involvement and cartilage more precisely and avoids ionizing radiation exposure, hence making it the preferred modality for evaluation in pediatric patients.

MRI of the hip in LCPD has a variable appearance based on the different stages of disease, which include the avascular, revascularization, and healing phases. Early on in the avascular phase, which is the most clinically apparent stage when the child presents with a limp, MRI may demonstrate areas of necrosis seen as low T1 signal in the femoral epiphysis which is typically in a subchondral location (Fig. 84.2). A crescent sign may be seen, which represents the subchondral fracture along the femoral head ossification nucleus (T1-hypointense and T2-hyperintense). Decreased or no enhancement of the femoral epiphysis may be seen. With the revascularization and healing phases, which last for years, the marrow usually shows heterogeneous signal. High T2 or STIR signal as well as enhancement of the lateral pillar provides prognostic information, as early reperfusion of the lateral column is a good prognostic indicator. Involvement of the physis may be subtle on MRI in children, as the normal physis appears T1-hypointense and T2-hyperintense. Morphologic changes of the femoral head such as undulation or cupping (Fig. 84.2b) convey a poorer prognosis, as many of these cases proceed to develop premature growth arrest. MRI signal changes may persist for up to six years after the healing phase.

The radiographic literature quotes multiple classification systems for the grading of LCPD of which the most widely used include the Catterall system, the Herring method, and the Stulberg method. The initial system by Catterall published in 1971 has been extensively studied; however, it has low inter-observer reliability. The Herring classification is based on the evaluation of the lateral pillar and has the highest reputed reliability among observers. The Stulberg classification focuses on the status of the femoral head and its relationship with the acetabulum at the completion of remodeling and skeletal maturity. The Stulberg classification is frequently used to classify the end result of patients with this disorder and has been shown to correlate with the age of onset of premature arthritis. It was modified by Herring in 2004.

The Herring classification splits the femoral head into three regions on an AP view of the pelvis, with the lateral third representing the "lateral pillar."

- Group A: No involvement of the lateral pillar. No density changes. No loss of height of the lateral pillar.
- Group B: Lucency in the lateral pillar with some loss of height but not exceeding 50%.
- Group B–C: A narrow lateral pillar of 2–3 mm, a lateral pillar with very little ossification, but at least 50% height, or a lateral pillar with exactly 50% loss of height that is depressed relative to the central pillar.
- Group C: Lucency in the lateral pillar with loss of height exceeding 50%.

Stulberg defined the classification as follows:

- Stage I: Normal hip joint.

- Stage II: Spherical with a larger than normal femoral head, a shorter femoral neck, or abnormally steep acetabulum.
- Stage III: Non-spherical femoral head with an ovoid, mushroom, or umbrella shape, but not flat.
- Stage IV: Flat femoral head and acetabulum.
- Stage V: Flat femoral head, neck, and acetabulum.

Typical clinical scenario

The classic presentation of LCPD is painless limping. The earliest clinical sign of LCPD is an intermittent limp, especially after exertion, with mild or intermittent pain radiating along anterior and medial aspects of the distal thigh and knee. Physical examination in cooperative children may reveal pain at the hip, with limited hip range of motion, typically during abduction and internal rotation. Treatment options include conservative measures with abduction stretching and bracing and surgical treatment with femoral and pelvic osteotomies.

Differential diagnosis

A child presenting with a limp raises several other diagnostic considerations including trauma, toxic synovitis, septic joint (Fig. 84.3a–c), juvenile idiopathic arthritis, ankylosing spondylitis), proximal focal femoral dysplasia, slipped capital femoral epiphysis, or osteoid osteoma. Other causes of avascular necrosis include sickle cell disease, Gaucher's disease thalassemia, steroids, prior infection, or arthritis. These may present with very similar radiologic findings to LCPD. Epiphyseal dysplasia may also be difficult to differentiate from LCPD, especially in younger children. Therefore, laboratory, clinical, and radiographic data along with joint aspiration may be necessary to help make a diagnosis.

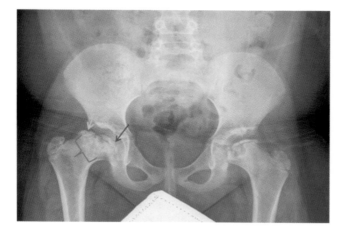

Teaching point

Radiographic findings help in establishing a specific diagnosis in a limping child. The initial evaluation should start with plain films, which are the mainstay for the diagnosis and follow-up of LCPD. MRI is a more sensitive exam, which enables better anatomic delineation and may help provide more prognostic information. Both imaging modalities have characteristic findings. Different classification systems are used for grading LCPD. Discussion with the local pediatric orthopedists regarding their classification method of preference is appropriate as the ultimate goal of management is to determine when containment procedures are necessary to reduce complications, including early onset osteoarthritis and leg length discrepancy.

REFERENCES

1. Barker DJ, Hall AJ. The epidemiology of Perthes' disease. *Clin Orthop Relat Res* 1986;**209**:89–94.

2. Daldrup-Link HE, Steinbach L. MR imaging of pediatric arthritis. *Magn Reson Imaging Clin N Am* 2009;**17**(3):451–67, vi.

3. Dillman JR, Hernandez RJ. MRI of Legg–Calve–Perthes disease. *AJR Am J Roentgenol* 2009;**193**(5):1394–407.

4. Herring JA, Kim HT, Browne R. Legg–Calve–Perthes disease. Part I: Classification of radiographs with use of the modified lateral pillar and Stulberg classifications. *J Bone Joint Surg Am* 2004;**86**-A(10):2103–20.

5. Kuo KN, Wu KW, Smith PA, *et al.* Classification of Legg–Calvé–Perthes disease. *J Pediatr Orthop* 2011;**31**(2 Suppl):S168–73.

6. Price CT, Thompson GH, Wenger DR. Containment methods for treatment of Legg–Calvé–Perthes disease. *Orthop Clin North Am* 2011;**42**(3):329–40.

Figure 84.1. A seven-year-old boy with bilateral LCPD. Red arrow points to sclerosis, flattening, and fragmentation of the femoral capital epiphysis, also referred to as coxa plana. The blue bracket points to the generalized enlargement and deformation of the femoral head which leads to lateral spreading and lack of containment, consistent with coxa magna. The yellow arrow points to involvement of the lateral pillar. There is slight lateral uncovering of the right femoral epiphysis. This is a Herring Group B classified hip as there is lucency in the lateral pillar with some loss of height but not exceeding 50%.

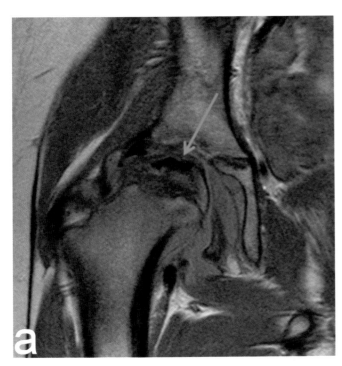
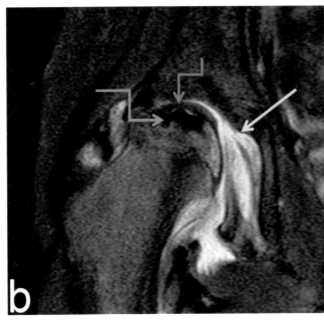

Figure 84.2. (a) T1-weighted MRI of the right hip in a nine-year-old female with LCPD demonstrates low T1 signal (green arrow) in the right femoral epiphysis superiorly, consistent with necrosis. **(b)** Additional T2-weighted image demonstrating the low T2 signal consistent with necrosis (green arrow), undulation of the femoral head, which portends a poorer prognosis (red arrow), and a joint effusion (yellow arrow).

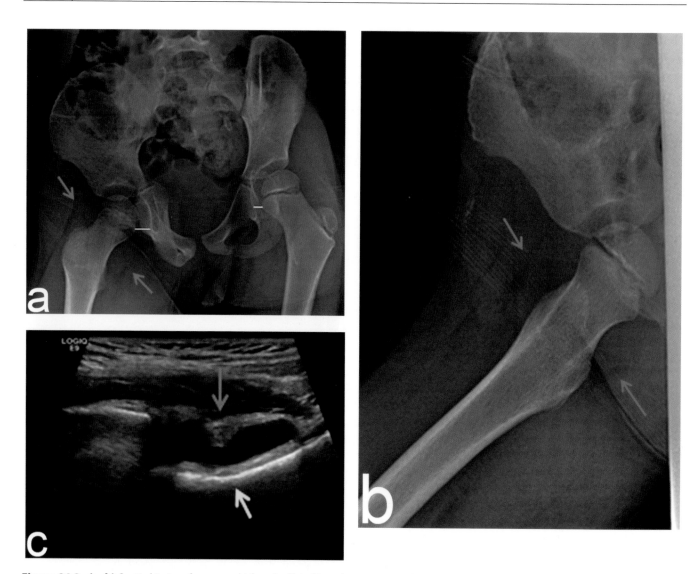

Figure 84.3. **(a, b)** Septic hip in a four-year-old female. Plain films demonstrating that the patient is slightly rotated; however, with widening of the right medial joint space compared to the left (yellow lines) and displacement of the gluteal and obturator fat planes from the underlying joint effusion (red arrows). **(c)** Ultrasound image of the same four-year-old girl with blue arrow demonstrating the anechoic right hip effusion. Yellow arrow points to the echogenic line with posterior shadowing consistent with the femoral metaphysis.

Slipped capital femoral epiphysis

Vy Thao Tran and Bo Yoon Ha

Imaging description

A 13-year-old boy presented with left groin pain. A radiograph of the pelvis was obtained and demonstrated widening and irregularity of the physis of the left proximal femur associated with demineralization of the femoral head. Klein's line, a line drawn along the tangent of the lateral margin of the femoral neck, did not intersect the left femoral head (Fig. 85.1a). Findings were consistent with slipped capital femoral epiphysis (SCFE). In addition, a "metaphyseal blush," an area of increased density in the proximal metaphysis was seen, representing bony healing (Fig. 85.1c). The affected left femoral epiphysis appeared smaller compared to the right side due to the posterior slippage (Fig. 85.1c). The Southwick method for evaluating the head-shaft angle may be helpful for preoperative planning (Fig. 85.1b). Figure 85.2 shows a follow-up radiograph in a different 12-year-old boy, demonstrating surgical pinning of a left-sided SCFE.

An MRI of a 10-year-old girl with SCFE shows high T2 signal within the physis and posteromedial slippage of the right femoral capital epiphysis. There is also an associated joint effusion and bone marrow edema (Fig. 85.3).

Importance

SCFE is the most common hip abnormality in adolescence and a major cause of osteoarthritis in adulthood. SCFE involves anterior displacement of the femoral metaphysis and posteromedial displacement of the femoral epiphysis at the level of the physis. Biomechanical and biochemical factors including obesity and the surge of hormonal activity during adolescence may contribute to the etiology of SCFE. Most SCFE are said to be idiopathic; however, an association with endocrine disorders is noted. SCFE affects approximately 10.8 in 100 000 children. Males are more commonly affected, possibly related to the weakening effect of testosterone on the growth plate. The incidence of bilateral SCFE has been quoted as ranging from 20 to 80%. The peak age of involvement occurs at 13–14 years of age for boys and 11–12 years of age for girls. Radiography is the primary imaging modality used in the evaluation of patients with suspected SCFE. MRI may be more sensitive in the evaluation of SCFE, particularly in diagnosing pre-slip SCFE. MRI imaging in SCFE (Fig. 85.3) can show disruption of the physis with edema around the growth plate, an intra-articular effusion, or disruption of the joint capsule. MRI is also helpful in visualizing femoral head vascularization pre- and postoperatively and for evaluating chondrolysis.

Early diagnosis of SCFE is important because it allows prompt initiation of potential joint-preserving therapies and prevention of further slippage. The two most common complications of SCFE include avascular necrosis (AVN) and chondrolysis, both of which predispose to early osteoarthritis. Chondrolysis, or acute cartilage necrosis of the femoral epiphysis, can occur in treated and untreated SCFE. It can be associated with pin penetration into the joint space and hence this should be avoided.

Various classification systems are used for the staging of SCFE. Radiographically, the Wilson classification is based on the relative displacement of the epiphysis on the metaphysis:

- Mild slip: Less than 1/3 displacement of the epiphysis with respect to the metaphysis.
- Moderate slip: 1/3 to 1/2 displacement of the epiphysis with respect to the metaphysis.
- Severe slip: More than 1/2 displacement of the epiphysis with respect to the metaphysis.

Alternatively, the Southwick classification system measures the epiphyseal shaft angle. The difference between the normal and the affected hip can be used to grade severity using this system:

- Mild: Less than 30 degrees.
- Moderate: 30–50 degrees.
- Severe: Greater than 50 degrees.

SCFE used to be classified clinically as acute, acute on chronic, or chronic, based on the time at which the patient presented. However, this is no longer favored and most orthopedic surgeons refer to the Loder classification system of SCFE as being "stable" or "unstable." This system is based on whether the patient can bear weight. "Unstable" SCFE is when the patient cannot bear weight whereas a "stable" SCFE is when the patient can bear weight, even when using crutches.

The gold standard for stable SCFE is single screw fixation (Fig. 85.2). Unstable SCFE treatment is still controversial in the orthopedic community with respect to the timing of fixation, the type of fixation, and the role of reduction and decompression. Prophylactic fixation of the opposite hip is still controversial in North America, although commonly accepted in Europe.

Patients should be followed closely for AVN as this generally occurs in the first 12 months and continued plain film screening of bilateral hips is recommended until the physes are closed due to the increased incidence of bilaterality in SCFE.

Typical clinical scenario

An obese child with groin pain is the typical clinical presentation of SCFE. A history of antecedent trauma may be elicited in some cases. Limitation of hip internal rotation and hip flexion may be seen on physical examination. Often, an out-toeing gait is present. Similar to other hip conditions, knee pain may be the major presenting symptom.

Differential diagnosis

Fractures, AVN or Legg–Calve–Perthes disease (LCPD), osteomyelitis, septic arthritis, stress fractures, or a groin pull are possible differentials for a child presenting with groin/hip pain. However, each will have different clinical and radiographic presentations.

In patients with a history of acute trauma, cortical disruption and a clear clinical history may help differentiate a fracture from SCFE. LCPD presents typically in younger patients with radiographs demonstrating joint space widening, subchondral femoral epiphyseal crescenteric lucency, and, in the latter stages, with epiphyseal flattening and sclerosis. There is no slippage of the epiphysis in AVN occurring independently from SCFE. (AVN is discussed in Case 84.)

In children with osteomyelitis, the metaphysis is commonly involved, first with either focal osteopenia, deep soft tissue swelling, and in the latter stages, bone destruction and periosteal reaction. MRI may delineate a subperiosteal and/or intraosseous abscess. Typically, the growth plate acts as a barrier to the spread of infection in the case of osteomyelitis.

Stress fractures are classified as insufficiency fractures or fatigue fractures. Insufficiency fractures occur in patients with normal stress applied to abnormal bone as in the cases of osteopenia/osteoporosis, osteogenesis imperfecta, osteomalacia/rickets, hyperparathyroidism, or chronic steroid use. Fatigue stress fractures occur from abnormal stress applied to normal bone and in the femoral neck typically are seen in long distance runners, jumpers, or ballet dancers. Both may present with increased sclerosis in the metaphyseal region or disruption of the bony trabeculae in the region of the femoral neck on plain film; however, Klein's line will not be abnormal and the only finding seen on MRI may be focal marrow edema.

Teaching point

An adolescent child with hip pain, particularly if obese, should be suspected of having SCFE. In the presence of a new radiographic diagnosis of SCFE, the child should be advised not to bear weight on the hip and be promptly referred to an orthopedic surgeon. If the child is unable to bear weight and in severe pain, AP views of the hips and a lateral view should be obtained. Frog leg lateral views, although typically helpful, should be avoided in patients suspected of having unstable acute SCFE as it can worsen the degree of slippage. MRI can be performed for selected cases where there is a question of the vascular supply to the femoral head, need for assessment of the periosteum, or suspected early SCFE that is not conclusively demonstrated by plain films. Plain films are, however, the mainstay modality for the diagnosis of SCFE and for postoperative monitoring of the hips.

REFERENCES

1. Boles CA, el-Khoury GY. Slipped capital femoral epiphysis. *Radiographics* 1997;**17**(4):809–23.

2. Gholve PA, Cameron DB, Millis MB. Slipped capital femoral epiphysis update. *Curr Opin Pediatr* 2009;**21**(1):39–45.

3. Loder RT. Controversies in slipped capital femoral epiphysis. *Orthop Clin North Am* 2006;**37**(2):211–21, vii.

4. Miese FR, Zilkens C, Holstein A, *et al.* MRI morphometry, cartilage damage and impaired function in the follow-up after slipped capital femoral epiphysis. *Skeletal Radiol* 2010;**39**(6):533–41.

5. Tins B, Cassar-Pullicino V, McCall I. The role of pre-treatment MRI in established cases of slipped capital femoral epiphysis. *Eur J Radiol* 2009;**70**(3):570–8.

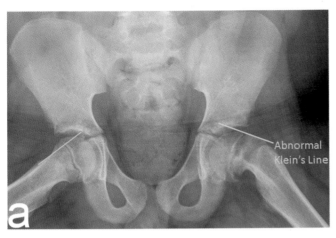

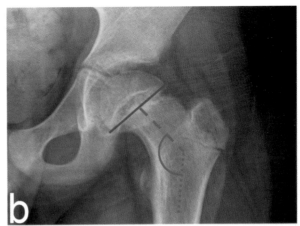

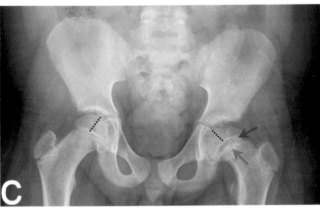

Figure 85.1. A 13-year-old boy with left groin pain and slipped capital femoral epiphysis (SCFE). **(a)** Frog lateral radiograph of the pelvis. There is an abnormal Klein's line (yellow) on the left which does not cross through the left femoral epiphysis due to left-sided SCFE. Note a normal Klein's line on the right which crosses through a portion of the femoral epiphysis. **(b)** Frontal radiograph of the left hip. The Southwick angle method is shown through the left hip. The solid blue line is drawn first at the margins of the femoral epiphysis. Then the dashed line is drawn perpendicular to that line. The last line is the dotted line drawn through the center of the shaft of the left femur. The angle between the dashed and dotted lines is the Southwick angle. A comparison between the two sides is made to ascertain the severity of the slip. **(c)** Frontal radiograph of both hips. Typical radiographic features of SCFE. The left femoral epiphysis appears smaller compared to the right side. The blue arrow points to widening and irregularity of the left physis. The red arrow points to the "metaphyseal blush" sign.

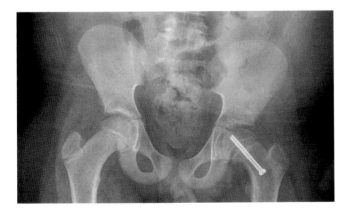

Figure 85.2. Frontal pelvic radiograph demonstrates surgical pinning of left-sided SCFE in a different 12-year-old boy. The right hip is normal. Follow-up plain films are obtained of the bilateral hips until growth plate fusion is complete.

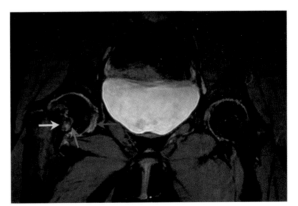

Figure 85.3. T2-weighted MRI of a 10-year-old girl with right-sided SCFE. Note the abnormal fluid signal seen at the level of the physis (red arrow) which may be the only finding present in early SCFE. There is an associated joint effusion (blue arrow) and adjacent marrow edema along the physis (yellow arrow) suggestive of an acute slip.

Langerhans cell histiocytosis: MRI/PET for diagnosis and treatment monitoring

Wolfgang P. Fendler, Eva Coppenrath, Klemens Scheidhauer, and Thomas Pfluger

Imaging description

A 12-year-old boy presented with chronic pain of the right knee. The pain became gradually worse over a three-month period and increased with pressure and after long walks. There was no history of trauma. On physical examination, no swelling or redness of the right knee was noted. Mild external rotation of the right hip as well as limited active and passive internal rotation was seen on examination.

An X-ray of the right knee was unremarkable. An X-ray of the right hip showed a focal, well-defined, round osteolytic lesion with a diameter of approximately 1 cm in the inferior acetabulum (Fig. 86.1). An MRI and ^{18}F-FDG PET were performed for further evaluation. T2 STIR images demonstrated a more extensive hyperintense lesion in the right ischium and an additional hyperintense lesion in the right femur (Fig. 86.2). These lesions showed enhancement on contrast-enhanced T1-weighted MR scans (not shown) and increased metabolic activity on ^{18}F-FDG PET (Fig. 86.2). The diagnosis of Langerhans cell histiocytosis (LCH) was established by CT-guided biopsy and histopathology. Chemotherapy according to the LCH-III protocol was initiated and well tolerated by the patient. Follow-up simultaneous ^{18}F-FDG PET/MR scans performed after treatment showed complete remission of both lesions. However, a new T2-hyperintense lesion was noted in the right ilium, which demonstrated normal ^{18}F-FDG uptake (Fig. 86.3). It was assumed that this lesion had occurred after the initial ^{18}F-FDG PET/MR scans and had been successfully treated as well. Thus, a conservative strategy without further systemic chemotherapy was chosen and a follow-up MRI after six months confirmed reduced lesion size.

Importance

LCH refers to a group of disorders involving clonal proliferation and activation of bone marrow derived dendritic cells. The current clinical classification stratifies patients into single-system LCH with one organ system involved (unifocal or multifocal, e.g. bone, skin, lymph node, lungs, central nervous system) or multisystem LCH with two or more organ systems involved.

Indications for treatment of single-system LCH include pain, restriction of mobility, and risk of fracture. Systemic treatment is indicated for patients with multisystem LCH. Patients with multisystem LCH and involvement of specific "risk organs" (hematopoietic system, liver, spleen) receive intensified treatment. Mortality is further determined by response to initial therapy. Patients who respond to initial therapy have survival outcomes similar to initial low-risk patients. Patients without response to initial treatment have a poor prognosis. Therefore, accurate initial staging and treatment monitoring is essential in order to determine the type of therapy chosen, identify non-responders and/or disease reactivation as early as possible, and change the treatment strategy as needed.

Plain radiographs, radiographic skeletal surveys, and ^{99m}Tc bone scans have traditionally been used for staging and re-staging of LCH. More recently, cross-sectional imaging studies have demonstrated a higher sensitivity and are now used at many centers for primary staging and post-therapy follow-up.

On MRI, active LCH lesions are typically hyperintense on T2-weighted and hypointense on T1-weighted images, with variable enhancement after the administration of gadolinium contrast agent. After successful treatment, the hyperintense signal on T2-weighted images and the contrast enhancement gradually resolve.

^{18}F-FDG PET detects the metabolic activity of viable LCH lesions with higher sensitivity than standard staging procedures. A decrease in standardized uptake value (SUV) is an early and accurate indicator of treatment response. After successful treatment, ^{18}F-FDG uptake decreases early whereas edema on MRI may persist for several months. PET/MR combines the advantages of high anatomic resolution and high soft tissue contrast, provided by MR, and high sensitivity and specificity, provided by PET.

Typical clinical scenario

LCH usually affects children between the ages of one and 15 years, with a minor preference for boys. Epidemiologic studies have revealed an incidence of 1.08 per 200 000 children a year in Europe. Thirty-seven percent of the LCH patients had disseminated disease which was mostly seen at a young age (< two years) and was associated with a mortality rate of 27% due to organ failure.

Differential diagnosis

LCH has a highly variable appearance, which can mimic many other pathologies. Differential diagnoses include osteomyelitis, other benign bone tumors such as bone cysts, non-ossifying fibromas and fibrous dysplasia, as well as malignant bone tumors such as Ewing's sarcoma, osteosarcoma, and metastases. Bone marrow infiltration by lymphoma cells may create a PET/MR image very similar to histiocytic lesions.

Teaching point

The prognosis of LCH patients is determined by organ system involvement at primary staging and by treatment response on follow-up studies. MRI and PET provide highly accurate information for primary staging and follow-up evaluations of patients. Active lesions show contrast enhancement on T1-weighted images, edema on T2-weighted images, and increased ^{18}F-FDG uptake on PET. After successful treatment, ^{18}F-FDG uptake decreases early whereas edema on MRI may persist for several months. A decreased ^{18}F-FDG uptake on PET is an early and accurate indicator of treatment response.

REFERENCES

1. Abla O, Egeler RM, Weitzman S. Langerhans cell histiocytosis: current concepts and treatments. *Cancer Treat Rev* 2010;**36**(4):354–9.
2. Broadbent V, Gadner H. Current therapy for Langerhans cell histiocytosis. *Hematol Oncol Clin North Am* 1998;**12**:327–38.
3. Carstensen H, Ornvold K. [Langerhans-cell histiocytosis (histiocytosis X) in children]. *Ugeskr Laeger* 1993;**155**(23):1779–83.
4. Carstensen H, Ornvold K. The epidemiology of Langerhans cell histiocytosis in children in Denmark. *Med Pediatr Oncol* 1993;**21**:387–8.
5. Gadner H, Grois N, Arico M, *et al.* A randomized trial of treatment for multisystem Langerhans' cell histiocytosis. *J Pediatr* 2001;**138**(5): 728–34.
6. Howarth DM, Gilchrist GS, Mullan BP, *et al.* Langerhans cell histiocytosis: diagnosis, natural history, management, and outcome. *Cancer* 1999;**85**:2278–90.
7. Kaste SC, Rodriguez-Galindo C, McCarville ME, *et al.* PET-CT in pediatric Langerhans cell histiocytosis. *Pediatr Radiol* 2007;**37**(7): 615–22.
8. Minkov M, Grois N, Heitger A, *et al.* Response to initial treatment of multisystem Langerhans cell histiocytosis: an important prognostic indicator. *Med Pediatr Oncol* 2002;**39**(6):581–5.
9. Phillips M, Allen C, Gerson P, *et al.* Comparison of FDG-PET scans to conventional radiography and bone scans in management of Langerhans cell histiocytosis. *Pediatr Blood Cancer* 2009;**52**(1):97–101.

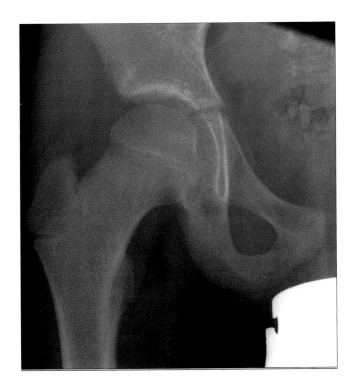

Figure 86.1. A 12-year-old boy with LCH. Frontal radiograph of the right hip shows a well-demarcated, focal osteolytic lesion in the inferior acetabulum.

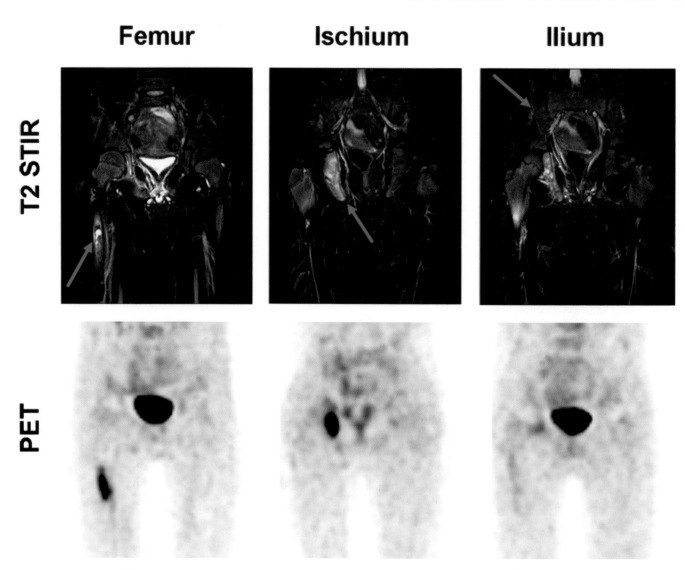

Figure 86.2. MRI and ^{18}F-FDG PET images of the pelvis and thighs at primary diagnosis. Coronal MRI and ^{18}F-FDG PET images of the pelvis and thighs were obtained in two separate investigations. Bone marrow edema was revealed on T2 STIR-weighted images in the right femur diaphysis and the right ischium. Both lesions show increased ^{18}F-FDG uptake (SUV$_{max}$: 8.3 and 10.1). The right ilium had a normal appearance in both studies.

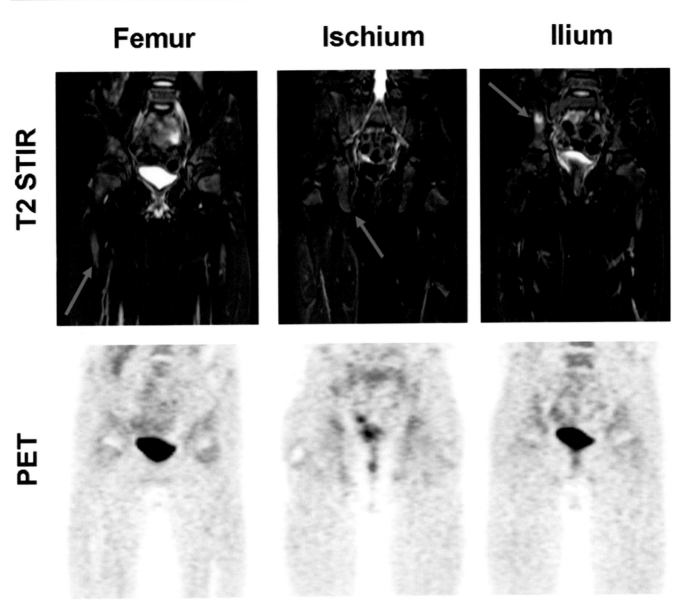

Figure 86.3. Simultaneous MRI and ^{18}F-FDG PET images of the pelvis and thighs at follow-up. Simultaneous MRI/PET acquisition of pelvis and thighs was performed one year after treatment. The previously diagnosed lesions have resolved. However, a new hyperintense lesion of the right ilium was seen on T2-weighted images, which did not show increased ^{18}F-FDG metabolism on PET. A conservative treatment strategy was pursued and the lesion resolved spontaneously.

Congenital syphilis

Vanessa Starr and Bo Yoon Ha

Imaging description

AP and lateral radiographs of the right lower extremity in a young infant demonstrated diffuse exuberant periosteal reaction, diaphyseal sclerosis, and metaphyseal irregularity with horizontal metaphyseal lucent lines (Fig. 87.1a,b), suggestive of bony changes of congenital syphilis. AP radiograph of the bilateral lower extremities in a different infant with congenital syphilis demonstrated irregular, focal lucencies of the medial proximal metaphyses of the bilateral tibiae, the Wimberger sign (Fig. 87.2). AP radiographs of bilateral upper extremities in another infant demonstrated metaphyseal lucencies and diaphyseal sclerosis (Fig. 87.3).

Importance

Congenital syphilis is transferred through the placenta in the second or third trimester in mothers with untreated or recently treated primary or secondary syphilis. The pathogenesis of this disease is transplacental migration of *Treponema pallidum* bacteria. Bony changes are thought to result mostly from trophic effects rather than direct osteomyelitis. There is inhibition of osteogenesis and disturbance of active endochondral ossification. Symmetric involvement of the sites of endochondral ossification leads to bony changes at the epiphyseal-metaphyseal junctions, costochondral junctions, and endochondral ossification sites in the sternum and spine. A baby born to a mother with untreated syphilis in the primary or secondary stage has a nearly 100% chance of acquiring the infection. Radiographic changes occur approximately six to eight weeks after initial infection, so that they may not be present at birth but only manifest subsequently. Direct clinical examination, treponemal tests, VDRL (venereal disease research laboratory [test for syphilis]), and rapid plasma reagin are used to confirm the diagnosis. Results are considered conclusive when the infant's titer is at least four times higher than that of the mother.

Osseous involvement has been reported to occur in 95% of symptomatic infants. Long bones are predominantly affected, manifesting as periostitis and osteitis as well as osteochondritis. Osteitis can result in lytic destructive lesions with reactive sclerosis in the diaphysis. Periostitis is related to infiltration of the periosteum by syphilitic granulation tissue. Osteochondritis is the result of symmetric involvement of endochondral ossification. In growing long bones, metaphyseal irregularity and widening of the zone of provisional calcification occurs with a characteristic "sawtooth" appearance. Erosive-lytic lesions in the medial proximal tibia are called the Wimberger sign, which is a characteristic finding in congenital syphilis, occurring in 20% of early cases (Fig. 87.2). Other classic radiographic findings include horizontal lucent bands at the metaphyses. The bones appear to be relatively fragile and pathologic fractures may occur.

Typical clinical scenario

The incidence of congenital syphilis in the USA is 10 in every 100 000 live births. Risk factors include low socioeconomic status, maternal age less than 30 years, history of maternal cocaine exposure, and inadequate prenatal care, amongst others. Currently, it is recommended that all pregnant women be screened for syphilis. Repeat tests in high-risk mothers can be performed before delivery. It is associated with a high rate of stillbirths and premature delivery. Treatment is intravenous penicillin.

Babies most commonly present with non-specific signs and symptoms such as fever, failure to thrive, and irritability. Presentation is divided into early and late onset. Babies with early onset syphilis, evident at two to 24 weeks of age, often have rhinorrhea, erythematous maculopapular rashes on the hands and feet as well as fissures near mucosal surfaces such as the mouth, nares, and anus. Clinical examination may reveal splenomegaly with or without associated hepatomegaly. Nearly a quarter of the patients will present with pseudoparalysis, or refusal to move an extremity secondary to pain. This clinically presents as a flaccid, bilateral, and symmetric paralysis. Laboratory abnormalities include anemia, leukopenia, thrombocytopenia, or leukocytosis. *Treponema pallidum* can also affect solid organs including kidneys, where glomerulonephritis ensues, lungs, liver, and gastrointestinal tract. Late onset congenital syphilis is typically diagnosed in patients beyond two years of age. The pathognomonic findings consist of interstitial keratitis, Hutchinson teeth, and deafness, also known as Hutchinson's triad. Osseous findings in late onset congenital syphilis include saddle nose deformity, frontal bossing, maxillary hypoplasia, saber shin, and other areas of focal or diffuse cortical thickening with occasional focal bony destructive lesions. Symmetric painless joint effusions typically involving the knees are named Clutton's joints; however, this is a relatively rare manifestation of late congenital syphilis.

Differential diagnosis

Congenital syphilis has an extensive differential diagnosis. Other congenital infections such as rubella and cytomegalovirus can also have metaphyseal irregularity or even destructive changes but more typically demonstrate irregular vertical lucencies of the metaphysis (celery stalking) and diffuse bony sclerosis in congenital rubella. Hematogenous osteomyelitis can occur in the first few weeks of life and is most frequently caused by Group B *Streptococcus*, the predominant cause of perinatal sepsis, acquired in the birth canal (Fig. 87.4a,b) or staphylococcal organisms. Metaphyseal involvement is typical, with variable deep soft tissue swelling, metaphyseal destructive changes, and periosteal reaction. Septic arthritis is almost invariable in association with neonatal osteomyelitis (Fig. 87.4a,b) because of the presence of transphyseal sinusoidal connections between the metaphyseal and epiphyseal vessels that disappear later in life.

Birth trauma and non-accidental injury are important differential diagnoses for the osseous manifestations of congenital syphilis. Clinical history should be elicited to help distinguish them.

Rickets (vitamin D deficiency) and copper deficiency are particularly prevalent in premature infants and are also in the differential for congenital syphilis. Rickets causes loss of the zone of provisional calcification, metaphyseal cupping and fraying, physeal widening, pathologic fractures, and periosteal reaction as well as diaphyseal bowing. Secondary hyperparathyroidism is associated with rickets in renal osteodystrophy and produces subperiosteal resorption that can sometimes mimic infection. This is unlikely to be present in a neonate. However, both congenital hyperparathyroidism and lytic bone changes in infantile myofibromatosis can mimic the Wimberger sign when the proximal medial tibia is affected. Laboratory values, infectious serologic testing, and clinical exam findings such as the classic maculopapular rash in syphilis can distinguish these entities.

Leukemia can cause symmetrical metaphyseal lucent bands, osteopenia, and periosteal reaction and is also a differential consideration.

Teaching point

Osseous abnormalities are common manifestations of congenital syphilis. Common radiographic findings include periostitis, osteitis, and osteochondritis, which result in prominent periosteal reaction, metaphyseal irregularity or lucency, and erosions. Osteochondritis affecting the medial proximal tibia is called the Wimberger sign and is a characteristic but not exclusive radiologic finding in congenital syphilis. Clinical examination and laboratory findings should be correlated for confirmation.

REFERENCES

1. Laird SM. Late congenital syphilis: an analysis of 115 cases. *Br J Vener Dis* 1950;**26**(3):143–5.
2. Mabey D, Richens J. Sexually transmitted diseases (excluding HIV). In: Cook GC, ed. *Manson's Tropical Diseases*, 20th edition. London, UK: W.B. Saunders Company, 1996; 336–40.
3. Sharma M, Solanki RN, Gupta A, *et al.* Different radiological presentations of congenital syphilis: four cases. *Indian J Radiol Imaging* 2005;**15**:53–7.
4. Swischuk LE. Skeletal system and soft tissues. In: Swischuk LE, ed. *Imaging of the Newborn, Infant and Young Child*, 4th edition. Philadelphia: Williams and Wilkins, 1997; 736–80.
5. Torchinsky MY, Shulman H, Landau D. Special feature: radiological case of the month. Congenital syphilis presenting as osteomyelitis with normal radioisotope bone scan. *Arch Pediatr Adolesc Med* 2001;**155** (5):613–14.

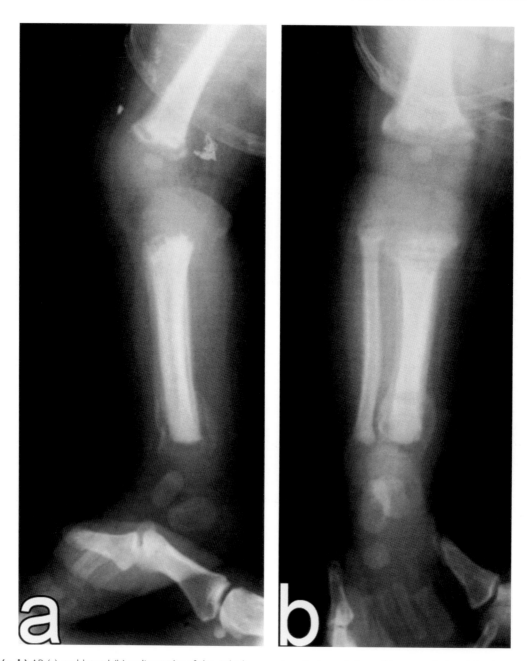

Figure 87.1. (a, b) AP (a) and lateral (b) radiographs of the right lower extremity in an infant with congenital syphilis demonstrate diffuse exuberant periosteal reaction, diaphyseal sclerosis, and metaphyseal irregularity with horizontal metaphyseal lucent lines.

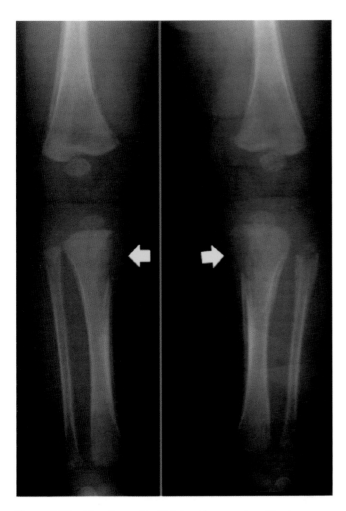

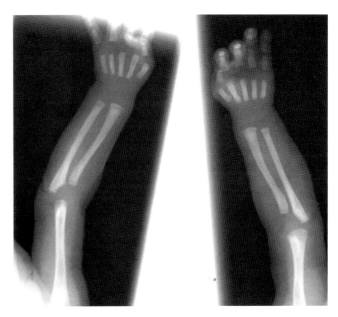

Figure 87.3. An AP radiograph of bilateral upper extremities in a different infant with congenital syphilis demonstrates metaphyseal lucencies and diaphyseal sclerosis of the long bones.

Figure 87.2. AP radiograph of bilateral lower extremities in a different infant with congenital syphilis demonstrates marked periosteal reaction of both distal femurs, proximal tibiae, and the proximal left fibula along with typical irregular lytic defects of the medial aspects of the bilateral proximal tibiae (Wimberger sign– arrows) and a lytic defect of the left proximal fibula.

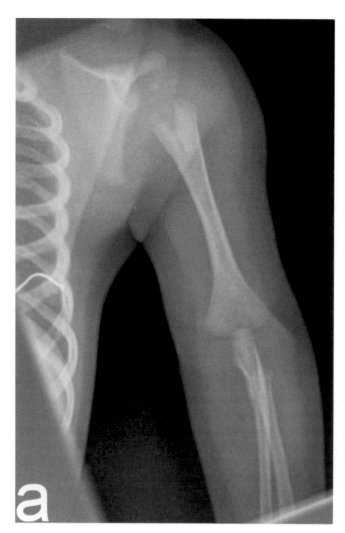
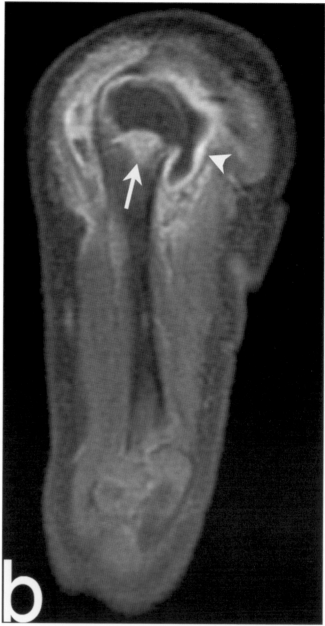

Figure 87.4. A two-week-old infant with fever and irritability, not using left arm. Blood cultures were positive for Group B *Streptococcus*. **(a)** Frontal radiograph demonstrates a lytic lesion of the left humeral metaphysis and probable joint space widening, likely related to an effusion. Findings are suggestive of osteomyelitis and septic arthritis. **(b)** Sagittal postcontrast MRI confirms the presence of osteomyelitis and septic arthritis. There is an area of metaphyseal enhancement (arrow) corresponding to the lytic lesion on plain film as well as a joint effusion with thickened enhancing synovium, marked surrounding soft tissue inflammation, and a small soft tissue abscess (arrowhead).

Medial malleolus avulsion fracture

Vanessa Starr and Bo Yoon Ha

Imaging description

A 13-year-old male patient had a twisting injury of the right ankle. Radiographs of the right ankle (in temporary cast) demonstrated a fracture of the right medial malleolus with a medially displaced fracture fragment (Fig. 88.1a). The fracture was noted to have metaphyseal, physeal, and epiphyseal components consistent with a Salter–Harris type IV injury. In addition, there was mild separation of the distal tibia and fibula, suggesting an injury of the tibiofibular syndesmosis. The patient was referred to orthopedic surgery for surgical fixation. A postsurgical radiograph of the right ankle demonstrated anatomic alignment of tibia and fibula with stabilizing screws in the medial malleolus and through the distal tibiofibular syndesmosis (Fig. 88.1b).

Importance

In 1931, McFarland described a pediatric fracture of the medial malleolus of the distal tibia that extended across the physis and sometimes into the metaphysis. These fractures were therefore previously described as McFarland fractures. The Salter–Harris classification has since become more frequently used to characterize pediatric fractures (Fig. 88.2). Salter–Harris I fractures extend through the physis. Type II fractures pass through the physis and metaphysis. Type III fractures extend through the physis and epiphysis. Type IV fractures pass through the epiphysis, physis, and metaphysis. Salter–Harris type V injury is a compression or crush injury of the physeal plate, associated with growth disturbance at the physis (Fig. 88.2). An avulsion fracture of the medial malleolus of the distal tibia that extends through the physis and epiphysis is therefore characterized as a Salter–Harris III or IV fracture depending upon whether there is extension of the fracture line into the metaphysis. The medial collateral ligament (MCL) of the ankle, also called the deltoid ligament, can be involved. The MCL is a strong ligamentous complex that is an important stabilizer of the ankle. The MCL components include a deep layer which courses from the medial malleolus to the talus and a deltoid-shaped superficial layer that extends from the medial malleolus to the navicular, the spring ligament, and the calcaneus. The importance of this fracture is that it often occurs in children and any disruption or damage to the developing growth plate can result in growth arrest. The incidence of associated growth arrest ranges from 13 to 50%. Leary *et al.* reported a statistically significant correlation between the amount of initial fracture displacement and the rate of premature physeal closure (PPC) with a relative risk of 1.15 (p < 0.01) in their multivariate analysis, indicating that for each 1 mm of displacement, there was a 15% increase of PPC.

These initial radiographic measurements of the displacement of the medial epiphyseal avulsed fragment can be useful for surgical planning as well as predicting prognostic outcome. Serial follow-up radiographs should be obtained at regular intervals until growth is properly assessed. Growth arrest is manifested by an angular deformity or limb-length discrepancy. Some orthopedic surgeons have described using a line drawn parallel to the lateral border of the tibial shaft and a second line drawn parallel to the tibial plafond on an AP radiograph to measure angular deformity of the ankle mortise. CT or MR imaging is useful to evaluate the location and size of physeal bars in areas of growth plate premature fusion.

Typical clinical scenario

These fractures occur in children before physeal closure and are typically related to an adduction or pronation injury. A factor that treating physicians can control in affecting PPC is the number of reduction attempts. Past literature has suggested that multiple reduction maneuvers may increase the risk of PPC due to further traumatic injury to an already damaged physis. One retrospective review of 48 cases of children with Salter–Harris III or IV fractures of the medial malleolus reported that open surgical arthrotomy resulted in improved anatomic reduction when compared to closed reduction. Currently, there are variable thoughts as to how much displacement is necessary for surgical intervention; however, the general consensus is that near anatomic alignment should be the goal irrespective of the chosen method of treatment. If growth arrest occurs, additional surgeries such as tibial lengthening, osteotomies, or excision of the physeal bar may be required.

Differential diagnosis

Pediatric ankle injuries include other types of fractures although each one has its own characteristic radiographic findings. The incisural ankle fracture is an avulsion of the lateral distal tibia by the intraosseous ligament, which does not extend into the anterior cortex. The juvenile tillaux fracture is a Salter–Harris type III injury and the triplane fracture is a Salter–Harris type IV injury of the anterolateral aspect of the distal tibia in adolescents with a partially closed growth plate. An adolescent pilon fracture involves the tibial plafond and is characterized by variable comminution with articular and physeal involvement.

Teaching points

An avulsion fracture of the medial malleolus of the distal tibia is characterized as a Salter–Harris III or Salter–Harris IV fracture depending upon whether the fracture line extends into the metaphysis or just involves the physis and epiphysis. The importance of these fractures is the potential complication of premature physeal closure and resultant growth arrest, which needs to be evaluated on serial follow-up radiographs. Near anatomic alignment obtained by surgical or closed reduction is of utmost importance for an optimal outcome.

REFERENCES

1. Cass JR, Peterson HA. Salter-Harris Type-IV injuries of the distal tibial epiphyseal growth plate, with emphasis on those involving the medial malleolus. *J Bone Joint Surg Am* 1983;**65**(8):1059–70.
2. Cottalorda J, Béranger V, Louahem D, et al. Salter-Harris Type III and IV medial malleolar fractures: growth arrest: is it a fate? A retrospective study of 48 cases with open reduction. *J Pediatr Orthop* 2008;**28**(6):652–5.
3. Leary JT, Handling M, Talerico M, et al. Physeal fractures of the distal tibia: predictive factors of premature physeal closure and growth arrest. *J Pediatr Orthop* 2009;**29**(4):356–61.
4. McFarland B. Traumatic arrest of epiphyseal growth of the lower end of tibia. *Br J Surg* 1931;**19**:78–82.
5. Mengiardi B, Pfirrmann CW, Vienne P, et al. Medial collateral ligament complex of the ankle: MR appearance in asymptomatic subjects. *Radiology* 2007;**242**(3):817–24.

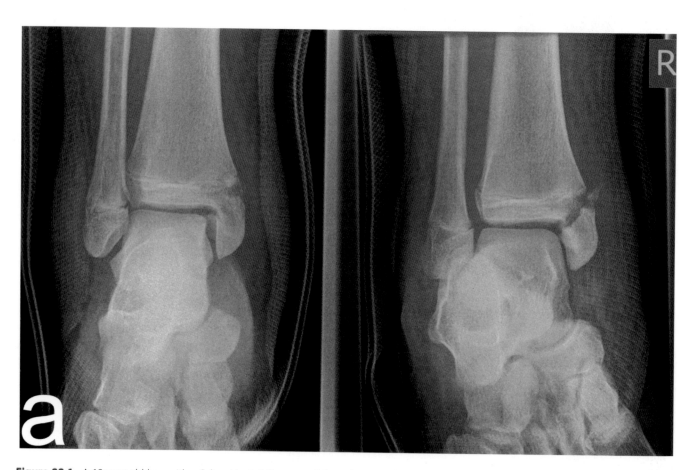

Figure 88.1. A 13-year-old boy with a Salter–Harris IV fracture of the right ankle. **(a)** Frontal and oblique casted radiographs of the right ankle demonstrate a displaced avulsed medial malleolar fracture with metaphyseal, physeal, and epiphyseal components. There is also mild separation of the distal tibia and fibula, suggesting injury of the distal tibiofibular syndesmosis.

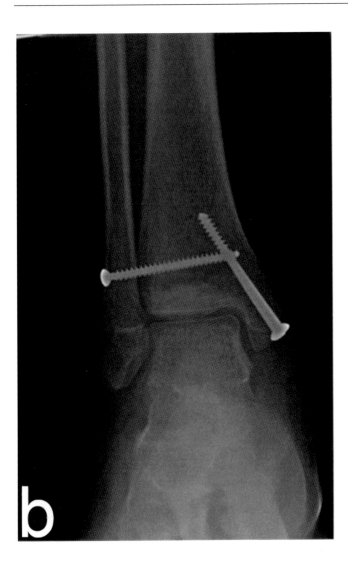

Figure 88.1. (cont.) **(b)** Postsurgical oblique radiograph of the right ankle demonstrates anatomic alignment of tibia and fibula with stabilizing screws in the medial malleolus and through the distal tibiofibular syndesmosis.

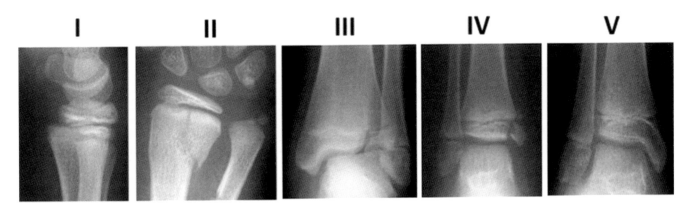

Figure 88.2. Salter–Harris fractures. Type I = physeal fracture. Type II = physeal and metaphyseal fractures. Type III = physeal and epiphyseal fractures. Type IV = physeal, metaphyseal, and epiphyseal fractures. Type V = crush injury of the physis.

Triplane fracture

Bo Yoon Ha

Imaging description

A 12-year-old female presented with a history of injury to the left ankle. An AP radiograph of the left ankle demonstrated a fracture in the distal lateral metaphysis of the left tibia with associated widening at the lateral aspect of the physis and probable epiphyseal fracture also, suggesting a Salter–Harris type IV fracture (Fig. 89.1a). The lateral radiograph more clearly demonstrated an extension of the fracture into the epiphysis (Fig. 89.1b), suggesting a complex triplane Salter–Harris type IV fracture with the epiphysis fractured in the sagittal plane, the physis separated in the axial plane, and the metaphysis fractured in the coronal plane. A CT scan better demonstrated the extent of the fracture with an anterolateral bony fragment of the tibial epiphysis and intra-articular extension into the tibiofibular syndesmosis and tibiotalar joint (Fig. 89.1c). Coronal and sagittal CT reformats clearly demonstrated the fractures of the posterolateral metaphysis, anterolateral physis, and central epiphysis (Fig. 89.1d–f) with involvement of the tibial plafond. The intra-articular extension into the tibiotalar joint was characterized by wide separation of the epiphyseal fragments at the joint surface with a displaced anterolateral epiphyseal fragment. The medial malleolus was intact.

Importance

The triplane fracture is a complex injury of the distal tibia in adolescents that does not entirely fit into the more simple Salter–Harris classification of physeal injuries. The triplane fracture accounts for 5–10% of all pediatric intra-articular ankle fractures and occurs due to external rotation forces during a specific time window of partial closure of the distal tibial epiphysis. The name derives from the three-dimensional involvement of the physis, epiphysis, and metaphysis in the frontal, transverse, and lateral planes. CT, with its excellent spatial resolution and multiplanar reconstruction capability, is usually used to delineate the exact extent of the fractures and the articular involvement, including the tibial plafond and the medial malleolus. The amount of separation and displacement of the epiphyseal fragments at the tibiotalar joint is crucial in deciding between conservative versus surgical management. Epiphyseal separation >2 mm is most often treated with surgical fracture fixation rather than casting.

The occurrence of the triplane fracture during adolescence is directly related to the physiologic pattern of distal tibial physeal closure (physiologic epiphysiodesis). Physeal closure starts at a central tibial bump (Kump's bump) anteromedially, then progresses medially and posterolaterally and finishes anterolaterally. The entire process of distal tibial physeal closure usually spans 18 months. It occurs around the age of

12–15 years (mean age: 13.5 years, range of age: 10–18 years), with complete closure occurring earlier in girls than in boys. The triplane fracture classically presents during the time period of medial physeal closure and before lateral physeal closure occurs. This explains the typical involvement of the anterolateral physis by this fracture.

There are eight different configurations of the triplane fracture described in the literature, including classic types and variants. The most common types are two- and three-fragment fractures. The different types have been categorized by the presence of epiphyseal and physeal involvement, the number of fragments, the appearance of the Salter–Harris fracture in each plane, and the degree of separation of the epiphyseal fragments. Articular involvement with extension to the tibial plafond is more common than a fracture of the medial malleolus. The triplane fracture may have a coexisting fibular fracture, which is not counted as a component of the triplane fracture. Associated deltoid ligament rupture and syndesmotic disruption have also been reported.

Typical clinical scenario

The triplane fracture occurs most commonly in patients 12–15 years of age, before complete closure of the distal tibial physis. The incidence is slightly higher in boys than in girls. The patients usually present with pain and deformity of the ankle after injury. The classic mechanism of injury is an external rotation force applied to the ankle through a supinated foot.

Less frequent non-displaced or extra-articular triplane fractures can often be managed with immobilization in a long leg cast. More frequent displaced intra-articular fractures need to be treated with open reduction and internal fixation.

Differential diagnosis

Pediatric ankle injuries include other types of fractures. Both the incisural ankle fracture and the juvenile tillaux fracture are also forms of transitional ankle fractures related to the asymmetric pattern of distal tibial physeal closure. The incisural ankle fracture is a lateral tibiofibular syndesmotic injury with accompanying avulsion of the lateral distal tibia by the intraosseous ligament. The fracture does not extend into the anterior tibia. A juvenile tillaux fracture is a Salter–Harris type III intra-articular fracture of the anterolateral tibial epiphysis and physis at a relatively late time point of physeal closure. The adolescent pilon fracture involves the tibial plafond and is characterized by articular and physeal involvement, with significant comminution, multiple displaced fracture fragments, and variable talar and fibular involvement.

Teaching point

The triplane fracture is an injury of the distal tibia in adolescents, during the time of partial closure of the physis, which involves three planes of the epiphysis, physis, and metaphysis. Physiologic physeal closure starts at a central tibial bump (Kump's bump) anteromedially, progresses medially and posterolaterally, and finishes anterolaterally, which contributes to the classic configurations of this fracture including two- or three-fragment fracture types. CT is often needed to delineate the exact extent of the fracture and intra-articular involvement in order to guide proper management.

REFERENCES

1. Brown SD, Kasser JR, Zurakowski D, et al. Analysis of 51 tibial triplane fractures using CT with multiplanar reconstruction. *AJR Am J Roentgenol* 2004;**183**(5):1489–95.
2. Butt WP. Triplane fractures of the distal tibia. *Orthopedics* 2001;**24** (2):106.
3. Cummings RJ. Triplane ankle fracture with deltoid ligament tear and syndesmotic disruption. *J Child Orthop* 2008;**2**(1):11–14.
4. Schnetzler KA, Hoernschemeyer D. The pediatric triplane ankle fracture. *J Am Acad Orthop Surg* 2007;**15**(12):738–4.

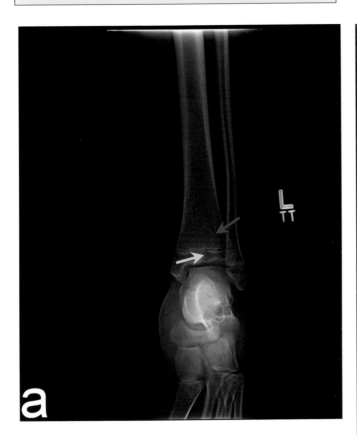

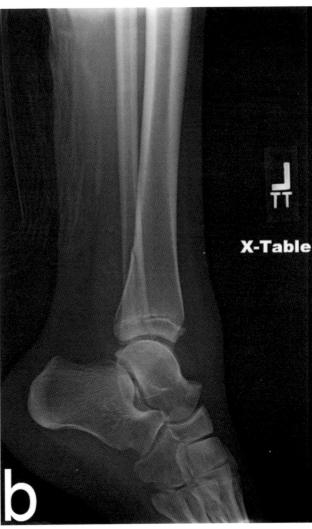

Figure 89.1. A 12-year-old patient with ankle injury, triplane fracture. **(a)** Ankle AP radiograph demonstrates a fracture of the lateral distal metaphysis of the tibia (blue arrow) with widening of the lateral aspect of the physis. There is probable extension of the fracture into the mid epiphysis (yellow arrow). **(b)** Ankle lateral radiograph demonstrates a triplane Salter–Harris type IV fracture involving mid epiphysis, anterior physis, and posterior metaphysis.

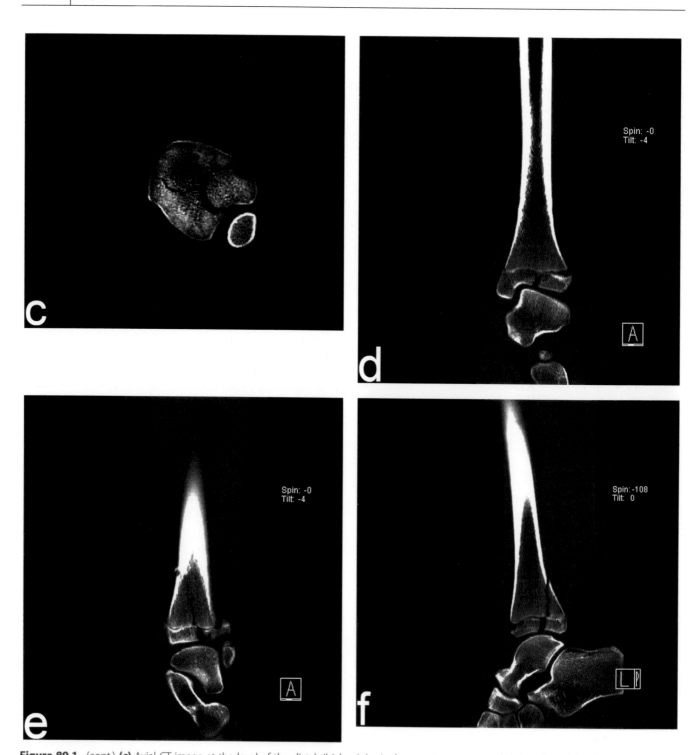

Figure 89.1. (cont.) **(c)** Axial CT image at the level of the distal tibial epiphysis demonstrates improved delineation of the fracture with an anterolateral bony fragment of the distal tibial epiphysis and intra-articular extension into the tibiofibular syndesmosis and tibiotalar joint. **(d, e)** Coronal CT reformats further clarify the anatomy of the fracture with metaphyseal, physeal, and epiphyseal components. There is intra-articular extension of the epiphyseal fracture into the tibiotalar joint with wide separation of the fracture fragments visible at the joint surface and a displaced anterolateral bony epiphyseal fragment. **(f)** Sagittal CT reformat redemonstrates the extent of the fracture with wide epiphyseal separation and a slight step off of the epiphyseal fragments at the joint space.

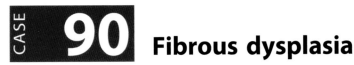

90 Fibrous dysplasia

Vy Thao Tran, Aman Khurana, and Bo Yoon Ha

Imaging description

A 17-year-old girl presented with progressive asymmetric left eye swelling. CT images through the left orbit demonstrated a mass centered in the left superior orbital rim, extending through the left cribriform plate and into the posterior ethmoidal air cells. The internal matrix of this mass had a ground glass appearance (Fig. 90.1a, b). The orbital apex appeared to be spared (Fig. 90.1). T2-weighted MR images through the orbit demonstrated a homogeneous hypointense signal of the mass (Fig. 90.1c, d). The mass displaced rather than invaded adjacent soft tissue structures. It displaced the frontal lobe superiorly and extended into the conus of the orbit, with mass effect on the superior and medial rectus muscles. The optic nerve did not appear to be encased. There was homogeneous enhancement of the mass on the T1-weighted MR images after intravenous administration of gadolinium (Gd)-DTPA (Fig. 90.1d). Additional CT (Figs. 90.2 and 90.3b) and plain film (Fig. 90.3a) images of two other children with fibrous dysplasia (FD), one of whom has McCune–Albright syndrome (MAS) (Fig. 90.3), demonstrate the classic ground glass bony matrix.

Importance

FD is a slow growing, benign disease process where the normal bone is replaced by various degrees of immature woven and fibrous bone. FD accounts for 5–10% of all bone tumors. The disease can be monostotic or polyostotic. Bone involvement is typically unilateral with relatively common involvement of the ribs and femur. Craniofacial involvement is reported in up to 25% of monostotic and in 50–100% of polyostotic forms. Among patients with skull lesions, the most commonly involved bones are the frontal, ethmoid, and sphenoid bones. Bone scans may demonstrate increased ^{99m}Tc-MDP tracer uptake and can be used to assess the overall disease burden throughout the body. The CT appearance of FD is variable, with a study by Brown et al. reporting a ground glass pattern in 56%, a homogeneously dense pattern in 23%, and a cystic variety in 21%. On MRI, FD is characteristically hypointense on T1- and T2-weighted images, due to its high cellularity, fibrous tissue content, and internal bony trabeculae. Cystic varieties of FD may present as T2-hyperintense lesions. In these cases, FD can be mistaken for a soft tissue neoplasm. In patients with sphenoid bone involvement, optic canal involvement occurs in 50–90%. MR interpretation should involve detailed evaluation of optic canal involvement and/or optic nerve encasement.

Typical clinical scenario

Most patients present before 30 years of age. The monostotic form is more common and typically affects the 20- to 30-year-old age group. Multiple bone FD usually presents before

10 years of age and stabilizes after puberty. There is no gender predilection. It may be a part of systemic syndromes such as Jaffe–Lichtenstein syndrome (JLS) or MAS (Fig. 90.3). JLS is characterized by polyostotic FD and café-au-lait pigmented skin lesions, while MAS includes hyperfunctional endocrinopathies manifesting as precocious puberty, hyperthyroidism, or acromegaly. The pathophysiology of FD is a somatic mutation, which results in abnormal osteoblast differentiation and production of dysplastic bone.

The clinical presentation of FD is variable and dependent on the mass effect of the affected bone on adjacent structures. When presenting in an extremity, bony contour abnormalities, pain, and pathologic fractures have been commonly noted. The diagnosis is usually made based on medical history as well as clinical and radiographic findings. Bone biopsy is reserved for patients with an atypical imaging appearance, with polyostotic disease, or concern for malignant degeneration, which occurs in about 0.4–4% of cases. Sarcomatous degeneration into osteosarcoma or fibrosarcoma is notably seen in patients who have undergone radiation therapy.

Since progression of FD stops after puberty, surgical intervention in children should be delayed as long as possible. For patients with symptomatic FD, bisphosphonate therapy can be utilized, which is reported to decrease bone pain, increase bony density to minimize fractures, and in some patients stabilize the lesion and prevent additional areas of involvement. DEXA scans have been found in some studies to be more consistent than serial radiographs for monitoring the effects of treatment. Patients with major disfigurement and neuropathies tend to undergo surgical rather than medical treatment although there are no randomized controlled clinical trials comparing the efficacy of bisphosphonate therapy to surgery. Because FD is a benign disease process, the goal of surgery is to preserve existing function and to prevent additional progressive deformity or neurologic compromise. Current studies recommend that patients with skull base involvement who are asymptomatic be managed with repeated ophthalmologic evaluation and long-term radiologic follow-up. If signs of optic nerve dysfunction develop, symptoms should be managed with partial decompression of the optic canal.

Differential diagnosis

The differential for FD can vary based on the diverse range in appearance of FD, which includes sclerosis or lucency. Potentially similar appearing bony lesions in the skull base include ossifying fibromas, metastatic disease, chondrosarcoma, meningioma, and less likely, Paget disease in a pediatric population.

Teaching point

An expansile bony lesion with an internal ground glass matrix should suggest the diagnosis of FD, particularly with unilateral involvement of the long bones, ribs, or skull base. Monostotic FD is more common and has an excellent prognosis. Poly-ostotic disease may be seen with MAS in childhood.

REFERENCES

1. Amit M, Fliss DM, Gil Z. Fibrous dysplasia of the sphenoid and skull base. *Otolaryngol Clin North Am* 2011;**44**(4):891–902.

2. Brown EW, Megerian CA, McKenna MJ, *et al.* Fibrous dysplasia of the temporal bone: imaging findings. *AJR Am J Roentgenol* 1995;**164**(3):679–82.

3. Cai M, Ma L, Xu G, *et al.* Clinical and radiological observation in a surgical series of 36 cases of fibrous dysplasia of the skull. *Clin Neurol Neurosurg* 2011;**114**(3):254–9.

4. Kos M, Luczak K, Godzinski J, *et al.* Treatment of monostotic fibrous dysplasia with pamidronate. *J Craniomaxillofac Surg* 2004;**32**(1):10–15.

5. Kransdorf MJ, Moser RP Jr, Gilkey FW. Fibrous dysplasia. *Radiographics* 1990;**10**(3):519–37.

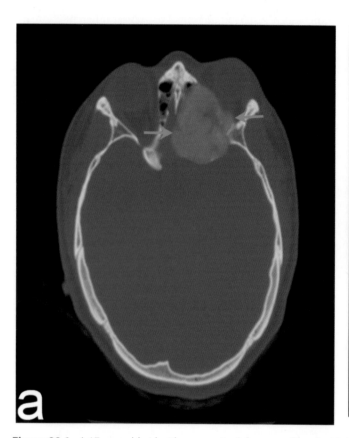
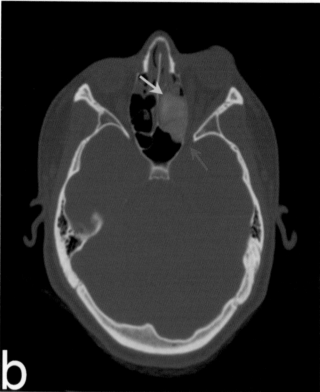

Figure 90.1. A 17-year-old girl with progressive left eye swelling. **(a, b)** Axial non-contrast CT images through the left orbit demonstrate a mass centered in the left superior orbital rim (green arrows), extending through the left cribriform plate into the posterior ethmoidal air cells (yellow arrow). The internal matrix of this mass has a ground glass appearance. The orbital apex appears to be spared (red arrow).

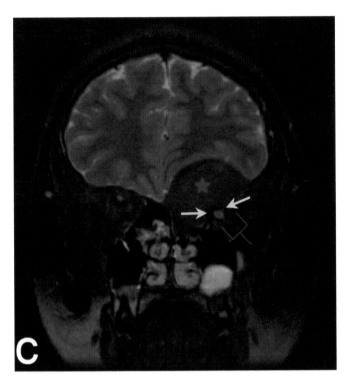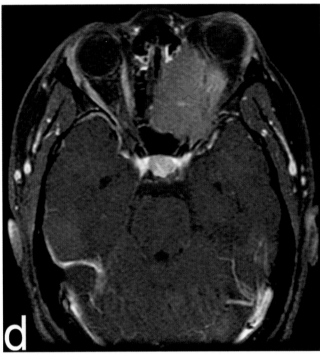

Figure 90.1. (cont.) **(c)** Coronal T2-weighted MR image through the orbit demonstrates the mass (purple star) appearing homogeneously hypointense, displacing the frontal lobe superiorly without extension into the cerebral parenchyma. There is intraconal orbital extension of the mass and mass effect on the superior and medial rectus muscles, which are compressed (yellow arrows). The optic nerve does not appear to be encased. The blue bracket points to the normal extraocular muscles. **(d)** Axial T1-weighted MR image after Gd-DTPA administration demonstrates homogeneous enhancement of the mass (red star).

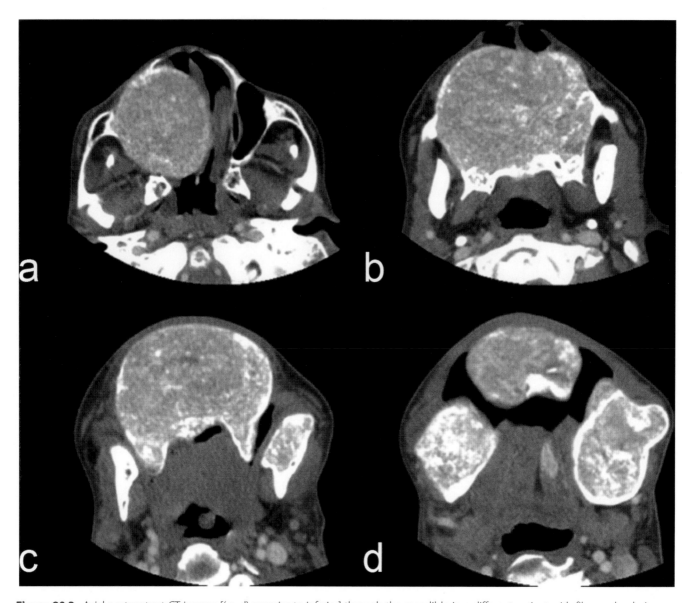

Figure 90.2. Axial postcontrast CT images [(a–d) superior to inferior] through the mandible in a different patient with fibrous dysplasia demonstrate a very large, expansile mass with ground glass appearance, involving the mandible and extending into the bilateral maxillary sinuses.

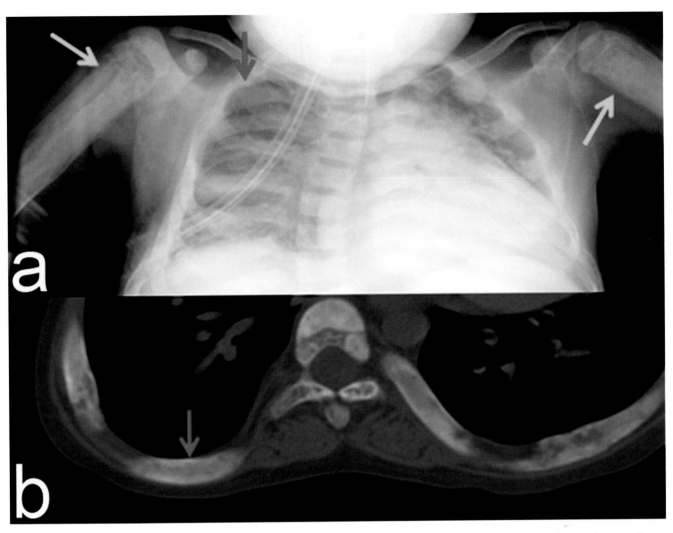

Figure 90.3. Chest radiograph **(a)** and axial CT slice **(b)** (bone window) in a nine-year-old boy with MAS who has diffuse polyostotic fibrous dysplasia with greater bone involvement on the right than the left. Red arrows point to the classic sclerotic ground glass internal matrix seen within the ribs on both plain film and non-contrast CT. Yellow arrows point to expanded proximal humeri with sclerotic ground glass, which relates to the amount of immature woven and fibrous bone. Long bones such as the humeri and femurs may develop varus deformities with time. (Case courtesy of Dr. Beverley Newman, Lucile Packard Children's Hospital, Stanford University.)

Vanessa Starr and Bo Yoon Ha

Imaging description

A 15-year-old boy presented with left-sided chest pain and a palpable chest wall mass. PA radiograph of the chest demonstrated osseous expansion and periosteal reaction in the left mid 8th rib and a large associated soft tissue mass (Fig. 91.1a). Axial contrast-enhanced CT of the chest demonstrated a heterogeneous soft tissue mass along the left chest wall. There was expansion, destruction, and periosteal reaction of the involved rib (Fig. 91.1b, c). An MRI of the abdomen, obtained to evaluate for metastases, was negative and also included the lower chest (Fig. 91.1d, e, f). This demonstrated a large heterogeneous T2 bright mass surrounding the left lower rib. The mass and marrow of the affected rib demonstrated restricted diffusion (bright signal on diffusion-weighted imaging [DWI] with dark signal on ADC map). Bone scan (not shown) did not demonstrate any metastases. Ewing's sarcoma of the chest wall was suggested as the most likely diagnosis. Subsequent pathology defined the lesion as an undifferentiated sarcoma of the chest wall.

An eight-year-old girl presented with right-sided chest pain and mass. CT findings were similar to the first case, with CT demonstrating a large lower chest wall soft tissue mass with adjacent rib destruction (Fig. 91.2). Pathology confirmed the diagnosis of Ewing's sarcoma of the chest wall.

Importance

The Ewing's sarcoma family of tumors comprise Ewing's sarcoma of bone, extraosseous Ewing's sarcoma, and primitive neuroectodermal tumor (PNET – have neural differentiation) and are all characterized by a typical chromosomal translocation (11:22)(q24;q12).

Peripheral neuroectodermal tumor of the chest wall or Ewing's sarcoma of the chest wall was previously known as Askin's tumor.

Ewing's sarcoma is a malignant tumor that was first described by James Ewing in 1921. It is a highly aggressive tumor of bone and soft tissue with characteristic radiologic, histologic, and cytogenetic findings. Pathology demonstrates small blue round cells, which stain positive for CD99 and have the EWS gene rearrangement. The most common bony sites are the long bones of the extremities, pelvis, chest wall, and spine. If in the long bones, the lesion is typically located in the diaphysis and very rarely crosses the growth plate or involves the epiphysis. The tumor typically arises from the medullary cavity.

The classic Ewing's sarcoma of bone presents radiographically as a permeative metadiaphyseal lesion with a wide zone of transition, aggressive lamellar "onion skin" periosteal reaction, and a large associated soft tissue mass. Nearly half of these tumors demonstrate a sclerotic or mixed lytic-sclerotic pattern. The lesion can invade the cortex; however, it can also traverse the haversian system, causing a large soft tissue mass with minimal cortical destruction. When centered in a vertebral body, it can cause vertebra plana. However, Ewing's sarcoma can have a myriad of radiographic appearances and in the Intergroup Ewing Sarcoma Study, nearly 27% of cases had at least one atypical component to their lesions. One such atypical appearance of Ewing's sarcoma is origin from the surface of the bone, resembling other periosteal-based malignancies such as parosteal osteosarcoma. Similar to parosteal osteosarcoma, patients with this surface-based Ewing's sarcoma have a relatively favorable prognosis.

MRI is currently considered the imaging study of choice in the evaluation of musculoskeletal mass lesions such as Ewing's sarcoma because of the lack of ionizing radiation and superior definition of tissue planes. CT or MR will demonstrate a permeative intramedullary mass, sometimes with subtle cortical destruction. The soft tissue component is often heterogeneously enhancing, with areas of central necrosis. On MRI, marrow involvement is seen as low signal, isointense to muscle on T1-weighted images and intermediate to high signal intensity on T2-weighted images. For the initial staging exam, it is important to cover the whole bone from proximal to distal joint, in order to evaluate for skip lesions, followed by closer evaluation of the primary tumor. It is difficult to discern tumor from peritumoral edema on T2-weighted images. Post-contrast images will demonstrate moderate heterogeneous enhancement, with kinetic studies demonstrating more rapid contrast enhancement of tumor compared to peritumoral edema. Previous trials of the Children's Oncology Group (COG) for patients with metastatic Ewing's sarcoma have relied upon technetium-based radionuclide whole body bone scans to detect and evaluate bone metastases. Since the inception of those previous trials, multiple studies have been published that suggest the superior performance of FDG PET scans for the diagnosis and evaluation of bone metastases in patients with Ewing's sarcoma. Both the primary tumor and metastases demonstrate increased FDG uptake; therefore, PET +/− CT or MRI can be used for staging and follow-up after treatment.

Typical clinical scenario

Ewing's sarcoma is the second most common bone tumor in children, after osteosarcoma, typically occurring between ages three and 25 years with a mean age of 13 years. It is rarely seen in patients older than 30 years of age. Pain is the most common presenting symptom. Males are twice as likely to be affected. The classic clinical presentation is a young boy presenting with fever, anemia, leukocytosis, elevated erythrocyte sedimentation rate (ESR), and a painful mass. As the symptoms are non-specific and may initially be misdiagnosed as infection, there could be a delay in diagnosis. At the time of initial diagnosis, 15–30% of patients have metastatic disease; the most common sites are local nodes, bone, and bone marrow.

Treatment usually consists of preoperative radiation or chemotherapy with vincristine, dactinomycin, and cyclophosphamide (VAC). After surgical excision, adjuvant chemotherapy is usually given, decreasing the risk of recurrence. Unresectable tumors may be treated with chemotherapy and local irradiation. Post-treatment contrast-enhanced MRI and follow-up PET/CT scans can be used to assess for recurrence.

Differential diagnosis

The most common differential diagnosis based on both clinical presentation and radiographic appearance is osteomyelitis. Chest wall infection is uncommon, with unusual organisms such as tuberculosis, actinomycosis (Fig. 91.3), and aspergillus being considerations, especially in immunosuppressed individuals. Chronic recurrent multifocal osteomyelitis (CRMO) may also be a differential consideration although the most common sites of involvement are long bones and clavicle. This entity is thought to be either an autoimmune disorder or related to occult infection and produces lytic/sclerotic expansile bony changes but without much associated soft tissue mass. Langerhans cell histiocytosis can have a myriad of appearances, including periosteal reaction and a prominent soft tissue mass; involvement of ribs is not uncommon. Primary bone lesions such as aneurysmal bone cyst and fibrous dysplasia are also differential possibilities for an expansile lytic or sclerotic rib lesion without a soft tissue mass. Other benign lesions with both bony and soft tissue components that can mimic more aggressive lesions include lymphangioma and osteoblastoma as well as trauma with fracture and/or soft tissue hematoma.

A sclerotic Ewing's sarcoma can have the appearance of an osteosarcoma although osteosarcoma typically affects a slightly older age group. Other sarcomas including chondrosarcoma, fibrosarcoma, and soft tissue sarcomas such as rhabdomyosarcoma and synovial sarcoma are in the differential diagnosis; however, these also usually affect older patients. Metastases to the chest wall (mostly bone) are more common than primary tumors and include neuroblastoma, hepatoblastoma, and leukemia/lymphoma; they are less likely to be associated with a large soft tissue mass. Intrapulmonary, mediastinal, and pleural neoplasms such as pleuropulmonary blastoma and neuroblastoma may spread directly to the chest wall.

Teaching point

The Ewing's sarcoma family comprises aggressive bone and/or soft tissue tumors affecting young children, pathologically characterized by small blue round cells and an *EWS* gene translocation. The majority arise from the pelvis or diaphysis of long bones or chest wall. The classic radiographic appearance is a permeative bony lesion with aggressive periosteal reaction and a large soft tissue mass. MRI should be used for initial and post-treatment evaluation of Ewing's sarcoma lesions as well as other bony and soft tissue masses of the chest wall, as it can better define the extent of disease, particularly with regard to the soft tissue mass. CT is helpful when additional lung or bone detail is needed.

REFERENCES

1. Erlemann R, Sciuk J, Bosse A, et al. Response of osteosarcoma and Ewing sarcoma to preoperative chemotherapy: assessment with dynamic and static MR imaging and skeletal scintigraphy. *Radiology* 1990;**175**(3):791–6.

2. Jedlicka P. Ewing Sarcoma, an enigmatic malignancy of likely progenitor cell origin, driven by transcription factor oncogenic fusions. *Int J Clin Exp Pathol* 2010;**3**(4):338–47.

3. Kaste SC, Strouse PJ, Fletcher BD, et al. Benign and malignant bone tumors. In: Slovis TL, ed. *Caffey's Pediatric Diagnostic Imaging*, 11th edition. Philadelphia: Mosby Elsevier, 2008; 2912–69.

4. Reinus WR, Gilula LA. Radiology of Ewing's sarcoma: Intergroup Ewing's Sarcoma Study (IESS). *Radiographics* 1984;**4**:929–44.

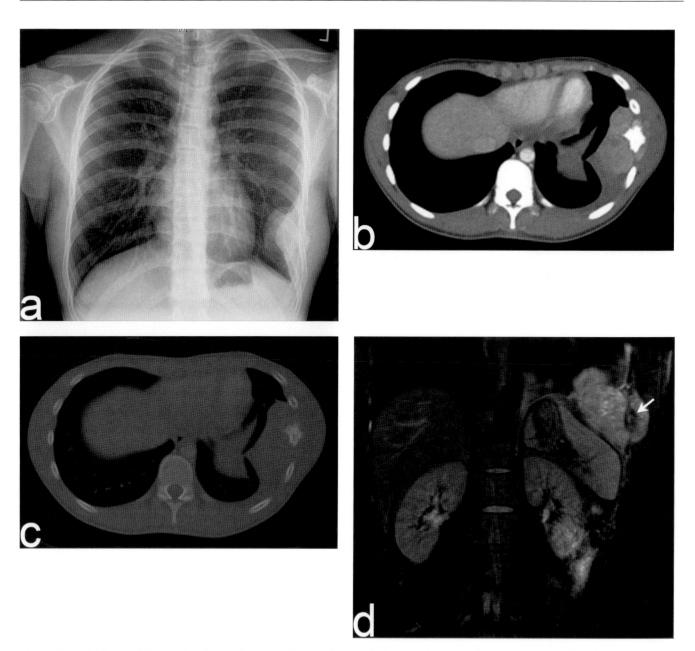

Figure 91.1. A 15-year-old boy with a chest wall mass, pathologically an undifferentiated sarcoma. **(a)** PA radiograph of the chest demonstrates osseous expansion and periosteal reaction in the left 8th rib and a large associated soft tissue component along the left chest wall and projecting over the left lower lung. **(b, c)** Axial contrast-enhanced CT images of the chest (b: soft tissue, c: bone window) demonstrate a heterogeneous soft tissue mass along the left chest wall. There is focal rib expansion, destruction, and periosteal reaction as well as pleural effusion. **(d)** Coronal T2-weighted image demonstrates a hyperintense heterogeneous left lower chest wall mass surrounding the expanded left 8th rib (arrow) with abnormal bright marrow signal. Adjacent pleural fluid is also evident.

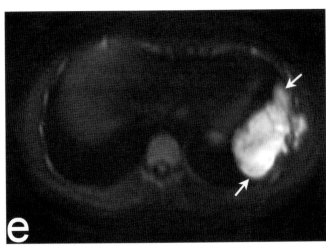

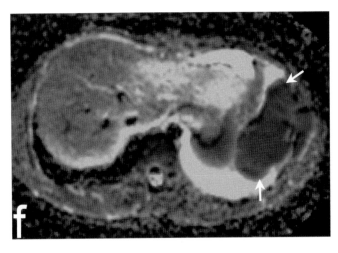

Figure 91.1. (cont.) **(e)** Axial diffusion-weighted MR image demonstrates bright signal in the mass. **(f)** ADC map shows dark signal in the mass and marrow of the affected rib, confirming that the bright signal on DWI is truly due to restricted diffusion rather than T2 shine through effect.

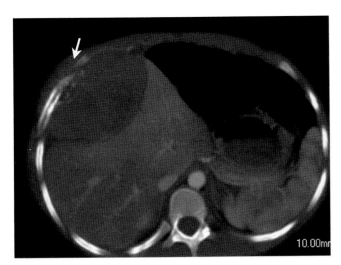

Figure 91.2. An 8-year-old female with Ewing's sarcoma of the chest wall. CT contrasted image at the thoraco-abdominal junction shows a large, slightly heterogeneous chest wall soft tissue mass centered around the anterior rib with bony destructive changes (arrow). The posterior component of the soft tissue mass exerts external mass effect on the liver. (Reprinted from *Radiologic Clinics of North America*, Vol. **49**(4), Newman B. Thoracic neoplasms in children, Pages 633–64, Copyright 2011, with permission from Elsevier.)

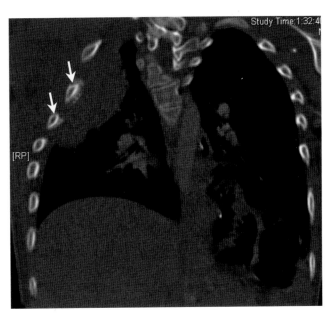

Figure 91.3. A 17-year-old with chest pain and fever several weeks after multiple dental extractions. Pathology – actinomycosis of the chest wall. Coronal contrast-enhanced CT demonstrates peripheral consolidation/mass extending to the chest wall. There is periosteal reaction in two ribs (arrows), with associated rib splaying. Incidental note is made of a left hiatal hernia.

Campomelic dysplasia

Ralph Lachman

Imaging description

A full-term newborn with polyhydramnios on third trimester ultrasound appeared dysmorphic with a cleft palate. On the AP chest radiograph the infant is noted to be intubated. The chest is slightly small with normal rib length (Fig. 92.1). The scapular bodies are absent. The midthoracic pedicles are unossified. The iliac wings are tall and narrow.

The femurs are disproportionately long compared to the shortened tibias. The skull is dolichocephalic and facial hypoplasia is present. The cervical spine has an S-shaped configuration with vertebral body hypoplasia (Fig. 92.1). These features are typical of acampomelic campomelic dysplasia.

Importance

Fetal and newborn presenting skeletal dysplasias are quite common and diverse. Campomelic dysplasia often presents in utero with short extremities (including femoral length) and bent femurs. It therefore is considered as one of the neonatal bent bone dysplasias. It usually represents a *SOX9* gene mutation. Some clinical signs and symptoms are important yet none are diagnostic.

On the other hand these four specific radiographic findings are pathognomonic (Fig. 92.2):

- Absent/hypoplastic scapular body
- Absent midthoracic vertebral pedicle ossification in the newborn period
- High/narrow iliac wings
- Bent femurs that appear disproportionately long.

At times the femurs will not be significantly bent (as in the described case). Then the entity has been termed "Acampomelic Campomelic Dysplasia." This represents clinical variability as they are also *SOX9* mutation abnormalities. As occurred in the described case, this can lead to diagnostic confusion.

Typical clinical scenario

More recently, many cases are picked up in utero by second trimester ultrasound. Careful fetal ultrasound analysis can perhaps identify one or other of the aforementioned pathognomonic findings. In the newborn there are some clinical findings. Short stature is evident. There is a rather typical facial dysmorphism. Laryngo-tracheo-malacia is quite common, leading to newborn respiratory distress. Neonatal death occurs in about three-quarters of the patients. The cervical lordosis (S-shaping of the cervical spine) is also a significant problem. Sex reversed (XY) females are seen. However, none of the aforementioned clinical findings are specifically diagnostic. Obviously a skeletal survey will allude to the diagnosis, so important for genetic counseling, prognostication, and management. Molecular analysis may be obtained if the diagnosis is questionable.

Differential diagnosis

Bent bone dysplasias (angulated femurs) including especially:

- Kyphomelic dysplasia (a heterogeneous group)
- Schwartz–Jampel syndrome
- Stüve–Wiedemann dysplasia
- Antley–Bixler syndrome
- Larsen and Larsen-like syndromes
- Osteogenesis imperfecta
- Cumming syndrome
- Scapuloiliac dysplasia.

> ### Teaching point
>
> A combination of findings including:
>
> - Absent/hypoplastic scapular bodies
> - Thoracic pedicle ossification defects
> - High narrow iliac wings
> - Disproportionately long (bent) femurs
>
> in a newborn (or late gestational fetus) is diagnostic of campomelic dysplasia.

REFERENCES

1. Alanay Y, Krakow D, Rimoin DL, *et al.* Angulated femurs and the skeletal dysplasias: experience of the International Skeletal Dysplasia Registry (1988–2006). *Am J Med Genet A* 2007;**143A**(11):1159–68.
2. Lachman RS. *Taybi and Lachman's Radiology of Syndromes, Metabolic Disorders and Skeletal Dysplasias*, 5th edition. St Louis: Mosby Inc, 2007; 720–1, 722–4, 881–3, 920–1, 972–3, 1018–24, 1089–90.

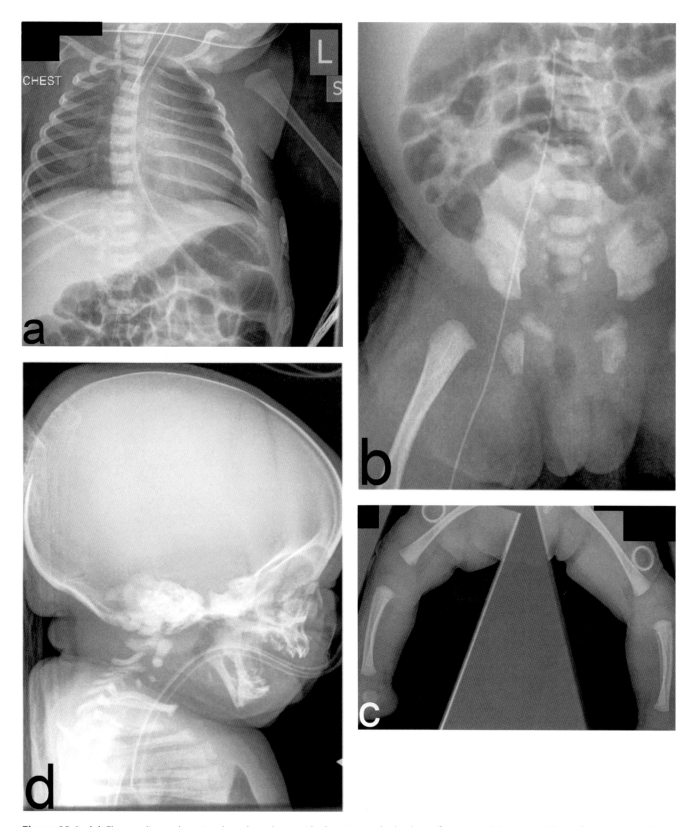

Figure 92.1. **(a)** Chest radiograph: an intubated newborn with absent scapular body ossification and absent pedicle ossification in the thoracic region. **(b)** The iliac wings are tall and narrow, other pelvic and hip structures are normal. **(c)** The femurs are disproportionately elongated, and not significantly bent, yet the tibias are short and bent. Fibulae are somewhat hidden and are also short. **(d)** A dolichocephalic-shaped skull, with both facial and mandibular hypoplasia; the cervical spine is S-shaped with marked vertebral body hypoplasia.

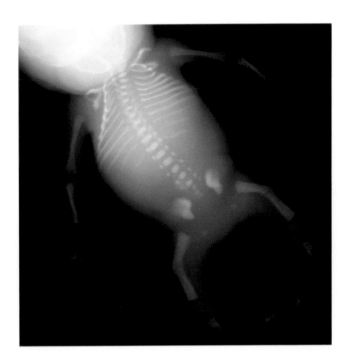

Figure 92.2. A 22-week fetus with similar findings as in the above newborn but with *bent* disproportionately long femurs. Also note: absent scapular bodies and lack of thoracic vertebral pedicle ossification. Diagnosis: classic campomelic dysplasia.

Type II collagenopathy (hypochondrogenesis)

Ralph Lachman

Imaging description

This 37-week gestational newborn infant was noted to be short statured and disproportionate. A midline cleft palate was identified. The hands seemed to be proportionately large compared to the other arm segments.

Radiographically, the thorax was quite small and the ribs were moderately shortened. The spine revealed lack of vertebral ossification in the cervical and lower lumbar and sacral regions (Fig. 93.1). In the pelvis the acetabular roofs were flat, the sacrosciatic notches were widened, and pubic bone ossification was absent. The lateral view of the spine, thorax, and skull base revealed ovoid, hypoplastic vertebral bodies and a large occipital ossification defect at the skull base. A film of the lower extremities revealed no epiphyseal ossification at the knees (as expected) and no ossification centers for talus and calcaneus. The radiograph of the hand and lower arm showed normal for age hand bone ossification but suggested that the hand was at least as long as the meso-bones.

All long bones had proportional diaphyseal shortening and otherwise normal metaphyseal/diaphyseal configuration (Fig. 93.1).

The radiographic findings are typical of a type II collagen defect and are closest to hypochondrogenesis in that spectrum of disorders.

Importance

The skeletal dysplasia that presents in the perinatal/newborn period must be diagnosed as early as possible in order to ascertain inheritance pattern for genetic counseling to the parents as well as prognostication and management. The radiographic evaluation is the most important part of the clinical workup of these disorders.

The type II collagenopathies are a spectrum of allelic disorders that share common radiographic and clinical features. Type II collagen is important for eye vitreous formation (early onset myopia); for palate formation (cleft palate); and for epiphyseal/epiphyseal equivalent ossification (epiphyseal ossification abnormalities).

The type II collagenopathies are a spectrum of disorders that extend from (severe to mild): achondrogenesis II (lethal), hypochondrogenesis (not immediately lethal but generally demise before 9 months), spondylo-epiphyseal dysplasia congenita (SEDC), spondylo-epi-metaphyseal dysplasia (SEMD)–Strudwick, Kniest dysplasia, and Stickler dysplasia type I (mildest phenotype). As mentioned, these are allelic conditions and need to be sorted out radiologically as the molecular abnormalities do not separate out the entities clearly from a clinical viewpoint. This is helpful for management. These disorders share common distinct radiologic changes. These

consist of absent or delayed basi-occipital ossification, poor vertebral ossification/formation, and epiphyseal/epiphyseal equivalent ossification delay. The "epiphyseal equivalent" bones are the talus, calcaneus, ischia, and pubic bones. The ischium ossifies at about 17 weeks, pubis at about 24 weeks, talus at 26 weeks, and the calcaneus at 23 weeks of gestation.

The presentation in the newborn of a type II collagen disorder makes a specific diagnosis at times quite difficult. Patients with SEDC, Kniest, and SEMD–Strudwick often look quite similar radiographically in the newborn period and may need to be sorted out after a year or two at follow-up. The similarity of hypochondrogenesis to SEDC is remarkable and only differs in severity of involvement in the former. One must be very careful about prognostication.

Typical clinical scenario

More and more infants/fetuses are discovered at second trimester ultrasound to have short femurs and other long bones. At delivery a comprehensive exam might uncover a cleft palate and short stature. A skeletal dysplasia is often suspected. A complete skeletal survey is required. If the films reveal the following findings, the diagnosis of a type II collagen disorder should be made:

- Occipital ossification defect of the skull base
- Epiphyseal and/or epiphyseal equivalent ossification delay
- Absent/hypoplastic/ovoid vertebral body ossification (especially in the cervical and lower lumbar-sacral regions).

Then the radiographs should be perused to try to ascertain the actual clinical diagnosis if possible.

Differential diagnosis

The differential diagnosis rests with other lethal and non-lethal, preterm and neonatal skeletal dysplasias. The well-described ones are easily radiographically diagnosed. They include thanatophoric dysplasias I and II, achondroplasia, diastrophic dysplasia, several bent bone dysplasias including campomelic dysplasia and cartilage–hair hypoplasia, and some forms of osteogenesis imperfecta (OI).

Teaching point

The films of a newly delivered fetus or newborn revealing poor vertebral ossification, epiphyseal (epiphyseal equivalent) ossification defects, and a skull base occipital ossification defect indicate a type II collagenopathy.

REFERENCES

1. Lachman RS. *Taybi and Lachman's Radiology of Syndromes, Metabolic Disorders and Skeletal Dysplasias*, 5th edition. St Louis: Mosby Inc, 2007; 915–16, 961–3, 1069–71, 969–71, 1072–5.

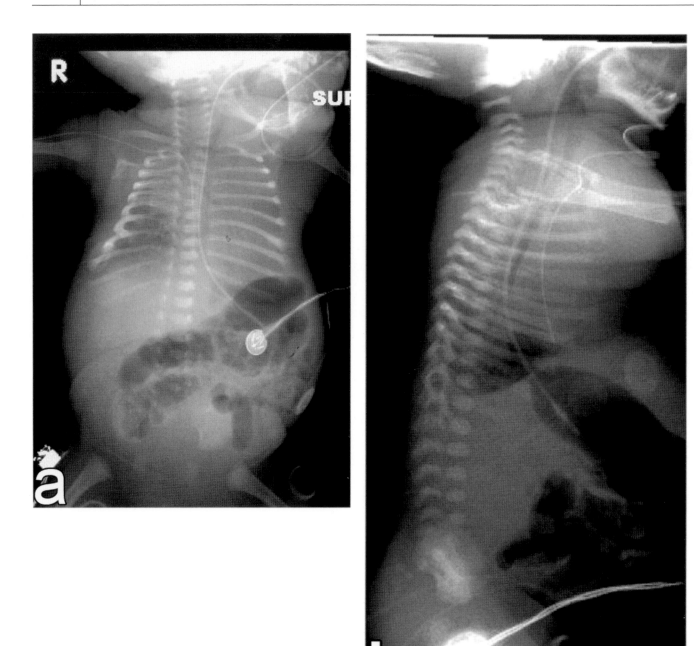

Figure 93.1. A 37-week gestation newborn. **(a)** AP thorax, spine, and pelvis. Small thoracic cage, not intubated, absent vertebral body ossification in cervical/lumbar-sacral spine region, flat acetabular roofs, wide sacrosciatic notches, absent pubic bone ossifications. **(b)** Lateral skull base, spine, thorax. Large ossification defect at skull base posterior to foramen magnum; deficient ossification at spine ends and hypoplastic, ovoid vertebral bodies in the thoracolumbar region; moderately shortened ribs.

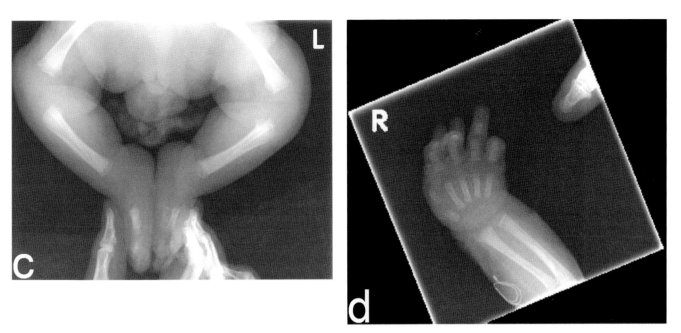

Figure 93.1. (cont.) **(c)** AP of lower extremities and feet. Absence of distal femur and proximal tibia ossification (normal for this gestational age); absent talus and calcaneal ossification (abnormal). **(d)** AP hand and forearm. Hand and wrist size is same as or greater than radius.

Morel-Lavallée lesions

Justin Boe

Imaging description

A 17-year-old presented with a rapidly enlarging right hip mass after a fall while skateboarding. An MRI was obtained which demonstrated a fluid collection between the subcutaneous tissues and underlying fascia of the right hip. The fluid collection was hypointense on T1-weighted images and contained a hyperintense lobule of fat (Fig. 94.1a). On T2-weighted images with fat suppression, the fluid was hyperintense and the lobule of fat demonstrated suppressed, hypointense signal (Fig. 94.1b). The appearance was considered to be compatible with a Morel-Lavallée lesion. Conservative management was offered, with eventual resolution of the lesion.

A two-year-old male presented with a left thigh mass two weeks after having his left thigh pinned beneath a wheel of a truck. Initial radiographs were negative for osseous fractures. An ultrasound demonstrated an anechoic fluid collection with debris and septations (Fig. 94.2a). A subsequent MRI revealed a fluid collection beneath the subcutaneous tissues and overlying the fascia of the medial left thigh, compatible with a Morel-Lavallée lesion. The fluid collection was noted to be hypointense on T1-weighted images (Fig. 94.2b) and hyperintense on T2-weighted sequences (Fig. 94.2c, d). Rim enhancement was noted (Fig. 94.2e). This lesion similarly resolved with conservative management.

Importance

The Morel-Lavallée lesion is a rare condition that was first described by the French physician Maurice Morel-Lavallée in the 1800s. It is described as an internal degloving in which the skin and subcutaneous tissues separate from the underlying fascia, resulting in a cavity containing blood, lymph, fat, and debris. Other names associated with this lesion are pseudocyst, post-traumatic soft tissue cyst, pseudolipoma, Morel-Lavallée hematoma, Morel-Lavallée effusion, and Morel-Lavallée extravasation. Lesions are commonly found around the thigh over the greater trochanter, often secondary to blunt trauma with associated hip and pelvic fractures. Other locations described include the abdominal wall, buttocks, lower lumbar spine, scapular region, and calf. The greater trochanteric region is particularly prone to this injury given the fixed attachment of the fascia, relative mobility of the overlying skin, and rich vascularity piercing the fascia in this region.

Plain radiographs are non-specific and may or may not show a soft tissue mass. With ultrasound, lesions can have a variable appearance but are usually hypoechoic to anechoic with no obvious relationship between the age of the fluid collection and its echogenicity. The shape varies from lobular in the acute phase to ovoid or flat and more well-defined with chronicity. Echogenic nodules may be present in the lesion, representing fat remnants, and echogenic septa can be seen. With CT, lesions may appear as well-defined fluid collections with fluid–fluid levels and a capsule. On MRI, signal characteristics are those of hemorrhage which can change to a seroma depending on the chronicity of the lesion. Lesions have been described as hypo- or hyperintense on T1- but usually hyperintense on T2-weighted images and often with a pseudocapsule in later stages. Internal or peripheral enhancement may be demonstrated and septations can be seen. A capsule, hypointense on all sequences, is frequently found to surround the lesion, which histologically consists of fibrous tissue and occasionally inflammatory infiltrate. A classification scheme based on the appearance of the lesions on MRI has been proposed.

Typical clinical scenario

The Morel-Lavallée lesion is typically a result of trauma; however, a history of trauma may be absent in up to one-third of cases. Patients may present with a thigh mass typically over the greater trochanteric region hours to days after the trauma. The lesion may present as a fluctuant area of the skin, swelling, or deformity and may remain stable in size, decrease in size, or slowly enlarge. Infection and necrosis of overlying skin may occur. These lesions may be missed in up to one-third of patients and be detected months to years after the trauma. If missed initially and slow growing, lesions can be mistaken for a soft tissue tumor. The lesion can be treated conservatively; however, the pseudocapsule may make lesions refractory to conservative treatment. Surgery or percutaneous drainage may be needed.

Differential diagnosis

The differential diagnosis for a Morel-Lavallée lesion includes fat necrosis, soft tissue tumor, and hematoma related to coagulopathy. Fat necrosis has a variable appearance on MRI with variable configurations, but often with a nodular appearance. A soft tissue tumor is possible; however, a careful search for a history of trauma should be elicited. A soft tissue cystic lesion such as a lymphangioma might also be a differential consideration but is likely to be more infiltrative and involve the subcutaneous tissues and less likely to have a temporal relationship to trauma. However, spontaneous or post-traumatic hemorrhage may occur in a lymphangioma or other underlying lesion.

> ### Teaching point
>
> A Morel-Lavallée lesion is a form of internal degloving injury with separation of the subcutaneous tissues from the underlying fascia, usually over the greater trochanteric region and usually with a clear history of trauma. Without a history of trauma, this lesion can be mistaken for a soft tissue tumor.

REFERENCES

1. Blacksin MF, Ha DH, Hameed M, *et al.* Superficial soft-tissue masses of the extremities. *Radiographics* 2006;**26**(5):1289–304.

2. Gilbert BC, Bui-Mansfield LT, Dejong S. MRI of a Morel-Lavallée lesion. *AJR Am J Roentgenol* 2004;**182**(5): 1347–8.

3. Mellado JM, Bencardino JT. Morel-Lavallée lesion: review with emphasis on MR imaging. *Magn Reson Imaging Clin N Am* 2005;**13**(4):775–82.

4. Mukherjee K, Perrin SM, Hughes PM. Morel-Lavallee lesion in an adolescent with ultrasound and MRI correlation. *Skeletal Radiol* 2007;**36**(Suppl 1):S43–5.

5. Neal C, Jacobson JA, Brandon C, *et al.* Sonography of Morel-Lavallee lesions. *J Ultrasound Med* 2008;**27**(7):1077–81.

6. Parra JA, Fernandez MA, Encinas B, *et al.* Morel-Lavallée effusions in the thigh. *Skeletal Radiol* 1997;**26**(4):239–41.

7. Tseng S, Tornetta P III. Percutaneous management of Morel-Lavallee lesions. *J Bone Joint Surg Am* 2006;**88**(1):92–6.

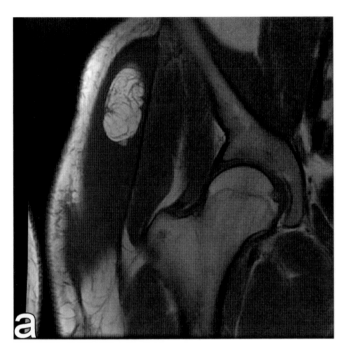
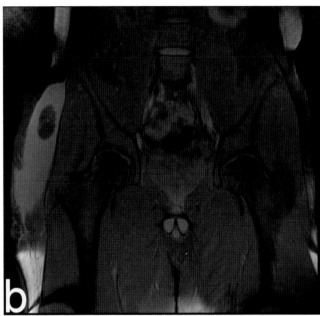

Figure 94.1. (a) T1-weighted coronal MRI image in a 17-year-old male demonstrates a fluid collection beneath the subcutaneous tissues and overlying the fascia compatible with a Morel-Lavallée lesion. The fluid is hypointense and contains a lobule of hyperintense fat. **(b)** T2-weighted MRI image with fat suppression demonstrates a hyperintense fluid collection beneath the subcutaneous tissues, containing a lobule of fat which is hypointense due to fat suppression.

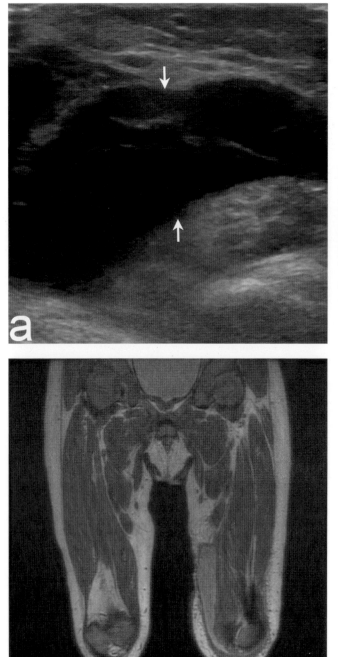

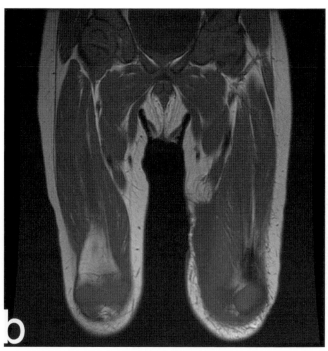

Figure 94.2. A two-year-old male with recent left thigh trauma and Morel-Lavallée lesion. **(a)** Ultrasound image of a fluid collection with septations in the region of the medial left thigh (arrows). **(b)** T1-weighted image demonstrates a hypointense fluid collection beneath the subcutaneous tissues of the medial left thigh. **(c)** Coronal T2-weighted image demonstrates a hyperintense fluid collection beneath the subcutaneous tissues of the medial left thigh.

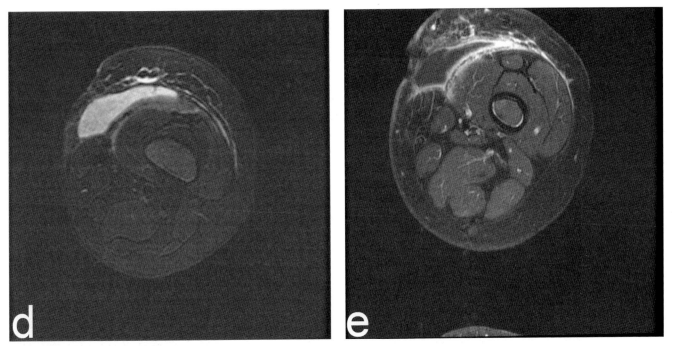

Figure 94.2. (cont.) **(d)** T2-weighted MR image with fat saturation demonstrates a hyperintense fluid collection beneath the subcutaneous tissues overlying the muscular fascia. **(e)** Axial T1-weighted postcontrast image with fat saturation demonstrates a rim-enhancing fluid collection beneath the subcutaneous tissues and overlying the fascia of the medial left thigh.

Infantile myofibromatosis

Justin Boe and Heike E. Daldrup-Link

Imaging description

A four-month-old male infant presented with a soft tissue mass of his upper back. There was no evidence of pain or other symptoms. A CT scan revealed a soft tissue mass involving the left paraspinal soft tissues of the lower thoracic spine with peripheral enhancement and central low attenuation relative to muscle (Fig. 95.1a). Additional bony lesions were demonstrated involving the thoracic spine at multiple levels. An example of a lytic lesion involving the right posterior elements of the lower thoracic spine (Fig. 95.1b) demonstrated peripheral enhancement (Fig. 95.1c). On MRI, multiple enhancing lesions were seen involving multiple vertebral bodies with collapse of several vertebral bodies (Fig. 95.1d). In addition, a homogeneously enhancing mass was discovered involving the extradural spinal canal (Fig. 95.1e). Radiographs performed as part of a skeletal survey demonstrated multiple lytic lesions primarily involving the metaphyses (Fig. 95.1f, g). Infantile myofibromatosis was confirmed histologically.

Importance

Infantile myofibromatosis is part of a group of soft tissue lesions known as the fibromatoses. These lesions are composed histologically of spindle-shaped fibrous cells surrounded by collagen. Lesions may be well-circumscribed or infiltrative. They can be multifocal and potentially involve multiple organ systems. Approximately 50% are solitary and 30–50% multiple. Metaphyses of long bones are often involved in those patients with osseous myofibromatosis. Radiographs display a lytic lesion sometimes with a sclerotic margin, and often in an eccentric location (Fig. 95.1f, g). Extremity lesions can be bilateral and symmetric (Fig. 95.1f). On CT, lesions have soft tissue attentuation often greater than muscle on precontrast images with peripheral enhancement postcontrast (Fig. 95.1a, c). Calcification within lesions has been observed. Signal intensity on MRI is variable with lesions described as being isointense to hypointense to muscle on T1-weighted images and hyperintense on T2-weighted images (unlike adult fibrous tumors, which usually appear hypointense). Hemorrhage, calcification, necrosis, and fat all can give a varied, heterogeneous appearance on MRI and CT. Tumors typically enhance avidly following contrast administration and often in a peripheral distribution.

Typical clinical scenario

Males are affected slightly more often than females. About half of the patients present with a mass at birth or shortly after, with 90% presenting with a mass or complications from a mass by the age of two years. Infantile myofibromatosis is considered to be a benign entity and solitary lesions often undergo spontaneous resolution. Unlike other forms of fibromatosis, the recurrence rate is low after surgery, at approximately 10%. In multifocal disease, spontaneous resolution is seen in roughly 30% of patients. Prognosis depends on complications from organ involvement, particularly if the cardiac or gastrointestinal systems are involved, with a mortality rate of approximately 15%.

Differential diagnosis

Infantile myofibromatosis can resemble other processes, including several with lytic bony lesions; thus the differential diagnosis is broad. Lesions to be considered include: metastatic neuroblastoma, Langerhans cell histiocytosis, enchondromatosis, multifocal osteomyelitis, congenital syphilis, fibrous dysplasia, soft tissue sarcoma, neurofibromatosis, leiomyomas, hemangiomas, lymphangiomatosis, and angiomatosis.

Teaching point

Infantile myofibromatosis is a proliferation of fibrous tissue in children primarily less than two years of age, presenting as a solitary mass or multifocal masses. Awareness of this disease process is important in young patients with single or multifocal soft tissue, bony, or visceral lesions involving one or many organ systems.

REFERENCES
1. Counsell SJ, Devile C, Mercuri E, et al. Magnetic resonance imaging assessment of infantile myofibromatosis. Clin Radiol 2002;57(1):67–70.
2. Eich GF, Hoeffel JC, Tschäppeler H, et al. Fibrous tumours in children: imaging features of a heterogeneous group of disorders. Pediatr Radiol 1998;28(7):500–9.
3. Koujok K, Ruiz RE, Hernandez RJ. Myofibromatosis: imaging characteristics. Pediatr Radiol 2005;35(4):374–80.
4. Meyer J, Fletcher B. Soft tissue neoplasms. In: Slovis T, ed. Caffey's Pediatric Diagnostic Imaging, 11th edition. Philadelphia: Mosby Elsevier, 2007; Chapter 160.
5. Robbin MR, Murphey MD, Temple HT, et al. Imaging of musculoskeletal fibromatosis. Radiographics 2001;21(3):585–600.

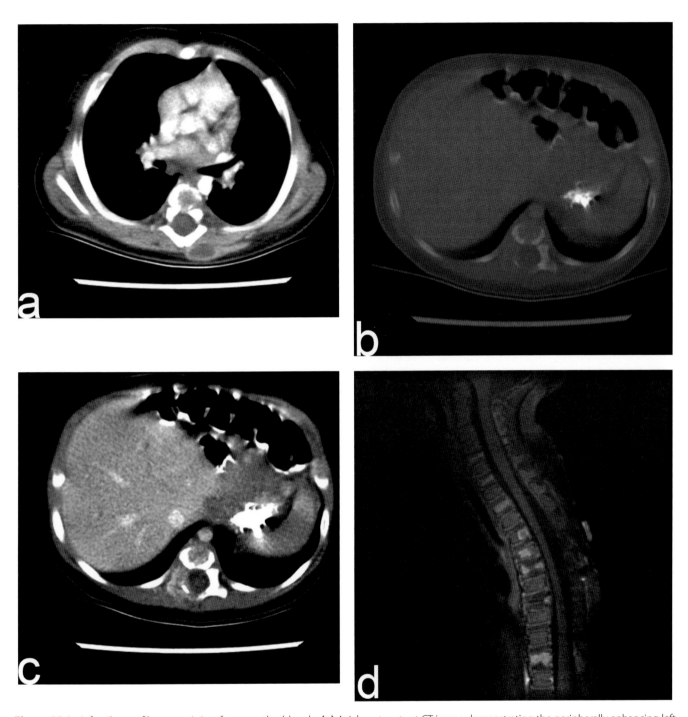

Figure 95.1. Infantile myofibromatosis in a four-month-old male. **(a)** Axial postcontrast CT image demonstrating the peripherally enhancing left paraspinal lesion discovered on clinical exam. **(b)** Axial CT image at the same level as Figure 95.1c with a bone window demonstrating the lytic nature of the lesion involving the right posterior elements of the lower thoracic spine. **(c)** Axial postcontrast CT image demonstrates a peripherally enhancing destructive lesion involving the right posterior elements of the lower thoracic spine. **(d)** Postcontrast T1-weighted MR image with fat saturation reveals multiple enhancing lesions throughout the thoracic spine with collapse of several vertebral bodies.

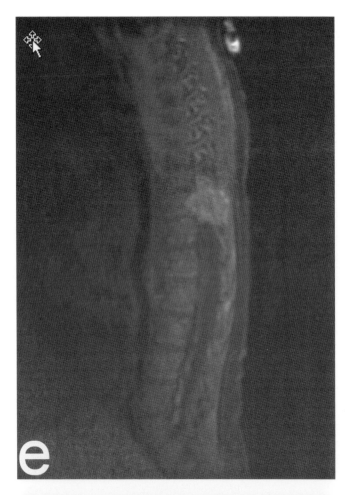

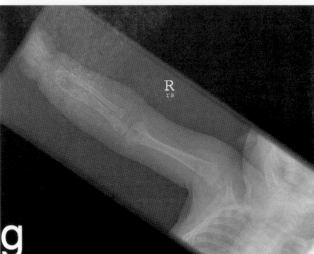

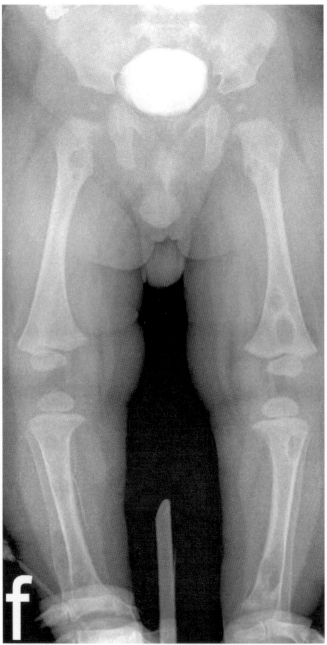

Figure 95.1. (cont.) **(e)** Postcontrast T1-weighted MR image with fat saturation demonstrating an enhancing intraspinal lesion. **(f)** Radiograph of the bilateral lower extremities demonstrates multiple lytic lesions primarily involving the metaphyseal regions. **(g)** Radiograph of the right upper extremity demonstrates multiple lytic lesions, some with sclerotic borders.

Osteochondritis dissecans of the capitellum

Rakhee Gawande

Imaging description

AP and lateral elbow radiographs (Fig. 96.1) of an 11-year-old girl with elbow pain demonstrated a small subarticular lucency in the lateral capitellum with surrounding sclerosis and subtle flattening of the capitellum. Based on these imaging findings a diagnosis of osteochondritis dissecans (OCD) of the capitellum was made.

Radiographs are the most common initial modality for screening patients with suspected OCD. In the elbow, supplemental views such as 45 degrees flexion or oblique views may help to demonstrate the lesion. Elbow radiographs may be normal in the early stages of OCD of the capitellum. With disease progression, flattening of the capitellum is noted with focal rarefaction and non-displaced subchondral fragmentation. In late stages, a focal defect of the articular surface may be noted, with presence of a loose body.

A radiographic classification of OCD has been described based on AP radiographs. A grade I lesion demonstrates cystic change in the lateral or middle capitellum, a grade II lesion shows a gap between the lesion and the underlying subchondral bone, and a grade III lesion is characterized by the presence of a loose body.

Importance

OCD of the capitellum is a disabling condition that affects young athletes. Successful treatment depends on an early diagnosis. Since radiographs are the initial screening modality, the described, sometimes subtle radiologic features must be carefully looked for in a young athlete with elbow pain.

Typical clinical scenario

OCD usually occurs in young athletes involved in sports that place repetitive valgus stress on the elbow. Most patients are young male baseball players or young female gymnasts who present with pain, swelling, and tenderness on the lateral aspect of the elbow. In the later stages there may be loss of extension and intermittent catching and locking of the elbow. The exact etiology is unknown but repetitive trauma and ischemia of the poorly vascularized capitellum are believed to play a major role.

While plain radiographs are almost invariably obtained first, MRI is currently the gold standard for the diagnosis and classification of OCD. MRI delineates both cartilage and bone and provides a better estimate of the size of the lesion and its stability, which are important for treatment planning.

Early lesions are seen as a focal hypointensity on T1-weighted and proton density images with variable T2 signal. Unstable lesions are characterized by the presence of a line of high signal intensity at the interface between the osseous fragment and adjacent bone. An articular fracture is indicated by joint fluid of high signal intensity passing through the subchondral bone, a focal osteochondral defect filled with joint fluid, or a 5 mm or larger fluid-filled cyst deep to the lesion. Ultimately an unstable lesion may invert or detach with loose body formation.

Differential diagnosis

OCD has to be distinguished from a self-limiting condition, osteochondrosis of the capitellum or Panner's disease, seen in young children between seven and 12 years of age. This condition is caused by ischemia and necrosis of the capitellar epiphysis (usually post-traumatic) followed by regeneration and recalcification and usually resolves with rest.

> ### Teaching point
>
> OCD of the elbow is a post-traumatic repetitive stress disorder of the lateral capitellum occurring in young athletes. Radiographic features may be subtle and need to be carefully looked for in evaluating a young athlete with elbow pain. MRI may be helpful for diagnosis and the detailed evaluation and classification used to assist with management decisions in OCD of the elbow as well as other locations.

REFERENCES

1. Jans LB, Ditchfield M, Anna G, Jaremko JL, Verstraete KL. MR imaging findings and MR criteria for instability in osteochondritis dissecans of the elbow in children. *Eur J Radiol* 2012;**81**(6):1306–10.
2. Kijowski R, De Smet AA. MRI findings of osteochondritis dissecans of the capitellum with surgical correlation. *AJR Am J Roentgenol* 2005;**185**(6):1453–9.
3. Kijowski R, De Smet AA. Radiography of the elbow for evaluation of patients with osteochondritis dissecans of the capitellum. *Skeletal Radiol* 2005;**34**(5):266–71.
4. Ruchelsman DE, Hall MP, Youm T. Osteochondritis dissecans of the capitellum: current concepts. *J Am Acad Orthop Surg* 2010;**18**(9):557–67.
5. van den Ende KI, McIntosh AL, Adams JE, Steinmann SP. Osteochondritis dissecans of the capitellum: a review of the literature and a distal ulnar portal. *Arthroscopy* 2011;**27**(1):122–8.

(a)

(b)

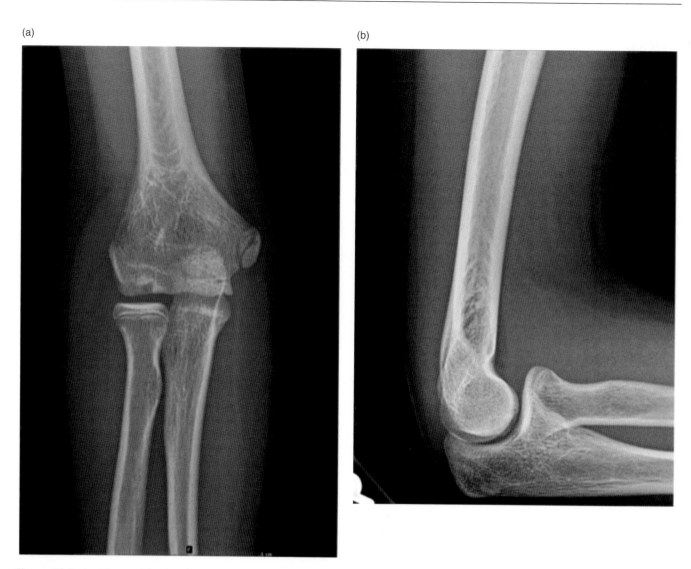

Figure 96.1. An 11-year-old girl with elbow pain and osteochondritis dissecans. **(a, b)** AP and lateral radiographs of the elbow demonstrate a small subarticular lucency in the capitellum with surrounding sclerosis.

Index

abdominal abscess, 177
abdominal distension, 229, 238
abdominal mass, 211, 269, 276
abdominal pain, 193, 196, 205, 234, 278, 297–8, 300
abdominal wall deficiency, 248, 250
    anterior, 322–3
Abernethy malformation, 111–13
aberrant left coronary artery arising from the
      pulmonary artery (ALCAPA), 141–3, 145
aberrant right coronary artery arising from the
      pulmonary artery (ARCAPA), 141, 144
abscesses, inaccessible, 183–4
acetabular roof coverage, 339–41
achondrogenesis, 326, 377
achondroplasia, 326
actinomycosis, 373
acute appendicitis, 183
acute lymphocytic leukemia (ALL), 56, 60
acute phase fibromatosis colli, 7
acute pneumonia, 62–4
acute scrotum, 307
ADC value, 270, 273
Addison disease, 23
adrenal abscess, 291
adrenal hematoma, 291
adrenal hemorrhage, 291–2, 313
adrenal insufficiency, 23
adrenal mass, 81, 294–5
adrenal neuroblastoma, 291–3
adrenoleukodystrophy, 23–4
adventitial hyperplasia, 158
agenesis, 30
air bronchograms, 56–9
air trapping, 44
airway obstruction, 79
Alagille syndrome, 208
alpha-fetoprotein, 307
alveolar proteinosis, 40, 42
alveolar ridge, 27
Amplatz guidewire, 183
amputation, forefoot, 147, 150
anal atresia, 316–17
anaplasia, 269
aneuploidy, 330
aneurysm, 117, 121
angel's wings appearance, 72, 75
angiocatheter, large bore, 170
angiomyolipomas, 245–6, 270
anterior abdominal wall defect, 322–3
antibiotics, 33, 255
aortic arch
    interrupted, 117–19
    right-sided, 94
aortic arch variant, 102, 104
aortic coarctation, 102, 117–19, 224
appendicitis, 298
    acute, 183
    lymphoid follicular hyperplasia and, 215
    perforated, 170, 177–8, 196–8
appendicolith, 177–8, 184, 196
appendix epididymis, 303

appendix testis torsion, 303–4
arterial switch procedure, 127–8, 130
arteriovenous fistulae, 162–8
arteriovenous malformations (AVMs), 112
arthritis, 205
    septic, 355, 358
arthrotomy, 359
aspiration pneumonia, 62
aspiration, causes of, 33
asplenia, 135, 138
asthma, 44, 48–9
atelectasis, 44, 47
    neonatal atypical peripheral, 73, 77
atrial septal defect (ASD), 107, 127, 129, 135
atrial switch procedure, 127, 131
attention-deficit/hyperactivity disorder, 23
atypical pneumonia, 62, 65
autoimmune disease, 66, 285
autoimmune hepatitis, 181
autosomal dominant disorders, 16, 245
autosomal dominant osteogenesis imperfecta, 328
autosomal dominant polycystic kidney disease
      (ADPCKD), 247, 319
autosomal recessive osteogenesis imperfecta, 328
autosomal recessive polycystic kidney disease
      (ARPCKD), 245, 247, 319
avascular necrosis, 343–4, 347
avascular phase LCPD, 343
avascularity, 308

bacterial meningitis, 14
bacterial pneumonias, 62, 65
bacterial pyelonephritis, 255–6
barium enema reduction, 170
barium upper GI study, 215–16, 218–19
Beckwith–Wiedemann syndrome, 260, 269
behavioral abnormalities, 23
bent bone dysplasias, 374
beta human chorionic gonadotropin, 307
beveled edges, 25, 28
bicuspid aortic valve, 117
bilateral hearing loss, 14, 16–17
bilateral overinflation, 40–1
bilateral renal dysplasia, 319–20
bilateral retinoblastoma, 1
bile ducts, 201–3
biliary atresia, 111, 113, 207–8
bilious vomiting, 218–19
bilirubin levels, 207–8, 334
Bioglue adhesive, 177, 179
biopsy
    Langerhans cell histiocytosis, 25
    lung, 40
bi-parietal calvarial lytic lesions, 25, 28
bisphosphonates, 365
bladder exstrophy, 322
Blalock–Taussig shunt, 95
Bland–White–Garland syndrome, 141
blunt pancreatic trauma, 234
Bochladek hernia, 329
bone biopsy, 365

bone fragility, 326–7
bone marrow, 294, 296
bone marrow edema, 352
bone marrow infiltration, 25
bone marrow transplantation, 23, 231
bone scintigraphy, 25
bony remodeling, 173
Botulinum toxin type A, 7
bowel atresia. *See* small bowel atresia
bowel loops, dilated, 237–8, 240
bowel malrotation, 218, 237
box-shaped heart, 122
brain tumors, 1–2
    craniopharyngioma, 10–12
    medulloblastoma, 18–19
branchial cleft cyst, 287
branchio-oto-renal syndrome, 16–17
bremsstrahlung images, 12
bronchial atresia, 79, 83, 330
bronchiectasis, 40, 43, 87
bronchiolitis, 44, 62
    chronic idiopathic, 40
bronchiolitis obliterans, 40, 43–4
bronchitis, 44
bronchoalveolar carcinomas, 80
bronchoalveolar lavage (BAL), 33
bronchogenic cyst, 79, 81, 330
bronchopulmonary malformation, 79–86
bronchoscopy, 44, 47
bullet fragments, 162, 164

calcium oxalate, 281
caliceal diverticulum, 245
calvarium, 25–6, 28, 327
campomelic dysplasia, 374–5
canal of Nuck, 297, 299
Candida albicans, 255
capitellum, osteochondritis dissecans, 387–8
cardiac dextroposition, 107–9
cardiac echocardiography, 141
cardiac obstructive lesions, 87
cardiomegaly, 112, 122–3, 141
cardiomyopathy, 122
carotid arteries
    internal, 32
    nasopharyngeal angiofibroma, 173
catheter embolization, 151, 155
Catterall system, 343
cavovarus foot deformity, 337
CD14 marker, 25
center-edge (CE) angle, 340, 342
cerebellar ataxia, 53
cerebral palsy, 336–7, 340
cerebral tumors, 270
cerebrovascular disease, 30
cervical extension of mediastinal thymus, 8
cervical lymphadenopathy, 8
cervical spine injuries, 162, 168
cervical teratoma, 8
cervicofacial hemangiomas, 30
cheek pain and swelling, 25, 27

chemotherapy
  Ewing's sarcoma, 371
    pleuropulmonary blastoma, 36
    trilateral retinoblastoma, 1
    Wilms' tumor, 269
chest wall sarcoma, 370-2
chest, lymphatic abnormalities, 87-93
cholangiography, 201, 208-9
choledochal cyst, 201-2
cholelithiasis, 334
cholestasis, 207-8, 334
chondrolysis, 347
chondrosarcoma, 36
chromosomal deletion syndrome, 339, 341
chronic idiopathic bronchiolitis, 40
chronic recurrent multifocal osteomyelitis
    (CRMO), 371
chylothorax, 87-8, 90
cirrhosis of the liver, 181
clear cell sarcoma, 270
cleft palate, 374, 377
cloaca, 316
Cloquet canal, 2, 5
Clostridium difficile, 228
clubfoot, 336-7
coarctation syndrome, 117
Coats' disease, 1
cochlea calcification, 14-15
cochlear implantation, 14
coeur en sabot, 94-6
coil embolization, 162-3, 165
COL1A1/2 genes, 326
collagenopathy, 377-8
colonic perforation, 169-71
colonic pneumatosis, 226, 228
colonic tumors, 215
comet tail artifact, 289-90
common bile duct, 201-3
confluent consolidation, 33-4
congenital chloride diarrhoea, 316
congenital diaphragmatic hernia, 329-31
congenital heart disease, 66-7, 94-5, 102, 127, 138
    cyanotic, 222
congenital lobar emphysema, 73, 78
congenital lobar overinflation, 79, 330
congenital neck cyst, 287
congenital rubella, 354
congenital syphilis, 354-6
congenital UPJ obstruction, 276, 278
congenital vertical talus, 336, 338
congenitally corrected transposition of the great
    arteries (CCTGA), 128, 133
congestive heart failure, 117, 125
    ALCAPA, 141-2
constipation, 226-7
contrast enema, 196, 199, See also water-soluble
    contrast enema
controlled ventilation techniques, 40
contusion, 234
copper deficiency, 355
corkscrew appearance, 218-19
coronary reimplantation, 142
corpus callosum, 23-4
cortical nephrocalcinosis, 281
coxa valga, 340
crackles, 40
craniopharyngioma, 10-12

crescent sign, 343
Crohn's disease, 205
croup, 48-50
cryptorchidism, 248
CSF space, leaks to, 10-12
curettage, 25
curved needle, 183-4
cyanosis, 112, 127-8, 136
cystic craniopharyngiomas, 10-11
cystic dysplasia, 79, 310
    kidneys, 319-20
cystic fibrosis, 226-7, 231
    meconium ileus and, 237-8, 316
cystic neuroblastoma, 319
cystic pleuropulmonary blastoma, 36, 39, 80
cystic pulmonary airway malformation (CPAM),
    36-7, 79-80, 82, 84, 330
cystic pulmonary lesion, 36
Cysto-Conray II, 237-8

dancing eye syndrome, 53
Dandy-Walker malformation, 30
demyelination, 23
Denys-Drash syndrome, 269, 272
dermoid cyst, 287
desmoplastic small round cell tumor, 229-30
desquamative interstitial pneumonitis (DIP), 40
developmental dysplasia of the hip (DDH),
    340-1
Di George syndrome, 66, 95
diabetes insipidus, 26
diaphragmatic hernia, congenital, 329-31
diaphyseal sclerosis, 354, 356
diarrhea, 53, 316
DICER1 gene mutation, 36, 270, 275
dietary modification, 23
Dietl's crisis, 276
diffuse follicular hyperplasia, 215
diffuse nephroblastomatosis, 260
distal ileal atresia, 316
distal intestinal obstruction syndrome (DIOS), 238
distal tibia fracture, 362-3
distal tibial physeal closure, 362
double bubble sign, 218-19
Down syndrome, 87, 95, 313
Drash syndrome, 260
D-transposition, 127-9
ductal ligament, 102
ductus venosus, 188
duodenal lymphoma, 205
duodenal obstruction, 218-19
duodenal thumbprinting, 205-6
duodenojejunal junction, 219, 221
duplicated collecting system, 257-8
duplication cysts, 201
dysmorphic facial features, 66-7, 374

Ebstein-Barr virus infection, 231
Ebstein's anomaly, 122-3
echogenic bowel, 316
echogenic streaks, 252
ectopia cordis, 322
ectopic cervical thymus, 20-1
ectopic thymus, 66, 69
ectopic ureterocele, 257-8
egg on a string appearance, 127, 129
embolization, nasopharyngeal angiofibroma, 173-5

embryonal mesenchymal neoplasm, 36
embryonal sarcoma of the liver, 211, 214
emphysema, 44
    pulmonary interstitial, 72, 76
end-stage renal disease (ESRD), 281
end-stage renal failure (ESRF), 281
endobronchial foreign bodies, 44-5
endochondral ossification, 354
endocrine dysfunction, 10
endovascular techniques, 151, 157
enema reduction, 169-70, 172
enterocolitis, 170, 200
enteroliths, 316-17
eosinophilic granuloma, 25
Eovist, 207, 210
epidermoid cysts, 307, 312
epididymo-orchitis, 303, 308
epidural masses, 294-5
epidural venous plexus, 162, 164, 166
epiphyseal ossification, 377
epiphyseal separation, 362, 364
epistaxis, 173-4
Escherichia coli, 255, 291
esophageal foreign body, 48-50
esophagrams, 44
Ewing's sarcoma, 229, 370-1, 373
extracorporeal membrane oxygenation (ECMO),
    329
extrahepatic biliary obstruction, 207-8
extrahepatic collateral arteries, 181-2
extralobar pulmonary sequestration, 292-3
extralobar sequestration, 80, 85
extraosseous Ewing's sarcoma, 370
extrapulmonary sequestration, 80
extratesticular lesions, 307-8
extrinsic lesions, left pulmonary artery, 98
ex utero intrapartum treatment (EXIT), 313, 329
eye
    extraocular extension, 1
    trilateral retinoblastoma, 1-3
eye swelling, 365-6

facial angiofibromas, 245
facial dysmorphism, 66-7, 374
facial hemangiomas, 30-1
fat necrosis, 380
fatigue stress fractures, 348
fatty acids, 23
femoral artery occlusion, 147-8
femoral epiphysis, 343-4
    slipped capital, 347-9
femoral head, 339, 341, 343-4
femoral head ossification, 340, 343
femoral venous line, 188, 191
femurs, bent, 374-5
fetal anal atresia, 316-17
fetal congenital diaphragmatic hernia, 329-31
fetal lung interstitial tumor, 80
fetal lymphatic malformation, 313-15
fetal osteogenesis imperfecta, 326-8
fetal renal dysplasia, 319-20
fibrolamellar carcinoma, 181
fibromatoses, 384
fibromatosis
    neurofibromatosis, 2, 158
fibromatosis colli, 7-8
fibromuscular dysplasia, 158-9

fibrotic phase fibromatosis colli, 7
fibrous dysplasia, 365–6, 371
fine-needle aspiration, 289
floating teeth, 25, 27
fluorine-18 positron emission tomography (PET), 350, 352
focal follicular hyperplasia, 215
focal nephroblastomatosis, 260, 262
focal pneumonia, 62
focal stenoses/occlusions, 30
follicular adenomas, 289
Fontan conduit, 112
foramen cecum, 287
forefoot varus deformity, 336–7
foveolar hyperplasia, 222–3
French method, 336
fungal disease, 62
fungal renal infections, 255

gadolinium, 88, 207, 210
gallbladder, 207
gallbladder ghost triad, 207
gallstones, 334–5
ganglioneuroblastoma, 53–4
ganglioneuroma, 53
gangrene, 147
gas cyst, 226
Gastrografin, 237–8, 242
gastroschisis, 322–3
germ cell tumor, 26, 66, 69, 297, 307–8, 310
Ghon complex, 63
Graf alpha angle, 339, 341
Graf beta angle, 339
Graf grading classification, 339
granulation tissue, 48
granulomatous disease, 57
Graves' disease, 285–6
greater trochanteric region, 380
groin pain, 347, 349
ground glass appearance, 365–6
ground glass opacity (GGO), 40–2
growth arrest, 359
guidewire embolization, 151, 153
gunshot wounds, 162

Haemophilus influenzae, 14
Hand–Schuller–Christian syndrome, 25
Harcke method, 339
Hashimoto's thyroiditis, 285
head-shaft angle, 347, 349
hearing loss, 14, 16–17, 23
hemangioendotheliomas, 211–12
hemangiomas, 31
    cervicofacial, 30
    facial, 30
    infantile, 211
hemangiomatosis, 112, 116
hematoma, 234
    adrenal, 291
hematuria, 252
hemidiaphragm inversion, 36, 38
hemihypertrophy, 260
hemithorax mass, 36–7 See also left hemithorax
hemoptysis, 44
Henoch–Schönlein purpura, 205–6
heparin, 147
hepatic abscess, 189

hepatic cyst, 189
hepatic encephalopathy, 112
hepatic neoplasm, 188
hepatitis
    autoimmune, 181
    neonatal, 208
hepatobiliary imino diacetic acid (HIDA) scan, 207–8
hepatoblastoma, 181, 189, 211, 213
hepatocellular carcinoma, 181–2
hepatopulmonary syndrome, 111–13
hereditary hemorrhagic telangiectasia (HHT), 112
herniation of bowel, 322–3
Herring classification, 343–4
heterotaxia, 138
Hilgenreiner's line, 340, 342
hindfoot equinus deformity, 336–7
hindfoot varus deformity, 336–7
hip dislocation, 339–40
hip dysplasia, 7
Hirschsprung's disease, 53, 237–40, 244, 317
histiocytes, 25
Hodgkin's lymphoma, 56–7, 59, 70
homocystinuria, 147–8
horseshoe kidney, 278
horseshoe lung, 107, 109
Houndsfield units, 35
Hutchinson's triad, 354
hybrid lesions, bronchopulmonary, 79–81, 86
hydrocele, 307
hydronephrosis, 245, 257–8
    renal cystic dysplasia and, 319
    ureteropelvic junction obstruction and, 276–7
hydrops fetalis, 313–14, 334–5
hydroureteronephrosis, 248
hyoid bone, 287–8
hyperalimentation, 88
hyperbilirubinemia, 207
hyperdense tumors, 18–19
hyperlucency, 44–5
hyperoxaluria, 281, 283
hyperparathyroidism, 281, 355
hyperpigmentation, 23
hypertension, 117–18
    pulmonary, 127, 329
    renovascular, 158
    Wilms' tumor, 269
hyperthyroidism, 285
hypervascularity, 308
hypochondrogenesis, 377–8
hyponatremia, 23
hypophosphatasia, 326
hypoplasia, 30, 374–5
hypoplastic left heart, 107, 117, 145
hypoplastic lung, 98
hypoplastic right lung, 107, 109
hypotonia, 66–7
hypovolemic shock, 238, 291
hypoxemia, 112

iatrogenic pathology, 151–7
idiopathic intussusception, 170, 196
ileocolic intussusception, 200
ileoileal intussusception, 170–1
iliac wings, 374–5
immune hydrops, 334
immunosuppression, 231

imperforate anus, 239, 316–17
incisural ankle fracture, 359, 362
infantile myofibromatosis, 384–5
inferior vena cava, drainage to, 107, 109
inflammation, thyroglossal duct cyst, 287
inguinal hernia, 298, 303, 306
insufficiency fractures, 348
interlobular septal thickening, 33, 40, 42
internal carotid artery, 32
internal degloving, 380
interrupted aortic arch, 117–19
interstitial pneumonia, 40
intestinal lymphangiectasia, 87
intestinal perforation, 237
intimal fibroplasia, 158
intracranial Berry aneurysms, 117
intracranial hemangiomas, 30
intracranial tumors, 1, 10, 18
intrahepatic ducts, 202–3
intrahepatic portal vein, 112
intralobar nephroblastomatosis, 260
intraluminal gas, 226
intramural gas, 226
intraocular hemorrhage, 2
intraocular mass, 1
intrapulmonary mass, 36
intrapulmonary sequestrations, 80
intratesticular neoplasms, 307–12
intrathoracic thymus, 20
intravascular foreign bodies, 151–7
intrinsic lesions, left pulmonary artery, 98
intussusception mimicry, 196–8, 205
intussusception reduction, 169–71
iodine-123 MIBG scan, 294, 296
iodine-123 uptake, 285–6
ischemia, lower extremity, 147–8
ischemic hemorrhagic infarction, 291

Jaffe–Lichtenstein syndrome, 365
jaundice, 207–8
joint laxity, 339–40
juvenile granulosa cell tumors, 307–8
juvenile myelomonocytic leukemia (JMML), 227
juvenile nasopharyngeal angiofibroma, 173–5
juvenile tillaux fracture, 362

Kasai portoenterostomy, 207
Kawasaki disease, 118
kidneys, enlarged, 252–3
Klebsiella pneumoniae, 255
Klein's line, 347, 349
Klippel–Trenaunay–Weber syndrome, 313
Kniest dysplasia, 377
Knudson's two-hit hypothesis, 1
Kommerell diverticulum, 102, 105
Kump's bump, 364

labial mass, 297–9
labyrinthitis ossificans, 14–15
laceration, 234
Langerhans cell histiocytosis (LCH), 25–9, 57, 61
    chest wall sarcoma and, 371
    classification, 25
    MRI/PET, 350–1
Langerhans cells, 25
lateral pillar, 343–4
Le Compte maneuver, 127, 130

left coronary artery, aberrant, 141–3, 145
left hemithorax, 37
  opacification, 87–8, 90
left isomerism, 112–13
left pulmonary artery sling, 98–9
left ventricular dilatation, 141
left ventricular failure, 142
Legg–Calve–Perthes disease (LCPD), 343–4, 348
lethal skeletal dysplasias, 326
Letterer–Siwe disease, 25
leukemia, 355
  acute lymphocytic, 56, 60
leukocoria, 1–2
Leydig cell tumors, 307–8
limb-body wall complex, 322
limping, 344
Lipiodol, 88, 181–2
lipoid pneumonia, 33–4
liver
  cirrhosis, 181
  mesenchymal hamartoma, 211–12
  umbilical venous catheter, 188–9, 192
liver dysfunction, 111, 113
liver herniation, 329–30
liver transplantation, 111, 113, 181, 208
lobectomy, 80
Loder classification, 347
lower extremity ischemia, 147–8
L-transposition, 128, 133
lumbar vein malposition, 188
lung cysts, 37–8
lung to head ratio (LHR), 329, 333
lung transplantation, 231, 233
lung volumes, 329, 333
lymph nodes
  enlarged, 287
  mediastinal and hilar, 56, 58
lymphangiectasia, 87–8, 91
lymphangiography, 88
lymphangioleiomyomatosis, 88
lymphangioma, 66, 69, 313, 380
lymphangiomatosis, 87, 93
lymphatic abnormalities, 87–93
lymphatic dysplasia syndrome, 87
lymphatic malformation, 315
  fetal, 313–14
lymphatic obstruction, 87, 91
lymphocytic hypophysitis, 26
lymphoid follicular hyperplasia, 215–16
lymphoma, 56–7, 59
  desmoplastic small round cell tumor, 230
  desmoplastic small round cell tumor and, 229
  PTLD and, 231
  thymus and, 66, 68, 70
lymphoproliferative disorders, 231
lymphoscintigraphy, 88
lytic expansion of ribs, 87, 90
lytic lesions, 25–6, 28–9
  myofibromatosis, 384–5

major aorticopulmonary collaterals (MAPCAs), 94–5, 97
malacia, 98
maxilla, 27
maxillary sinus walls, 27
McCune–Albright syndrome, 365, 369
McFarland fractures, 359

meconium, 316
  calcification, 316–17
meconium aspiration, 72, 76
meconium ileus, 237–44, 316
meconium peritonitis, 237–8, 242, 316
meconium plug syndrome, 239
medial collateral ligament, 359
medial fibroplasia, 158, 161
medial hyperplasia, 158
medial malleolus avulsion fracture, 359–60
mediastinal lymphadenopathy, 56–8, 61
mediastinal mass, 36, 48–50
  Hodgkin's lymphoma, 56
  lymphatic abnormalities and, 87
  lymphoma, 60
mediastinal shift, 36–7
mediastinal thymus, 20–1, 66, 71
medullary nephrocalcinosis, 281–2
medulloblastoma, 18–19
megacystis-microcolon syndrome, 248
meningitis, 14
  subacute, 62
mental retardation, 245
mesenchymal hamartoma, 211–12
mesoblastic nephroma, 269, 273, 319
metanephric stromal tumor, 270
metanephros, 260, 262
metaphyseal blush, 347, 349
metaphyseal lucencies, 354–6
metastases
  desmoplastic small round cell tumor, 229–30
  Ewing's sarcoma, 370–1
  neuroblastoma, 294–5
  Wilms' tumor, 269
metatarsus adductus, 336
methicillin resistant *Staphylococcus aureus* (MRSA), 212
methylprednisolone, 25
microcolon, 237–9, 244, 316
micromelia, 326
microphthalmos, 2, 30
middle aortic syndrome, 193–4
midgut volvulus, 218–19, 237–8
midline intracranial tumor, 1
miliary pneumonia, 62–3
mitral regurgitation, 142
monostotic disease, 365
monostotic EG, 26
Morel-Lavallée lesion, 380–1
Morgagni hernia, 329
mucoid impacted bronchus, 79, 83
Mucomyst, 237–8, 242
mucosal fold thickening, 205–6
multicystic dysplastic kidney, 276–7, 319–20
multifocal retinoblastoma, 1
multilocular cystic nephroma, 270, 275
multinodular goiter, 285
multiple polyposis, 215
multisystem LCH, 350
mycobacteria, atypical, 62–3, 65
mycobacterial infection, 57
myofibromatosis, 385
  infantile, 384

nasogastric tube placement, 151, 154
nasopharyngeal angiofibroma, 173–5

Neisseria meningitidis, 14, 291
neonatal airleak, 72–8
neonatal atypical peripheral atelectasis (NAPA), 73, 77
neonatal bent bone dysplasias, 374
nephrectomy, 270
nephroblastomatosis, 260–1
  Wilms' tumor and, 269
nephrocalcinosis, 281–2
nephrogenic rests, 260, 262, 269
nephrolithiasis, 281, 298
nephromegaly, 245
Neuhauser's sign, 238
neuroblastoma, 7–8, 29, 53, 189, 193–4, 294–5
  adrenal, 291–3
  ganglioneuroblastoma, 53–4
  lymphatic malformation and, 313
  Wilms' tumor and, 270
neurocristopathy, 53
neuroendocrine cell hyperplasia of infancy (NEHI), 40–1
neurofibromatosis, 2, 158
neurologic impairment, 23
nodes, lungs, 62
nodular pneumonia, 62
nodules, lungs, 56–7, 64
non-Hodgkin's lymphoma, 56
non-immune hydrops, 334
non-specific interstitial pneumonia (NSIP), 40
Noonan's syndrome, 87, 313
no-way valve, 44

obstructive hydrocephalus, 18–19
oligohydramnios, 76, 248
Ommaya device, 10, 12
Omnipaque, 183, 185, 238
omphalocele, 322, 324
Ondine's curse, 53
one-way valve, 44
opsoclonus myoclonus, 53–4, 294
optic nerve, 3
optic nerve atrophy, 30
optic-hypothalamic astrocytoma, 26
oral lithium, 122
orbitopathy, 285
orchiectomy, 307, 311
Osler–Rendu–Weber syndrome, 112
osteitis, 354
osteoarthritis, 347
osteochondritis, 354
osteochondritis dissecans, 387–8
osteochondrosis, 387
osteogenesis imperfecta, 326–8
osteolytic lesion, 350–1
osteomyelitis, 26, 348, 354, 358
  chest wall sarcoma and, 371
  chronic recurrent multifocal, 371
osteonecrosis, 343, 345
osteopenia, 355
osteosarcoma, 370–1
osteosclerosis, 281
ovarian cystic teratoma, 297, 301
ovarian cysts, 297–8, 300
ovarian torsion, 297–302
ovarian tumor, 297
oxalosis, 281–2

P chromic phosphate colloid, 10–12
P sodium phosphate, 11
pancreatic duct, 201
pancreatic trauma, 234–5
pancreatitis, acute, 234–6
Panner's disease, 387
papillary thyroid carcinoma, 290
parieto-occipital white matter, 23
parosteal osteosarcoma, 370
patchy air trapping, 40, 42
patent ductus arteriosus (PDA), 94–6, 107, 117–18
patent ductus venosus, 115
patent foramen ovale (PFO), 135
Pavlik harness, 340
peel, 322–3
pelvic inflammatory disease (PID), 298, 300
pelvicalyceal distortion, 269, 271
pelvocaliectasis, 276
penetrating neck injury, 163
penicillin, 354
pentobarbital, 207
percent predicted lung volume (PPLV), 329
percutaneous sclerosis, 88
peribronchial myofibroblastic tumor, 80
pericardial effusion, 56, 122, 125
perihilar markings, 40–1
perilobar nephroblastomatosis, 260
perimedial fibroplasia, 158
perinatal sepsis, 354
periostitis, 354–6
peripancreatic fluid, 234–6
peripherally inserted central catheter (PICC), 151, 153
peritumoral edema, 370
Perkin's line, 340, 342
peroxisome disorders, 23
persistent hyperplastic primary vitreous, 1, 5
Peyer's patches, 169, 196
PHACES syndrome, 30–1
pharyngitis, 205
pigment stones, 334
pigtail catheter, 169–70, 172, 177–8
pilocytic astrocytoma, 18
pilon fracture, 359, 362
pinch off syndrome, 151
pineal gland, 1
pineal gland tumor, 1
pituitary hormone, 10
pituitary infundibulum, 26
plain film skeletal survey, 25
planovalgus foot deformity, 337
plasma homocysteine level, 147
pleural effusion, 36, 56, 87–8, 91, 334–5
pleuropulmonary blastoma, 36–7, 80
  subtypes, 36
pneumatic enema reduction, 169–70, 172
pneumatocele, 81
pneumatosis intestinalis cystoides, 226–7, 238
pneumomediastinum, 72–4
pneumonia, 44
  acute and subacute, 62–4
  adenopathy and, 62
  bronchopulmonary malformation and, 81
  interstitial, 40
  lipoid, 33–4
  lymphoma and, 56–7
  TAPVR and, 136, 138

pneumopericardium, 73, 77
pneumoperitoneum, 73, see also tension pneumoperitoneum
pneumothorax, 72–3, 76–7
point-of-care (POC) ultrasound, 169
polycystic ovarian syndrome, 298, 300
polyhydramnios, 374
polyostotic disease, 365, 369
polysplenia, 111, 207–8
Ponseti method, 336
popliteal artery occlusion, 147–8
portal vein, 188
portopulmonary syndrome, 111–13
portosystemic shunt, 113–16
posterior fossa anomalies, 30
posterior fossa tumor, 18–19
post-transplantation lymphoproliferative disorder (PTLD), 56, 61, 231–3
Potter's syndrome, 76
pouch of Douglas, 297
pre-auricular pits, 16–17
premature physeal closure (PPC), 359
primary renal insufficiency, 283
primitive neuroectodermal tumor (PNET), 370
prostaglandin therapy, 94–5, 222–3
proximal focal femoral deficiency, 340
prune belly syndrome, 248–9
pseudocapsule, 269
pseudocoarctation, 118
pseudocysts, 234, 236, 238
Pseudomonas aeruginosa, 255
pseudoparalysis, 354
pthisis bulbi, 2
pulmonary arteries, 94–5, see also left pulmonary artery sling
  ALCAPA, 141–3, 145
pulmonary atresia, 94–6, 122, 125, 135
pulmonary edema, 136, 141, 143
pulmonary hyperplasia, 79
pulmonary hypertension, 329
pulmonary hypoplasia, 72, 76, 122, 326, 329
pulmonary interstitial emphysema, 72, 76
pulmonary interstitial glycogenosis (PIG), 40
pulmonary lymphangiectasia, 87, 92
pulmonary sequestration, 79–80, 82
pulmonary valve leaflets, 95
pulmonary vascular resistance, 141–2, 329
pulmonary vasculature, 112–13
pulmonary venous drainage, 135, 137, 140
pulmonary venous obstruction, 136
pulmonic stenosis, 122, 128
purpura, 205
pyelonephritis, 247, 255–6
pyloric stenosis, 222, 225
pyogenic abscesses, 211
pyohydronephrosis, 257–8
pyramidal tract symptoms, 23

radiotherapy
  craniopharyngioma, 10–11
  pleuropulmonary blastoma, 36
  Wilms' tumor, 269
Ranke's complex, 63
Rashkind procedure, 127
Rastelli operation, 128, 132
re-coarctation, 117, 121

reimplantation
  coronary, 142
  left pulmonary artery, 98
renal abscess, 255–6
renal artery stenosis, 118, 158, 160, 193–4
renal cell carcinoma, 245, 270
renal cortex, 260
renal cysts, 245–6, 260
renal dysplasia
  cystic, 319–20
  obstructive, 76
renal hamartoma, 269
renal malformations, 16
renal medullary carcinoma, 270, 275
renal osteodystrophy, 281, 283
renal parenchyma, 260, 272
renal pelvis dilatation, 276–7
renal vein thrombosis, 252–3, 292
renovascular hypertension, 158
resection
  craniopharyngioma, 10–11
  desmoplastic small round cell tumor, 229
  pleuropulmonary blastoma, 36
  Wilms' tumor, 269
respiratory distress syndrome, 136
reticuloendothelial system, 25
retinal astrocytic hamartomas, 2
retractions, 40–1
retrocardiac pneumomediastinum, 72, 74
revascularization, 30, 343
Rh immunoglobulin, 334
rhabdoid tumors, 270, 274
rhabdomyosarcoma, 8, 36
rickets, 281, 355
right atrial dilatation, 122–3
right middle lobe syndrome, 63
rockerbottom foot, 337–8
ROHHADNET syndrome, 53
Roux-en-Y anastomosis, 207

Salter–Harris classification, 359, 361–2
Salter–Harris type IV fracture, 359–60, 362–3
scapular body ossification, 374–5
scimitar syndrome, 107–9, 145
scrotal mass, 307, 309
  differential diagnosis, 308
scrotal pain, 303–4
scrotolith, 303
secundum ASD, 127
seizures, 23, 245
sensorineural hearing loss, 14, 16, 23
septic arthritis, 355, 358
septic arthritis of infancy, 340
Sertoli cell tumors, 307–8
sex cord-stromal tumors, 307–8
Shenton's line, 340
Shone syndrome, 117
short gut syndrome, 322
short stature, 377
sickle cell disease, 270, 275
single screw fixation, 347
single-system LCH, 350
sinus tract, 177, 179
skeletal dysplasias, 326, 374, 377
slipped capital femoral epiphysis (SCFE), 347–9
small bowel atresia, 237–9, 243, 322
small bowel fistula, 177–8

small bowel follow through (SBFT), 215–16, 219
small bowel obstruction, 237–44
small left colon syndrome, 239
snare-wire, 151, 157
snowman appearance, 135, 138
soap-bubble appearance, 238
soft tissue mass, 370, 372, 384
soft tissue swelling, 334–5
soft tissue tumor, 380
Southwick method, 347, 349
SOX9 gene mutation, 374
spermatic cord torsion, 307–8
spinal tumor seeding, 18
splenogonadal fusion, 311
splenorenal shunt, 111–13
spondylo-epi-metaphyseal dysplasia (SEMD)–Strudwick, 377
spondylo-epiphyseal dysplasia congenita, 377
spontaneous pneumothorax, 36
sporadic aniridia, 260, 269
standardized uptake value (SUV), 350
Staphylococcus aureus, 212, 255
steno-occlusive disease, 32
sternocleidomastoid muscle, 7–9
steroids, 329
Stickler dysplasia type I, 377
Streptococcus, 291, 354, 358
Streptococcus pneumonia, 14, 62, 72
stress fractures, 348
string of beads appearance, 158, 161
string of pearls sign, 298
Stulberg classification, 343
Sturge–Weber syndrome, 30, 32
subacute pneumonia, 62–4
subchondral fracture, 343
subcortical cysts, 319–20
superior mesenteric vein/artery relationships, 218–20
suprasellar mass, 10–11
surfactant disorders, 40, 42, 72, 74, 77
surgery, see also resection
    aortic coarctation, 117
    fibromatosis colli, 7
    scimitar syndrome, 108
    tetralogy of Fallot, 95
    transposition of the great arteries (TGA), 127
    vascular ring, 102
swallowing difficulty, 48–9
syndromal cysts, 319
syphilis, congenital, 354–6

T cell ALL, 56, 60
T lesions, 128
T lymphocytes, 66
tachypnea, 33–4, 40–1
Takayasu arteritis, 118, 158, 195
Takeuchi procedure, 142
talocalcaneal angles, 336–7
talo-first metatarsal angles, 336–7

tardus and parvus pattern, 158
technetium-99, 88, 207
technetium-99 MAG3 renography, 276
technetium-99 MDP scan, 294, 296
technetium-99 sulfur colloid scan, 10–11
Temno needle, 183, 186
tension pneumoperitoneum, 169–70, 172
teratoma, 313
terminal ileum, 215–16
testicular appendix torsion, 303–4
testicular cancer, 229
testicular torsion, 303, 308, 312
testis-preserving surgery, 308
tetralogy of Fallot, 94–6, 102–3
thanatophoric dysplasia, 326
Thibierge–Weissenbach syndrome, 281
thoracic duct, 87
thoracic pedicle ossification, 374–5
thrombocytopenia, 252
thromboembolism, 147
thymic cysts, 20, 22
thymic sail sign, 66, 68, 73
thymic wave sign, 66–7
thymolipoma, 66, 69
thymopharyngeal duct, 20
thymus, 66–71, 123, 126 see also mediastinal thymus
thyroglossal duct cyst, 287–8
thyroid acropathy, 285
thyroid colloid cyst, 289–90
thyroid nodules, 289–90
tibial artery, 147–8
tibiofibular syndesmosis, 359, 361
tissue adhesives, 177, 179
tissue plasminogen activator (tPA), 147, 150
torsion
    ovarian, 297–302
    testicular appendix, 303–4
torticollis
    fibromatosis colli, 7–8
total anomalous pulmonary venous return (TAPVR), 135–40
tracheal bronchus, 98
tracheal diverticulum, 98, 100
tracheal stenosis, 98, 101
tracheoplasty, 98
transarterial hepatic chemoembolization (TACE), 181–2
transection, 234–5
transposition of the great arteries (TGA), 127–8, 134
traumatic arteriovenous fistulae, 162–8
traumatic pancreatic injury, 234–5
tree-in-bud appearance, 62–4
Treponema pallidum bacteria, 354
triangular cord sign, 207
tricuspid regurgitation, 122, 124
trilateral retinoblastoma, 1–3
triplane fracture, 362–3
trisomy 13, 326
trisomy 18, 260, 269, 326

trisomy 21, 122, 326
Truncus arteriosus, 102–3
tube placement, traumatic, 72, 75
tuberculosis, 57, 62–3
tuberculous pneumonia, 62–4
tuberous sclerosis, 2, 245–6, 270
tumor thrombus, 269, 271
Turner's syndrome, 87, 117, 313
two-way valve, 44
type II collagenopathy, 377–8

umbilical arterial line (UAL), 192
umbilical venous catheter (UVC), 188–94
unilateral unifocal retinoblastoma, 1
upper respiratory tract infection
    viral, 36
ureterocele, 257–8
ureteropelvic junction obstruction, 276–7
urinary stasis, 276
urinary tract abnormalities, 248
urinary tract infections, 257–8
urorectal fistula, 316–17
usual interstitial pneumonia (UIP), 40

VAC chemotherapy, 371
von Hippel–Lindau disease, 245
vanillylmandelic acid (VMA), 292
vascular abnormalities, 30
vascular embolization, 80
vascular ring, 102–4
vascular stenosis, 193
vasculitis, 117–19
vasoactive intestinal peptide (VIP) tumor, 53
vegetable oils, 33
ventriculomegaly, 10
vertebra plana, 25, 29
vertebral arteriovenous fistulae, 162–8
vertebral ossification, 377
vesicoureteral reflux, 257, 276–7
vestibule calcification, 14–15
viral pneumonias, 62
vision loss, 1
visual deficits, 23
vitamin supplementation, 147
vitiligo, 285
von Hippel–Lindau syndrome, 270

WAGR syndrome, 269
wall to wall heart, 122–3
water-soluble contrast enema, 237–8, 241
Weigert–Meyer rule, 257
whirlpool sign, 218, 220, 298, 300
white matter demyelination, 23
Wilms' tumor, 269–75
    nephroblastomatosis and, 260, 263
Wilson classification, 347
Wimberger sign, 354–5, 357

yolk sac tumors, 307, 309

zonal phenomenon, 23